Essentials of Human Physiology and Pathophysiology for Pharmacy and Allied Health

D0144891

Essentials of Human Physiology and Pathophysiology for Pharmacy and Allied Health

Laurie K. McCorry
Martin M. Zdanowicz
Cynthia Y. Gonnella

To Dennis,
Laurie McCorry

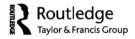

Routledge
Taylor & Francis Group

First published 2019
by Routledge
711 Third Avenue, New York, NY 10017

and by Routledge
2 Park Square, Milton Park, Abingdon, Oxon, OX14 4RN

Routledge is an imprint of the Taylor & Francis Group, an informa business

ISBN: 978-0-367-00046-2 (hbk)
ISBN: 978-0-367-00048-6 (pbk)

Typeset in Palatino LT Std
by Lumina Datamatics

Contents

Preface..xxv
Authors..xxvii

Chapter 1 The cell 1
1.1 Plasma membrane...2
    1.1.1 Structure and function of the plasma membrane 2
    1.1.2 Membrane transport 6
1.2 Membrane potential..11
    1.2.1 Development of the resting membrane potential.....................12
1.3 Electrical signals 15
    1.3.1 Graded potentials 15
    1.3.2 Action potentials...17
    1.3.3 Conduction of the action potential 20
1.4 Synaptic transmission..26
    1.4.1 Chemical synapses 26
    1.4.2 Summation 30
    1.4.3 Interconnections between neurons 32
    1.4.4 Factors affecting synaptic transmission 33
        1.4.4.1 Altered release of a neurotransmitter 33
        1.4.4.2 Altered interaction of a neurotransmitter with
               its receptor 34
        1.4.4.3 Altered removal of a neurotransmitter from the
               synaptic cleft..35
        1.4.4.4 Replacement of a deficient neurotransmitter 35
1.5 Cell injury..35
    1.5.1 Cellular adaptation..36
    1.5.2 Mechanisms of cell injury...38
    1.5.3 Manifestations of cellular injury 40
    1.5.4 Cell death..41
    1.5.5 Tissue repair 43
    1.5.6 Steps in tissue (wound) repair..44
Medical terminology 47
Bibliography 49

Chapter 2   Homeostasis..**51**
2.1   Homeostasis 51
     2.1.1   Negative feedback..54
     2.1.2   Positive feedback...55
Medical terminology 56
Bibliography 57

Chapter 3   The immune system...**59**
3.1   Overview of immune function...59
     3.1.1   Agents of infectious disease..60
     3.1.2   Effector cells of the immune system 62
     3.1.3   Immune responses..62
     3.1.4   Innate immune system 63
     3.1.5   Adaptive immune system 65
          3.1.5.1   Classification of antibodies 66
          3.1.5.2   Structure of antibodies....................................67
          3.1.5.3   Actions of antibodies.......................................68
          3.1.5.4   Clonal selection theory 70
          3.1.5.5   Primary versus secondary responses...............71
          3.1.5.6   Active versus passive immunity 72
          3.1.5.7   Types of T cells 74
          3.1.5.8   Actions of T cells...75
          3.1.5.9   MHC molecules 77
3.2   Alterations in immune function...78
     3.2.1   Hypersensitivity reactions 78
          3.2.1.1   Type I hypersensitivity reaction 78
          3.2.1.2   Type II hypersensitivity reaction....................80
          3.2.1.3   Type III hypersensitivity reaction...................83
          3.2.1.4   Type IV hypersensitivity reaction 83
     3.2.2   Autoimmune disease 84
Medical terminology 85
Bibliography 87

Chapter 4   Inflammation **89**
4.1   Inflammatory mediators 95
     4.1.1   Histamine and mast cells 95

Chapter 5   Blood and hemostasis...**99**
5.1   Blood 100
     5.1.1   Plasma 100
     5.1.2   Erythrocytes 101
     5.1.3   Leukocytes..105
     5.1.4   Platelets...107

Contents

5.2   Hemostasis 108
5.3   Alterations in hemostasis 114
       5.3.1   Conditions associated with decreased coagulation 114
                5.3.1.1   Hemophilia 114
                5.3.1.2   von Willebrand disease 114
                5.3.1.3   Vitamin K deficiency 115
                5.3.1.4   Liver disease 115
       5.3.2   Conditions affecting platelets 115
                5.3.2.1   Thrombocytopenia 115
                5.3.2.2   Immune thrombocytopenia purpura 116
                5.3.2.3   Antiphospholipid syndrome 116
       5.3.3   Conditions leading to increased blood coagulation
                (hypercoagulability) 116
       5.3.4   Disseminated intravascular coagulation (DIC) 117
                5.3.4.1   Manifestations of DIC 117
                5.3.4.2   Treatment of DIC 117
5.4   Alterations in hematologic function and oxygen transport 118
       5.4.1   Hematopoiesis 118
       5.4.2   Anemia 119
                5.4.2.1   General manifestations of anemia 119
       5.4.3   Types of anemia 120
                5.4.3.1   Hemolytic anemia 120
                5.4.3.2   Blood loss anemia 120
       5.4.4   Inherited anemia 121
                5.4.4.1   Sickle cell disease 121
                5.4.4.2   Thalassemia 125
                5.4.4.3   Glucose-6-phosphate dehydrogenase deficiency 126
                5.4.4.4   Aplastic anemia 126
                5.4.4.5   Polycythemia 127
Medical terminology 128
Bibliography 128

Chapter 6   The circulatory system 131
6.1   Blood vessels 133
6.2   Blood pressure 137
6.3   Blood flow 139
6.4   Regulation of arterial pressure 141
       6.4.1   Vasomotor center 145
       6.4.2   Baroreceptors 146
       6.4.3   Chemoreceptors 148
       6.4.4   Low-pressure receptors 149
       6.4.5   Vasoconstrictors 150
       6.4.6   Vasodilators 154

6.5   Venous regulation..155
        6.5.1   Blood volume...157
        6.5.2   Sympathetic stimulation of the veins 158
        6.5.3   Skeletal muscle activity 158
        6.5.4   Respiratory activity...158
6.6   Effects of gravity on the circulation..............................159
6.7   Regulation of blood flow through tissues......................160
        6.7.1   Active hyperemia 160
        6.7.2   Autoregulation...161
6.8   Effects of acute exercise on the circulatory system...........161
6.9   Capillary exchange..163
6.10   Disease of blood vessels 168
        6.10.1 Arterial disease...168
        6.10.2 Atherosclerosis and dyslipidemia.......................169
        6.10.3 Inflammatory disease of arteries.........................173
        6.10.4 Aneurysm...175
                6.10.4.1   Clinical manifestations of aneurysm 175
                6.10.4.2   Treatment of aneurysms 176
        6.10.5 Disease of the veins..176
                6.10.5.1   Venous thrombosis 176
                6.10.5.2   Embolism 179
                6.10.5.3   Anticoagulant and thrombolytic drug therapy...179
                6.10.5.4   Varicose veins...180
                6.10.5.5   Chronic venous insufficiency................180
6.11   Disorders of blood pressure..180
        6.11.1 Primary (Essential) hypertension 181
        6.11.2 Secondary hypertension..182
        6.11.3 Malignant hypertension 183
        6.11.4 Hypertension in pregnancy 183
        6.11.5 Effects of chronic hypertension 184
        6.11.6 Diagnosis and treatment of essential hypertension 185
        6.11.7 Treatment of hypertension...................................186
        6.11.8 Hypotension...187
                6.11.8.1   Manifestations of hypotension 187
                6.11.8.2   Treatment of hypotension....................188
6.12   Shock..188
        6.12.1 Hypovolemic shock 188
                6.12.1.1   Physiologic responses to hypovolemic shock 189
                6.12.1.2   Stages of symptoms of hypovolemic shock.........190
                6.12.1.3   Treatment of hypovolemic shock 190
        6.12.2 Distributive shock 191
                6.12.2.1   Symptoms of distributive shock...........191
                6.12.2.2   Treatment of distributive shock...........191

6.12.3   Cardiogenic shock..193
                6.12.3.1   Symptoms of cardiogenic shock..................194
                6.12.3.2   Treatment of cardiogenic shock..................194
6.12.4   Complications of shock 194
Medical terminology 195
Bibliography 196

Chapter 7   The heart **199**
7.1   Functional anatomy of the heart 202
    7.1.1   Myocardial wall..205
7.2   Electrical activity of the heart 209
7.3   Electrocardiogram 215
7.4   Cardiac cycle..218
    7.4.1   Ventricular filling..219
    7.4.2   Isovolumetric contraction 219
    7.4.3   Ejection...221
    7.4.4   Isovolumetric relaxation...................................221
7.5   Cardiac output 222
7.6   Control of heart rate 224
7.7   Control of stroke volume..227
7.8   Effect of exercise on cardiac output 232
7.9   Diseases of the heart..233
    7.9.1   Disorders of the pericardium, myocardium, and
                endocardium 233
                7.9.1.1   Disorders of the pericardium..................233
    7.9.2   Diseases of the myocardium..............................235
                7.9.2.1   Myocarditis..235
                7.9.2.2   Cardiomyopathies 236
    7.9.3   Disorders of the endocardium and heart valves 239
                7.9.3.1   Infectious endocarditis............................239
                7.9.3.2   Rheumatic heart disease 240
    7.9.4   Disorders of the heart valves...........................241
                7.9.4.1   Mitral valve prolapse 243
                7.9.4.2   Congenital heart defects.........................245
7.10   Myocardial ischemia 246
    7.10.1   Manifestations of myocardial ischemia 247
    7.10.2   Acute coronary syndromes...............................248
                7.10.2.1   Rational for treatment of myocardial ischemia....248
                7.10.2.2   Treatment of myocardial ischemia 249
7.11   Myocardial infarction..250
    7.11.1   Coronary blood flow and myocardial infarction.................250
    7.11.2   Clinical manifestations of myocardial infarction................252
    7.11.3   Compensatory mechanisms for myocardial infarction 252
    7.11.4   Complications of myocardial infarction 254

7.11.5   Rationale for therapy 254
                7.11.5.1   Treatment for myocardial infarction...................255
7.12   Heart failure...256
        7.12.1   Classification of heart failure...............................256
        7.12.2   Left heart failure 257
                7.12.2.1   Manifestations of left-heart failure....................257
        7.12.3   Right heart failure 258
                7.12.3.1   Manifestations of right-heart failure...................259
        7.12.4   Physiologic compensation for heart failure..........259
        7.12.5   Diagnosis of heart failure 264
        7.12.6   Rationale for treatment of heart failure...............265
7.13   Cardiac arrhythmia 266
        7.13.1   Factors that may contribute to the development of a
                cardiac arrhythmia 267
        7.13.2   Inherited arrhythmias..267
        7.13.3   Mechanisms of cardiac arrhythmia 267
        7.13.4   Types of arrhythmia...269
                7.13.4.1   Sinus node arrhythmia 270
                7.13.4.2   Atrial arrhythmia...............................270
                7.13.4.3   Ventricular arrhythmia 271
        7.13.5   Heart block...272
                7.13.5.1   First-degree heart block......................272
                7.13.5.2   Second-degree heart block 272
                7.13.5.3   Third-degree heart block 273
                7.13.5.4   Stokes-Adams syndrome.....................273
                7.13.5.5   Bundle branch block 273
        7.13.6   Diagnosis of arrhythmia......................................273
        7.13.7   Rationale for the treatment of cardiac arrhythmia 273
        7.13.8   Treatment of cardiac arrhythmia.........................274
                7.13.8.1   Pharmacologic....................................274
                7.13.8.2   Non-pharmacologic treatment of arrhythmia.....275
Medical terminology 275
Bibliography 277

Chapter 8   The respiratory system 279
8.1   Blood-gas interface 281
8.2   Airways..282
        8.2.1   Cartilage...282
        8.2.2   Epithelium...283
8.3   The pleura..284
8.4   Mechanics of breathing...284
        8.4.1   Thoracic volume...284
        8.4.2   Inspiration 284
        8.4.3   Expiration 285

	8.4.4	Lung volume	285
	8.4.5	Pulmonary pressures	286
8.5	Interdependence		293
8.6	Airway resistance		293
	8.6.1	Lung volume	294
	8.6.2	Airway obstruction	294
	8.6.3	Bronchial smooth muscle tone	295
8.7	Ventilation		297
	8.7.1	Standard lung volumes	297
	8.7.2	Total ventilation	300
	8.7.3	Alveolar ventilation	300
	8.7.4	Dead space	301
8.8	Diffusion		302
8.9	Partial pressures		304
8.10	Gas transport		309
	8.10.1	Transport of oxygen	309
	8.10.2	Factors affecting the transport of oxygen	312
	8.10.3	Transport of carbon dioxide	314
8.11	Regulation of ventilation		315
	8.11.1	Chemoreceptor response to decreased arterial PO_2	319
	8.11.2	Chemoreceptor response to increased arterial PCO_2	320
		8.11.2.1 Chemoreceptor response to increased arterial hydrogen ion concentration	321
8.12	Ventilatory response to exercise		321
8.13	Disorders of the respiratory system		322
	8.13.1	Respiratory infections	323
		8.13.1.1 Infections of the upper respiratory tract	323
		8.13.1.2 Infections of the lower respiratory tract	326
	8.13.2	Cancers of the respiratory tract	331
		8.13.2.1 Laryngeal cancer	331
		8.13.2.2 Lung cancer	331
	8.13.3	Obstructive and restrictive pulmonary disorders	332
	8.13.4	Obstructive pulmonary disorders	333
		8.13.4.1 Asthma	333
	8.13.5	Chronic obstructive pulmonary disease (COPD)	337
		8.13.5.1 Bronchitis	337
		8.13.5.2 Emphysema	338
	8.13.6	Cystic fibrosis	342
		8.13.6.1 Manifestations of cystic fibrosis	342
		8.13.6.2 Diagnosis of cystic fibrosis	343
		8.13.6.3 Treatment of cystic fibrosis	343
	8.13.7	Restrictive pulmonary disorders	344
		8.13.7.1 Pleuritis, pleural effusion	344
		8.13.7.2 Pneumothorax	344

                  8.13.7.3   Atelectasis...346

                  8.13.7.4   Bronchiectasis..347

       8.13.8   Acute respiratory distress syndrome 348

                  8.13.8.1   Manifestations of ARDS 349

                  8.13.8.2   Treatment of ARDS..349

       8.13.9   Respiratory distress syndrome of the newborn...................349

                  8.13.9.1   Manifestations of respiratory distress

                                  syndrome in the newborn 350

                  8.13.9.2   Treatment of respiratory distress syndrome

                                    in the newborn..350

       8.13.10   Interstitial lung diseases...350

                  8.13.10.1 Manifestations of interstitial lung disease 350

                  8.13.10.2 Treatment of interstitial lung diseases...............351

       8.13.11   Respiratory failure..351

                  8.13.11.1 Manifestations of respiratory failure 351

                  8.13.11.2 Treatment of respiratory failure 352

Medical terminology 352

Bibliography 354

Chapter 9   The digestive system...355

9.1   Digestive tract wall..357

       9.1.1   Mucosa...357

       9.1.2   Submucosa 358

       9.1.3   Muscularis externa...358

       9.1.4   Serosa 359

9.2   Regulation of gastrointestinal function 360

       9.2.1   Intrinsic nerve plexuses...360

       9.2.2   Extrinsic autonomic nerves..361

       9.2.3   Gastrointestinal hormones...361

9.3   Mouth...363

9.4   Pharynx 365

9.5   Esophagus...366

9.6   Stomach...366

       9.6.1   Gastric motility 367

       9.6.2   Gastric secretion 369

9.7   Liver...373

9.8   Gallbladder 375

9.9   Pancreas..376

9.10   Transport of bile and pancreatic juice...................................376

9.11   Small intestine 377

       9.11.1   Motility of the small intestine..378

       9.11.2   Digestion and absorption in the small intestine 378

       9.11.3   Carbohydrates 378

       9.11.4   Proteins 380

	9.11.5	Lipids	381
	9.11.6	Water and electrolytes	382
9.12	Large intestine		382
	9.12.1	Motility of the large intestine	383
	9.12.2	Secretion of the large intestine	384
9.13	Gastrointestinal disorders		384
	9.13.1	Abnormalities of the esophagus	384
		9.13.1.1 Swallowing disorders—dysphagia	384
		9.13.1.2 Manifestations of GERD	385
		9.13.1.3 Treatment of GERD	387
	9.13.2	Disorders of the stomach	387
		9.13.2.1 Gastritis	387
		9.13.2.2 Peptic ulcers	388
	9.13.3	Disorders of the intestines	390
		9.13.3.1 Irritable bowel syndrome (IBS)	390
		9.13.3.2 Inflammatory bowel disease	390
	9.13.4	Disorders of intestinal motility and absorption	396
		9.13.4.1 Diarrhea	396
		9.13.4.2 Constipation	396
		9.13.4.3 Intestinal malabsorption	397
	9.13.5	Gastrointestinal cancers	398
		9.13.5.1 Esophageal cancer	398
		9.13.5.2 Stomach cancer	398
		9.13.5.3 Colorectal cancer	398
9.14	Hepatobiliary disorders		398
	9.14.1	Tests of liver function	399
	9.14.2	Infectious disease of the liver	399
		9.14.2.1 Viral hepatitis	399
	9.14.3	Alcoholic liver disease	402
	9.14.4	Cirrhosis	403
		9.14.4.1 Manifestations of cirrhosis and liver failure	403
		9.14.4.2 Treatment of cirrhosis	405
	9.14.5	Liver cancer	405
	9.14.6	Disorders of the gallbladder	406
		9.14.6.1 Gallstone formation (Cholelithiasis)	406
		9.14.6.2 Cholecystitis	407
	9.14.7	Disorders of the pancreas	407
		9.14.7.1 Pancreatitis	407
		9.14.7.2 Pancreatic cancer	408
		9.14.7.3 Clinical manifestations of pancreatic cancer	409
Medical terminology			409
Bibliography			410

Chapter 10   The renal system **413**
10.1   Functional anatomy of the kidneys..415
          10.1.1   Vascular component..417
          10.1.2   Tubular component 418
10.2   Basic renal processes 419
10.3   Glomerular filtration..420
          10.3.1   Filtration barrier..420
          10.3.2   Determinants of filtration 421
10.4   Tubular reabsorption...423
          10.4.1   Sodium reabsorption...425
          10.4.2   Chloride reabsorption 427
          10.4.3   Water reabsorption 427
          10.4.4   Production of urine of varying concentrations 428
          10.4.5   Potassium ion secretion 434
          10.4.6   Hydrogen ion secretion..434
10.5   Plasma clearance..434
10.6   Renal blood flow...436
          10.6.1   Autoregulation..437
          10.6.2   Myogenic mechanism 437
          10.6.3   Tubuloglomerular feedback 438
          10.6.4   Resistance of the afferent arteriole 439
          10.6.5   Sympathetic nerves 439
          10.6.6   Angiotensin II...441
          10.6.7   Prostaglandins...442
10.7   Control of sodium excretion..443
10.8   Control of water excretion..445
10.9   Disorders of the kidney and urinary tract 448
          10.9.1   Evaluation of renal function..448
          10.9.2   Disorders of the glomerulus..449
                       10.9.2.1   Acute glomerulonephritis 449
                       10.9.2.2   Rapidly progressing glomerulonephritis...............449
                       10.9.2.3   IgA nephropathy (Berger's disease) 449
          10.9.3   Nephrotic syndrome 450
          10.9.4   Pyelonephritis 451
          10.9.5   Urinary tract infections 451
                       10.9.5.1   Manifestations of urinary tract infection 451
                       10.9.5.2   Treatment of urinary tract infection.....................452
          10.9.6   Renal calculi (kidney stones)...452
                       10.9.6.1   Manifestations of renal calculi.............................452
                       10.9.6.2   Diagnosis of renal calculi.....................................453
                       10.9.6.3   Treatment of renal calculi 453
          10.9.7   Renal tumors 453
                       10.9.7.1   Manifestations of renal tumors............................453
                       10.9.7.2   Treatment of renal tumors....................................453

10.9.8   Polycystic kidney disease.......................................454
           10.9.8.1   Manifestations of polycystic kidney
                        disease..454
           10.9.8.2   Treatment of polycystic kidney disease 454
10.9.9   Renal failure 454
           10.9.9.1   Acute renal failure..............................455
           10.9.9.2   Manifestations of acute renal failure 455
           10.9.9.3   Treatment of acute renal failure................455
10.9.10   Chronic renal failure 455
           10.9.10.1   Manifestations of chronic renal failure........456
           10.9.10.2   Treatment of renal failure 456
10.10   Disorders of the bladder and urethra..............................459
           10.10.1   Urine reflux 459
           10.10.2   Neurogenic bladder 460
           10.10.3   Urinary incontinence 461
                       10.10.3.1   Treatment of overactive bladder ...461
           10.10.4   Bladder cancer 461
Medical terminology 461
Bibliography 462

Chapter 11   The endocrine system...465
11.1   Biochemical classification of hormones 467
11.2   Transport of hormones 469
11.3   Functional classification of hormones.............................470
11.4   Hormone interactions..471
11.5   Mechanisms of hormone action 471
11.6   The pituitary gland 476
11.7   Relationship between the hypothalamus and the pituitary
        gland...477
11.8   Negative feedback control 479
11.9   Neurohypophysis...479
           11.9.1   Antidiuretic hormone 479
           11.9.2   Oxytocin..482
11.10   Adenohypophysis 483
           11.10.1   Gonadotropins....................................483
           11.10.2   Thyroid-stimulating hormone (TSH) 484
           11.10.3   Adrenocorticotropic hormone (ACTH) 484
           11.10.4   Prolactin..484
           11.10.5   Growth hormone (GH)..............................485
11.11   Thyroid gland 486
           11.11.1   Thyroid hormones.................................486
           11.11.2   Calcitonin 489
11.12   Parathyroid glands..489

11.13   Adrenal glands 491
      11.13.1   Adrenal medulla...491
      11.13.2   Adrenal cortex 491
      11.13.3   Mineralocorticoids 491
      11.13.4   Glucocorticoids..493
      11.13.5   Adrenal androgens...495
11.14   Pancreas 495
      11.14.1   Insulin 496
      11.14.2   Glucagon..497
11.15   Endocrine disorders...498
      11.15.1   Abnormalities of the hypothalamus/pituitary glands.....498
               11.15.1.1   Hypopituitarism......................................499
      11.15.2   Disorders of the anterior pituitary gland.........................499
               11.15.2.1   Alterations of growth hormone
                                secretion 499
      11.15.3   Disorders of the posterior pituitary...............................502
               11.15.3.1   Syndrome of inappropriate ADH
                                (SIADH).......................................502
               11.15.3.2   Diabetes insipidus 502
      11.15.4   Alteration of thyroid function 503
               11.15.4.1   Tests of thyroid function...........................503
               11.15.4.2   Hypothyroidism 504
               11.15.4.3   Hyperthyroidism.......................................506
      11.15.5   Disorders of the adrenal glands 507
               11.15.5.1   Hyposecretion of adrenal hormones 507
      11.15.6   Disorders of the adrenal medulla 512
               11.15.6.1   Pheochromocytoma 512
               11.15.6.2   Diagnosis of pheochromocytoma................512
               11.15.6.3   Manifestations of pheochromocytoma.........512
               11.15.6.4   Treatment of pheochromocytoma 512
11.16   Diabetes 512
      11.16.1   The endocrine pancreas...513
      11.16.2   Diabetes mellitus 514
               11.16.2.1   Types of diabetes 514
               11.16.2.2   Type 1 diabetes...516
      11.16.3   Long-term complications of diabetes 518
               11.16.3.1   Diabetic neuropathy..................................519
               11.16.3.2   Diabetic nephropathy 520
               11.16.3.3   Vascular disease..521
               11.16.3.4   Diabetic retinopathy..................................521
               11.16.3.5   Impaired healing and increased
                                infections risk..521
               11.16.3.6   Increased risk of infection 522

11.16.4   Diabetes in pregnancy 522
            11.16.4.1   Gestational diabetes 522
Medical terminology 522
Bibliography 524

Chapter 12   The reproductive system..**527**
12.1   Gametogenesis 528
        12.1.1   Spermatogenesis...528
        12.1.2   Oogenesis 528
12.2   Male reproductive system 529
        12.2.1   Testes 529
        12.2.2   Epididymides..529
        12.2.3   Vas deferens 530
        12.2.4   Ejaculatory ducts 530
        12.2.5   Penis 530
        12.2.6   Prostate 530
        12.2.7   Seminal vesicles...530
        12.2.8   Bulbourethral glands 531
12.3   Female reproductive system 532
        12.3.1   Ovaries..532
        12.3.2   Fallopian tubes...533
        12.3.3   Uterus..533
        12.3.4   Vagina..533
        12.3.5   Follicular phase..534
        12.3.6   Luteal phase 535
        12.3.7   Hormonal regulation of the ovarian cycle.....535
12.4   Disorders of the male reproductive system 539
        12.4.1   Disorders of the penis....................................539
                    12.4.1.1   Peyronie's disease.............................539
                    12.4.1.2   Priapism 539
                    12.4.1.3   Impotence 540
        12.4.2   Disorders of the testis and scrotum 540
                    12.4.2.1   Spermatocele 540
                    12.4.2.2   Varicocele...540
                    12.4.2.3   Testicular cancer 540
        12.4.3   Disorders of the prostate 541
                    12.4.3.1   Prostatitis 541
                    12.4.3.2   Benign prostatic hyperplasia (BPH) 541
                    12.4.3.3   Prostate cancer 543
12.5   Disorders of the female reproductive system...............544
        12.5.1   Disorders of the vagina, cervix, and uterus....544
                    12.5.1.1   Vaginitis 544
                    12.5.1.2   Cervical lesions and cervical cancer 544
                    12.5.1.3   Endometriosis 545

          12.5.1.4 Endometrial (Uterine) cancer.............................546
          12.5.1.5 Uterine fibroids 547
          12.5.1.6 Uterine prolapse 547
     12.5.2 Disorders of the ovaries...547
          12.5.2.1 Polycystic ovary syndrome 547
          12.5.2.2 Ovarian cancer 548
     12.5.3 Menstrual disorders...549
          12.5.3.1 Amenorrhea..549
          12.5.3.2 Dysmenorrhea..549
          12.5.3.3 Menopause 550
          12.5.3.4 Symptoms 550
          12.5.3.5 Treatment 550
     12.5.4 Disorders of the breast..550
          12.5.4.1 Mastitis...550
          12.5.4.2 Fibrocystic changes 551
          12.5.4.3 Proliferative changes..................................551
     12.5.5 Breast cancer 551
          12.5.5.1 Risk factors for breast cancer 551
          12.5.5.2 Diagnosis 552
          12.5.5.3 Treatment 552
          12.5.5.4 Prognosis...552
12.6 Sexually transmitted diseases 552
     12.6.1 Diagnosis 553
     12.6.2 Risk factors 553
          12.6.2.1 Bacterial STDs 553
          12.6.2.2 Viral STDs 554
          12.6.2.3 Other STDs 554
          12.6.2.4 Long-term consequences of STDs 555
Medical terminology 555
Bibliography 556

Chapter 13 The nervous system 559
13.1 Neurons...561
13.2 Level of CNS function..562
13.3 The brain 563
13.4 Blood-brain barrier 578
13.5 Cerebrospinal fluid 580
13.6 The spinal cord...581
     13.6.1 Functions of the spinal cord.....................................583
          13.6.1.1 Composition of the spinal cord 583
          13.6.1.2 Ascending tracts 586
          13.6.1.3 Descending tracts 587

13.6.2   Spinal reflexes 590
          13.6.2.1   Withdrawal reflex 591
          13.6.2.2   Crossed-extensor reflex.............................593
13.7 Disorders of the nervous system 593
      13.7.1   Disorders of the brain 593
                13.7.1.1   Brain injury...593
                13.7.1.2   Traumatic brain injury 594
                13.7.1.3   Intracranial hematoma...............................594
                13.7.1.4   Increased intracranial pressure.................596
                13.7.1.5   Symptoms of increased ICP 596
                13.7.1.6   Treatment of increased ICP 596
                13.7.1.7   Brain ischemia and hypoxia.....................597
                13.7.1.8   Causes of brain ischemia or hypoxia.................597
                13.7.1.9   Manifestations of cerebral ischemia or
                            hypoxia.. 597
      13.7.2   Stroke...598
                13.7.2.1   Symptoms of stroke....................................599
                13.7.2.2   Complications of stroke...............................600
                13.7.2.3   Diagnosis of stroke 600
                13.7.2.4   Treatment of stroke.....................................600
      13.7.3   CNS infections 600
                13.7.3.1   Manifestations of CNS infections.......................602
                13.7.3.2   Diagnosis of CNS infections 602
                13.7.3.3   Treatment of CNS infections 602
      13.7.4   CNS tumors...602
                13.7.4.1   Type of CNS tumors...................................603
                13.7.4.2   Manifestations of CNS tumors 603
                13.7.4.3   Diagnosis of CNS tumors...........................604
                13.7.4.4   Treatment of CNS tumors..........................604
      13.7.5   Seizure disorders 604
                13.7.5.1   Epilepsy...604
                13.7.5.2   Type of seizures 604
                13.7.5.3   Focal seizures 604
                13.7.5.4   Generalized seizures 605
                13.7.5.5   Diagnosis of seizure disorders..................606
                13.7.5.6   Treatment of seizure disorders 607
      13.7.6   Headache 607
                13.7.6.1   Primary headaches 607
                13.7.6.2   Secondary headaches..................................608
      13.7.7   Degenerative disorders of the brain and CNS 608
                13.7.7.1   Parkinson's disease 608
                13.7.7.2   Alzheimer's disease 611
                13.7.7.3   Huntington's disease 615

13.7.7.4   Amyotrophic lateral sclerosis 616
13.7.7.5   Multiple sclerosis..617
13.7.8   Spinal injury...618
13.7.8.1   Manifestations of spinal cord injury..................619
13.7.8.2   Treatment of spinal cord injury 619
Medical terminology 619
Bibliography 621

Chapter 14 The autonomic nervous system 623
14.1   Regulation...624
14.2   Pathways...625
14.3   Divisions 626
14.4   Neurotransmission 630
14.5   Receptors...633
14.6   Functions...636
Medical terminology 641
Bibliography 642

Chapter 15 Pain..645
15.1   Nociceptors...646
15.2   Hyperalgesia...648
15.3   Neurotransmission 649
15.4   Pain pathways..649
15.5   Types of pain 654
15.5.1   Tissue ischemia 654
15.5.2   Muscle spasm...654
15.5.3   Visceral pain...655
15.5.4   Referred pain...655
15.6   Treatment of pain..657
15.6.1   Nonnarcotic analgesics...657
15.6.2   Opioid analgesics 658
15.6.3   Adjuvant analgesics 659
Medical terminology 659
Bibliography 659

Chapter 16 Muscle...661
16.1   Smooth muscle...662
16.1.1   Structure of smooth muscle 662
16.1.2   Calcium and the mechanism of contraction.......664
16.1.3   Smooth muscle contraction is slow and prolonged 665
16.1.4   Types of smooth muscle 666
16.1.5   Factors influencing the contractile activity of
smooth muscle...668

16.1.6   Length–tension relationship 669
16.1.7   Hyperplasia...670
16.2   Skeletal muscle...670
16.2.1   Muscle tension and movement 671
16.2.1.1   Isometric versus isotonic contraction 672
16.2.2   Structure of skeletal muscle..672
16.2.2.1   Sarcomeres...673
16.2.2.2   Thick filaments..673
16.2.2.3   Thin filaments 675
16.2.3   Neuromuscular junction 675
16.2.4   Mechanism of contraction...676
16.2.4.1   Sources of ATP for muscle contraction..............680
16.2.5   Muscle fatigue..681
16.2.6   Oxygen debt..682
16.2.7   Types of muscle fibers...682
16.2.8   Muscle mechanics 684
16.2.8.1   Number of muscle fibers contracting 685
16.2.8.2   Amount of tension developed by each
contracting muscle fiber 686
16.3   Disorders of skeletal muscle 688
16.3.1   Metabolic disorders of skeletal muscle 688
16.3.1.1   McArdle's disease..689
16.3.1.2   Pompei disease 689
16.3.2   Cerebral palsy 690
16.3.2.1   Symptoms 690
16.3.2.2   Treatment 690
16.3.3   Muscular dystrophy (MD) 690
16.3.3.1   Duchenne muscular dystrophy 691
16.3.3.2   Becker muscular dystrophy 692
16.3.3.3   Facioscapulohumeral muscular dystrophy 692
16.3.3.4   Limb girdle muscular dystrophy 692
16.3.4   Myasthenia gravis 693
16.3.4.1   Symptoms...693
16.3.4.2   Diagnosis 693
16.3.4.3   Treatment 694
Medical terminology 694
Bibliography 695

Chapter 17 The skeletal system...697
17.1   Bone as a tissue and an organ 698
17.2   Hemopoiesis...698
17.2.1   Erythropoiesis..698
17.2.2   Thrombopoiesis 698
17.2.3   Leukopoiesis 699

17.3   Mineral deposition 699
17.4   Mineral resorption..699
17.5   Calcium homeostasis...700
17.6   Disorders of the skeletal system 700
       17.6.1   Osteoporosis..701
             17.6.1.1   Manifestations of osteoporosis 702
             17.6.1.2   Diagnosis of osteoporosis....................................702
             17.6.1.3   Treatment of osteoporosis 702
       17.6.2   Paget's disease 702
             17.6.2.1   Clinical manifestations of Paget's disease 702
       17.6.3   Osteomalacia..703
             17.6.3.1   Clinical manifestations of osteomalacia.............703
       17.6.4   Rheumatoid arthritis (RA) 704
             17.6.4.1   Manifestations of rheumatoid arthritis 704
             17.6.4.2   Diagnosis of rheumatoid arthritis.......................705
             17.6.4.3   Treatment of rheumatoid arthritis.......................706
       17.6.5   Systemic Lupus Erythematosus 706
             17.6.5.1   Manifestations of SLE 706
             17.6.5.2   Diagnosis and treatment of SLE..........................706
       17.6.6   Ankylosing spondylitis 707
       17.6.7   Osteoarthritis 707
             17.6.7.1   Manifestations of OA...707
             17.6.7.2   Treatment of OA 709
       17.6.8   Gout..709
             17.6.8.1   Manifestations of gout 709
             17.6.8.2   Treatment of gout 710

Chapter 18 Cancer 711
18.1   Introduction...711
18.2   Cancer terminology 711
       18.2.1   Specific nomenclature examples 713
18.3   Theories of oncogenesis...714
       18.3.1   Mutation of DNA 714
       18.3.2   Hereditary 715
18.4   Local effects of cancer 715
18.5   Systemic effects of cancer 716
18.6   Tumor staging 717
18.7   Cancer detection 717
       18.7.1   Tumor cell markers 717
       18.7.2   Tumor grading...718
       18.7.3   Visualization 719
       18.7.4   Biopsy..719

18.8   Rationale for cancer therapy 719
      18.8.1   Treatment of cancer..719
      18.8.2   Hormonal therapy...719
      18.8.3   Radiation therapy..720
      18.8.4   Immune-based therapies ("biologic response
                modifiers") 720

Chapter 19 HIV 721
19.1   Introduction...721
19.2   HIV structure and lifecycle 722
19.3   Stages in an HIV infection...725
      19.3.1   Acute illness stage...725
      19.3.2   Asymptomatic stage 725
      19.3.3   Symptomatic or AIDS stage................................725
19.4   Epidemiology of HIV infection.....................................726
19.5   Laboratory of diagnosis of HIV....................................726
19.6   Rationale for treatment of HIV 727
      19.6.1   Treatment of HIV..727

Index 731

Preface

The presentation of material within the chapters was designed to maximize clarity and facilitate conveyance of key points to the students. Numerous subheadings, bulleted lists, tables, and definitions of key terms are included in each chapter along with study objectives that are designed to focus students on important concepts within each chapter. The word "pathophysiology" is derived from the Greek word "pathos" which means "suffering, disease" and "physiology" which is the science of the normal function of living things." Pathophysiology content in this text is specifically designed to build upon the information provided in the sections related to the normal physiology. We also believe that pathophysiology is a bridge between physiology and pharmacology. As a result of the authors' experience in teaching both pathophysiology and pharmacology it has become clear that the time to introduce health science students to therapeutics is in pathophysiology where the mechanism and effects of disease are explored in detail and the application of the drugs makes the most sense. A rationale for drug therapy section is therefore included in each chapter to allow students to correlate information they have learned on selected diseases to the clinical application of drugs.

Authors

Laurie K. McCorry, PhD, was a professor for 18 years teaching courses that included human physiology, pathophysiology, cardiovascular physiology, and exercise physiology at the Massachusetts College of Pharmacy and Health Sciences, Boston, Massachusetts, as well as anatomy and physiology at Bay State College, Boston, Massachusetts. She is currently the dean of science, engineering and mathematics at Bunker Hill Community College in Boston, Massachusetts.

Martin M. Zdanowicz received a BS in biology from NYU-Polytechnic, Brooklyn, New York, an MA in biology/physiology from S.U.N.Y. Binghamton, Vestal, New York, and a PhD in pharmaceutical sciences (Pharmacology) from St. John's University, New York. After completing his doctorate, he went on to work as a research scientist at North Shore University Hospital-Cornell Medical College, New York, in the area of endocrinology and metabolism. He assumed a full-time faculty appointment with the Massachusetts College of Pharmacy and Health Sciences, Boston, Massachusetts, and served as chair of pharmaceutical sciences and director of graduate studies. Dr. Zdanowicz moved to the South University School of Pharmacy in Savannah, Georgia where he served as chair of pharmaceutical sciences. He was promoted to full professor in January 2008. Teaching areas include pharmacology, pathophysiology, and pharmacogenomics. Dr. Zdanowicz has received the Trustee's Award for teaching excellence and was voted teacher of the year seven times by students at three institutions. His current research interests include pharmacogenomics, drug addiction, cardiovascular pharmacology, and curriculum development. Dr. Zdanowicz holds membership in a number of professional societies and has published numerous peer-reviewed articles and several textbooks. He is currently completing an MPH online from the University of South Florida, Tampa, Florida. Dr. Zdanowicz currently serves as the associate dean for health studies at the University of Miami School of Nursing and Health Studies, Coral Gables, Florida, where he oversees programs in public health, health science, and health informatics.

Cynthia Y. Gonnella has been teaching anatomy and physiology, general biology, and nutrition at Bunker Hill Community College in Boston, Massachusetts, for the past 25 years. She also teaches at Middlesex Community College in Lowell, Massachusetts. She earned her degree from the University of Massachusetts and has designed numerous web-based courses for life sciences. When she is not teaching, she enjoys a successful writing career, and also paints and explores the land along the Concord River in Massachusetts.

chapter one

The cell

Study objectives

- Describe the function of each of the components of the plasma membrane
- Understand the physiological importance of the permeability barrier created by the plasma membrane
- Describe the factors that affect diffusion
- Explain how osmosis takes place
- Understand the clinical significance of the osmotic pressures of solutions
- Describe the factors that affect mediated transport
- Compare and contrast facilitated diffusion and active transport
- Define membrane potential
- Compare the distribution and permeability differences of ions across the cell membrane
- Describe how differences in ion distribution and permeability contribute to the resting membrane potential
- Describe how a cell's resting membrane potential is developed and maintained
- Explain the role of the Na^+-K^+-ATPase pump in the process of ion exchange across the cell membrane
- Distinguish between depolarization, hyperpolarization, and repolarization
- Compare and contrast graded potentials and action potentials
- Describe the process of local current flow
- Explain the mechanism by which action potentials are generated
- Understand the function of sodium and potassium voltage-gated channels
- Distinguish between the absolute refractory period and the relative refractory period
- Describe the process of saltatory conduction
- Explain the functional significance of myelin
- Explain why the conduction of the action potential is unidirectional
- Describe the mechanism by which chemical synapses function
- Describe the effects of a neurotransmitter binding to its receptors on the postsynaptic neuron
- Compare and contrast excitatory synapses and inhibitory synapses
- Distinguish between an EPSP and an IPSP
- Describe how neurotransmitters are removed from the synaptic cleft
- Explain how temporal summation and spatial summation take place
- Distinguish between convergence and divergence

- Understand how pH and hypoxia affect synaptic transmission
- Describe the potential mechanisms by which drugs, toxins and diseases affect synaptic transmission
- Explain why synaptic transmission is unidirectional
- Distinguish between an agonist and an antagonist
- Compare and contrast the various forms of cellular adaptation. What is the purpose of these adaptive changes?
- Discuss the underlying mechanisms by which cellular injury can occur
- Describe the major manifestations that present when cells are injured. Why does each of these manifestations occur?
- Define apoptosis and necrotic cell death. How do they differ?
- List the specific types of cellular necrosis that may occur and their distinct characteristics
- Define gangrene and gas gangrene
- Discuss the two mechanisms by which tissue repair occurs. Give examples of specific cell types that will utilize each repair mechanism
- List the steps involved in wound repair along with the key features of each step
- List various factors that can impair wound healing
- What is a keloid scar? Why does it occur?

1.1   Plasma membrane

Each cell is enclosed within a plasma membrane that separates the cytoplasmic contents of the cell, or the intracellular fluid (ICF), from the fluid outside of the cell, the extracellular fluid (ECF). An important homeostatic function of this plasma membrane is to serve as a *permeability barrier* that insulates or protects the cytoplasm from immediate changes in the surrounding environment. Furthermore, it allows the cell to maintain a cytoplasmic composition that is very different from that of the ECF. The functions of neurons (nerve cells) and muscle cells depend on this difference. The plasma membrane also contains many enzymes and other components such as antigens and receptors. These structures allow cells to interact with other cells, neurotransmitters, blood-borne substances such as hormones, and various other chemical substances, such as drugs.

1.1.1   Structure and function of the plasma membrane

The major components of the plasma membrane include:

- Phospholipids
- Cholesterol
- Proteins
- Carbohydrates

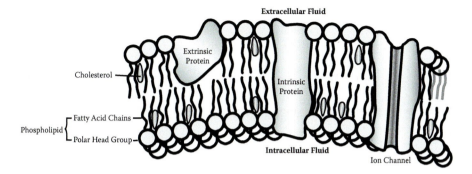

Figure 1.1 Structure of the plasma membrane. The plasma membrane is composed of a bilayer of phospholipid molecules. Associated with this bilayer are intrinsic proteins, which are embedded within and span the membrane, and extrinsic proteins, which are found on the external or internal surface of the membrane. Molecules of cholesterol are found in the inner, nonpolar region of the membrane.

The basic structure of the plasma membrane is formed by *phospholipids* (see Figure 1.1). These molecules are one of the more abundant of the membrane components. Phospholipids are *amphipathic* molecules that have both polar (water-soluble) and nonpolar (water-insoluble) regions. They are composed of a phosphorylated glycerol backbone, which forms a polar head group that is hydrophilic, and a nonpolar region containing two hydrophobic fatty acid chains. In an aqueous environment, such as the body, these molecules are arranged in a formation referred to as the *lipid bilayer* consisting of two layers of phospholipids. The polar region of the molecule is oriented toward the outer surface of the membrane where it can interact with water; and the nonpolar, hydrophobic fatty acids are in the center of the membrane away from the water. The functional significance of this lipid bilayer is that it creates a *semipermeable barrier*. Lipophilic, or non-water-soluble, substances can readily cross the membrane by simply passing through its lipid core. Important examples of these substances include gases, such as oxygen and carbon dioxide, and fatty acid molecules, which are used to form energy within muscle cells.

Most hydrophilic, or water-soluble, substances are repelled by this hydrophobic interior and cannot simply diffuse through the membrane. Instead, these substances must cross the membrane using specialized transport mechanisms. Examples of lipid-insoluble substances that require such mechanisms include proteins, nutrient molecules such as glucose and amino acids, and all species of ions (Na^+, Ca^{++}, H^+, Cl^-, and HCO_3^-). Therefore, the plasma membrane plays a very important role in determining the composition of the ICF by selectively permitting substances to move in and out of the cell.

**PHARMACY APPLICATION:
LIPID SOLUBILITY AND DRUG ELIMINATION**

The lipid solubility of many substances can change when physiological conditions vary. For example, the surrounding pH can determine whether a molecule is in a protonated form (positively charged, lipid-insoluble) or in an unprotonated form (uncharged, lipid-soluble). As discussed, charged substances do not readily cross the membrane, as do uncharged substances. This principle regarding lipid solubility is used in the treatment of an overdose of phenobarbital, a barbiturate used for sedation and seizure disorders. Phenobarbital is normally 30% removed by urinary excretion. In the case of an overdose, it would be advantageous to enhance urinary excretion. Alkalization of the urine to a pH of 7.5–8 helps to promote excretion. In fact, by alkalinizing the urine, the amount of phenobarbital excreted increases 5- to 10-fold. After alkalization, more phenobarbital would be ionized in the urine and, therefore, become lipid-insoluble and, therefore, the drug would not be reabsorbed from the kidney, but would instead be eliminated in the urine.

Another important aspect of the lipid bilayer is that the phospholipids are not held together by chemical bonds. This enables the molecules to move about freely within the membrane, resulting in a structure that is not rigid in nature, but instead, is very fluid and pliable. Another substance contributing to membrane fluidity is *cholesterol*. Cholesterol has a steroid nucleus that is lipid-soluble. Therefore, these molecules are found in the interior of the membrane lying parallel to the fatty acid chains of the phospholipids (see Figure 1.1). As such, they prevent the fatty acid chains from packing together and crystallizing, which would decrease membrane fluidity.

Membrane fluidity is very important in terms of function in many cell types. For example, skeletal muscle activity involves the shortening and lengthening of the muscle fibers. Furthermore, as white blood cells leave the blood vessels and enter the tissue spaces to fight infection, they must squeeze through tiny pores in the wall of the capillary, requiring significant deformation of the cell and its membrane. Finally, in all cells, many processes that transport substances across the plasma membrane require the embedded proteins to change their conformation and move about within the bilayer. In each case, for the cell membrane, or the entire cell, to change its shape, the membrane must be very fluid and flexible.

Proteins are also associated with the lipid bilayer and essentially float within it. Intrinsic, or transmembrane, proteins are embedded within and span the membrane. These proteins are like phospholipids in that they are amphipathic with the polar regions of the molecule extending beyond the lipid bilayer and the nonpolar region embedded within it. Extrinsic, or peripheral, proteins are found on either the internal or the external surface of the membrane (see Figure 1.1). These proteins are not amphipathic and do not associate with the internal region of the membrane. The membrane proteins provide a variety of important cellular functions by forming the following structures:

- Channels
- Carrier molecules
- Enzymes
- Chemical receptors
- Antigens

Some proteins may form *channels* through the cell membrane, which allow small water-soluble substances, such as ions, to enter or leave the cell. These channels are quite specific and allow only one type of ion to pass through it (e.g., sodium channels, calcium channels). Other proteins may serve as *carrier molecules* that selectively transport larger water-soluble molecules, such as glucose or cellular products, across the membrane. *Enzymes*, which regulate specific chemical reactions, are extrinsic proteins and are found on either the internal (e.g., adenylate cyclase) or the external (e.g., acetylcholinesterase) surfaces of the membrane. *Chemical receptors* are found on the outer surface of the cell membrane and selectively bind with various endogenous molecules such as neurotransmitters and hormones as well as drugs. Many substances that are unable to enter the cell and cause a direct intracellular effect may indirectly influence intracellular activity without crossing the membrane through receptor activation. Other proteins found on the external surface of the plasma membrane are *antigens*. These molecules serve as cell "markers" that allow the body's immune system to distinguish between our own cells and foreign cells or organisms, such as bacteria and viruses.

The plasma membrane contains a small amount of *carbohydrate* (2%–10% of the mass of the membrane) found predominantly on the outer surface. This carbohydrate is found attached to most of the protein molecules, forming glycoproteins, and to some of the phospholipid molecules (<10%), forming glycolipids. Consequently, the external surface of the cell has a carbohydrate coat, or glycocalyx.

These carbohydrate moieties have several important functions including the following:

- *Repel negatively charged substances*: many of the carbohydrates are negatively charged creating an overall negative charge on the surface of the cell that repels negatively charged extracellular molecules and helps to keep red blood cells apart from each other

- *Cell-to-cell attachment*: the glycocalyx of one cell may attach to the glycocalyx of another cell, which causes the cells themselves to become attached
- *Receptors*: carbohydrates may also serve as specific membrane receptors for extracellular substances, such as hormones
- *Immune reactions*: carbohydrates play a role in the ability of cells to distinguish between "self" cells and foreign cells

**PHARMACY APPLICATION:
HYDROPHILIC DRUGS BIND TO RECEPTORS**

Many substances within the body, including neurotransmitters and hormones, are hydrophilic and, therefore, are incapable of entering the cells to carry out their effects directly. Instead, they bind to their specific receptors on the cell surface. This receptor binding then elicits a series of intracellular events that alter cell function and cell metabolism. As such, there are many instances where it would be clinically advantageous to either enhance or inhibit these activities. Therefore, drugs may be designed to bind to these specific receptors. A drug that binds to and stimulates a receptor, mimicking the action of the endogenous chemical substance, is referred to as a receptor *agonist*. An example is albuterol sulfate, a selective β_2-adrenergic receptor agonist. Stimulation of β_2-adrenergic receptors on airway smooth muscle causes dilation of the airways in a patient experiencing an asthmatic attack and relieves the patient's wheezing. Conversely, a drug that binds to and blocks a receptor, preventing the action of the endogenous substance, is referred to as a receptor *antagonist*. An example in this case is cimetidine hydrochloride, which inhibits histamine H_2 receptors on parietal cells in the stomach. Because histamine H_2 receptor stimulation leads to gastric acid secretion, blockade of these receptors with an antagonist reduces acid secretion. While cimetidine hydrochloride is the active ingredient in Pepcid®, ranitidine hydrochloride, another histamine H_2 receptor antagonist, is found in Zantac® and works in much the same way. These drugs may be used to treat patients with a peptic ulcer or gastroesophageal reflux disease (GERD).

1.1.2   Membrane transport

The lipid bilayer arrangement of the plasma membrane renders it semipermeable. Uncharged or nonpolar molecules, such as oxygen, carbon dioxide and fatty acids, are lipid soluble and may permeate through the membrane quite readily. Charged or polar molecules, such as glucose, proteins, and ions, are water soluble and are impermeable and unable to cross the membrane unassisted. These substances require protein channels or carrier molecules to enter or leave the cell.

Mechanisms by which substances may cross the plasma membrane include:

- Passive diffusion
- Osmosis
- Mediated transport

The movement of molecules and ions from one place to another, under the power of molecular motion, is referred to as *passive diffusion*. Molecules and ions are in constant motion, and the velocity of their motion is proportional to their concentration. When a molecule is unevenly distributed across a permeable membrane with a higher concentration on one side and a lower concentration on the opposite side, there is said to be a *concentration gradient* or a concentration difference. Although all the molecules are in motion, there will be a tendency for a greater number of molecules to move from the area of high concentration toward the area of low concentration. This uneven movement of molecules is referred to as *net diffusion*. The net diffusion of molecules continues until the concentrations of the substance on both sides of the membrane are equal and the subsequent movement of molecules through the membrane is in a *dynamic equilibrium*. In other words, the number of molecules moving in one direction across the membrane is equal to the number of molecules moving in the opposite direction. At this point, although the diffusion of molecules continues, there is no further *net* diffusion.

Many molecules diffuse across membranes in our body moving from one compartment to another. For example, oxygen and glucose diffuse from the ECF (higher concentration) into the ICF (lower concentration) where the cell uses these substances to make ATP (energy). The movement of a substance across a membrane is also referred to as *flux*. Specifically, the movement of a substance *into* the cell is referred to as *influx* and the movement of a substance *out of* the cell is referred to as *efflux*.

The rate of diffusion of a substance is influenced by several factors (see Table 1.1). It is proportional to the concentration gradient, the permeability of the membrane, and the surface area of the membrane. For example, as the permeability of the membrane increases, the rate of diffusion of a given substance across the membrane increases. Diffusion is inversely

Table 1.1 Factors that influence the rate of diffusion of a substance

Factor	Rate of diffusion
↑ Concentration gradient	↑
↑ Permeability of the membrane	↑
↑ Surface area of the membrane	↑
↑ Molecular weight of the substance	↓
↑ Thickness of the membrane	↓

proportional to the molecular weight of the substance and the thickness of the membrane. Larger molecules diffuse more slowly.

The movement of ions depends not only on a concentration gradient but also on an *electrical gradient*. Opposite charges are attracted to each other. Therefore, positively charged ions (cations) are attracted to a negatively charged area and negatively charged ions (anions) are attracted to a positively charged area. This electrical attraction enhances diffusion of the ions, while ions of a similar charge tend to repel each other and oppose diffusion. These two forces, the concentration gradient and the electrical gradient, may work together to cause a greater diffusion of ions. Alternatively, these forces may oppose each other and, thereby, limit the net diffusion of the ion (see Figure 1.2).

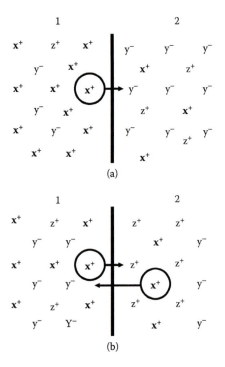

Figure 1.2   Diffusion of ions. The solutions on both side 1 and side 2 contain X^+, Y^-, and Z^+. Assume that the membrane is permeable only to X^+. (a) The concentration of X^+ is greater on side 1 than on side 2. The number of negative charges is greater on side 2 than on side 1. Therefore, there will be net diffusion of X^+ from side 1 to side 2 due to both the concentration gradient and the electrical gradient. Both gradients work together, promoting the diffusion of X^+ across the membrane. (b) The concentration of X^+ is greater on side 1 than on side 2. The number of negative charges is greater on side 1 than on side 2. Therefore, X^+ will tend to diffuse from side 1 to side 2 due to the concentration gradient. However, X^+ will also tend to diffuse from side 2 to side 1 due to the electrical gradient. In this case, the two forces promoting diffusion oppose each other and limit the net diffusion of X^+ across the membrane.

Osmosis is the net movement of water through a semipermeable membrane down its own concentration gradient from an area of high water concentration to an area of low water concentration. Water is a small, polar molecule that can easily diffuse across plasma membranes through small intermolecular spaces. This movement of water across cell membranes in some tissues (e.g., kidney) may be significantly facilitated by the presence of a group of membrane proteins that form channels referred to as *aquaporins.*

In other words, water moves toward an area of higher *solute* concentration. The solute particles may be thought of as "drawing" the water toward them. Therefore, the *osmotic pressure* of a solution is the pressure or force by which water is drawn into the solution through a semipermeable membrane. The magnitude of this pressure depends on the number of solute particles present. An increase in the number of particles in the solution results in an increase in the osmotic pressure and, therefore, an increase in the movement of water toward it.

The plasma membrane is *semipermeable,* meaning it is not permeable to all solute particles and, therefore, maintains a concentration difference for many ions and molecules across itself. Water, however, crosses the membrane freely in either direction. The movement of water in and out of the cell will occur whenever there is a difference in osmotic pressure between the ICF and the ECF. For example, an increase in the osmotic pressure of the ECF (more solute, lower water concentration) will cause water to leave the cell by osmosis. The resulting decrease in the fluid volume of the cell may lead to cellular dehydration. On the other hand, a decrease in the osmotic pressure in the ECF (less solute, higher water concentration) will cause water to enter the cell by osmosis. The increase in the fluid volume of the cell may lead to an increase in *hydrostatic pressure* within the cell. An excessive increase in hydrostatic pressure may cause the cell to burst.

PHARMACY APPLICATION: INTRAVENOUS SOLUTIONS

Intravenous (i.v.) solutions are commonly administered to patients in hospitals, long-term care facilities and ambulances. They are used primarily to replace body fluids and to serve as a vehicle for injecting drugs into the body. The advantages of this pharmaceutical dosage form include the rapid onset of action, the ability to treat patients unable to take medication orally and the ability to administer a medication unavailable in any other dosage form.

(Continued)

PHARMACY APPLICATION: INTRAVENOUS
SOLUTIONS (Continued)

Intravenous solutions must be isotonic (same osmotic pressure) with red blood cells. If red blood cells were to be exposed to a hypotonic (lower osmotic pressure) i.v. solution, water from this solution would move into the cells causing them to swell and possibly lyse. If red blood cells were to be exposed to a hypertonic (higher osmotic pressure) i.v. solution, water would move out of the cells causing them to dehydrate and shrink. Both conditions would damage the red blood cells and disrupt function. Intravenous injections are often prepared with 0.9% sodium chloride or 5% dextrose, both of which are approximately isotonic with red blood cells. These solutions prevent any unwanted osmosis, or movement of water, into or out of the red blood cells.

Patient discomfort is another important consideration. The stinging caused by a hypotonic or hypertonic i.v. solution is not experienced with one that is isotonic.

In the process of *mediated transport*, carrier proteins embedded within the plasma membrane assist in the transport of larger, polar molecules into or out of the cell. When a substance attaches to a specific binding site on the carrier protein, the protein undergoes a conformational change such that this site with the bound substance moves from one side of the plasma membrane to the other. The substance is then released.

Mediated transport displays three important characteristics influencing its function:

- Specificity
- Competition
- Saturation

Carrier proteins display a high degree of *specificity*. In other words, each of these proteins may bind only with select substances that "fit" into its binding site. Another characteristic is *competition*. Different substances that have similar chemical structures may be able to bind to the same carrier protein and, therefore, compete for transport across the membrane. The third characteristic displayed by mediated transport is *saturation*. The greater the number of carrier proteins being utilized at any given time, the greater the rate of transport. Therefore, initially as the concentration of a substance increases, the number of active carrier molecules increases, and the rate of transport increases. However, there are a finite number of carrier proteins in the cell membrane. Once all these proteins are being utilized in the transport process, any further increase in the concentration of the substance no longer increases the rate of transport because it has reached its maximum. At this point, the process is saturated.

There are two forms of mediated transport:

- Facilitated diffusion
- Active transport

With *facilitated diffusion*, carrier proteins move across the membrane in either direction and will transport a substance down its concentration gradient. In other words, substances are moved from an area of high concentration to an area of low concentration. This process is passive and requires no energy. An example of a substance transported by facilitated diffusion is glucose, which is a large, polar molecule. Because cells are constantly utilizing glucose to form ATP, there is a persistent concentration gradient for diffusion into the cell.

With *active transport*, energy is expended to move a substance against its concentration gradient from an area of low concentration to an area of high concentration. This process is used to accumulate a substance on one side of the plasma membrane or the other. The most common example of active transport is the sodium-potassium pump that involves the activity of Na^+-K^+-ATPase, an intrinsic, enzymatic membrane-bound protein. For each ATP molecule hydrolyzed by the Na^+-K^+-ATPase, the pump moves 3 Na^+ ions out of the cell and 2 K^+ ions into the cell. As will be discussed, the activity of this pump contributes to the difference in the composition of the ECF and the intracellular fluid, which is necessary for nerve cells and muscle cells to function.

1.2   Membrane potential

Both ICF and the ECFs are electrically neutral solutions, meaning each has an equal number of positively charged ions and negatively charged ions. A simple but important concept is that oppositely charged ions are attracted to each other and ions of the same charge repel each other. In an unstimulated or resting cell, there is a slight accumulation of negatively charged ions (–) on the internal surface of the plasma membrane. These negatively charged ions are attracted to an equal number of positively charged (+) ions that have accumulated on the external surface of the membrane. Therefore, at rest, all cells are defined as electrically *polarized*—the inside of the cell is slightly negative relative to the outside. This separation of charges across the plasma membrane is referred to as *membrane potential*. The degree of the membrane potential depends primarily on the number of opposite charges that are separated by the membrane. The greater the separation of charge, the greater the membrane potential.

Because the actual number of charges involved is quite small, the potential is measured in millivolts (mV). Furthermore, the sign (+ or −) of the potential is defined by the predominant charge on the internal surface of the cell membrane. Therefore, the membrane potential under resting conditions is negative. Recall that a resting cell has a higher concentration of negatively charged ions on the inside of the membrane. As will be discussed, nerve cells and muscle cells rely on changes in membrane potential for their functions. Nerve cells use changes in the membrane potential to transmit nerve impulses and muscle cells use changes in the membrane potential to shorten (contract).

1.2.1   Development of the resting membrane potential

In a typical unstimulated neuron (nerve cell), the *resting membrane potential* is approximately −70 mV. The development of this potential depends on the *distribution* and *permeability* of three ions: sodium (Na^+), potassium (K^+), and anions (A^-) (see Table 1.2 and Figure 1.3). These ions are unevenly distributed between the ICF and the ECF and they each have a different degree of permeability across the plasma membrane. Sodium ions are found in a greater concentration in the ECF, K^+ ions are found in a greater concentration in the ICF, and A^- refers to large anionic proteins found solely within the cell. Under resting conditions, most mammalian plasma membranes are approximately 50–75 times more permeable to K^+ ions than they are to Na^+ ions. However, the membrane is always impermeable to anions. In other words, anionic proteins (proteins that carry a negative charge) remain within the cell while Na^+ and K^+ ions pass through. It is due to this separation of charged particles that the resting membrane potential is created and maintained.

The passage of Na^+ and K^+ ions in and out of the cell depends on two factors:

- Concentration gradient
- Electrical gradient

Consider the condition where the membrane is permeable only to potassium. Because potassium is in greater concentration inside the cell, the K^+ ions initially diffuse down their *concentration gradient* and out of the cell,

Table 1.2   Concentration and permeability of ions responsible for the membrane potential in a resting nerve cell

Ion	Concentration (mM/L)		Relative permeability
	Extracellular fluid	Intracellular fluid	
Na^+	150	15	1
K^+	5	150	50–75
A^-	0	65	0

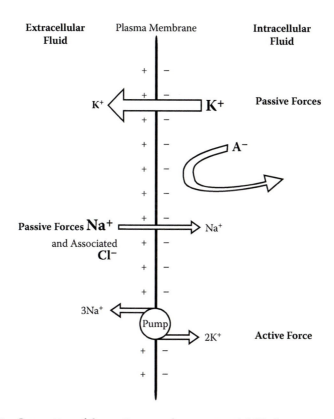

Figure 1.3 Generation of the resting membrane potential. Under resting conditions, potassium (K+) is significantly more permeable than sodium (Na+) and the negatively charged intracellular anions (A−) are impermeable. Therefore, the abundant outward movement of K+ ions down their concentration gradient exerts a powerful effect, driving the membrane potential toward the equilibrium potential for potassium (−90 mV). However, the slight inward movement of Na+ ions, which would tend to drive the membrane potential toward the equilibrium potential for sodium (+60 mV), renders the membrane potential somewhat less negative than −90 mV. The balance of these two opposing effects results in a resting membrane potential in a typical neuron of −70 mV. The maintenance of the concentration differences for sodium and potassium is due to the continuous activity of the Na+-K+ pump.

resulting in an excess of positively charged ions accumulating in the ECF, along the external surface of the membrane. The impermeable A− ions, which remain inside the cell along the internal surface of the plasma membrane, are attracted to these (+) charges. This outward movement of positively charged ions creates an internal environment that is more negative relative to the outside. However, as the positively charged K+ ions continue to diffuse outward, an electrical gradient begins to develop, which influences the diffusion of additional K+ ions. Recall that the K+ ions that had moved out of the cell, down their concentration gradient, have caused an excess of (+) charges to accumulate on the external surface of the membrane. Because like charges repel each other, the initial K^+ ions would begin to repel any additional K^+ ions and oppose further movement of (+) charges outward. Instead, the positively charged K^+ ions are now electrically attracted to the negatively charged A^- ions remaining inside the cell. At this point, K^+ ions diffuse back into the cell down their *electrical gradient*. Eventually, the subsequent force that moves K^+ ions inward, exactly balances the initial force that moved K^+ ions outward, and there is no further net diffusion of potassium. The membrane potential at this point has reached the *equilibrium potential for K^+ (E_K^+)* and is equal to -90 mV. Therefore, when the permeability of the plasma membrane to potassium is high compared to that of sodium, the membrane potential approaches -90 mV.

Next consider the condition where the membrane is permeable only to sodium. Because sodium is in a greater concentration outside of the cell, the Na^+ ions initially diffuse into the cell down their concentration gradient. An excess of these positively charged ions accumulate in the ICF along the internal surface of the plasma membrane and an excess of negative charges, in the form of impermeable extracellular chloride (Cl^-) anions, remain outside the cell, along the external surface of the plasma membrane. This inward movement of positively charged ions creates a membrane potential that is positive because the inside of the cell is now positive relative to the outside. However, as the positively charged Na^+ ions continue to diffuse inward, once again an electrical gradient develops. The initial (+) charges that have accumulated in the ICF begin to repel any additional Na^+ ions and oppose the further movement of (+) charges inward. Instead, the positively charged Na^+ ions are now attracted to the negatively charged Cl^- ions remaining outside the cell. Eventually, the initial force moving Na^+ ions inward down their concentration gradient is balanced by the subsequent force moving Na^+ ions outward down their electrical gradient and there is no further net diffusion of sodium. The membrane potential at this point has reached the *equilibrium potential for Na^+ (E_{Na}^+)* and is equal to $+60$ mV. Therefore, when the permeability of the plasma membrane to sodium is high compared to that of potassium, the membrane potential approaches $+60$ mV.

At any given time, the membrane potential is closer to the equilibrium potential of the ion that is more permeable. Under normal resting conditions, both Na^+ ions and K^+ ions are permeable; however, potassium is significantly (50–75 times) more permeable than sodium and a high amount of K^+ ions diffuse outward while a very small number of Na^+ ions diffuse inward, down their respective concentration gradients. This comparatively copious outward movement of K^+ ions exerts a powerful influence on the value of the resting membrane potential, driving it toward its equilibrium potential of -90 mV. However, the slight inward movement of Na^+ ions, which would tend to drive the membrane potential toward its equilibrium potential of

+60 mV, renders the membrane potential slightly less negative than −90 mV. The balance of these two opposing effects results in a resting membrane potential in a typical neuron of −70 mV (see Figure 1.3).

The Na⁺-K⁺ pump also plays a vital role in the process outline above. For each molecule of ATP expended, three Na⁺ ions are pumped out of the cell into the ECF and two K⁺ ions are pumped into the cell into the ICF. The result is the unequal transport of positively charged ions across the membrane such that the outside of the cell becomes more positive compared to the inside of the cell or, in other words, the inside of the cell is more negative compared to the outside of the cell. Therefore, the activity of the pump has a small direct contribution to the generation of the resting membrane potential.

The other even more important effect of the Na⁺-K⁺ pump is that it maintains the concentration differences for sodium and potassium by accumulating Na⁺ ions outside of the cell and K⁺ ions inside of the cell. As previously discussed, the passive diffusion of these ions down their concentration gradients is predominantly responsible for generating the resting membrane potential. Sodium diffuses inward and potassium diffuses outward. The continuous activity of the pump returns the Na⁺ ions to the ECF and the K⁺ ions to the ICF. Therefore, it can be said that the pump also has an indirect contribution to the generation of the resting membrane potential due to the maintenance of the concentration differences for the relevant ions.

1.3   Electrical signals

Both nerve cells and muscle cells rely on changes in their membrane potentials to carry out their activities. In this chapter, the focus is on nerve cells or *neurons*; however, many of the same principles also apply to muscle cells.

The function of neurons is to convey information to other cells in the form of electrical signals. There are two types of electrical signals transmitted by neurons: graded potentials and action potentials. These signals occur due to ion flux (movement) across the plasma membrane. A given stimulus will cause its effect by altering the permeability of the plasma membrane to one or more ions. The involved ions will then diffuse into or out of the cell according to their concentration and electrical gradients. The result of this movement causes a change in the membrane potential.

1.3.1   Graded potentials

Graded potentials are short-distance signals (see Table 1.3). They are local changes in the membrane potential that occur at *synapses*, where one neuron connects with another neuron. The magnitude of these signals varies with the strength of the stimulus. As the intensity of the stimulus increases, the number

Table 1.3   Distinguishing features of graded potentials and action potentials

Graded potentials	Action potentials
Short-distance signals	Long-distance signals
Magnitude is stimulus dependent	Magnitude is constant (all-or-none phenomenon)
Signal travels by local current flow	Signal travels by local current flow or by saltatory conduction
Magnitude of signal dissipates as it moves away from the site of stimulation	Magnitude of signal is maintained along entire length of neuron
Initiated at synapses (where one neuron comes into contact with another neuron)	Initiated at axon hillock
Result in depolarization or hyperpolarization	Depolarization only

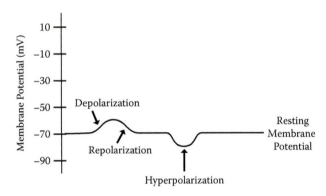

Figure 1.4   Types of changes in membrane potential. The resting membrane potential in a typical neuron is −70 mV. Movement of the membrane potential toward zero (less negative) is referred to as depolarization. The return of the membrane potential to its resting value is referred to as repolarization. Movement of the membrane potential farther away from zero (more negative) is referred to as hyperpolarization.

of ions diffusing across the cell membrane increases and the magnitude of the change in the membrane potential increases. This change may be in either direction such that the membrane potential may become more negative or less negative compared to the resting membrane potential (see Figure 1.4). *Depolarization* occurs when the membrane potential becomes less negative, moving toward zero. As will be discussed, depolarization makes the neuron more excitable. *Hyperpolarization* occurs when the membrane potential becomes more negative, moving farther away from zero. Hyperpolarization tends to make the neuron less excitable. These signals are transient or short-lived. Once the stimulus has been removed, the membrane potential returns to its resting state. Following a depolarization, the membrane is said to undergo *repolarization* and a return to its resting potential.

The mechanism by which the signal is transmitted along the cell membrane is referred to as *local current flow*, or the movement of positively charged ions. Around a stimulus causing a depolarization, the inside of the cell becomes positive (less negative) relative to the outside of the cell. Because opposite charges attract, the (+) charges in this area are attracted to and move toward the negative charges on the adjacent areas of the internal surface of the cell membrane and, thus, these adjacent areas become depolarized due to the presence of these (+) charges. This process continues and the electrical signal travels along the cell membrane away from the initial site of the stimulus. However, these graded or local potentials travel only short distances. The cell membrane is not well insulated and the current (positive charges) tends to drift away from the internal surface of the cell membrane. Consequently, as the signal travels along the membrane, the number of (+) charges causing the depolarization of the next region of membrane continually decreases and, therefore, the magnitude of the depolarization also decreases. The farther away from the initial site of stimulation, the smaller the magnitude of the signal until it eventually dies out.

1.3.2 Action potentials

Action potentials are long-distance electrical signals (see Figure 1.4). These signals travel along the entire neuronal membrane. Unlike graded potentials where the magnitude of the signal steadily dissipates, the magnitude of an action potential is maintained throughout the length of the axon. Furthermore, in contrast to graded potentials whose magnitude is stimulus dependent, action potentials are always the same size. If a stimulus is strong enough to depolarize the membrane to a critical level referred to as the *threshold*, then the membrane continues to depolarize on its own, independent of the stimulus. Typically, the threshold potential is approximately 20 mV less negative than the resting membrane potential. Once threshold is reached, the continued depolarization takes place automatically. This is due to the diffusion of ions based on their concentration and electrical gradients and not due to the original stimulus itself.

Given that action potentials are always of a similar magnitude, how can stimuli of varied strengths be distinguished? A suprathreshold stimulus, one that is larger than necessary to depolarize the membrane simply to threshold, does not produce a larger action potential, but it does increase the *frequency* at which action potentials are generated. In other words, a stronger stimulus will trigger a greater number of action potentials per second.

The generation of an action potential involves changes in permeability to both Na^+ ions and K^+ ions through *voltage-gated ion channels*. However, these permeability changes take place at slightly different times (see Figure 1.4). Voltage-gated ion channels open and close in response to changes in membrane potential. Initially, some stimulus will cause the membrane to depolarize toward threshold. When this occurs, voltage-gated Na^+ channels begin to open and Na^+ ions enter the cell down their concentration and electrical gradients. (Recall that at this point, Na^+ is not only in a greater concentration outside the cell, the inside of the cell is negative relative to the outside.) The influx of Na^+ ions causes further depolarization resulting in the opening of more voltage-gated Na^+ channels, the continued influx of Na^+ ions and so on. This is an example of a positive-feedback mechanism (Chapter 2). This process of depolarization and opening of voltage-gated Na^+ channels continues until the membrane is depolarized to threshold. At this point, all the Na^+ channels are open and there is a very rapid and abundant influx of Na^+ ions and the permeability to Na^+ ions is approximately 600 times greater than normal. This ion flux causes the upward swing or the "spike" of the action potential. During this phase of the action potential, the membrane reverses polarity due to the marked influx of (+) charges and the membrane potential at the peak of the action potential is +30 mV.

Approximately 1 ms after the Na^+ channels open, they close. This prevents any further diffusion of (+) charges into the cell. At the same time, voltage-gated K^+ channels open and K^+ ions leave the cell down their concentration and electrical gradients. (At this point, K^+ is not only in a greater concentration inside the cell, the inside of the cell is positive relative to the outside.) During this phase of the action potential, the permeability to K^+ ions is approximately 300 times greater than normal. This efflux of (+) charges causes the membrane to repolarize back toward the resting membrane potential.

Sodium channels open more rapidly than the K^+ channels because they are more voltage-sensitive and just a small depolarization is sufficient to open them. Larger changes in membrane potential associated with further cell excitation are required to open the less voltage-sensitive K^+ channels. Therefore, the increase in the permeability to K^+ ions occurs later than that of Na^+ ions. This is functionally significant because if both types of ion channels opened concurrently, then the change in membrane potential that would occur due to Na^+ ion influx would be cancelled out by K^+ ion efflux and the action potential could not be generated.

To more fully understand the mechanism by which the action potential is generated, further explanation concerning the structure and activity of the voltage-gated ion channels is necessary. A *voltage-gated Na^+ channel* has two different gates: the *activation gate* and the *inactivation gate*. At the resting membrane potential of −70 mV in an unstimulated neuron, the activation gate is closed and the permeability to Na^+ ions is very low. In this resting state, the channel is closed but capable of opening in response to a stimulus. When stimulated by depolarization to threshold, the activation gates open very rapidly and Na^+ ions diffuse into the cell causing the upward swing of the action potential. Once these activation gates open, the inactivation gates begin to close although the closure of these gates takes place more slowly. Approximately 1 ms after the gates open, they begin to close. At the peak of the action potential when the inactivation gates are now all closed, these channels are no longer permeable to Na^+ ions and they are incapable of opening regardless of further stimulation. Therefore, the Na^+ channels cannot reopen, Na^+ ions cannot enter the cell and another action potential cannot be generated. In fact, these voltage-gated channels cannot return to their resting position and become capable of opening until the neuron has first repolarized to −70 mV from the existing action potential. This period, beginning when all the Na^+ channels are open and lasting through the inactivation phase of the Na^+ channels, is referred to as the *absolute refractory period*. Regardless of the strength of the stimulus, no new action potentials can be generated. The length of this period, approximately 2 ms, limits the number of action potentials that neurons can generate to up to 500 per second.

The *voltage-gated K^+ channel* has only one gate, which is typically closed at the resting membrane potential. This gate also opens in response to depolarization of the membrane toward zero. However, unlike the activation gate of the voltage-gated Na^+ channel that opens very quickly, this gate opens very slowly so that the permeability to K^+ ions is delayed. In fact, they begin to open at approximately the same time that the inactivation gates in the Na^+ channels close. Therefore, there is a simultaneous decrease in Na^+ ion permeability and an increase in K^+ ion permeability, resulting in the outward movement of (+) charges and a rapid repolarization.

The voltage-gated K^+ channels not only open slowly, they close slowly as well. Therefore, the increase in permeability to K^+ ions is prolonged. Potassium ions continue to exit the cell and the membrane potential approaches the equilibrium potential for potassium. This phase of the action potential is referred to as the *after-hyperpolarization*. Because the membrane potential is now farther away from threshold, a larger than normal stimulus is necessary to cause depolarization to threshold. During this phase of hyperpolarization, it is possible but more difficult for the neuron to generate another action potential. This *relative refractory period* lasts from the end of the absolute refractory period until the voltage-gated K^+ channels have returned to their resting state and the membrane once again returns to its resting potential.

During the action potential, Na^+ ions entered the cell and K^+ ions exited the cell. To prevent the eventual dissipation of the concentration gradients for Na^+ ions and K^+ ions across the cell membrane over time, these substances must be returned to their original positions. The slow but continuous activity of the Na^+-K^+ pump is responsible for this function and returns Na^+ ions to the ECF and K^+ ions to the ICF.

PHARMACY APPLICATION: SEIZURES

Epilepsies affect approximately 2.5 million patients in the United States. This debilitating disease is characterized by seizures that involve the sudden discharge of electrical activity in specific populations of brain neurons. This inappropriate electrical activity is thought to arise from the cerebral cortex. Accordingly, the symptoms experienced by a given patient are related to the region of the cortex involved.

Phenytoin (Dilantin®), along with recently FDA-approved medications, is useful in the treatment of all types of partial and tonic-clonic (grand mal) seizures. Its mechanism of action involves the slowed rate of recovery of voltage-gated Na+ channels and, thus, these channels remain in their inactivation state longer and the absolute refractory period is prolonged. This effect limits the sustained, repetitive firing of the neurons and, therefore, prevents the seizures.

1.3.3   Conduction of the action potential

A typical neuron consists of four functional regions:

- Cell body
- Axon hillock
- Axon
- Axon terminal

First is the *cell body* with its *dendrites*, which are projections from the cell body that greatly increase the surface area. This is the site of communication and input from other neurons. These inputs result in the generation of graded potentials that travel a short distance to the *axon hillock*, the region of the cell body from which the axon arises. Following sufficient stimulation of the neuron, an action potential is generated at the axon hillock. This action potential must then be propagated or regenerated along the third portion of the neuron, the axon. The *axon*, or nerve fiber, is an elongated projection that transmits the action potential away from the cell body toward other cells. The final component of the neuron is the *axon terminal* where the neuron communicates, by way of this action potential, with another cell or cells. The conduction of the action potential along the length of the axon is the subject of this section. Communication between a neuron and another cell is discussed in Chapter 13.

The action potential is initiated at the axon hillock (see Figure 1.5). This region is particularly excitable due to the presence of an abundance of voltage-gated Na+ channels. As the axon hillock is stimulated by excitatory

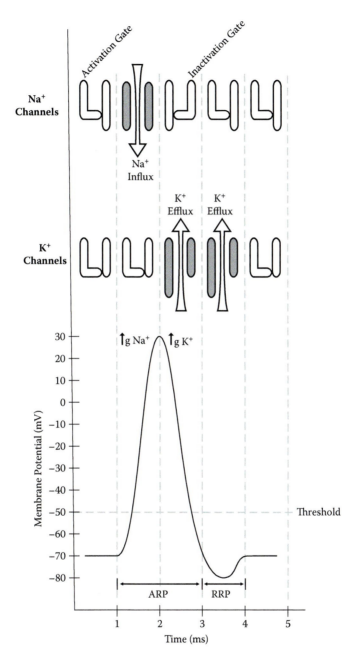

Figure 1.5 The action potential. At the resting membrane potential (−70 mV), most ion channels are in their resting state, that is, closed but capable of opening. When the neuron is stimulated and depolarized, the activation gates of the voltage-gated

(Continued)

inputs, there is a marked influx of Na+ ions and this region of the cell membrane becomes positive inside, resulting in an action potential. The rest of the axon is still at its resting membrane potential and is negative inside. As with graded potentials, this electrical signal also travels by local current flow (see Figure 1.6). The (+) charges in the region of the action potential are attracted to the negative charges in the immediately adjacent region of the axonal membrane. This current flow depolarizes the new region, causing an increase in the permeability of the cell membrane to Na+ ions through the voltage-gated ion channels. The subsequent influx of Na+ ions further depolarizes the membrane so that it reaches threshold and a *new action potential* is generated in this region. At the same time, the original site of action potential generation at the axon hillock repolarizes due to the efflux of K+ ions. This process of generating new action potentials sequentially along the membrane enables the signal to maintain its strength as it travels the distance to the axon terminal.

Another mechanism of conduction of an action potential along the length of a neuron is *saltatory conduction*, and it occurs in *myelinated* axons (see Figure 1.7). Myelin is a lipid sheath wrapped around the axon at regular intervals. The myelin is not actually part of the axon itself, but instead it comes from other cells. In the central nervous system (CNS; brain and spinal cord), the myelin-forming cell is the *oligodendrocyte*, one of several types of support cells for centrally located neurons. In the peripheral nervous system (all neurons that lie outside of the CNS and communicate with various body parts), myelin is formed by the *Schwann cells*. The lipid of the myelin in each

Figure 1.5 (Continued) Na+ channels open, permitting the influx of Na+ ions and further depolarization toward threshold. At the threshold potential, all voltage-gated Na+ channels are open, resulting in the "spike" of the action potential. Approximately 1 ms after the activation gates open, the inactivation gates of the Na+ channels close. In addition, the activation gates of the K+ channels open, resulting in the efflux of K+ ions and the repolarization of the neuron. The protracted increase in K+ ion permeability results in the after-hyperpolarization. It is during this time when the membrane potential in the neuron is farther away from threshold that the cell is in its relative refractory period (RRP) and a larger than normal stimulus is needed to generate an action potential. The absolute refractory period (ARP) begins when the voltage-gated Na+ channels have all become activated and continues through the inactivation phase. During this time, there can be no further Na+ ion influx and no new action potentials can be generated. Voltage-gated Na+ channels return to their resting state (activation gates closed, inactivation gates open) when the membrane potential approaches the resting membrane potential of the neuron.

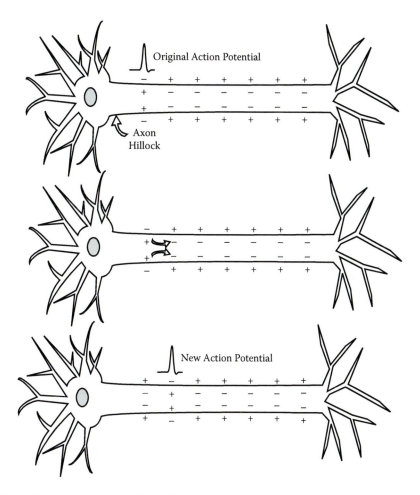

Figure 1.6 Conduction of the action potential along an axon by local current flow. Upper panel: Action potentials are generated at the axon hillock. When stimulated to threshold, this region of the membrane becomes positive (+30 mV) inside relative to the outside due to the influx of Na+ ions. The remainder of the axon is at its resting membrane potential (–70 mV). Middle panel: Because opposite charges attract, the (+) charges in the stimulated area are attracted to the (–) charges in the adjacent region of the membrane. This movement of (+) charges, or local current flow, depolarizes this adjacent region. Lower panel: The depolarization of the adjacent region causes the activation of voltage-gated Na+ channels, the influx of Na+ ions, and the generation of a new action potential. The original area of stimulation, meanwhile, has repolarized back to the resting membrane potential. This process, which is unidirectional, continues along the length of the axon.

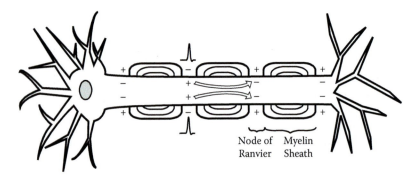

Figure 1.7 Saltatory conduction. Transmission of electrical impulses in a myelin-ated axon occurs by way of saltatory conduction. The myelin sheath, which is composed primarily of lipid, insulates the axon and prevents the generation of mem-brane potentials. Membrane potentials occur only at the gaps in the myelin sheath, referred to as the nodes of Ranvier or myelin sheath gaps. Therefore, transmission of the impulse, or the generation of action potentials, occurs.

case comes from multiple layers of the plasma membrane of these cells as they wrap around and around the axon. This lipid provides good insula-tion, preventing the movement of current across the cell membrane. Without ion flux, action potentials cannot be generated in the regions covered with myelin. Instead, action potentials occur only at the breaks in the myelin sheath referred to as the *nodes of Ranvier*. These nodes are located about 1–2 mm apart. The flow of current from an active node "skips" down the axon to the adjacent node to cause depolarization and generate a new action potential. This transmission of the impulse from node to node is referred to as saltatory conduction, from the Latin word *saltare*, meaning "to leap."

Saltatory conduction results in a significant increase in the *velocity of con-duction* of the nerve impulse down the axon compared to that of local current flow in an unmyelinated axon (see Table 1.4). The speed of conduction is directly correlated to the urgency of the information that is being conveyed by a given neuron. Nerve fibers carrying less important information, such as those regulating slow digestive processes, are unmyelinated. An example

Table 1.4 Factors that affect the velocity of conduction

Factor	Velocity of conduction
Myelination of axon (saltatory conduction)	↑
↑ Diameter of axon	↑

of a nerve fiber with myelin is one that innervates skeletal muscle so that movements can be executed rapidly.

The functional significance of the myelin is revealed by the neurological deficits observed in patients with *multiple sclerosis*. This disorder is caused by the demyelination of neurons in the brain, the spinal cord and the optic nerve. The loss of myelin disrupts the normal conduction of impulses along the axons of these neurons and results in weakness, numbness, loss of bladder control, and visual disturbances.

Another advantage of the presence of myelin along an axon is that the conduction of the impulse is energetically more efficient. Because action potentials occur only at the nodes of Ranvier, fewer Na^+ ions and K^+ ions move in and out of the cell. Therefore, less metabolic energy is required to return these ions to their original positions along the cell membrane and to maintain the proper concentration gradients. In unmyelinated axons, action potentials and, therefore, ion flux occur along the entire length of the axon. These neurons expend more energy returning these ions to their original positions.

A second factor that influences the velocity of conduction of the action potential is the *diameter of the axon*. The greater the diameter then, the lower the resistance to current flow along the axon. Therefore, the impulse is conducted along large nerve fibers more rapidly. Large myelinated nerve fibers, such as those innervating skeletal muscle, exhibit the highest conduction velocity. Small unmyelinated fibers, such as those of the autonomic nervous system innervating the heart, smooth muscle of the blood vessels and the gastrointestinal tract, and glands, conduct nerve impulses more slowly.

Conduction of the action potential along the axon is *unidirectional*. In other words, the nerve impulse travels away from the cell body and the axon hillock and toward the axon terminal only. As the current flows from the initial area of activity to the adjacent region of the axon, the new region becomes depolarized and generates an action potential. Simultaneously, the initial area has entered its absolute refractory period due to the inactivation of the voltage-gated Na^+ channels. Then, as the current flows away from the second active area, it has no effect on the original site of activity. Instead, the current continues forward and depolarizes the next adjacent region of the axon. By the time the original site has recovered from the refractory period and is capable of being restimulated, the action potential has traveled too far along the axon to affect this site by way of local current flow. This unidirectional conduction ensures that the signal reaches the axon terminal where it can influence the activity of the innervated cell as opposed to traveling back and forth along the axon ineffectively.

PHARMACY APPLICATION: LOCAL ANESTHETICS

Pain is a protective mechanism that alerts an individual to the occurrence of tissue damage. Stimulation of nociceptors (pain receptors) alters the membrane permeability to ions, the predominant effect of which is the influx of Na^+ ions down their electrical and chemical gradients. Sufficient Na^+ ion influx results in the generation of an action potential that is then propagated along the afferent neuron to the CNS where the painful stimulus is perceived. Local anesthetics, such as lidocaine and procaine (also known as Novocain™) prevent or relieve the perception of pain by interrupting the conduction of the nervous impulse. These drugs bind to a specific receptor site on the voltage-gated Na^+ channels and block ion movement through them. Without Na^+ ion influx, an action potential cannot be generated in the afferent neuron and the signal fails to reach the CNS. In general, the action of these drugs is restricted to the site of application and becomes less effective upon diffusion of the drug away from the site of action in the nerve.

1.4   Synaptic transmission

Most neurons, particularly in the CNS, receive thousands of inputs. The function of a neuron is to communicate or relay information to another cell by way of an electrical impulse. A *synapse* is the site where the impulse is transmitted from one cell to the next. A neuron may terminate on a muscle cell, a glandular cell or another neuron. The discussion in this chapter will focus on neuron-to-neuron transmission. At these types of synapses, the *presynaptic neuron* transmits the impulse *toward* the synapse and the *postsynaptic neuron* transmits the impulse *away* from the synapse. Specifically, it is the axon terminal of the presynaptic neuron that synapses with the cell body or the dendrites of the postsynaptic neuron. As will become evident, the transmission of the impulse at the synapse is *unidirectional* and the presynaptic neuron influences the activity of the postsynaptic neuron only.

1.4.1   Chemical synapses

Most of the synapses in the nervous system are *chemical synapses* where the presynaptic neuron and the postsynaptic neuron are not in direct contact but instead are separated by a narrow (20–50 nm) space called the *synaptic cleft*. This space prevents the direct spread of the electrical impulse from one cell to the next. Instead, a chemical referred to as a *neurotransmitter* is released by the presynaptic neuron. The neurotransmitter diffuses across

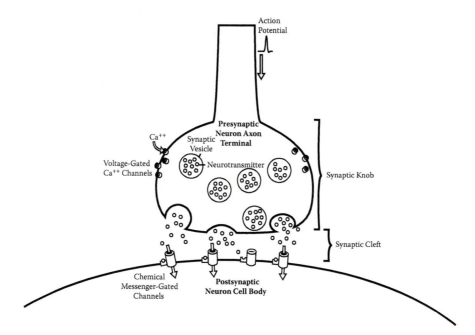

Figure 1.8 Mechanism of action at a chemical synapse. The arrival of an action potential at the axon terminal causes voltage-gated Ca^{++} channels to open. The resulting increase in concentration of Ca^{++} ions in the ICF facilitates the exocytosis of the neurotransmitter into the synaptic cleft. Binding of the neurotransmitter to its specific receptor on the postsynaptic neuron alters the permeability of the membrane to one or more ions, thus causing a change in the membrane potential and the generation of a graded potential in this neuron.

the synaptic cleft, binds to specific receptors in the postsynaptic membrane and alters the electrical activity of the postsynaptic neuron.

The mechanism of action of a chemical synapse is shown in Figure 1.8. The axon terminal broadens to form a swelling referred to as a *synaptic knob*. Within the synaptic knob are many mitochondria that supply the energy for synaptic function and many *synaptic vesicles* that store the pre-formed neurotransmitter. Also, found in the membrane of the synaptic knob are *voltage-gated Ca^{++} channels*. When the electrical impulse, or action potential, has been transmitted along the length of the axon and reaches the axon terminal (synaptic knob), the accompanying change in voltage, or depolarization, causes the voltage-gated Ca^{++} channels to open. Ca^{++} ions, which are in greater concentration in the ECF compared to the ICF, move down their concentration gradient and enter through the synaptic knob's plasma membrane. The influx of Ca^{++} ions induces the release of the neurotransmitter by triggering the movement of the synaptic vesicles to the membrane. Using the process of exocytosis, the vesicles fuse with the membrane and the neurotransmitter is released into the synaptic cleft. The region of the synaptic knob where there is an abundance of voltage-gated Ca^{++} channels and where the vesicles tend to fuse with the membrane is referred to as the *active zone*. The neurotransmitter molecules diffuse across the cleft and bind to specific receptors on the membrane of the postsynaptic neuron. This binding of the neurotransmitter may alter the permeability of the postsynaptic neuron to one or more ions or it may elicit biochemical changes within the cell by way of G proteins. The activation of G proteins also opens or closes ion channels. As always, a change in ion permeability results in a change in the membrane potential of the cell. This change in membrane potential at the synapse, which represents the information as received by the postsynaptic neuron, is in the form of a *graded potential* only. At any given synapse, the change in membrane potential is not great enough to reach threshold and generate an action potential. Instead, many graded potentials generated at one or more synapses are conducted over the cell membrane toward the axon hillock. If the depolarization caused by multiple graded potentials added together is sufficient for the axon hillock to reach threshold, then an action potential is generated here.

There are two important characteristics of synaptic function. First, the transmission of the electrical impulse is *unidirectional*, from the presynaptic neuron to the postsynaptic neuron. This is because only the presynaptic neuron releases neurotransmitter and only the postsynaptic neuron possesses the receptor that will elicit the expected response. Second, the strength of the response is variable and depends on the amount of neurotransmitter released into the synaptic cleft. As mentioned previously, the neurotransmitter is preformed and stored in vesicles within the synaptic knob. Each vesicle contains a fixed amount of neurotransmitter that is referred to as a *quantum*. The amount of neurotransmitter released depends on the number of vesicles that fuse with the membrane in response to the stimulating action potential. As more neurotransmitter is released to bind with its receptors, the greater the response in the postsynaptic neuron.

There are two types of synapses:

- Excitatory synapses
- Inhibitory synapses

At an *excitatory synapse*, binding of the neurotransmitter to its receptor causes an increase in the permeability of the membrane to Na^+ ions and K^+ ions through *chemical messenger-gated channels* that are closely associated with the receptor. Na^+ ions enter the cell down both their concentration and electrical gradients, and K^+ ions leave the cell down their concentration gradient only. Because there are two forces causing the inward diffusion of sodium and only one force causing the outward diffusion of potassium, the influx of Na^+ ions is significantly greater than the efflux of K^+ ions. This greater movement

PHARMACY APPLICATION: ALZHEIMER'S DISEASE

Alzheimer's disease (AD) is a common, chronic progressive neurologic disorder. Early-onset AD occurs in patients younger than 65 years of age. However, late-onset AD is more prevalent accounting for 70% of the cases. This disorder affects approximately 4 million Americans, yet the cause remains unknown. It is characterized by the loss of neurons in the cerebral cortex as well as the presence of neurofibrillary tangles and plaques. Neurochemically, AD is associated with a decrease in the level of choline acetyltransferase in the brain. This enzyme is needed for the synthesis of the neurotransmitter, acetylcholine, which is associated with memory. In patients with AD, the deficiency in choline acetyltransferase (and, therefore, acetylcholine) is directly correlated to the severity of the dementia.

Currently there is no cure for AD. However, medications are available to slow the progression of the disease. These drugs have been designed to enhance the level of available acetylcholine in the brain. Long-lasting acetylcholinesterase inhibitors are drugs that inhibit the enzyme that degrades acetylcholine, resulting in more acetylcholine being available in the synapse to carry out its effects. Three prescribed medications currently in use are Aricept® (donepezil), Excelon® (rivastigmine), and Razadyne® (galantamine).

of (+) charges into the cell results in a small depolarization of the neuron and is referred to as an *excitatory postsynaptic potential (EPSP)*. An EPSP is a graded potential only. A single action potential occurring at a single excitatory synapse opens too few Na^+ channels to depolarize the membrane all the way to threshold; however, it does bring the membrane potential closer toward it. This increases the likelihood that subsequent stimuli will continue the depolarization to threshold and that an action potential will be generated by the postsynaptic neuron.

At an *inhibitory synapse,* binding of the neurotransmitter to its receptor causes an increase in the permeability of the membrane to either K^+ ions or, more commonly, Cl^- ions through chemical messenger-gated channels (sodium channels are not affected). As a result, K^+ ions may leave the cell down their concentration gradient carrying (+) charges outward or Cl^- ions may enter the cell down their concentration gradient carrying (–) charges inward. In either case, the neuron becomes more negative inside relative to the outside and the membrane is now hyperpolarized. This small hyperpolarization is referred to as an *inhibitory postsynaptic potential (IPSP)*. The movement of the membrane potential farther away from threshold decreases the likelihood that an action potential will be generated by the postsynaptic neuron.

Almost invariably, a neuron is genetically programmed to synthesize and release only a single type of neurotransmitter. Therefore, a given synapse is either always excitatory or always inhibitory. Once a neurotransmitter has bound to its receptor on the postsynaptic neuron and has caused its effect, it is important to inactivate it or remove it from the synapse to prevent it from continuing its activity indefinitely. Several mechanisms to carry this out have been identified:

- Passive diffusion of the neurotransmitter away from the synaptic cleft
- Destruction of the neurotransmitter by enzymes located in the synaptic cleft or in the plasma membranes of the presynaptic or postsynaptic neurons
- Active re-uptake of the neurotransmitter into the synaptic knob of the presynaptic neuron for reuse or enzymatic destruction

1.4.2   Summation

As previously mentioned, a single action potential at a single synapse results in a graded potential only, either an EPSP or an IPSP. Therefore, the generation of an action potential in the postsynaptic neuron requires the addition or *summation* of a sufficient number of excitatory inputs to depolarize this neuron to threshold. Two types of summation may occur:

- Temporal summation
- Spatial summation

Temporal summation occurs when multiple EPSPs (or IPSPs) produced by a *single* presynaptic neuron in close sequence exert their effect on the membrane potential of the postsynaptic neuron. For example, an action potential in the presynaptic neuron produces an EPSP and partial depolarization of the postsynaptic neuron (see Figure 1.9). While the postsynaptic neuron is still depolarized, a second action potential in the presynaptic neuron produces another EPSP in the postsynaptic neuron that adds to the first EPSP and further depolarizes this neuron. As more and more EPSPs add together, the membrane depolarizes closer and closer toward threshold until an action potential is generated. Although temporal summation is illustrated in Figure 1.8 with the summation of relatively few EPSPs, the addition of up to 50 EPSPs may be necessary to reach threshold. Because a presynaptic neuron may generate up to 500 action potentials per second, temporal summation occurs quite readily. The strength of the signal to the postsynaptic neuron is, therefore, influenced by the *frequency of nerve impulses* generated by the presynaptic neuron.

Spatial summation occurs when multiple EPSPs (or IPSPs), produced by *many* presynaptic neurons, exert their effects on the membrane potential of the postsynaptic neuron simultaneously. For example, Figure 1.10 depicts a single

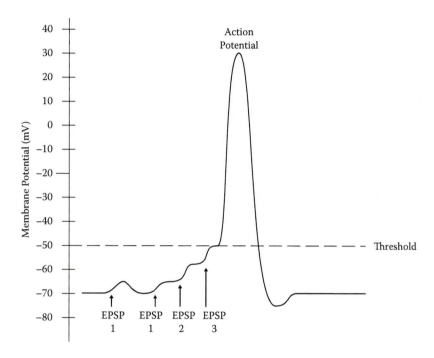

Figure 1.9 Temporal summation. Multiple excitatory postsynaptic potentials (EPSPs) produced by a single presynaptic neuron in close sequence may add together to depolarize the postsynaptic neuron to threshold and generate an action potential.

postsynaptic neuron that is innervated by three presynaptic neurons. Inputs from presynaptic neurons A and B are excitatory and the input from presynaptic neuron C is inhibitory. Once again, single action potentials in either neuron A or B produce individual EPSPs that are insufficient to depolarize the postsynaptic neuron to threshold. However, if EPSPs from neurons A and B are produced at the same time, the depolarizations add together and the membrane potential of the postsynaptic neuron reaches threshold, resulting in the generation of an action potential. Inputs from neurons A (excitatory) and C (inhibitory) occurring simultaneously may, in effect, cancel each other out, resulting in little or no change in the membrane potential of the postsynaptic neuron. As with temporal summation, this example has been simplified to clearly illustrate the concept. In actuality, a large number of excitatory inputs from different presynaptic neurons are necessary to depolarize the postsynaptic neuron to threshold. Because a typical neuronal cell body receives thousands of presynaptic inputs, spatial summation also occurs quite readily. The number of presynaptic neurons that are active simultaneously, therefore, influences the strength of the signal to the postsynaptic neuron. Under normal physiological conditions, temporal summation and spatial summation may occur concurrently.

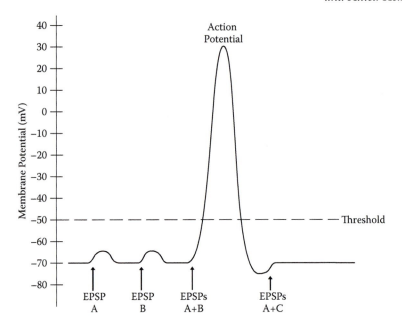

Figure 1.10   Spatial summation. Multiple excitatory postsynaptic potentials (EPSPs) or inhibitory postsynaptic potentials (IPSPs) produced by many presynaptic neurons simultaneously may add together to alter the membrane potential of the postsynaptic neuron. Sufficient excitatory input (A and B) will depolarize the membrane to threshold and generate an action potential. The simultaneous arrival of excitatory and inhibitory inputs (A and C) may cancel each other so that the membrane potential does not change.

1.4.3   Interconnections between neurons

The interconnections or communication among neurons in humans is very extensive. Imagine the complexity of the electrical activity that may occur among 100 billion neurons in the human brain where each of these neurons provides input to and receives input from hundreds of other neurons. The diversity of these interconnections accounts for the uniqueness of many abstract neurological phenomena in individuals such as intellect, personality, and memory. There are two types of interconnections:

- Convergence
- Divergence

Convergence occurs when the axon terminals of many presynaptic neurons all synapse with a single postsynaptic neuron. As discussed previously, spatial summation of nerve impulses relies on the presence of convergence. *Divergence* occurs when the axon of a single presynaptic neuron branches and synapses with multiple postsynaptic neurons. In this way, activity in a single nerve fiber can affect several regions of the nervous system, each with a different function, at the same time.

1.4.4   Factors affecting synaptic transmission

Several factors influence the synaptic transmission of electrical impulses:

- pH of the interstitial fluid
- Hypoxia
- Drugs, toxins, and diseases

Neurons are very sensitive to changes in the *pH of the interstitial fluid* surrounding them. Normally the pH of arterial blood is 7.4. Under conditions of *alkalosis*, in which the pH increases, the excitability of neurons also increases, rendering them more likely to generate action potentials. This inappropriate stimulation of the nervous system may lead to seizures, particularly in epileptics who are predisposed to having them. Under conditions of *acidosis*, in which the pH decreases, the excitability of neurons is depressed, rendering them less likely to generate action potentials. This lack of stimulation of the nervous system may lead to a comatose state. Severe diabetic acidosis or acidosis associated with end-stage renal failure will often lead to coma.

Neuronal function depends on a constant supply of oxygen. *Hypoxia,* a decrease in oxygen availability, depresses neuronal activity. Interruption of blood flow to the brain for only a few seconds leads to unconsciousness. A prolonged lack of blood flow, which is characteristic of stroke, leads to permanent brain damage in the affected area.

Many *drugs, toxins*, and *diseases* also exert their clinical effects by altering some phase of synaptic activity. In fact, drugs can alter literally every level of neuronal and synaptic function. There are four mechanisms by which these effects may occur:

- Altered release of a neurotransmitter
- Altered interaction of a neurotransmitter with its receptor
- Altered removal of a neurotransmitter from the synaptic cleft
- Replacement of a deficient neurotransmitter

1.4.4.1   Altered release of a neurotransmitter

Tetanus is an infectious disease caused by the bacterium, *Clostridium tetani.* This bacterium produces a neurotoxin active on inhibitory synapses in the spinal cord. Motor neurons, the neurons that supply skeletal muscle and cause contraction, have cell bodies that lie in the spinal cord. Under normal circumstances, these motor neurons receive both excitatory and inhibitory inputs from various sources. The balance of these inputs results in the appropriate degree of muscle tone or muscle contraction. Tetanus toxin prevents the release of gamma amino butyric acid (GABA), an important neurotransmitter active at the inhibitory synapses. Elimination of the inhibitory inputs results in unchecked or unmodulated excitatory input to the motor neurons. The resulting uncontrolled muscle spasms initially occur in the muscles of the jaw, giving rise to the expression *lockjaw*. The muscle spasms eventually affect the respiratory muscles, which prevents inspiration and leads to death due to asphyxiation.

1.4.4.2   Altered interaction of a neurotransmitter with its receptor

The interaction of a neurotransmitter with its receptor may be altered pharmacologically in several ways. One such mechanism involves the administration of *antagonists*, drugs that bind to a given receptor and prevent the action of the neurotransmitter but, by classical definition, initiate no other effect. An interesting clinical example of this form of therapy involves schizophrenia, a severe mental disorder characterized by delusions, hallucinations, social withdrawal, and disorganized speech and behavior. While the precise cause of schizophrenia is unknown, its pathophysiology appears to involve neuronal pathways that release excessive amounts of the neurotransmitter dopamine. Antipsychotic drugs, such as Thorazine® (chlorpromazine) and Haldol® (haloperidol), minimize the symptoms of schizophrenia by blocking dopamine receptors, thereby preventing the excess dopamine from exerting its effects. However, these first-generation drugs have potentially harmful neurological side effects. Newer, second-generation medications pose lower risks of serious side effects. These drugs include Abilify® (aripiprazole), Rexulti® (brexpiprazole), cariprazine® (Vraylar), and Clozaril® (clozapine).

An *agonist* is a drug that binds to a given receptor and stimulates it. In other words, agonists mimic the effect of endogenous neurotransmitters. Albuterol, the active ingredient in medications such as Ventolin®, is a β_2-adrenergic receptor agonist. Stimulation of these receptors in the lungs causes the airways to dilate. Therefore, albuterol is effective in reversing the bronchospasm and dyspnea (difficulty in breathing) associated with asthma.

Another mechanism by which neurotransmitter/receptor interaction may be altered involves the administration of drugs that *facilitate* the binding of the endogenously produced neurotransmitter to its receptor. Once again, the neurotransmitter used as an example is GABA, the most prevalent inhibitory neurotransmitter in the nervous system. Not only does it contribute to the regulation of skeletal muscle tone by inhibiting the activity of motor neurons, it is involved in the regulation of mood and emotions by acting as a CNS depressant. The benzodiazepines, which are anti-anxiety drugs and include Valium® (diazepam) and Ativan® (lorazepam), act by binding to a specific site on the GABA receptor. This binding causes a conformational change in the receptor protein that enhances the binding of GABA. As more GABA binds to the receptors, its effectiveness in the CNS is increased and anxiety is decreased.

1.4.4.3   Altered removal of a neurotransmitter from the synaptic cleft

The third mechanism by which drugs may alter synaptic activity involves changes in neurotransmitter re-uptake or degradation. Very well-known examples of drugs in this category are Prozac® (fluoxetine) and the more recently prescribed Cymbalta® (duloxetine) and Wellbutrin® (bupropion), which are used to treat depression. While the complete etiology is unknown, it is widely accepted that depression involves a deficiency of monoamine neurotransmitters (e.g., norepinephrine and serotonin) in the CNS. Prozac, a selective serotonin re-uptake inhibitor, prevents the removal of serotonin from the synaptic cleft. Cymbalta prevents the re-uptake of both serotonin and norepinephrine, whereas Wellbutrin prevents the re-uptake of dopamine and norepinephrine. Therefore, the concentration and activity of these neurotransmitters in the brain are enhanced and the symptoms of depression are relieved.

1.4.4.4   Replacement of a deficient neurotransmitter

Finally, synaptic activity may be altered by the replacement of a deficient neurotransmitter. This form of drug therapy is effective in the treatment of Parkinson's disease. The pathophysiology of Parkinson's involves the progressive destruction of dopaminergic (dopamine-releasing) neurons, resulting in a deficiency of dopamine in certain areas in the brain. In addition to neuronal pathways involved in the regulation of mood and emotion, dopamine is released by neurons that inhibit skeletal muscle contraction. Because motor neurons normally receive both excitatory and inhibitory inputs, the inhibition provided by the dopaminergic pathways results in smooth, precise muscle contractions. In the patient with Parkinson's disease, this loss of inhibition leads to increased muscle tone, or muscle rigidity, and resting tremors. These symptoms are alleviated by administering levodopa (L-dopa), a precursor for dopamine. L-dopa is taken up by the axon terminals of dopaminergic neurons and used to form dopamine. Interestingly, in some patients, a side effect of this dopamine replacement therapy is the development of symptoms characteristic of schizophrenia. Recall that this mental disorder is caused by overactive dopaminergic neurons. On the other hand, drugs used to treat schizophrenia, dopamine receptor antagonists, may elicit the symptoms of Parkinson's disease.

1.5   Cell injury

Cellular injury can occur as a result of trauma, infection, ischemia, and exposure to toxins. Many disease processes begin with cellular injury. The environment around cells is dynamic and constantly changing. In this fluid environment, cells are exposed to numerous stimuli and stresses, some of which may be injurious. In order for cells to survive, they must have the ability to adapt to variable conditions. This process of adaptation can involve changes in cellular size, cell number or cell type. Adaptive changes may be physiologic and benefit the individual or be pathologic and detrimental to the individual.

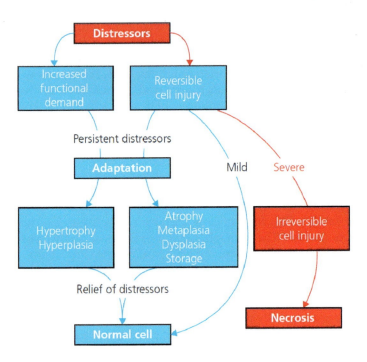

1.5.1 Cellular adaptation

Cellular adaptation occurs when cells change in response to changes in their environment (see Figure 1.11).

1. *Atrophy*:
   - Atrophy is characterized by a decrease in size of a cell or tissue
   - Causes of atrophy may include prolonged bed rest, disuse of limbs or tissue, poor tissue nutrition and ischemia
   - Decreased size results in decreased oxygen consumption and metabolic needs of the cells and may increase the overall efficiency of cell function

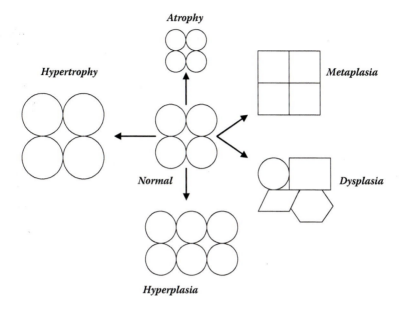

Figure 1.11   Adaptive changes in cells.

- Atrophy is generally a reversible process, except for atrophy caused by loss of nervous innervation to a tissue

2. *Hypertrophy*:
   - Hypertrophy is characterized by an increase in cell size and tissue mass but not cell number
   - Hypertrophy may be a normal physiologic response to increased workload, such as the increase in muscle mass that is seen with exercise. It may, however, be pathologic as in the case of the cardiac hypertrophy that is seen with prolonged hypertension. Such pathologic hypertrophy is often irreversible. Hypertrophy may also be a compensatory process. When one kidney is removed, for example, the remaining kidney hypertrophies to increase its functional capacity
   - Often occurs when a cell or tissue is exposed to an increased workload
   - Occurs in tissues that cannot increase cell number as an adaptive response

3. *Hyperplasia*:
   - Hyperplasia is characterized by an increase in the number of cells in an organ or tissue
   - Hyperplasia can only occur in cells capable of mitosis (therefore not in muscle or nerve cells)
   - Hyperplasia may be a normal process, as in the breast and uterine hyperplasia that occurs during pregnancy, or pathologic, such as gingival hyperplasia (overgrowth of gum tissues) that may be seen in certain patients receiving the drug phenytoin. As with hypertrophy, hyperplasia may also be a compensatory mechanism. For example, when a portion of the liver is surgically removed, the remaining hepatocytes (liver cells) increase in number to preserve functional capacity of the liver
4. *Metaplasia*:
   - Metaplasia is characterized by the conversion of one cell type to another that might have a better chance of survival under certain circumstances
   - Metaplasia often occurs in response to chronic irritation or inflammation
   - An example of metaplasia can be observed in the respiratory passages of chronic cigarette smokers. Following years of exposure to irritating cigarette smoke, the ciliated columnar epithelium lining the respiratory passages gradually converts to stratified squamous epithelium. Although the stratified squamous cells may be better able to survive the constant irritation of cigarette smoke, they lack the cilia of the columnar epithelial cells that are necessary for clearing particulates from the surfaces of the respiratory passages
5. *Dysplasia*:
   - Dysplasia is characterized by a derangement of cell growth that leads to tissues with cells of varying size, shape and appearance. It is not a true adaptive change but more so a pathologic change
   - Dysplasia generally occurs in response to chronic irritation and inflammation. Dysplastic changes may be a precursor to cancer in certain instances such as in the cervix, GI or respiratory tract

1.5.2   Mechanisms of cell injury

Cell injury can occur in a number of different ways. The extent of injury that cells experience is often related to the intensity and duration of exposure to the injurious event or substance. Cellular injury may a reversible process, in which case the cells can recover their normal function, or irreversible and lead to cell death. Although the causes of cellular injury are many (see Table 1.5), the underlying mechanisms of cellular injury usually fall into one of two categories, *free radical injury* or *hypoxic injury*.

Table 1.5   Causes of cellular injury

Physical Injury:
  • Mechanical trauma
  • Temperature extremes (e.g., burn injury, frostbite)
  • Electrical current
Chemical Injury:
  • Chemicals, toxins, heavy metals, solvents, smoke, pollutants, drugs, gases
Radiation Injury:
  • Ionizing radiation (e.g., gamma rays, X-rays)
  • Nonionizing radiation (e.g., microwaves, infrared, laser)
Biologic Agents:
  • Bacteria, viruses, parasites
Nutritional Injury:
  • Malnutrition
  • Obesity

1. *Free Radical Injury*:

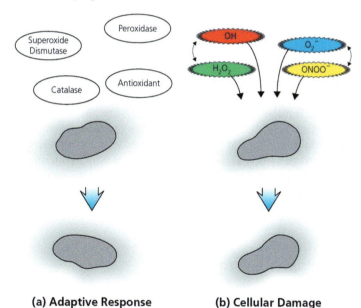

(a) Adaptive Response   (b) Cellular Damage

  • Free radicals are highly reactive chemical species that have one or
    more unpaired electrons in their outer shell.
  • Examples of free radicals include *superoxide* (O_2^-), *hydroxyl radicals*
    (OH), and *hydrogen peroxide* (H_2O_2).

- Free radicals are generated as by-products of normal cell metabolism and are inactivated by free radical scavenging enzymes within the body such as *catalase* and *glutathione peroxidase*. When excess free radicals are formed from exogenous sources or the free radical protective mechanisms fail, injury to cells can occur
- Free radicals are highly reactive and can injure cells through:
  - Peroxidation of membrane lipids
  - Damage of cellular proteins
  - Mutation of cellular DNA
- Exogenous sources of free radicals include tobacco smoke, organic solvents, pollutants, radiation, and pesticides
- Free radical injury has been implicated as playing a key role in the normal aging process as well as in a number of disease states such as diabetes mellitus, cancer, atherosclerosis, Alzheimer's disease, and rheumatoid arthritis

2. *Hypoxic Cell Injury*:
  - Hypoxia is a lack of oxygen in cells and tissues that may result from ischemia, or poor oxygenation of blood
  - During periods of hypoxia, aerobic metabolism of the cells begins to fail. This loss of aerobic metabolism leads to dramatic decreases in ATP production within the cells. Hypoxic cells begin to swell as energy-driven processes (such as ATP-driven ion pumps) begin to fail. The pH of the extracellular environment begins to decrease as waste products such as lactic acid, a product of anaerobic metabolism, begin to accumulate. The cellular injury process may be reversible, if oxygen is quickly restored; or irreversible, and lead to cell death. Certain tissues such as the brain are particularly sensitive to hypoxic injury. Death of brain tissues can occur only 4–6 minutes after hypoxia begins
  - The loss of ionic balance in hypoxic cells can also lead to the accumulation of intracellular calcium, which is normally closely regulated within cells. There are a number of *calcium-dependent protease* enzymes present within cells that become activated in the presence of excess calcium and begin to digest important cellular constituents

1.5.3 Manifestations of cellular injury

1. *Cellular Swelling*:
  - Caused by an accumulation of water due to the failure of ATP-driven ion pumps. Breakdown of cell membrane integrity and accumulation of cellular electrolytes may also occur
  - Cellular swelling is considered to be a reversible change

2. *Cellular Accumulations*:
   - In addition to water, injured cells can accumulate a number of different substances as metabolic and transport processes begin to fail.
   - Substances that can be accumulated in injured cells may include fats, proteins, glycogen, calcium, uric acid and certain pigments such as melanin
   - These accumulations are generally reversible but can indicate a greater degree of cellular injury. Accumulation of these substances can be so marked that enlargement of a tissue or organ may occur. An example of this is the fatty accumulation (*steatosis*) that can develop in the liver of an alcoholic as the liver becomes injured and its function impaired

1.5.4 Cell death

Cells death falls into two main categories, *apoptosis* and *necrotic cell death*.
   1. *Apoptosis*:
      - Apoptosis is a controlled, genetically "preprogrammed" cell death that occurs with aging and normal wear and tear of the cell. Apoptosis may be a mechanism to eliminate worn out or genetically damaged cells. Certain viral infections (e.g., the Epstein-Barr virus) may activate apoptosis within an infected cell, thus killing both the host cell and infecting virus
      - Apoptosis may involve the activation of "suicide genes" that turn on in response to certain chemical signals and lead to cell lysis and destruction through the activation of cellular enzymes called *caspases*
      - It has been theorized that cancer may arise as a failure of normal apoptosis in damaged or mutated cells
      - A physiologic example of normal apoptosis would be the sloughing of the endometrium during the menstrual cycle
   2. *Necrotic Cell Death*:
      - Involves the unregulated, enzymatic digestion ("autolysis") of a cell and its components
      - Occurs as a result of irreversible cellular injury
      - Different types of tissues tend to undergo different types of necrosis. Three main types of necrosis have been identified (see Table 1.6)
   3. *Gangrene*:
      Gangrene is the clinical term used when a large area of tissue undergoes necrosis (see Figure 1.12). Gangrene may be classified as being *"dry gangrene"* or *"wet gangrene."* With dry gangrene, the skin

Table 1.6   Types of cellular necrosis

Liquefaction Necrosis:

- Digestive enzymes released by necrotic cells soften and liquefy dead tissue
- Occurs in tissues, such as the brain, that are rich in hydrolytic enzymes

Caseous Necrosis:

- Dead tissue takes on a crumbly, "cheese-like" appearance; dead cells disintegrate, but their debris is not fully digested by hydrolytic enzymes
- Occurs in conditions like tuberculosis where there is prolonged inflammation and immune activity

Coagulative Necrosis:

- Dead tissues appear firm, gray, and slightly swollen
- Often occurs when cell death results from ischemia and hypoxia; the acidosis that accompanies ischemia denatures cellular proteins and hydrolytic enzymes
- E.g., seen with myocardial infarction

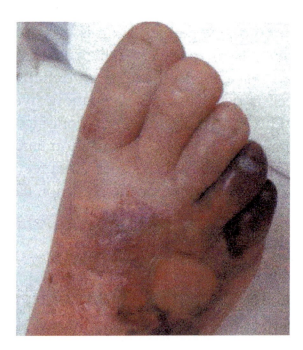

Figure 1.12   Gangrene. (a) Dry Gangrene; (b) Wet Gangrene; and (c) Gas Gangrene.

surrounding the affected area shrinks, wrinkles and turns black. There is generally a clear line of demarcation between living and dead tissue. In contrast, wet gangrene presents with an area that is cold, wet from tissue exudates and swollen. Wet gangrene often occurs when venous return from the affected tissue is lacking and a clear line of demarcation is generally not evident between living and dead tissue. A *gas gangrene* may also occur if the area of necrosis becomes infected with bacteria (often *Clostridium*) that produce hydrogen sulfide gas as a by-product

1.5.5   *Tissue repair*

Injured or damaged tissues can be repaired in one of two ways, by *regeneration* or through *connective tissue replacement*. The mechanism used for repair will depend upon the type of cells that were injured. Certain cells in the body are fully or partially capable of regenerating after an injury, whereas other cells types are not and can only be replaced with connective (scar) tissue.

1. *Repair by Regeneration*
   - With regeneration, the injured tissue is repaired with the same tissue that was lost. A full return of function occurs and afterwards there is little or no evidence of the injury.
   - Repair by regeneration can only occur in *labile cells* (cells that continue to divide throughout life) or *stable cells* (cells that have stopped dividing but can be induced to regenerate under appropriate conditions of injury). Examples of labile cells include those of the skin, oral cavity and bone marrow. Examples of stable cells include hepatocytes of the liver. Certain cell such as nerve cells and cardiac muscle cells are *fixed* cells and cannot undergo regeneration under any circumstances. These cell types are only capable of repairing injuries through connective tissue replacement.
2. *Repair by Connective Tissue Replacement*
   - Involves the replacement of functional tissue with nonfunctional connective tissue (collagen).
   - Full function does not return to the injured tissue.
   - Scar tissue remains as evidence of the injury.

1.5.6   Steps in tissue (wound) repair

Clean, neat wounds such as surgical incisions are said to heal by *primary intention* because they tend to heal quickly and evenly with a minimum of tissue loss. *Sutures* are used to bring the edges of wounds together to facilitate the process of healing by primary intention. Larger, open types of wounds may take considerably longer to heal and are said to heal by *secondary intention*. In secondary intention, the edges of the wound are not able to come into contact with one another and, as a result, the gap must be filled by granulation tissue (see below). These larger wounds often require a significant amount of tissue replacement, take longer to heal and tend to be associated with more obvious scar formation. In general, tissue repair involves three stages, the *inflammatory* stage, the *proliferative* stage, and the *maturational/remodeling* stage:

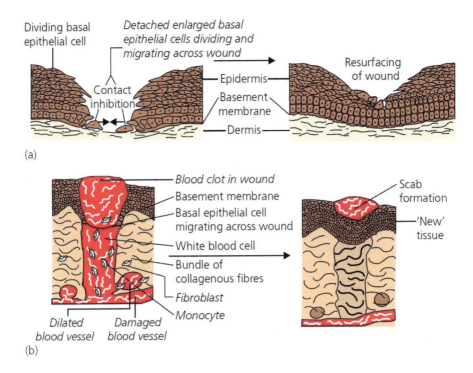

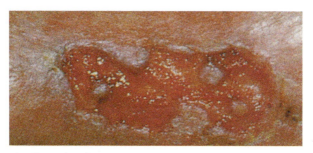

(a) Inflammatory Stage

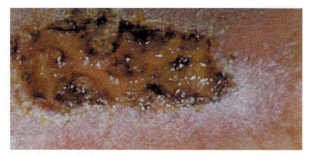

(b) Proliferative Stage

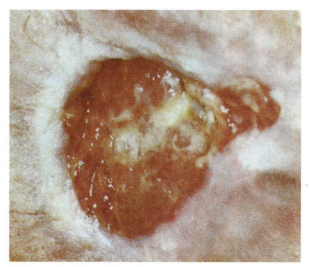

(c) Maturational/Remodeling Stage

1. *Inflammatory Stage*
   - Starts with the formation of a fibrin blood clot to stem bleeding from the injury.
   - Infiltration of phagocytic white blood cells occurs. Neutrophils tend to arrive first followed by larger macrophages. The arriving macrophages produce *growth factors* that stimulate growth of epithelial cells around the wound as well as *angiogenesis* (the formation of new blood vessels).

2. *Proliferative Stage*
   - Over the first 1–3 days after the initial injury, *fibroblasts* in and around the injured tissue proliferate in response to growth factors such as *fibroblast-activating factor* produced by infiltrating macrophages. These activated fibroblasts produce the collagen that will repair the bulk of the wound. Epithelial cells at the margins of the wound also proliferate in response to macrophage-produced growth factors. Angiogenesis is likewise occurring at this point. The soft, pink tissue that forms during this phase of wound healing is referred to as *granulation tissue.*
   - Over time, the collagen that is laid down adds mechanical strength to the repaired area. *Contraction* of the wound occurs over the course of 1–2 weeks as the edges of the wound grow closer to one another.
   - *Suturing* a wound can facilitate healing by primary intention and minimize scar tissue formation by bringing the margins of the wound into close contact with one another.

3. *Maturation and Remodeling*
   - Over the course of one to several months following the injury, there is continued synthesis of collagen in conjunction with removal of old collagen by *collagenase* enzymes. This *remodeling* of the collagen is designed to maximize strength of the repair. Capillaries that were present in the repaired area begin to disappear, leaving an avascular scar. The maturation and remodeling phase of the healed wound may continue for a number of years; however, for larger wounds, the final healed scar will never have the full tensile strength that the original tissue had prior to the injury.
   - A number of factor can impair the wound healing process (see Table 1.7)

KELOID SCARS

Large, raised scars that result from oversynthesis of collagen and decreased collagen breakdown. Keloid scars are often unsightly and may extend beyond the original boundaries of the wounds. A familial tendency for keloid scar formation has been observed with a greater occurrence in blacks than whites.

Table 1.7 Factors that impair wound healing

- Malnutrition
- Poor blood flow and hypoxia (*hyperbaric oxygen* may be used to facilitate wound healing)
- Impaired immune response (immunosuppressive drugs, diseases affecting immune function such as HIV and diabetes)
- Infection of wound
- Foreign particles in the wound
- Old age (decreased immune activity, poor circulation, poor nutrition)

Medical terminology

Absolute refractory period (rē-frăk′tō-rē): Condition where the neuron is completely resistant to any stimulus such that there is no change in membrane potential

Acidosis (ăs″ĭ-dō′sĭs): An increase in the concentration of hydrogen ions in the arterial blood such that the pH is less than 7.4

Action potential (ăk′shŭn pō-těn′shăl): Long-distance electrical signal that is transmitted nondecrementally along the entire length of the axon

Agonist (ăg′ŏn-ĭst): A chemical substance or drug that binds to a receptor and elicits the same effects as an endogenously produced substance or neurotransmitter

Alkalosis (ălk″ă-lō′sĭs): A decrease in the concentration of hydrogen ions in the arterial blood such that the pH is greater than 7.4

Amphipathic (ăm-fē-păth′ĭk): A molecule with a polar (hydrophilic) region and a nonpolar (hydrophobic) region

Antagonist (ăn-tăg′ŏn-ĭst): A chemical substance or drug that binds to a receptor and blocks or prevents the effects of an endogenously produced substance or neurotransmitter

Antigen (ăn′tĭ-jěn): A protein marker on the surface of a cell that identifies the cell as "self" or "non-self" (foreign)

Axon (ăk′sŏn): Elongated process of a neuron that transmits action potentials away from the cell body

Axon hillock (ăk′sŏn hĭl′ŏk): Small projection from the neuronal cell body from which the axon arises; initial site of action potential generation in a neuron

Convergence (cŏn-věr′gĕns): Condition where more than one presynaptic neuron synapses with and influences one postsynaptic neuron

Dendrite (děn′drīt): Process extending from the neuronal cell body that receives electrical signals from other neurons

Depolarization (dē-pō″lăr-ĭ-zā′shŭn): When the inside of the neuron becomes less negative; a decrease in the membrane potential or separation of charge

Diffusion (dĭ-fū′zhŭn): Movement of molecules or ions from a region of high concentration to a region of low concentration

Divergence (dī-vĕr′gĕns): Condition where one presynaptic neuron branches, synapsing with and influencing more than one postsynaptic neuron

Efflux (ē′flŭx): Outward movement of a substance

Equilibrium (ē-kwĭl-ĭ′brē-ŭm): A state of balance

Equilibrium potential (ē″kwĭ-lĭb′rē-ŭm pō-tĕn′shăl): State where the concentration and electrical gradients are balanced and, therefore, the efflux and influx of a given ion are also equal such that there is no further net diffusion

Facilitation (fă-sĭ″ĭ-tā′shŭn): Condition where a postsynaptic neuron has received a subthreshold stimulus and is, therefore, partially depolarized and more likely to generate an action potential upon subsequent stimulation

Graded potential (grād′ĕd pō-tĕn′shăl): Short-distance electrical signal; local change in membrane potential

Hydrophilic (hī-drō-fĭl′ĭk): Attracted to water

Hydrophobic (hī-drō-fō′bĭk): Repelled by water

Hydrostatic pressure (hī″drō-stăt′ĭk prĕsh′ŭr): Pressure exerted by fluid

Hyperpolarization (hī-pĕr-pō″lăr-ĭ-zā′shŭn): When the inside of the neuron becomes more negative; an increase in the membrane potential or separation of charge

Hypoxia (hī-pŏks′ē-ă): An abnormal decrease in oxygen in the tissues

Influx (ĭn′flŭx): Inward movement of a substance

Intravenous (ĭn-tră-vē′nŭs): Within a vein

Lipid bilayer (lĭp′ĭd bī′lā-er): The cell membrane, consisting of two layers of phospholipids oriented such that the hydrophilic portion of the molecules face outward and the hydrophobic portion of the molecules are in the center

Lipophilic (lī-pō-fĭl′-ĭk): Attracted to fats or lipids

Membrane potential (mĕm′brān pō-tĕn′shăl): The electrical difference between the inside and the outside of the cell

Myelin (mī′ĕ-lĭn): Plasma membranes of Schwann cells (peripheral nervous system) or oligodendrocytes (central nervous system) that wrap around an axon forming an electrically insulating sheath

Osmosis (ŏz-mō′sĭs): Movement of water through a semipermeable membrane from a region of high water concentration to a region of low water concentration

Osmotic pressure (ŏz-mŏt′ĭk prĕsh′ŭr): A measure of the tendency for a solution to gain water by osmosis when separated from another solution of lower osmolarity by a semipermeable membrane

Polarization (pō″lăr-ĭ-zā′shŭn): Condition of the resting cell in which the inside is negative relative to the outside; separation of charge

Quantum (kwŏn′tŭm): A fixed or definite amount

Relative refractory period (rē-frăk′tō-rē): Condition where the neuron requires a stronger stimulus to depolarize to threshold and generate an action potential

Repolarization (rē-pō″lăr-ĭ-zā′shŭn): Return to the resting membrane potential following the depolarization of the cell membrane

Saltatory conduction (săl′tă-tō″rē kŏn-dŭk′shŭn): Transmission of the action potential along a myelinated axon

Synapse (sĭn′aps): Point of contact between two neurons, typically including the axon terminal of one neuron and the cell body or dendrites of the second

Synaptic knob (sĭn-ăp′tĭc nŏb): Region of the presynaptic axon terminal that comes into close apposition with the postsynaptic neuron

Threshold (thrĕsh′ōld): Membrane potential at which an action potential may be generated

Unidirectional (ū″nē-dĭ-rĕk′shŭn-ŏl): In one direction only

Vesicle (vĕs′ĭ-kl): Membranous sac that stores preformed neurotransmitter in the synaptic knob

Bibliography

AHFS Drug Information 2000, American Society of Health-System Pharmacists, Bethesda, MD, 2000.

Baldessarini, R., Therapy of depression and anxiety disorders, in *Goodman and Gilman's: The Pharmacological Basis of Therapeutics*, 11th ed., Brunton, L. L., Lazo, J. S., Parker, K. L., Eds., McGraw-Hill, New York, 2006, chap. 17.

Baldessarini, R., and Tarazi, F. I., Pharmacotherapy of psychosis and mania, in *Goodman and Gilman's: The Pharmacological Basis of Therapeutics*, 11th ed., Brunton, L. L., Lazo, J. S., Parker, K. L., Eds., McGraw-Hill, New York, 2006, chap. 18.

Bear, M. F., Connors, B. W., and Paradiso, M. A., Chemical control of the brain and behavior, in *Neuroscience, Exploring the Brain*, 3rd ed., Lippincott Williams & Wilkins, Philadelphia, PA, 2007, chap. 15.

Bell, D. R., *Core Concepts in Physiology*, Lippincott-Raven Publishers, Philadelphia, PA, 1998.

Bloom, F., Neurotransmission and the central nervous system, in *Goodman and Gilman's: The Pharmacological Basis of Therapeutics*, 11th ed., Brunton, L. L., Lazo, J. S., Parker, K. L., Eds., McGraw-Hill, New York, 2006, chap. 12.

Boss, B. J., Concepts of neurological dysfunction, in *Pathophysiology, The Biologic Basis for Disease in Adults & Children*, Mosby, St. Louis, MO, 2002, chap. 15.

Buxton, I. L. O., Pharmacokinetics and pharmacodynamics: the dynamics of drug absorption, distribution, action and elimination, in *Goodman and Gilman's: The Pharmacological Basis of Therapeutics*, 11th ed., Brunton, L. L., Lazo, J. S., Parker, K. L., Eds., McGraw-Hill, New York, 2006, chap. 1.

Catterall, W., and Mackie, K., Local anesthetics, in *Goodman and Gilman's: The Pharmacological Basis of Therapeutics*, 11th ed., Brunton, L. L., Lazo, J. S., and Parker, K. L., Eds., McGraw-Hill, New York, 2006, chap. 14.

Costanzo, L., *Physiology*, 3rd ed., W. B. Saunders Company, Philadelphia, PA, 2006.

Diagnosis and treatment of schizophrenia. (2016, October 11). Retrieved from http://www.mayoclinic.org/diseases-conditions/schizophrenia/home/ovc-20253194.

Finley, P. R., Selective serotonin re-uptake inhibitors: pharmacologic profiles and potential therapeutic distinctions. *Annals of Pharmacotherapy*, 28(12): 1359–1369, 1994.

Fox, S., *Human Physiology*, 9th ed., McGraw-Hill, New York, 2006.

Garoutte, B., *Neuromuscular Physiology*, Mill Valley Medical Publishers, Millbrae, CA, 1996.

Guyton, A. C., and Hall, J. E., *Textbook of Medical Physiology*, 11th ed., W. B. Saunders Co., Philadelphia, PA, 2006.

Hanson, M., *Pathophysiology, Foundations of Disease and Clinical Intervention*, W. B. Saunders Co., Philadelphia, PA, 1998.

Hunt, M. L., Jr., *Training Manual for Intravenous Admixture Personnel*, 5th ed., Baxter Healthcare Corp., Deerfield, IL, 1995.

Kane, J. M., Schizophrenia. *New England Journal of Medicine*, 334(1): 34–41, 1996.

Lombard, J. H. and Rusch, N. J., Cells, nerves and muscles, in *Physiology Secrets*, Raff, H., Ed., Hanley and Belfus, Inc., Philadelphia, PA, 1999, chap. 1.

McNamara, J. O., Pharmacotherapy of the epilepsies, in *Goodman and Gilman's: The Pharmacological Basis of Therapeutics*, 11th ed., Brunton, L. L., Lazo, J. S., and Parker, K. L., Eds., McGraw-Hill, New York, 2006, chap. 19.

Pasch, S. K., Disorders of thought, mood, and memory, in *Pathophysiology, Concept of Altered Health States*, Porth, C. M., Ed., Lippincott Williams & Wilkins, Philadelphia, PA, 2005, chap. 53.

Rhoades, R., and Pflanzer, R., *Human Physiology*, 4th ed., Brooks/Cole, Pacific Grove, CA, 2003.

Rockhold, R. W., The chemical basis for neuronal communication, in *Fundamental Neuroscience for Basic and Clinical Applications*, Haines, D. E., Ed., Churchill Livingstone/Elsevier, Philadelphia, PA, 2006, chap. 4.

Sherwood, L., *Human Physiology from Cells to Systems*, 5th ed., Brooks/Cole, Pacific Grove, CA, 2004.

Silverthorn, D., *Human Physiology: An Integrated Approach*, 4th ed., Prentice Hall, Upper Saddle River, NJ, 2007.

Standaert, D. G., and Young, A. B., Treatment of central nervous system degenerative disorders, in *Goodman and Gilman's: The Pharmacological Basis of Therapeutics*, 11th ed., Brunton, L. L., Lazo, J. S., Parker, K. L., Eds., McGraw-Hill, New York, 2006, chap. 20.

Stedman's Medical Dictionary for the Health Professions and Nursing, 5th ed., Lippincott, Williams & Wilkins, Philadelphia, PA, 2005.

Taber's Cyclopedic Medical Dictionary, 20th ed., F. A. Davis Co., Philadelphia, PA, 2005.

Widmaier, E., Raff, H., and Strang, K., *Vander's Human Physiology, The Mechanisms of Body Function*, 10th ed., McGraw-Hill, New York, 2006.

chapter two

Homeostasis

Study objectives

- Define the internal environment
- Understand the importance of homeostasis
- Describe the overall function of each of the three major components of the nervous system
- Compare the general functions of the nervous system and the endocrine system
- Distinguish between negative feedback and positive feedback
- Describe the potential role of medications in the maintenance of homeostasis

2.1   Homeostasis

Physiology is the study of the functions of the human body. In other words, if anatomy describes the structure or morphology of the parts of the body, physiology describes how these parts work. This discipline considers the mechanisms by which each of the various tissues and organs carry out their specific activities. Emphasis is placed on the processes that control and regulate the physiological activities in the body.

For the body to function optimally, conditions within the body, referred to as the *internal environment*, must be very carefully regulated. Therefore, many important variables, such as body temperature, blood pressure, blood glucose, oxygen, and carbon dioxide content of the blood as well as electrolyte balance are actively maintained within narrow physiological limits.

This maintenance of relatively constant or steady-state internal conditions is referred to as *homeostasis*. It is important because the cells and tissues of the body will survive and function efficiently only when these internal conditions are properly maintained. This is not to say that the internal environment is fixed or unchanging. The body is constantly faced with a changing external environment as well as with events and activities occurring within the body that may alter the balance of important variables. For example, most metabolic reactions within our cells consume oxygen and glucose. These substances must then be replaced. In addition, these reactions produce metabolic wastes including carbon dioxide and urea, which must then be eliminated. Therefore, it is more accurate to say that the internal

Table 2.1 Contribution of organ systems to the maintenance of homeostasis

Organ system	Function
Nervous System	Regulates muscular activity and glandular secretion; responsible for all activities associated with the mind
Endocrine System	Regulates metabolic processes through secretion of hormones
Muscular System	Allows for body movement; contributes to thermoregulation
Circulatory System	Transports nutrients, oxygen, waste, carbon dioxide, electrolytes, and hormones throughout the body
Respiratory System	Obtains oxygen and eliminates carbon dioxide; regulates acid–base balance (pH)
Gastrointestinal Tract	Digests and absorbs food substances to provide nutrients to the body
Renal System	Eliminates waste products from the body; regulates blood volume and blood pressure; regulates acid–base balance (pH)

environment is in a *dynamic steady state*, one that is constantly changing, but where optimal conditions are physiologically maintained.

All the organ systems in the body, except the reproductive system, contribute to the maintenance of homeostasis (see Table 2.1). For example, the gastrointestinal tract digests foods to provide nutrients to the body. The respiratory system obtains oxygen and eliminates carbon dioxide. The circulatory system transports these materials and others from one part of the body to another. The renal system eliminates wastes and plays a role in regulating blood volume and blood pressure.

The study of physiology includes not only the study of how each of these systems carries out its functions, but also the mechanisms involved that regulate these activities to maintain homeostasis under a variety of conditions. For example, the body's needs are very different during a resting state compared with that of exercise. How do organ systems adjust their activities in response to varied levels of physical exertion or when confronted with altered internal and external environments? To maintain homeostasis, the body must first be able to monitor and sense changes in the internal environment. Second, it must be able to compensate, or adjust, for these changes.

There are two regulatory systems in the body that influence the activity of all the other organ systems so that homeostasis is ultimately maintained. These are:

- Nervous system
- Endocrine system

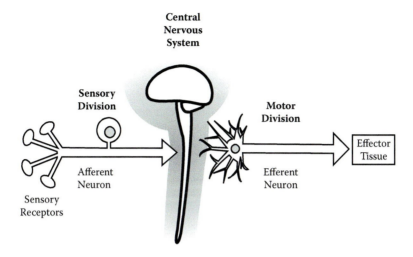

Figure 2.1 Functional components of the nervous system. The sensory division of the peripheral nervous system is sensitive to changes in the internal and external environment. The information gathered by this component of the nervous system is transmitted to the CNS where it is processed, integrated, and interpreted. The CNS then determines the appropriate response to this input. This response is carried out by the transmission of nerve impulses in the motor division of the peripheral nervous system to the effector tissues.

There are three functional components of the *nervous system* (see Figure 2.1):

- Sensory division of the peripheral nervous system
- Central nervous system
- Motor division of the peripheral nervous system

Many different types of sensory receptors are located throughout the body. These receptors monitor the status of the internal environment or that of the surroundings. *Sensory receptors* are sensitive to specific types of stimuli and measure the value of a physiological variable. For example, *arterial baroreceptors* measure arterial blood pressure and *chemoreceptors* measure the amount of oxygen and carbon dioxide in the arterial blood. The information detected by these sensors then travels by way of *afferent* neuronal pathways to the *central nervous system* (CNS).

The CNS is the *integrative portion* of the nervous system and consists of:

- Brain
- Spinal cord

The brain receives, processes, and stores sensory input; generates thoughts; and determines the reactions that the body should perform in response to this input. The spinal cord is important in processing reflexes. It is within this integration area of the nervous system that the actual value of a physiological variable as measured by a sensory receptor is compared with its set point or optimal value. One or more compensatory responses to the sensory input are then determined.

The third component of the nervous system is the *motor division*. Appropriate signals are transmitted from the CNS to various body parts or *effector tissues* by way of *efferent* neuronal pathways. These effector tissues include a variety of the body's tissues and organs, specifically, the muscles and glands within the tissues and organs. The effector tissues carry out the appropriate physiological responses to bring the variable back to within its normal limits.

The other regulatory system in the body contributing to the maintenance of homeostasis is the *endocrine system*, which carries out its effects by secreting *hormones*. These hormones are transported in the blood to the specific tissues upon which they exert their effects.

The following generalizations regarding the two regulatory systems may be made. The nervous system primarily regulates muscular activity and glandular secretion. The endocrine system primarily regulates metabolic activity in the body's cells. However, these two systems may not only work together in the regulation of many organs, they may also influence each other's activity.

2.1.1　Negative feedback

Most of the body's *compensatory homeostatic mechanisms* function by way of *negative feedback*. This is a response that causes the level of a variable to change in a direction opposite to that of the initial change. Because the response returns the variable back to its baseline level, it has a *stabilizing* effect on the body. For example, when blood pressure increases, the arterial baroreceptors are stimulated and an increased number of nerve impulses are transmitted to the CNS through afferent pathways. The region of the brain regulating the cardiovascular system responds to this sensory input by altering efferent nerve activity to the heart. The result is a decrease in heart rate and, therefore, a decrease in blood pressure back to its baseline value (see Figure 2.2). In general, when some physiological variable becomes too high or too low, a control system elicits a negative feedback response consisting of one or a series of changes that returns the variable to within its normal physiological range. These compensatory mechanisms operating via negative feedback allow the body to effectively maintain homeostasis.

Interestingly, one of the greatest stressors on the body and, therefore, challenges to the maintenance of homeostasis is increased physical activity or exercise. During intense exercise, glucose utilization can be increased

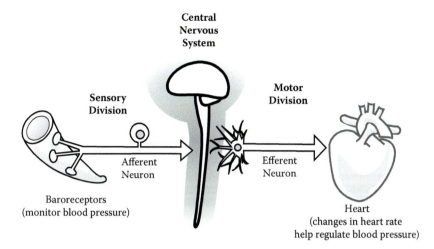

Figure 2.2 Negative feedback. Negative feedback responses are employed through-out the body to maintain homeostasis. In this example, any change in blood pressure, which is monitored within the circulatory system and processed or interpreted within the CNS, will cause reflex changes in heart rate. The change in heart rate will be in the opposite direction of the change in blood pressure. If blood pressure increases, then heart rate decreases. If blood pressure decreases, then heart rate increases. In this way, blood pressure is adjusted back to its normal value.

up to 20-fold, skeletal muscle pH drops dramatically, several liters of water can be lost in the form of sweat and core body temperature can increase to as high as 106°F. These profound disturbances must be compensated for to ensure cell survival. An important focus throughout this textbook will be how tissue and organ system functions are regulated under various normal physiological conditions and, where appropriate, under abnormal patho-physiological conditions. Furthermore, discussions of how basic physiologi-cal principles may be applied to the practice of pharmacy are included.

2.1.2 Positive feedback

Although there are fewer physiological examples, there are also processes in the body that utilize positive feedback responses. These responses *amplify* the initial change in a variable. In other words, if the level of a variable increases, positive feedback responses cause the level of the variable to increase fur-ther, which has a *destabilizing* effect on the body. An interesting example involves parturition, or childbirth. As labor begins and the uterus contracts, it pushes the baby downward and stretches the cervix. Consequently, sig-nals are transmitted to the hypothalamus of the brain, which stimulates the secretion of the hormone oxytocin. This hormone acts on the uterus to cause powerful muscular contractions, again pushing downward on the baby and

PHARMACY APPLICATION: HOMEOSTATIC FUNCTIONS OF DRUGS

Diseases are generally divided into two categories: those in which the pathophysiology involves the internal failure of some normal physiological process and those that originate from some external source such as bacterial or viral infection. In either case, the individual is unable to maintain homeostasis, and one or more variables in the internal environment will be disrupted and the tissue or organ function is impaired. Therefore, many of the medications currently in use are designed to assist the body in the maintenance of homeostasis when its own regulatory mechanisms fail to do so. For example, angiotensin-converting enzyme (ACE) inhibitors, such as enalapril and benazepril, and beta-blockers, such as propranolol and metoprolol, lower blood pressure in patients with idiopathic (unexplained) hypertension (elevated blood pressure). Another example is that a common complication in patients with type 1 diabetes mellitus is hyperglycemia (excess glucose in the blood). Insulin injections allow the cells of these patients to take up and store glucose, which effectively lowers the blood glucose to the normal range. As a final example, diuretics such as furosemide decrease blood volume and, therefore, reduce cardiac workload in patients with congestive heart failure. In each of these disorders, pharmacological intervention is necessary for the given organ system to function efficiently and effectively to maintain the health of the patient.

resulting in further stretch of the cervix. This stretch causes the secretion of more oxytocin and so on until the baby has been expelled from the uterus. Other examples of positive feedback involve voltage-gated sodium channels and the generation of electrical signals in nerve cells (discussed in Chapter 1) as well as the mechanism for blood clotting (discussed in Chapter 5).

Medical terminology

Afferent (ăf′ĕr-ĕnt): Carrying or transporting toward a central location

Efferent (ĕf′ĕr-ĕnt): Carrying or transporting away from a central location

Homeostasis (hō″mē-ō-stā′sĭs): The maintenance of an internal equilibrium or a dynamic steady state in an individual by altering appropriate physiological processes in the body's tissues and organs

Internal environment: Conditions within the body

Negative feedback: A response that opposes the original change in the system

Positive feedback: A response that amplifies the original change in the system

Bibliography

AHFS Drug Information 2000, American Society of Health-System Pharmacists, Bethesda, MD, 2000.

Papanek, P. E., Exercise physiology and the bioenergetics of muscle contraction, in *Physiology Secrets*, Raff, H., Ed., Hanley & Belfus, Philadelphia, PA, 1999, chap. 8.

Porterfield, S., *Endocrine Physiology*, Mosby, Inc., St. Louis, MO, 2001.

Sherwood, L., *Human Physiology from Cells to Systems*, 5th ed., Thomson Brooks/Cole, Pacific Grove, CA, 2004.

Silverthorn, D., *Human Physiology: An Integrated Approach*, 4th ed., Prentice Hall, Upper Saddle River, NJ, 2007.

Stedman's Medical Dictionary for the Health Professions and Nursing, 5th ed., Lippincott, Williams & Wilkins, Philadelphia, PA, 2005.

Taber's Cyclopedic Medical Dictionary, 20th ed., F. A. Davis Co., Philadelphia, PA, 2005.

Widmaier, E., Raff, H., and Strang, K., *Vander's Human Physiology, The Mechanisms of Body Function*, 10th ed., McGraw Hill, New York, 2006.

chapter three

The immune system

Study objectives

- Describe the functions and activities of the immune system
- Explain how interferon defends against invading viruses and tumor cells
- Describe the function of natural killer cells
- Describe how complement defends against invading bacteria
- Compare and contrast the general characteristics of the innate immune system and the adaptive immune system
- List the different types of antibodies and their functions
- Describe the two functional regions of the antibody molecule
- Explain how antibodies defend against invading bacteria
- Explain the clonal selection theory
- Compare and contrast primary responses and secondary responses
- Distinguish between active immunity and passive immunity
- List the three types of T cells and their functions
- Explain how cytotoxic T cells defend against invading viruses
- Distinguish between class I MHC glycoproteins and class II MHC glycoproteins
- Compare and contrast the four types of hypersensitivity reactions that can occur in terms of their etiology and major clinical manifestations.
- Define anaphylaxis. List the physiologic symptoms that accompany it and explain why each symptom occurs.
- Discuss possible factors that may be involved in the development of an autoimmune disease

3.1 Overview of immune function

Immunity is defined as the body's ability to eliminate foreign organisms or substances as well as abnormal cells. The immune system consists of tissues, cells, and molecules that work together to form an internal defense system. As such, the immune system is capable of recognizing and destroying, or neutralizing, pathogens and substances that are foreign to the "normal self." The immune system performs several functions and activities that are important in maintaining health or, as in the case of tissue rejection, causing disease. These include:

- Defense against infection
- Removal of cells and tissue debris
- Immune surveillance
- Allergies and autoimmune diseases
- Rejection of tissue grafts and newly introduced proteins

The immune system provides *defense against infection* by pathogenic microorganisms such as bacteria, viruses, fungi, and parasites. Immune deficiency results in an increased susceptibility to infections. This is exemplified by patients with AIDS or individuals taking chemotherapy or immunosuppressant drugs.

Another function of this system involves the *removal* of "worn out" cells, such as aged red blood cells, as well as tissue debris. Injury and disease cause tissue damage and cell death. The removal of the tissue debris is an important step in wound healing and the tissue repair process.

Immune surveillance involves the identification and destruction of abnormal or mutant cells that have originated within or invaded the body. For example, this function serves as the primary internal defense mechanism against tumor growth and cancer, or for a fight against bacterial pneumonia.

Allergies and autoimmune diseases are inappropriate immune responses that threaten an individual's health. An allergy, or type I hypersensitivity reaction, is a response to a seemingly harmless environmental agent (ragweed, dust, pet dander), food (nuts, shellfish), or drugs (penicillin). Symptoms may include nasal congestion, sneezing, runny nose, asthma, hives, diarrhea, and anaphylaxis. Autoimmune diseases occur when the immune system erroneously produces antibodies against the body's own cells and may result in damage to tissues and disruption of normal organ function. Examples of autoimmune diseases include rheumatoid arthritis, systemic lupus erythematosus, type 1 diabetes mellitus, and Crohn's disease. Symptoms of each of these diseases are related to the organ systems affected.

Tissues and organs transplanted from a donor are recognized by the immune system as being foreign to the body. The resulting immune responses, or type II hypersensitivity reactions, may damage and destroy these tissues. Therefore, the recipient of a transplant must inhibit these responses with the administration of immunosuppressive drugs such as tacrolimus, cyclosporine, rapamycin, mycophenolic acid, and leflunomide.

3.1.1   Agents of infectious disease

Many microorganisms, which are not visible to the human eye, can cause infectious disease and include bacteria, viruses, fungi, and parasites.

This chapter will focus on defense provided by the immune system against bacteria and viruses.

Bacteria are nonnucleated, single-celled organisms that consist of a single chromosome of DNA and a cytoplasm containing the reproductive and metabolic machinery of the cell. As such, bacteria can synthesize DNA, RNA, and proteins and can reproduce independently. These microorganisms cause disease primarily by releasing enzymes or toxins that physically injure or functionally disrupt cells and tissues.

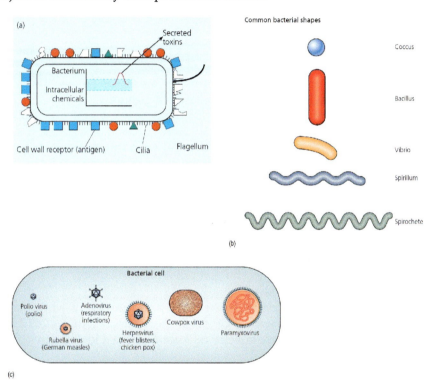

Viruses are pathogens consisting of nucleic acid (DNA or RNA) enclosed by a protein coat. These microorganisms lack the cellular machinery for protein synthesis and energy production and are, therefore, not classified as living cells. As such, they are incapable of reproducing outside of a living cell. Therefore, viruses must invade a susceptible living "host" cell and use the biosynthetic machinery of that cell to replicate. Viruses may damage tissues and cause disease in many ways including the following:

- Hijacking the host cell so that it produces additional viruses
- Depletion of essential cellular components
- Production by the cell of substances that are toxic to itself
- Transformation of the cell into a cancer cell

3.1.2   Effector cells of the immune system

Leukocytes (white blood cells) are the effector cells of the immune system and are responsible for the destruction of invading microorganisms, identification and destruction of cancer cells, and phagocytosis of tissue debris, including dead and injured cells. Leukocytes are present in the blood only transiently in that they leave the blood vessels and enter the tissues, moving toward areas of inflammation or infection, where they carry out their effects. Briefly, the primary characteristics and functions of the five types of leukocytes are as follows:

- *Neutrophils*: Highly mobile phagocytes that attack and destroy invading bacteria and remove tissue debris
- *Monocytes*: Immature leukocytes that leave the blood, enter the tissue and transform into large, tissue-bound phagocytes
- *Eosinophils*: Granulocytes that destroy parasitic worms and are involved in allergic reactions
- *Basophils*: Leukocytes that are structurally and functionally similar to connective tissue mast cells in that they release histamine and heparin; involved in allergic reactions
- *Lymphocytes*:
  - *B lymphocytes (B cells)*: Transform into plasma cells that produce antibodies; antibodies act in the indirect destruction or neutralization of bacteria and bacterial toxins
  - *T lymphocytes (T cells)*: Involved in the direct destruction of virus-invaded cells and mutant cells

A more detailed explanation of the structure and function of white blood cells can be found in Chapter 17. Other effector cells include *natural killer (NK) cells* and *mast cells*. These effector cells are discussed in detail in subsequent sections of this chapter.

3.1.3   Immune responses

The immune system can be divided into two systems:

- Innate immune system
- Adaptive immune system

Working together to protect the body from infection, these two types of immune systems elicit responses that differ in their timing and selectivity.

3.1.4   *Innate immune system*

Referred to as the *nonspecific immune system*, the innate immune system consists of inherent, built-in defense mechanisms that *nonselectively* defend the body against foreign material and substances. Because these responses are nonspecific, they are elicited *immediately* and are broadly reacting. These mechanisms provide a rapid, initial defense against infectious agents, chemical irritants, and tissue injury.

Neutrophils and macrophages play a key role in the innate immune system. These phagocytes contain *Toll-like receptors* (*TLRs*) on their plasma membranes. There are several different types of TLRs, each of which recognizes different molecular patterns expressed by pathogens (PAMPs). These PAMPs are shared by many infectious agents, which reduces the need for a large number of receptor types. Furthermore, PAMPs are clearly distinguishable from "self" molecular patterns on the surface of the body's own cells. Engagement of the PAMP with the TRL on the phagocyte triggers phagocytosis and the secretion of cytokines that stimulate inflammation.

In summary, the innate immune system elicits defense mechanisms that are rapid and nonspecific. However, the effectiveness of these mechanisms is limited because the responses tend to be weak. The benefit of the innate immune system is that it limits the spread of infection until the slower, but more powerful, adaptive immune system can be activated.

Innate immune responses include the following:

- Inflammation (discussed in Chapter 4)
- Interferon
- Natural killer cells
- Complement system

A second form of innate immune response involves the release of *interferon* from virus-infected cells. This protein helps to contain viral infection by interfering with the replication of viruses in other host cells. Interferon binds to specific receptors on uninfected cells. This receptor binding leads to the synthesis of over two dozen proteins that contribute to viral resistance via multiple mechanisms, including the inhibition of transcription, translation, protein processing, and virus maturation. Thus, when the virus enters the interferon-altered cell, it is unable to replicate.

Other functions of interferon include the following:

- Increase in macrophage activity
- Increase in production of antibodies

- Increasing in activity of NK cells and cytotoxic T cells
- Decreasing cell division and decreasing tumor growth

NK cells are lymphocytes that are distinct from B cells and T cells in their ability to nonspecifically destroy virus-infected cells and tumor cells. Referred to as *natural killer cells*, these cells are unlike cytotoxic T cells in that the recognition of a specific antigen is not necessary for their activation. However, the nature of the NK cell surface receptor that allows these cells to identify their targets remains largely unknown. The mechanism of NK cytotoxicity is similar to cytotoxic T cells in that they cause the direct lysis of virus-infected cells and tumor cells by the production and release of pore-forming proteins.

The fourth form of innate immune response involves the *complement system*. This family of proteins is typically found circulating in the blood in inactive forms. As with fibrinogen and the clotting factors, complement proteins leak into the tissue spaces during an inflammatory response.

The complement system may be activated by three pathways:

- Classical pathway
- Alternative pathway
- Lectin pathway

The *classical pathway* is elicited when complement protein C1 binds to an antibody. Activation of C1 leads to the activation of the other complement proteins in the system. This pathway is more rapid and efficient than the alternative and lectin pathways. The *alternative pathway* is triggered when complement protein C3b binds with proteins or polysaccharides on the surface of a microbe. This binding and activation of C3b leads to the activation of other complement proteins. Last, the *lectin pathway* is triggered when plasma mannose-binding lectin (MBL) attaches to a microbe. MBL is structurally similar to C1 and, therefore, serves to activate the complement system. It is important to note that the alternative and lectin pathways are components of the innate immune system, whereas the classical pathway is involved in the adaptive immune system. Regardless, the effects of complement activation are the same. The overall effects include:

- Direct lysis of the invading microbe
- Enhancement of the inflammatory response

Complement-mediated cytolysis of microbes involves the formation of the *membrane attack complex (MAC)*. Binding of C3b to the microbe leads to the activation of complement factors C5 through C9 in a stepwise fashion. These factors then aggregate and embed in the membrane of the microbe, forming a pore. The ensuing osmotic flux of water into the cell results in cell lysis.

Complement augments several steps in the inflammatory response, including the following:

- Enhanced release of histamine
- Vasodilation and increased permeability
- Chemotaxis
- Opsonization

Complement factors C3a and C5a stimulate the release of histamine from tissue mast cells. The histamine then promotes the vascular changes that result in increased delivery of phagocytes to the tissue. Complement factors C3a and C5a also serve as chemotaxins, drawing the phagocytes through the tissue to the site of injury. Finally, as described previously, C3b serves as an opsonic agent and enhances phagocytosis.

3.1.5   Adaptive immune system

Adaptive immunity, also referred to as *specific* or *acquired* immunity, responses develop more slowly than the innate immune responses. However, they are much more powerful and effective at eliminating infection. In addition, adaptive immunity responses are highly specific in that they are directed toward a specific microbial invader. As such, the immune system requires prior exposure to the infectious agent to elicit these responses. Adaptive immune responses are triggered by *antigens*. These molecules are large (mol. wt. >10,000), complex, and unique. Typically, antigens are foreign proteins and may include microbial cell surface receptors and bacterial toxins. Large polysaccharides may also be antigenic in nature.

There are two types of lymphocytes involved in adaptive immunity: B cells and T cells. Each type is derived from stem cells in the bone marrow. However, B cells differentiate and mature in the bone marrow; whereas T cells differentiate and mature in the thymus, a collection of lymphoid tissue located in the midline of the thoracic cavity, above the heart and between the lungs. Once matured, B cells and T cells are released into the blood. Some of these cells remain in the blood or enter the lymph and body tissues. In this way, they conduct immune surveillance and are on the constant search for invading microbes and tumor cells. However, most of the lymphocytes (approximately 2 trillion) establish colonies in peripheral lymphoid tissues such as the lymph nodes, spleen, adenoids, tonsils, and appendix. Regardless of location, exposure to a specific microbial protein, or antigen, stimulates cell division and the production of new generations of specific lymphocytes.

B cells and T cells have surface receptors that recognize a specific antigen. Binding of an antigen to its receptor elicits a specific immune response. There are two types of adaptive immune responses:

- Antibody-mediated immunity
- Cell-mediated immunity

Referred to as humoral immunity, *antibody-mediated immunity* involves the activation of B lymphocytes. These responses begin when an antigen binds to its specific B cell surface receptor. Under the influence of cytokines released from *helper T cells*, the B cell matures into a *plasma cell*, which, in turn, produces antibodies. These cells have an elaborate rough endoplasmic reticulum (the site of protein synthesis) and can produce as many as 2,000 antibodies per second. These antibodies eventually gain access to the blood and are referred to as *gamma globulins* or *immunoglobulins*. Under normal conditions, antibodies account for approximately 20% of all plasma proteins.

3.1.5.1 Classification of antibodies

There are five classes of antibodies:

- IgM: Serves as the B-cell surface receptor for antigen binding; is associated with the primary immune response; acts as an efficient activator of the complement system.
- IgG: Circulates as the predominant (75%) antibody in the serum; is produced in secondary immune responses; inactivates pathogens (e.g., opsonization) and activates the complement system; crosses the placenta and provides neonatal immunity.
- IgA: Protects sites of potential microbial invasion from infection due to its presence in the secretions and the mucus membranes of the digestive, respiratory, reproductive, and urinary systems; is found in saliva and tears; provides neonatal immunity due to its presence in maternal milk.
- IgE: Serves as the mediator for acute inflammatory responses and allergic responses due to its presence on the surface of mast cells; provides protection against parasitic worms.
- IgD: Serves as the B cell surface receptor for antigen binding; circulates in trace amounts; physiological activities unclear.

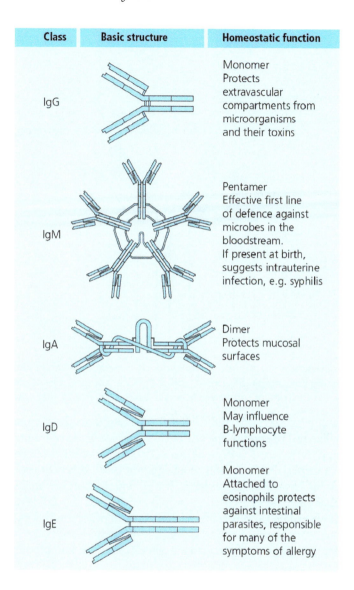

Class	Basic structure	Homeostatic function
IgG		Monomer Protects extravascular compartments from microorganisms and their toxins
IgM		Pentamer Effective first line of defence against microbes in the bloodstream. If present at birth, suggests intrauterine infection, e.g. syphilis
IgA		Dimer Protects mucosal surfaces
IgD		Monomer May influence B-lymphocyte functions
IgE		Monomer Attached to eosinophils protects against intestinal parasites, responsible for many of the symptoms of allergy

3.1.5.2   Structure of antibodies

Antibodies are composed of four interlinked polypeptide chains:

- 2 long, heavy chains
- 2 short, light chains

These chains are arranged so that the antibody molecule is in the shape of a "Y" (see Figure 3.1). The arm regions contain the *antigen-binding fragments (Fab)*

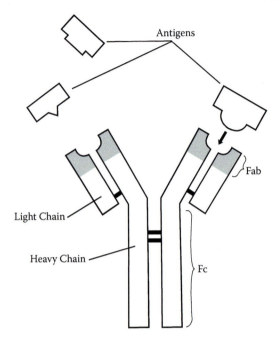

Figure 3.1 Structure of antibodies. The antibody molecule is shaped like a "Y." The antigen-binding fragments (Fab) bind with a specific antigen. The constant region (Fc) determines the type of protective action to be carried out by that antibody.

and are unique for each different antigen; the fragments determine antibody specificity. The tail portion of the antibody molecule is the *constant region (Fc)*. This region determines the type of protective action carried out by the antibody. For example, the Fc region of an IgG antibody binds to the surface of phagocytes; IgG serves as an opsonin. The Fc region of an IgE antibody binds to the surface of mast cells. After antigen binding to the IgE antibody, the mast cell degranulates and releases histamine and other mediators of allergic and inflammatory reactions. The Fc region of an IgM antibody binds with complement protein C1 and leads to the activation of the complement system.

3.1.5.3 *Actions of antibodies*

Antibodies exert their protective effects by several different mechanisms (see Figure 3.2):

- Neutralization
- Agglutination
- Activation of the complement system
- Opsonization
- Mast cell degranulation
- Stimulation of NK cells

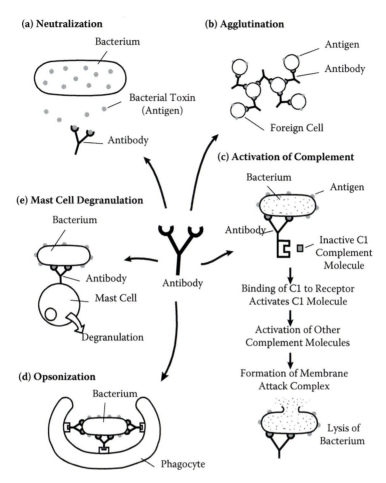

Figure 3.2 Actions of antibodies. Antibodies may physically hinder antigens by way of neutralization (a) or agglutination (b). Antibodies may also amplify innate immune responses including the activation of the complement system (c), opsonization (d), and mast cell degranulation (e).

Neutralization and *agglutination* are forms of *physical hindrance* of antigens, which, in fact, plays a relatively minor role in antibody protection against antigens. Specifically, neutralization involves the binding of bacterial toxins with their specific antibodies and the toxins are unable to interact with or damage susceptible cells. Agglutination involves the clumping of foreign cells such as bacteria or mismatched red blood cells. This process enhances the likelihood of phagocytosis. Agglutination reactions are also used clinically to identify bacteria and to type red blood cells. IgM and, to a lesser extent, IgG are effective agglutinating agents.

Activation of the complement system, opsonization, mast cell degranulation, and *stimulation of killer cells* all involve the amplification of innate immune responses. These are the most powerful protective actions of antibodies.

Antibodies, specifically IgM antibodies, are the most potent activators of the complement system. As discussed previously, the complement system causes the direct lysis of bacteria via the membrane attack complex. In addition, this system enhances every aspect of the inflammatory response including chemotaxis and opsonization.

Opsonization involves the binding of IgG antibodies to the surface of phagocytes as well as to invading bacteria. The linkage between the phagocyte, the IgG and the bacterium prevents the escape of the microbe and enhances phagocytosis.

Mast cells have IgE antibodies on their cell surfaces. Binding of specific antigens to the IgE molecules results in mast cell degranulation and the release of chemicals such as histamine that mediate the inflammatory response.

Killer cells are similar to NK cells, discussed previously, in that they cause the lysis of cells. However, to carry out their effects, killer cells require the target bacterium to be coated with antibodies. The antigen-bound antibody then binds to the surface of the killer cell by way of the Fc region and the killer cell is activated to release *perforin molecules*. These molecules aggregate and insert themselves into the bacterial cell membrane, forming a pore and causing cell lysis.

3.1.5.4   Clonal selection theory

There are literally millions of different types of antigens that may elicit an antibody-mediated immune response. However, each type of B lymphocyte with its specific IgM antibody as its cell surface receptor may respond to only one specific antigen. Therefore, millions of different types of B cells are needed to recognize each of these antigens. As such, a remarkably diverse population of B cells is produced during fetal development. Each of these B cells is capable of synthesizing antibodies against a specific antigen. All the offspring from a given B cell are identical to the original lymphocyte and form a *clone*. Furthermore, these cells produce the same specific antibody. Because millions of different B lymphocytes are required to produce so many different antibodies, it should be clear that the number of types of B cells must be limited. When exposed to an antigen, expansion of the clone, or increasing the number of antibody-producing cells, is necessary to achieve an effective immune response.

The *clonal selection theory* is illustrated in Figure 3.3. Exposure to an antigen causes the selective activation of a *naïve lymphocyte*, one that has not been previously exposed to the antigen. The B cell then proliferates forming two types of cells:

- Plasma cells
- Memory cells

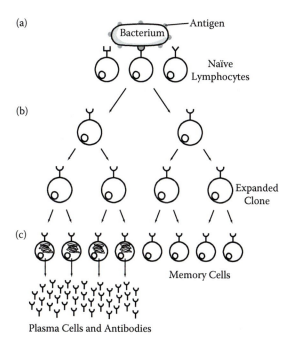

(a)

Antigen

Bacterium

Naïve Lymphocytes

(b)

Expanded Clone

(c)

Memory Cells

Plasma Cells and Antibodies

Figure 3.3 Clonal selection theory. (a) A naïve B cell is exposed to an antigen. (b) The now-activated B cell proliferates and expands the clone. (c) Some of the progeny become antibody-producing plasma cells and others become memory cells.

Most of the cellular offspring are plasma cells. As mentioned, these cells have an elaborate rough endoplasmic reticulum system and are the actual antibody-producing cells during an immune response. Although the newly produced antibodies have the same antigen-binding sites as the IgM cell surface receptors, they are, in fact, IgG molecules. These IgG antibodies then exert their protective effects against the foreign antigen by way of opsonization or activation of the complement system.

3.1.5.5 Primary versus secondary responses

The initial exposure to an antigen elicits the *primary response*. Characteristics of this antibody response include the following:

- The response is delayed several days until sufficient numbers of plasma cells are formed and antibody production is prolific.
- The peak of this response is reached in 2–3 weeks.
- Symptoms of infection occur.

Subsequent exposure to the same antigen elicits the *secondary response*. This response involves the activation of the long-lived memory cells, which were formed during the primary response. The presence of these memory cells expands the number of clone cells and, therefore, increases the number of lymphocytes available to respond to the antigen. In addition, memory cells are more readily stimulated by the antigen because the cell surface receptors have a greater affinity for the antigen than did the original B lymphocyte that produced the clone. The characteristics of the secondary response are quite different from those of the primary response and include the following:

- The response is more rapid (days vs. weeks), more potent (the magnitude of antibody production is 100 times greater), and longer-lasting (several weeks).
- This faster, more powerful response prevents or minimizes overt infection and the development of symptoms.
- This response provides long-term immunity against a specific disease.

The primary response to antigen exposure may occur by way of:

- Actual exposure to the microbe
- Vaccination

A microbe typically includes two components:

- Virulent portion
- Antigenic portion

The virulent portion of the microbe elicits disease. The antigenic portion elicits the immune response. Vaccine development involves stripping a microbe of its disease-inducing capability while leaving its antigenic nature intact, and the patient develops an immune response against this now harmless antigen and forms the memory cells necessary for long-lasting immunity. Once again, the development of overt disease is averted upon exposure to the actual microbial antigen.

Interestingly, some microbial infections do not elicit the formation of memory cells. In these cases, exposure to the antigen does not result in long-lasting immunity. An example of this phenomenon is streptococcal infection or "strep throat." The course of the disease and the intensity of the symptoms are the same following each exposure.

3.1.5.6 *Active versus passive immunity*

Active immunity involves the production of antibodies following exposure to an antigen. The discussion of antibody-mediated immunity thus far has described the active immune process.

Passive immunity involves the transfer of preformed antibodies from one individual (human or animal, such as horse and sheep) to another. Examples of passive immunity include the following:

- Transplacental passage of IgG from mother to fetus
- Acquisition of IgA from mother's colostrum and milk by a nursing infant
- Injection of human polyclonal antibodies to patients with tetanus infection (antitoxin)
- Administration of horse polyclonal antibodies to patients with botulism (antitoxin)
- Injection of human polyclonal antibodies to patients following a bite from an animal possibly infected with rabies (antiviral)

The clinical administration of preformed antibodies is very effective in providing immediate protection from virulent infectious agents or lethal toxins to which a patient may have been exposed. The transfer of antibodies from mother to offspring is quite beneficial because the maturity of an infant's immune system is incomplete for several months. Passively acquired antibodies are usually broken down within 1 month.

PHARMACY APPLICATION: ANTIBIOTIC AGENTS

The body's natural defense mechanisms are not always adequate in preventing microbial infection. However, it was not until after World War II that effective pharmacotherapies were developed. Antibacterial agents are generally referred to as antibiotics. Penicillin is one of the earliest discovered and widely used antibiotic agents. The use of penicillin began in the 1940s. Since that time, the development of new antibiotic agents has been explosive with different classes of drugs acting at different target sites in bacteria. Mechanisms of antibiotic action include:

- Inhibition of synthesis of the bacterial cell wall (e.g., penicillins, cephalosporins)
- Inhibition of bacterial protein synthesis (e.g., erythromycin, tetracyclines)
- Altered bacterial protein synthesis (e.g., aminoglycosides)
- Interruption of nucleic acid synthesis (e.g., fluoroquinolones)
- Interference with normal metabolism (e.g., sulfonamides)

The selection of an antibiotic agent may be made empirically, definitively or prophylactically.

(Continued)

PHARMACY APPLICATION: ANTIBIOTIC AGENTS (Continued)

Of significant concern is the increasing prevalence of bacterial resistance to antibiotic agents. There are three general categories of bacterial resistance including:

- Drug does not reach its target (e.g., loss of effective porin-channels decrease the rate of entry of drug into the bacterium)
- Drug is not active (e.g., production of drug-modifying enzymes by the bacterium)
- Target is altered (e.g., mutation of the natural target)

The responsible use of antibiotics is essential to avoid or minimize the development of resistance.

The second form of adaptive immunity is *cell-mediated immunity*, which involves the activation of T cells. This form of immunity provides defense against microbial invaders located within the host's cells where antibodies and the complement system are unable to reach and destroy them. Specifically, T lymphocytes cause the destruction of virus-infected cells and tumor cells.

Similar to B cells, T cells are clonal and antigen specific. In addition, receptors capable of recognizing foreign antigens are found on the surface of the T cell. Unlike B cells, T cells are activated only when their receptors bind with the foreign antigen as well as the self-antigen on the host cell surface. The exception to activation by way of the foreign antigen and self-antigen complex involves the immune response to whole transplanted foreign cells.

3.1.5.7 Types of T cells

There are three types of T lymphocytes produced by the body.

1. Cytotoxic T cells: Also referred to as killer T cells or CD8 cells, these lymphocytes destroy virus-infected cells, tumor cells, and transplanted cells.
2. Helper T cells: Also referred to as CD4 cells, these lymphocytes are more abundant and account for 60%–80% of circulating T cells. These are the lymphocytes that are selectively destroyed by the AIDS virus. The resulting loss of the numerous contributions of these cells to immune responses leaves the patient susceptible to infection.
3. Suppressor T cells: By inhibiting the activities of cytotoxic T cells and helper T cells, suppressor T cells prevent the development of an excessive immune reaction that may be harmful to the body.

3.1.5.8 Actions of T cells

Cytotoxic T cells *directly* destroy target cells. In contrast, the immune functions of the helper T cells are *indirect*. Helper T cells modulate the activities of other effector cells of the immune system and increase the overall magnitude of the immune response.

1. *Cytotoxic T cells*: These cells secrete chemicals that destroy their target cells (see Figure 3.4). The following mechanism describes how the cytotoxic T cell destroys a virus-infected cell, which is its most frequent target. As mentioned previously, viruses must invade a living host cell to replicate. As it enters the host cell, the virus leaves a portion of its antigenic protein coat on the cell surface in association with the host's self-antigen. (The viral DNA proceeds into the cell to carry on metabolism and reproduction.) The cytotoxic T cell with the appropriate receptor recognizes and binds to the foreign antigen and self-antigen complex. The now activated T cell releases granules containing *perforin molecules* into the extracellular fluid. These molecules aggregate and insert themselves into the membrane of the host cell forming a pore-like channel. This channel allows water and salt to enter the host cell and cause cell lysis.

   The activated cytotoxic T cell may also release chemicals referred to as *granzymes*. These enzymes enter the infected cell through the perforin channels and elicit self-destruction of the cell by way of *apoptosis*.

   Lysis of virus-infected cells causes the release of the viruses into the extracellular fluid. The now exposed viruses are engulfed and destroyed by macrophages.

2. *Helper T cells*: These cells secrete chemicals that amplify the activity of other effector cells of the immune system. These *cytokines* include all the chemicals (other than antibodies) that are secreted by leukocytes. Most of the cytokines are secreted by helper T cells. These cytokines and their immune actions include the following:

   - B-cell growth factor: enhances the development of antigen-stimulated B lymphocytes into antibody-secreting plasma cells (secreted by *T helper 2 cells*)
   - T-cell growth factor (interleukin 2, IL-2): enhances the activity of the T lymphocytes in the activated clone; enhances the activity of appropriate B lymphocytes (secreted by *T helper 1 cells*)
   - Chemotaxins: attract phagocytes to the infected area
   - Macrophage-migration inhibition factor: causes the accumulation of macrophages in the infected area by limiting their outward migration; enhances the phagocytic activity of macrophages

These chemicals and others that are active during immune responses are summarized in Table 3.1.

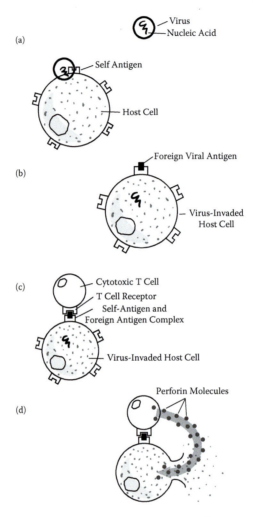

Figure 3.4   Mechanism of action of cytotoxic T cells. The lysis of virus-infected cells involves several steps including (a) viral invasion of the host cell, (b) incorporation of foreign antigen into the host cell membrane in association with the self-antigen, (c) binding of the specific cytotoxic T cell to the self-antigen and foreign antigen complex, and (d) release of perforin molecules that form channels in the host cell membrane, allow for the influx of water and salt into the cell and cause cell lysis. Viruses released from the lysed cell are then removed and destroyed by macrophages.

Table 3.1   Chemicals active during immune responses

Antibodies: Gamma globulins, immunoglobulins; secreted by plasma cells to
  defend against invading bacteria
B-Cell Growth Factor: Enhances the development of antigen-stimulated B cells into
  plasma cells
Chemotaxins: Molecules that attract phagocytes to an area of infection or
  inflammation
Complement: Family of proteins that cause lysis of invading bacteria and enhance
  the inflammatory response (e.g., chemotaxis, opsonization)
Cytokines: Proteins released by one type of immune cell that influence the growth
  and activity of other immune cells
Granzymes: Cytotoxic enzymes that initiate apoptosis in virus-infected cells
Histamine: Released from mast cells and basophils; initiates the inflammatory
  response by causing vasodilation and increased capillary permeability
Interferon: Protein released from virus-infected cells; inhibits replication of viruses
  in other host cells
Macrophage-Migration Inhibition Factor: Limits the outward migration of
  macrophages; enhances the phagocytic activity of macrophages
Membrane Attack Complex: Composed of complement proteins C5–C9; causes lysis
  of invading bacteria
Perforin: released from cytotoxic T cells and killer cells; causes lysis of
  virus-infected cells and tumor cells
T-Cell Growth Factor: Enhances the activity of T cells in an activated clone;
  enhances the activity of select B cells

3.1.5.9   MHC molecules

Self-antigens are also referred to as *MHC molecules* because their synthesis occurs by way of a group of genes called the *major histocompatibility
complex*. Everyone has their own unique pattern of MHC molecules or cell
markers. The presence of these glycoproteins on the surface of the body's
cells identifies the cells as "self" and, accordingly, T lymphocytes do not
respond to them.

There are two classes of MHC molecules:

- Class I MHC glycoproteins
- Class II MHC glycoproteins

Class I MHC glycoproteins are found on the surface of all nucleated cells in
the body. This includes virus-infected cells and tumor cells. These molecules
enable *cytotoxic T cells* to respond to foreign antigens remaining on the surface
of the infected cell. It is quite logical that cytotoxic T cells do not respond to
foreign antigens in the absence of MHC molecules. As described previously,
these T cells defend against foreign antigen only when it has become incorporated into the infected cell's membrane and not when it is in the free form.

Class II MHC glycoproteins are found on the surface of select immune cells including macrophages, B cells and cytotoxic T cells. These molecules are recognized by *helper T cells*. As such, helper T cells respond to foreign antigens only when they are present on the surface of the immune cells with which they interact.

In summary, class I MHC glycoproteins facilitate the interaction of cytotoxic T cells with virus-infected cells and class II MHC glycoproteins facilitate the interaction of helper T cells with the immune cells that they activate.

3.2   Alterations in immune function

A normal functioning immune system is designed to protect the body against invasion from foreign organisms and aids in the repair of damaged tissues. However, under certain circumstances, activation of the immune system may be excessive or inappropriate and lead to life-threatening hypersensitivity reactions. In the case of autoimmune disease, a malfunctioning immune system may also mistakenly target normal human tissues for destruction.

3.2.1   Hypersensitivity reactions

A hypersensitivity reaction is an enhanced and abnormal immune response. Hypersensitivity reactions may occur immediately or be delayed for one to several days. Hypersensitivity reactions often involve the activation of immune cells that can lead to the production of antibodies and cytokines. There are four types of hypersensitivity reactions:

3.2.1.1   Type I hypersensitivity reaction
- Type I hypersensitivity reactions are mediated by the antibody IgE. In susceptible individuals, exposure to an antigen leads to the inappropriate overproduction production of IgE molecules that attach now attach to the membranes of *mast cells*. When this occurs, an individual is said have become *sensitized* to a particular antigen. Mast cells are found throughout many tissues and contain large amounts of the pro-inflammatory mediator *histamine* as well as other substances that enhance inflammation. Upon a second exposure to the antigen, the antigen enters the system and binds to mast cell-bound IgE, which now causes the rupture of the mast cells and the release of inflammatory mediators.
- An example of a localized type I hypersensitivity reaction would be seasonal allergic rhinitis. The asthmatic response that occurs in the airways of susceptible individual also exhibits features that are characteristic of a type I hypersensitivity reaction.
- A very severe type I hypersensitivity reaction occurs with *anaphylaxis* (see anaphylaxis box).

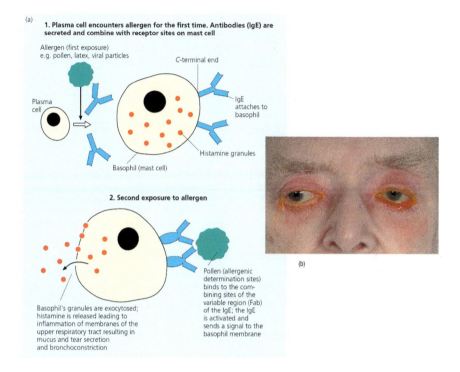

(a)

1. Plasma cell encounters allergen for the first time. Antibodies (IgE) are secreted and combine with receptor sites on mast cell

Allergen (first exposure)
e.g. pollen, latex, viral particles

C-terminal end

Plasma cell

IgE attaches to basophil

Histamine granules

Basophil (mast cell)

2. Second exposure to allergen

Basophil's granules are exocytosed; histamine is released leading to inflammation of membranes of the upper respiratory tract resulting in mucus and tear secretion and bronchoconstriction

Pollen (allergenic determination sites) binds to the combining sites of the variable region (Fab) of the IgE; the IgE is activated and sends a signal to the basophil membrane

(b)

ANAPHYLAXIS

- Anaphylaxis is a life-threatening phenomenon that involves the rapid and widespread release of histamine and other inflammatory mediators from IgE-coated mast cells.
- Occurs in individuals who have been previously "sensitized" or exposed to a specific antigen such as bee venom or certain foods such as nuts.
- Anaphylaxis is characterized by massive vasodilation caused by the release of inflammatory mediators. This widespread vasodilation can lead to marked hypotension and circulatory collapse. Increased vascular permeability also occurs and leads to a leakage of fluids into tissues.
- Inflammatory mediators such as histamine are also potent constrictors of bronchial smooth muscle and cause a marked narrowing of respiratory passages.
- Other manifestations of anaphylaxis may include itching, flushing of the skin, and gastrointestinal upset.

QUESTION BOX

What types of medication would be useful for treating a patient who is experiencing anaphylaxis?

3.2.1.1.1 Manifestations of type I hypersensitivity reaction (Figure 3.5) Many of the physiologic effects observed with a type I hypersensitivity reaction are due to the effects of histamine, which causes vasodilation, increased vascular permeability and bronchoconstriction. Effects on the eyes, nose and throat include conjunctivitis, rhinitis, excess mucus production, edema, swelling and bronchoconstriction. Systemic manifestations in the case of anaphylaxis include marked hypotension, circulatory collapse, severe GI symptoms, difficulty breathing, flushing, sweating, and generalized hives. Treatment of anaphylaxis involves the injection of *epinephrine*, which is a potent vasoconstrictor and bronchodilator. Antihistamines would also be useful. Patients who experience type I hypersensitivity reactions may be clinically "desensitized" by exposing them to very small quantities of the offending antigen over a prolonged period of time.

3.2.1.2 Type II hypersensitivity reaction

- Type II hypersensitivity reactions are tissue-specific reactions that involve the IgG or IgM antibodies interacting with specific antigens on the surface of cells.
- Binding of antibody to antigen can lead to the activation of the complement system and subsequent destruction of the target cell through lysis. Such examples would include blood transfusion mismatch (ABO) reactions and *hemolytic disease of the newborn* that occurs when the mother and infant's blood ABO or Rh proteins are incompatible.
- In the case of *Goodpasture disease*, antibodies are produced against basement membrane proteins in the glomerulus and the lungs. Binding of these antibodies leads to the infiltration and activation of neutrophils that in turn release their cytotoxic granules onto the tissue. The end result is marked inflammation and possible fibrosis of the tissue.
- The case of *Graves' disease* is unusual in that antibodies are produced that bind to the thyroid stimulating hormone (TSH) receptors on the thyroid gland. Binding of these antibodies stimulates the release of thyroid hormones and leads to hyperthyroidism. Graves' disease is the most common cause of hyperthyroidism (Figure 3.6).

3.2.1.2.1 Manifestations and treatment of type II hypersensitivity reaction
- The symptoms of a type II hypersensitivity reaction will depend upon the effect of the abnormal antibodies. In cases where antibodies activate complement proteins, there will be cell lysis and destruction.

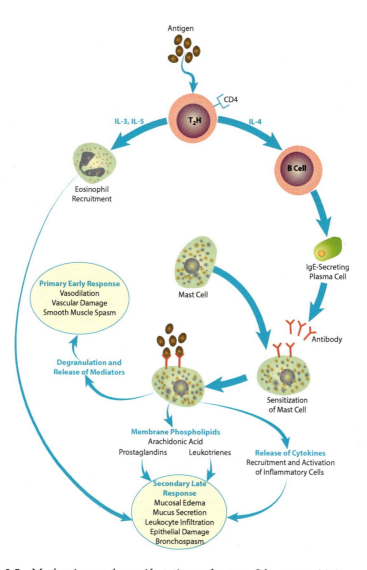

Figure 3.5 Mechanism and manifestations of a type I hypersensitivity reaction. The process begins with the activation of helper T-cells (T$_2$H) by antigen which in turn activate other immune cells such as B-cells. Activated B-cells produce IgE antibodies that attach to the surface of mast cells. Subsequent exposure to the antigen leads to the binding of IgE on the surface of mast cells which in turn causes mast cell degranulation. The release of various inflammatory mediatory from mast cells causes the physiologic symptoms of anaphylaxis. The "early" phase of anaphylaxis is mediated mainly though histamine and involves vasodilation and increases in vascular permeability. The secondary or "late" phase of anaphylaxis is slower to develop and is due to the release of inflammatory mediators such as cytokine, prostaglandins and leukotrienes.

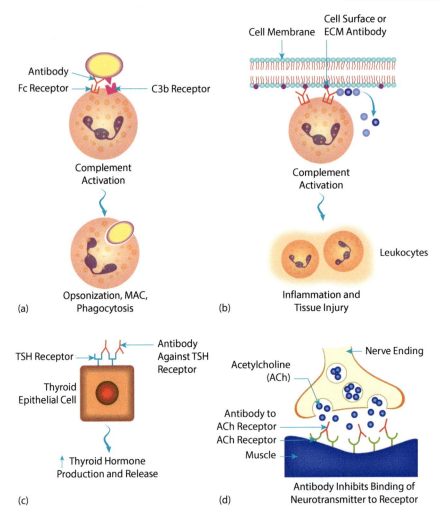

Figure 3.6 Type II hypersensitivity reactions: (a) Opsonization of antigen and complement or antibody-mediated phagocytosis, (b) Complement and antibody-mediated inflammation, (c) Antibodies developed against TSH receptors in Grave's Disease, (d) Antibodies directed against skeletal muscle acetylcholine receptors in myasthenia gravis.

When antibody binding leads to the recruitment of immune cells such as neutrophils, the effect will be tissue inflammation and possible damage. With Graves' disease, the antibodies mimic the stimulatory effects of TSH and lead to hyperthyroidism. Treatment for severe cases of type II hypersensitivity reactions may include corticosteroids or other immune-suppressing medications.

3.2.1.3   *Type III hypersensitivity reaction*

- Type III reactions occur when circulating antigen-antibody complexes precipitate out of circulation and lodge in the walls of a blood vessel or in a tissue. When immune complexes lodge in a tissue they can lead to the activation of complement proteins and subsequent tissue injury and destruction.
- Immune complexes themselves may also become trapped in the glomerulus of the kidney where they trigger a localized inflammatory reaction that can lead to glomerulonephritis.
- Conditions in which type III hypersensitivity reactions occur include severe infections, *systemic lupus erythematosus* (an autoimmune condition in which antigen-antibody complexes form against collagen in the body), and *serum sickness* (a condition in which antibodies form against foreign substances in the blood such as drugs, venoms and foreign blood antigens).
- *Arthus reaction* is a term used to describe localized vasculitis caused by a type III reaction. Such reactions can occur after injection of antigen (e.g., the site of vaccination or immunization) and lead to tissue ulceration.

3.2.1.3.1   *Manifestations and treatment of type III hypersensitivity reaction*

- Extensive edema, urticaria, vasculitis, glomerulonephritis, tissue or organ damage.
- Treatment for severe cases of type III hypersensitivity reactions may include corticosteroids or other immune-suppressing medications.

3.2.1.4   *Type IV hypersensitivity reaction*

- A type IV reaction is a delayed hypersensitivity reaction that is mediated by T lymphocytes and does not involve antibodies.
- Cytotoxic or helper T cells are activated by exposure to an antigen. Once activated, helper T cells release inflammatory cytokines that lead to activation of other immune cells as well as the activation of the coagulation cascade, whereas activated cytotoxic T cells will directly destroy the target tissue. The inflammation and damage that may take hours or days to occur because it takes time for the activation of lymphocytes to occur.
- Examples of type IV hypersensitivity reaction include delayed allergic reactions (poison ivy), contact dermatitis (latex allergy), many drug reactions and the reaction that occurs with the *tuberculin* skin test for tuberculosis. A hypersensitivity *pneumonitis* (pulmonary inflammation) may also occur in individuals that inhale antigens such as sawdust and animal dander (Figure 3.7).

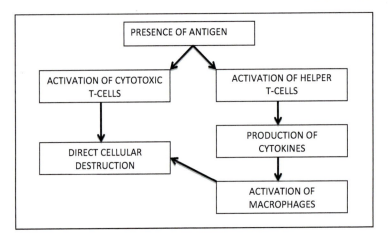

Figure 3.7   Mechanism of a type IV hypersensitivity reaction.

3.2.2 Autoimmune disease

Autoimmune diseases are a group of conditions that occur when an individual's immune system inappropriately targets their own tissues. Some common autoimmune diseases are shown in Table 3.2 along with the tissues they affect. For reasons that are unclear, the patient's immune system is no longer able to accurately distinguish "self" antigens, that is, normal tissue components that make up the body from "non-self" antigens, that is, foreign components that are not normally part of the body. Several theories have been proposed to explain how an autoimmune disease might develop:

1. *Genetic factors*: A number of autoimmune diseases such as *ankylosing spondylitis*, type I diabetes and rheumatoid arthritis have been associated with the presence of certain HLA alleles. The mechanism of this genetic predisposition is uncertain and all patients with these genetic susceptibilities do not go on to develop the disease. As with many diseases, genetic predisposition alone is not sufficient to cause the disease, and it is likely that some additional factor or environmental exposure (e.g., viral infection, antigenic exposure, toxin exposure) is also necessary in order to trigger the disease process.

2. *Infection*: It has been hypothesized that viral or bacterial infections might introduce antigens into the body that resemble or "mimic" particular proteins that are normally found in the body. This *molecular mimicry* can cause the immune system to mount an attack against normal body proteins that it mistakes for the similar foreign antigen that was introduced. An example of this occurs with rheumatic heart disease, a condition in which immune cells attack glycoproteins in the

Table 3.2   Some common autoimmune diseases

Disease	Tissue(s) affected
Addison's Disease	Adrenal gland
Ankylosing Spondylitis	Joints, spine
Churg Strauss Syndrome	Lungs, skin, nerves
Crohn's Disease	Intestines
Type I Diabetes Mellitus	Pancreas
Goodpasture Syndrome	Kidney, lungs
Graves' Disease	Thyroid
Hashimoto's Disease	Thyroid
Multiple Sclerosis	Nervous tissue
Myasthenia Gravis	Acetylcholine receptors in skeletal muscle
Rheumatoid Arthritis	Joints
Rheumatic Fever	Heart, joints
Sjögren's Syndrome	Tear and salivary glands
Systemic Lupus Erythematosus	Multiple tissues are affected throughout the body
Wegener's Granulomatosis	Blood vessels

heart and joint tissues that resemble a similar protein found on the infecting streptococci bacteria.

3. *Expression of sequestered antigens*: Autoimmune disease may also be triggered when antigens that are normally hidden from immune system surveillance become expressed or accessible to immune cells. Certain proteins in the body remain *sequestered* in anatomical locations such as the brain (protected by the blood-brain barrier), anterior portion of the eye (protected by the blood-ocular barrier), as well as the spermatozoa in testes, that are not normally scanned by the immune system. If there is a breakdown in the barriers protecting these tissues or if any of the sequestered proteins are released, the immune system will encounter new proteins that it will deem antigenic and mount a response against the tissue(s) in which they are found.

Medical terminology

Agglutination (ă-gloo″tĭ-nā'shŭn): Antigen-antibody reaction in which cells or particles are removed from solution

Antigenic (ăn-tĭ-jĕn'ĭk): Capable of inducing a specific immune response

Apoptosis (ă-pŏp-tō'sĭs): Programmed cell death

Calor (kā'lor): Heat

Chemotaxis (kē″mō-tăk'sĭs): Movement of phagocytes toward an area of inflammation

Clone (klōn): Group of lymphocytes all capable of recognizing and responding to a specific foreign antigen

Cytokine (sī′tō-kīn): Protein produced by an immune cell that regulates the immune response

Diapedesis (dī″ă-pĕd-ē′sĭs): Movement of phagocytes out of the capillary into the tissue during an inflammatory response

Dolor (dō′lor): Pain

Edema(ĕ-dē′mă): Accumulation of fluid in a tissue

Endoplasmic reticulum (ĕn-dō-plăs′mĭk rĕ-tĭk′ū-lŭm): Network of tubules within the cytoplasm where the synthesis and modification of molecules takes place

Functio laesa (fŭnk′shē-ō lē′să): Impaired function

Hypersensitivity (hī″pĕr-sĕn″sĭ-tĭv′ĭ-tē): Increased responsiveness to a stimulus

Immunity(ĭ-mū′nĭ-tē): Protection from disease, especially infectious disease

Immunoglobulin (ĭm″ū-nō-glŏb′ū-lĭn): Antibody

Innate (ĭn-nāt′): Inherent, intrinsic, existing at birth

Interferon (ĭn-tĕr-fēr′-ŏn): Glycoprotein released from virus-infected cells with anti-viral and anti-tumor effects

Lysosome (lī′sō-sōm): Cellular organelle containing digestive enzymes

Margination (măr″jĭ-nā′shŭn): Adhesion of phagocytes to the wall of the capillary during an inflammatory response

Naïve (nă-ēv′): Natural, unlearned, unaffected

Neutralization (nū″trăl-ĭ-zā′shŭn): Counteracting the effects of an agent that produces morbidity or disease

Opsonization (ŏp″sō-nī-zā′shŭn): Facilitation of phagocytosis

Perforin (pĕr′fōr-ĭn): Protein released by natural killer cells and cytotoxic T cells that causes the lysis of virus-infected cells

Phagocytosis (făg″ō-sī-tō′sĭs): Process in which phagocytes engulf and destroy microorganisms, particles or cellular debris

Polyclonal (pŏl″ē-klōn′ăl): Referring to proteins arising from multiple cell lines

Prolific (prō-lĭf-ĭk): Fruitful, productive

Pus (pŭs): Fluid containing dead phagocytes and cellular debris

Rubor (roo′bor): Redness

Transcription (trăn-skrĭp′shŭn): Synthesis of messenger RNA

Translation (trăns-lā′shŭn): Synthesis of proteins

Transplacental (trăns″plă-sĕn′tă): Across the placenta

Tumor (tū′mor): Swelling

Virulent (vĭr′ū-lĕnt): Infectious, pathogenic

Bibliography

Abbas, A. K. and Lichtman, A. H., *Basic Immunology, Functions and Disorders of the Immune System*, 2nd ed., Updated Edition 2006–2007, Saunders Elsevier, Philadelphia, PA, 2006–2007.

Chambers, H. F., Antimicrobial agents: general considerations, in *Goodman and Gilman's, The Pharmacological Basis of Therapeutics*, 9th ed., Brunton, L. L., Lazo, J. S., and Parker, K. L., Eds., McGraw Hill, New York, 2006, chap. 43.

Delves, P. J., Martin, S. J., Burton, D. R., and Roitt, I. M., *Roitt's Essential Immunology*, 11th ed., Blackwell Publishing, Malden, MA, 2006.

Dunne, Jr., W. M., Mechanisms of infectious disease, in *Pathophysiology, Concepts of Altered Health States*, 7th ed., Porth, C. M., Ed., Lippincott Williams & Wilkins, Philadelphia, PA, 2005, chap. 18.

Fox, S. I., *Human Physiology*, 9th ed., McGraw Hill, Boston, MA, 2006.

Guyton, A. C., and Hall, J. E., *Textbook of Medical Physiology*, 11th ed., W. B. Saunders, Philadelphia, PA, 2006.

http://www.fda.gov/CDER/Drug/advisory/nsaids.htm

Porth, C. M., Alterations of the immune response, in *Pathophysiology, Concepts of Altered Health States*, 7th ed., Porth, C. M., Ed., Lippincott Williams & Wilkins, Philadelphia, PA, 2005, chap. 21.

Roberts, L. J., and Morrow, J. D., Analgesic-antipyretic and anti-inflammatory agents and drugs employed in the treatment of gout, in *Goodman and Gilman's, The Pharmacological Basis of Therapeutics*, 9th ed., Brunton, L. L., Lazo, J. S., and Parker, K. L., Eds., McGraw Hill, New York, 2006, chap. 27.

Sherwood, L., *Human Physiology, From Cells to Systems*, 5th ed., Brooks/Cole, Pacific Grove, CA, 2004.

Silverthorn, D. U., *Human Physiology, An Integrated Approach*, 4th ed., Prentice Hall, Upper Saddle River, NJ, 2007.

Sommer, C., The immune response, in *Pathophysiology, Concepts of Altered Health States*, 7th ed., Porth, C. M., Ed., Lippincott Williams & Wilkins, Philadelphia, PA, 2005, chap. 19.

Stedman's Medical Dictionary for the Health Professions and Nursing, 5th ed., Lippincott Williams & Wilkins, Baltimore, MD, 2005.

Taber's Cyclopedic Medical Dictionary, 20th ed., F. A. Davis Co., Philadelphia, PA, 2005.

Widmaier, E. P., Raff, H., and Strang, K. T., *Vander's Human Physiology, The Mechanisms of Body Function*, McGraw Hill, Boston, MA, 2006.

chapter four

Inflammation

Study objectives

- List the symptoms of inflammation
- Explain the steps of the inflammatory response and how they protect against bacterial invasion
- Describe the role that mast cells play in inflammation
- List the major physiologic actions of histamine in the body
- Identify the major inflammatory mediators that are produced from arachidonic acid and describe the key physiologic effects of each

The inflammatory response is a complex, multistep reaction involving the accumulation of phagocytes and plasma proteins at a site of infection, toxin exposure, or tissue injury. The purpose of this response is to:

- Isolate, destroy or inactivate infectious microbes
- Remove tissue debris
- Promote tissue repair

The cardinal signs or symptoms of inflammation include:

- *Rubor*: redness due to increased blood flow to the affected area
- *Tumor*: swelling due to increased capillary permeability and fluid accumulation in the affected area
- *Calor*: increased temperature (heat) due to the increased blood flow
- *Dolor*: pain
- *Functio laesa*: altered or impaired function of the affected area

The inflammatory response involves a series of steps that are similar in most instances (see Figure 4.1).

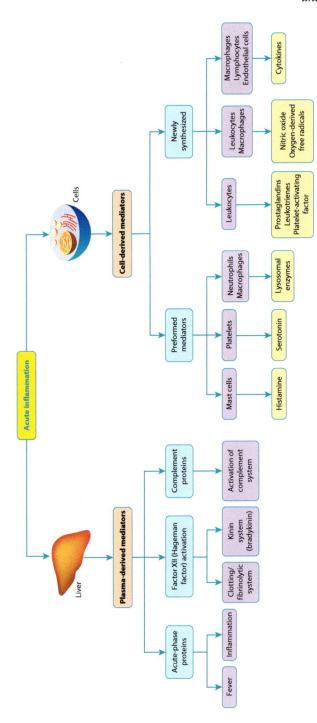

Figure 4.1   Steps in the inflammatory response.

Defense by tissue macrophages: A small number of macrophages can be found in the body's tissues at any given time. These macrophages provide the first step in protection from infection by phagocytizing invading microbes.

Localized vasodilation: Vasodilation of arterioles increases blood flow to the affected area, resulting in the increased delivery of phagocytes and plasma proteins, and is caused, primarily, by histamine released from activated mast cells as well as by activated bradykinin. Mast cells are found in connective tissues, particularly in areas of potential microbial entry to the body such as the lungs, skin, and gastrointestinal tract. Vasodilation in the inflamed area leads to redness and heat.

Increased capillary permeability: In addition to vasodilation, histamine and bradykinin cause the pores between the endothelial cells to increase in size, resulting in an increase of capillary permeability and the movement of plasma proteins into the tissue spaces.

Localized edema: Vasodilation and increased capillary permeability lead to localized edema. As will be discussed in Chapter 6, vasodilation and increased blood flow lead to an increase in capillary pressure (P_c). Furthermore, the presence of escaped plasma proteins within the tissue spaces leads to an increase in interstitial fluid colloid osmotic pressure (π_i). The increase in P_c and π_i increases the filtration and reduces the reabsorption of fluid. In other words, fluid moves out of the capillaries and accumulates in the tissue. In addition to redness and heat (due to increased blood flow), symptoms of edema include swelling and pain (due to distension of the tissue).

Walling-off the inflamed area: As mentioned above, several types of plasma proteins escape from the vascular compartment and enter the tissue spaces. Of interest in the inflammatory response, are the *clotting* and *anticlotting factors* (proteins) that circulate in the blood. As will be discussed in Chapter 5, the inactive plasma protein *fibrinogen* is converted into the active *fibrin*, which forms clots within the tissue spaces. This effectively walls off the injured area and prevents or delays the spread of infection. Subsequently, anticlotting factors, which are activated more slowly, dissolve these clots when they are no longer needed.

Infiltration of phagocytes: Increased numbers of phagocytes are needed to engulf and destroy infectious microbes, remove tissue debris, and prepare the injured area for healing and repair. This step is facilitated by the increase in blood flow and the increase in capillary permeability. Neutrophils arrive first, typically within 1 hour. Monocytes arrive within 8–12 hours and proceed to swell and mature into macrophages within the next 8–12 hours.

The emigration of phagocytes from the vascular compartment, toward the injured area, involves three steps:

- *Margination*: phagocytes adhere to the endothelial cells of the capillary wall.
- *Diapedesis*: phagocytes squeeze through the capillary pores and enter the tissue space.
- *Chemotaxis*: phagocytes move through the tissue up a concentration gradient of *chemotaxins* that are released at the site of injury.

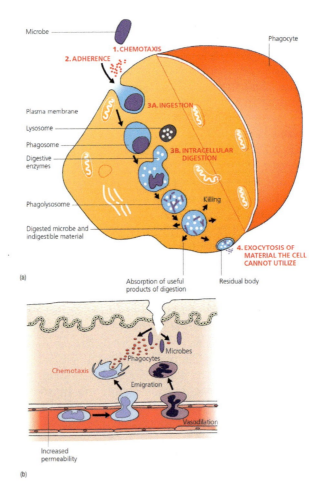

Opsonization: Opsonization is the process by which bacteria are marked for phagocytosis. The two most important *opsonins*, or chemicals, that bind to and label the bacteria, are *antibodies* and *complement*

protein C3b. Opsonization by way of antibodies will be discussed later in this chapter. Opsonization by way of C3b is a form of innate immunity. The concentration of C3b in the injured area is increased due to the increased capillary permeability and leakage of plasma proteins into the tissue space. This complement factor binds non-specifically with the invading bacteria. In addition, there are receptors specific for C3b on the surface of the phagocytes. Binding of the C3b with its receptor creates a linkage between the bacterium and the phagocyte that prevents the "escape" of the bacterium (see Figure 4.2). In this way, bacteria are more readily and more efficiently engulfed by phagocytes.

Phagocytosis: Phagocytosis is the process of ingestion and digestion of bacteria, foreign particles, and tissue debris. These substances are internalized within a vesicle formed from the plasma membrane, termed an endocytic vesicle. The vesicle will ultimately fuse with a *lysosome,* an organelle filled with hydrolytic enzymes. Phagocytes have an abundance of lysosomes. The enzymes degrade the substances within the vesicle. Inevitably, some amount of these destructive enzymes escapes into the cytoplasm and kills the phagocyte itself. Neutrophils are capable of engulfing 5–25 bacteria before they are killed by the enzymes. Macrophages engulf and destroy as many as 100 bacteria before they die. *Pus* is a fluid found in an infected wound that consists of living and dead phagocytes, necrotic tissue, and bacteria.

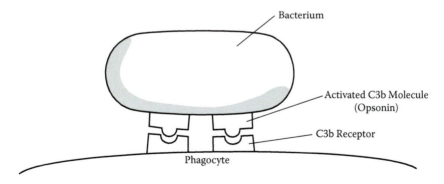

Figure 4.2 Opsonization. Activated complement factor C3b binds nonspecifically with an invading microbe such as a bacterium. C3b also binds with a receptor on the surface of a phagocyte. In this way, the bacterium and the phagocyte are linked and phagocytosis is facilitated.

PHARMACY APPLICATION: ANTI-INFLAMMATORY DRUGS

In some instances, the inflammatory response may be exaggerated, prolonged, or inappropriate. Inflammation in these situations is without benefit and may, in fact, cause serious injury to the tissue or impair the tissue's function. Nonsteroidal anti-inflammatory drugs (NSAIDs) include a chemically heterogeneous group of compounds with anti-inflammatory, analgesic, and antipyretic effects. The prototype drug in this class is aspirin. The major mechanism of action of these drugs involves the inhibition of cyclooxygenase, the enzyme involved in the synthesis of prostaglandins. This family of compounds contributes to and exacerbates the inflammatory response. Most over-the-counter medications, such as ibuprofen (Advil®, Motrin®) and naproxen (Aleve®), inhibit both cyclooxygenase-1 (COX-1) and cyclooxygenase-2 (COX-2). The inhibition of COX-2 mediates the therapeutic effects of these drugs. However, the inhibition of COX-1 may lead to undesired side effects such as gastric ulcers.

More recently, selective COX-2 inhibitors have been developed. These substances, which include celecoxib (Celebrex®), rofecoxib (Vioxx®), and valdecoxib (Bextra®), were effective therapeutically and caused fewer gastric side effects. However, it was not until these drugs were widely prescribed to patients that it was determined that they may be associated with an increased risk of serious cardiovascular events such as heart attack and stroke. Both rofecoxib and valdecoxib have been removed from the market.

Glucocorticoids can prevent or reduce inflammation in response to mechanical, chemical, infectious, and immunological stimuli. In fact, these drugs suppress almost every aspect of the inflammatory response. They are useful in treating inappropriate immune responses such as allergic reactions (poison ivy rash, asthma) and inflammation associated with arthritis. However, it should be noted that the use of glucocorticoids does not address the underlying cause of the inflammation, only the symptoms.

The mechanism of action of the glucocorticoids involves decreasing the release of substances that contribute to the inflammatory response—including histamine, prostaglandins, cytokines, and endothelial leukocyte adhesion molecule-1 (ELAM-1)—resulting in a reduction of vasodilation, leukocyte extravasation, and chemotaxis. In addition, the activation of T cells and antibody production is decreased. Therefore, an undesired effect of this immunosuppression is an accompanying increased risk of infection.

4.1 Inflammatory mediators

4.1.1 Histamine and mast cells

Mast cells are essentially sac-like cells filled with granules that contain various inflammatory mediators. Mast cells are located in numerous tissues and "degranulate" or release their contents in response to stimuli such as injury, chemical/toxin exposure, heat, or antibody binding in the case of anaphylaxis. Histamine is a major component of mast cell granules. Once released, the major effects of histamine include vasodilation, increased vascular permeability, and constriction of bronchial smooth muscle. Mast cell granules also contain two chemotactic factors, *neutrophil chemotactic factor* and *eosinophil chemotactic factor*, which help attract leukocytes to the inflamed or injured tissue. In addition to degranulation, activated mast cells will also synthesize a number of other inflammatory mediators such as cytokines, prostaglandins, and leukotrienes (see details below) as well as *platelet-activating factor*, which stimulates platelet aggregation and increases vascular permeability.

1. *Prostaglandins and Leukotrienes*: The prostaglandins and leukotrienes are *eicosanoid* inflammatory mediators derived from the 20-carbon unsaturated fatty acid *arachidonic acid* that is a component of the phospholipids found in cell membranes. Arachidonic acid is released from the mast cell membrane when there is tissue injury or damage. There are two key enzymes involved in the conversion of arachidonic acid, *cyclooxygenase (COX)*, and *lipoxygenase (LOX)*. COX converts arachidonic acid into the *prostaglandins* (e.g., PGD_2, PGI_2, PGE). The prostaglandins have numerous effects depending upon the tissue, but in general they enhance inflammation, contract smooth muscle, increase capillary permeability, and cause vasodilation. Certain prostaglandins are also *pyrogenic* and can raise body temperature. In platelets, COX converts arachidonic acid into *thromboxane A_2*, a potent platelet activator and enhancer of platelet aggregation. The lipoxygenase enzyme converts arachidonic acid in the *leukotrienes* (e.g., LTA_4, LTB_4, LTE_4). The *leukotrienes* also enhance inflammation, increase vascular permeability and cause vasodilation. They are also potent bronchoconstrictors that play a key role in asthma. LTB_4 is also involved in the chemotaxis of neutrophils. Aspirin and non-steroidal anti-inflammatories (e.g., ibuprofen) inhibit the production of prostaglandins and thromboxane through the inhibition of the enzyme cyclooxygenase. Corticosteroids exert a highly potent anti-inflammatory effect because they inhibit the release of arachidonic acid from the cell membrane, thus inhibiting the formation of all eicosanoid inflammatory mediators (see Figure 4.3).

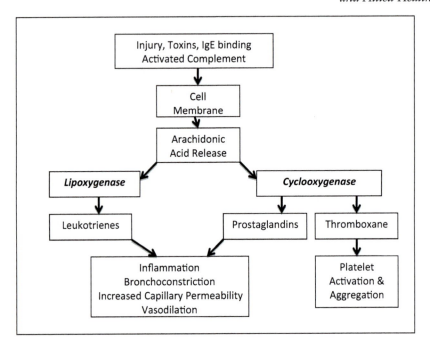

Figure 4.3   Eicosanoid pathway.

2. *Cytokines*: Cytokines are small proteins produced by a number of different cell types within the body. Three major cytokines are released by human cells: *interleukins (ILs), interferons (IFNs), and tumor necrosis factor-alpha (TNF-α)*:

QUESTION

Why is aspirin used to reduce the risk for blood clots in susceptible patients?

- *Interleukins*: Interleukins are produced primarily by activated macrophages and immune cells. Approximately two-dozen interleukins have been identified thus far. A number of interleukins such as IL-1 are pro-inflammatory. They can also cause fever and attract leukocytes through chemotaxis. A number of interleukins also act upon the bone marrow to stimulate the proliferation of immune cells.

- *Interferons*: Interferons are also small proteins produced primarily by cells that are infected with a virus. They function as endogenous antiviral proteins that help protect uninfected cells from viral infection. They may also enhance the inflammatory response by stimulating the activity of immune cells such as macrophages. There are three interferons produced in humans, IFN-α, IFN-β, and IFN-γ. The interferons are used clinically but have a number of significant side effects at pharmacologic doses that limit their overall usefulness.

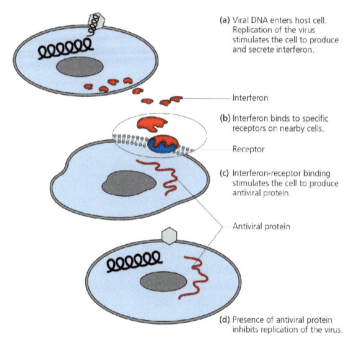

(a) Viral DNA enters host cell. Replication of the virus stimulates the cell to produce and secrete interferon.

Interferon

(b) Interferon binds to specific receptors on nearby cells.

Receptor

(c) Interferon-receptor binding stimulates the cell to produce antiviral protein.

Antiviral protein

(d) Presence of antiviral protein inhibits replication of the virus.

- *Tumor Necrosis Factor-alpha*: TNF-α is a very potent inflammatory mediator produced by activated macrophages. Release of TNF-α leads to increased expression of adhesion molecules in the vascular endothelium that in turn leads to neutrophil aggregation. In addition, TNF-α can stimulate the release of cytokines, eicosanoids and *chemokines* from the endothelium. TNF-α can exert systemic effects including fever, anorexia, and muscle wasting. Excess production of TNF-α is believed to play a key role in the development of the wasting syndrome *cachexia* that is observed in patients with metastatic cancer and AIDS.

3. *Chemokines*: Chemokines are a family of small peptides that mainly function as chemotactic substances for immune cells. They are produced by a number of cell types including endothelial cells, macrophages and fibroblasts in response to the release of pro-inflammatory cytokines.

Table 4.1   Cytokine actions

Interleukins (IL-1 to IL-17):
- Produced mainly by activated immune cells
- Inflammatory mediators
- Stimulate proliferation and differentiation of T cells, B cells, macrophages and natural killer cells
- Chemotactic factors for T cells and leukocytes

Interferons (α, β, γ):
- Produced by viral-infected cells
- Antiviral proteins that protect other cells from viral infection
- Activate macrophages

Tumor Necrosis Factors (α and β):
- Produced by activated macrophages
- Inflammatory mediators
- Cytotoxic to tumor cells
- Increase the activity of phagocytic cells

Transforming Growth Factor β:
- Produced by lymphocytes, macrophages and platelets
- Chemotactic for macrophages
- Stimulates the activity of fibroblasts for wound healing

---

4. *Nitric Oxide*: Nitric oxide (NO) is a short-lived substance produced by a number of tissues, including the vascular endothelium. NO causes vasodilation through the relaxation of vascular smooth muscle but is also a potent mediator of inflammation that can inhibit leukocyte aggregation, platelet adhesion and cytokine release. NO also exerts free-radical scavenging properties.

5. *Fever*: Fever is a systemic response to inflammation or infection. A number of endogenous substances such as the cytokines (e.g., IL-1) and prostaglandins are *pyrogenic*, meaning they increase body temperature. Exogenous pyrogens include bacteria and bacterial toxins. Both endogenous and exogenous pyrogens may raise body temperature through direct interaction with the thermoregulatory centers in the hypothalamus. Although the beneficial effects of fever are uncertain, there is some evidence that significant changes in body temperature may impair the activity of infectious microorganisms or their toxins that are sensitive to changes in temperature (see Table 4.1).

chapter five

Blood and hemostasis

Study objectives

- Discuss the major functions of the plasma proteins
- Describe the morphological characteristics and the function of erythrocytes
- Explain how various blood types are determined and what blood types are compatible for transfusion
- Describe how the Rh factor may lead to hemolytic disease of the newborn
- Discuss the major functions of each of the five types of leukocytes: neutrophils, eosinophils, basophils, monocytes, and lymphocytes
- Describe the origin of thrombocytes
- Discuss the role of platelets in the various aspects of hemostasis
- Describe the role of vascular constriction in hemostasis
- Explain how a platelet plug is formed
- Distinguish between the extrinsic pathway and the intrinsic pathway of blood coagulation
- Explain how blood clot growth is limited
- Explain how blood clots are dissolved
- Discuss the various genetic conditions that lead to abnormal bleeding
- Describe the various means by which acquired bleeding disorders might occur
- List drugs that might impair hemostasis and blood clotting
- List conditions that might lead to hypercoagulability
- Outline the process of erythropoiesis and discuss the role of hypoxia and erythropoietin release
- Compare and contrast sickle cell anemia and thalassemia in terms of their etiology and major manifestations
- Describe how different anemias may affect the size, shape and color of red blood cells
- Explain how iron deficiency can lead to anemia. What patient populations are at greatest risk for iron-deficiency anemia?
- Define aplastic anemia and list some possible causes
- What is polycythemia? Why might it occur?

5.1   Blood

Blood consists of cellular elements [*erythrocytes* (red blood cells), *leukocytes* (white blood cells), and *thrombocytes* (platelets)] as well as plasma, the fluid in which the blood cells are suspended. Normally, the total circulating blood volume is about 8% of the body weight (about 5 L in women and 5.5 L in men). Women have relatively more adipose tissue, which is relatively avascular, than men and that, therefore, accounts for the lower blood volume.

The cellular elements of the blood have a short life span and must be continuously replaced. Collectively, the formation of red blood cells, white blood cells, and platelets is referred to as *hematopoiesis*, which occurs within the red bone marrow. In adults, red bone marrow is found in the pelvis, the ribs, and the sternum.

5.1.1   Plasma

The fluid portion of the blood is called *plasma* and accounts for 55%–60% of the total blood volume. Plasma is about 90% water, with the remaining 10% comprises proteins (8%) and other substances (2%), including hormones, enzymes, nutrient molecules, gases, electrolytes, and excretory products (see Table 5.1), which are either dissolved in the plasma (e.g., gases) or exist as colloidal materials (dispersed solute materials that do not precipitate out, e.g., proteins). The three major plasma proteins are:

- Albumin
- Globulins
- Fibrinogen

Albumin is the most abundant (about 60%) of the plasma proteins and is synthesized in the liver. An important function of albumin is to bind with various molecules in the blood and serve as a *carrier protein*, transporting substances throughout the circulation. Substances that bind with albumin include hormones, amino acids, fatty acids, bile salts, and vitamins. Albumin also serves as an *osmotic regulator*. Because capillary walls are impermeable to plasma proteins, these molecules exert a powerful osmotic force on the water in the blood. In fact, the plasma colloid osmotic pressure exerted by plasma proteins is the only force that retains water within the vascular compartment and, therefore, maintains blood volume (see Chapter 6).

Globulins account for about 38% of the plasma proteins. There are three types of globulins: alpha (α), beta (β), and gamma (γ). The alpha and beta globulins are involved in several activities. They *transport substances* in the blood (e.g., hormones, cholesterol, iron), function as *clotting factors*, and serve as *precursor molecules* (e.g., angiotensinogen). Gamma globulins function as *antibodies*, which play an important role in the immune response. Alpha and

Table 5.1 Antiplatelet and anticoagulant drugs

Drugs that Inhibit Platelet Aggregation

NSAIDs, Aspirin

- Inhibit the production of thromboxane A_2 in platelets by blocking the enzyme cyclooxygenase

ADP Receptor Antagonists (e.g., Clopidogrel)

- Antagonize ADP receptors on platelets to block their activation

gpIIb-IIIa Antagonists (e.g., Abciximab)

- Antagonize the platelet gpIIb-IIIa receptors that platelets utilize to bind to one another

Drugs that Inhibit Coagulation Cascades

Warfarin

- Acts by preventing the reduction of *vitamin K*, which is an essential cofactor in the formation of clotting factors II, VII, IX and X

Heparin

- Enhances the actions of the endogenous anticoagulant *antithrombin III*, which is responsible for inactivating the clotting cascades

Direct Thrombin Inhibitors (e.g., Dabigatran)

- Block the activity of thrombin, which catalyzes the formation of fibrin

Factor Xa Inhibitors (e.g., Rivaroxaban)

- Blocks the activity of clotting factor Xa

The major unwanted effect of drugs that inhibit platelet activity or the coagulation cascades is unwanted bleeding and possible hemorrhage.

---

beta globulins are synthesized in the liver, and the gamma globulins are made by the lymphocytes (a type of white blood cell).

Fibrinogen also plays a role in the blood clotting process and is also synthesized in the liver. It serves as a precursor for *fibrin*, which forms the *meshwork* of a blood clot.

5.1.2 Erythrocytes

The most numerous of the cellular elements in the blood are the *erythrocytes* (*red blood cells*). On average, there are 5 million red blood cells per microliter (μL) of blood, or a total of about 25–30 trillion red blood cells in the adult human body. The percentage of the blood that is made up of red blood cells is referred to as the *hematocrit*. An average hematocrit is about 45% (42%, females; 47%, males). As such, the *viscosity* of the blood is determined primarily by these elements.

Red blood cells are small, flat, biconcave discs. Each cell is approximately 7.5 μm in diameter and 2 μm thick. This shape maximizes the surface area of the cell and facilitates the diffusion of oxygen across the cell membrane. Furthermore, red blood cells are very flexible and easily change shape. This feature allows them to squeeze through capillaries as narrow as 3 μm in diameter. The average life span of a red blood cell is about 120 days. As such, red blood cells must be replaced at a rate of 2–3 million cells per second. Red blood cell production is regulated by the hormone, *erythropoietin*. Low levels of oxygen stimulate the release of erythropoietin from the kidneys into the blood. As red blood cells age, their membranes become fragile and the cells are prone to rupture. Aged cells are removed by phagocytic cells in the *spleen, liver,* and *bone marrow.*

PHARMACY APPLICATION: RECOMBINANT HUMAN ERYTHROPOIETIN

Anemia may result from several pathophysiologic conditions or their treatments including:

- Hemodialysis
- Chronic renal failure
- AIDS
- Chemotherapy
- Surgery (e.g., cardiac procedures)

Epoetin alfa is a recombinant human erythropoietin. This compound, which was developed in the late 1980s, is administered by injection. Available preparations include Epogen® and Procrit®. Along with adequate iron intake, this therapy is highly effective in treating anemias by enhancing red blood cell production. More recently, a longer-acting derivative of Epoetin alfa, Darbepoetin (ARANESP®), has been developed and which remains in the circulation for 24–26 hours.

Some athletes misuse these drugs to try to increase hemoglobin levels and improve their physical performance, an illegal practice referred to as "blood doping."

The primary function of red blood cells is to transport oxygen to the tissues. The red, oxygen-carrying molecule within the red blood cell is *hemoglobin*. This molecule has two components: the *globin portion* and the *heme portion*. There are four globin proteins, each of which is bound to a heme group. Each heme group contains an *iron* atom that binds reversibly with oxygen. The average hemoglobin content in the blood is about 15 g/100 mL of blood, all of it within the red blood cells. In fact, because of their high hemoglobin content, each red blood cell has the capacity to transport more than one billion oxygen molecules. This hemoglobin/oxygen-carrying capacity of the red blood cell is facilitated by the lack of a nucleus or any other membranous organelles within these cells.

Red blood cells are labeled with *cell surface antigens* that determine *blood type*. There are two types of inherited antigens: A antigens and B

Table 5.2 Analysis of red blood cells

A sample of blood is collected by venipuncture. Tests performed may include:

- *Complete Blood Count (CBC)*—a count of red blood cells, white blood cells and platelets
- *White Blood Cell Differential Count*—determines the percent of each type of white cell present in the blood
- *Mean Corpuscular Hemoglobin Concentration (MCHC)*—measure of the amount of hemoglobin in each red blood cell
- *Mean Corpuscular Volume (MCV)*—measure of the size or volume of red blood cells
- *Hematocrit*—the volume of red blood cells expressed as a fraction of the total volume of the blood
- *Morphologic Examination*—to detect changes in blood cell shape or size
- *Erythrocyte Sedimentation Rate*—the rate at which red blood cells settle out of suspension; changes with alterations in plasma protein concentration, chronic infection, and malignancy

antigens. An individual obtains two genes, one from each parent, that determine the production of antigens. Accordingly, there are four possible blood types (see Table 5.2):

- Type A (A antigen)
- Type B (B antigen)
- Type AB (both A and B antigens)
- Type O (neither A nor B antigens)

Antibodies are specialized molecules produced by the immune system to attack foreign antigens. Blood antibodies act against a foreign blood type by attaching to the red blood cells' antigen and causing *agglutination* (clumping) or *hemolysis* (rupture) of the red blood cells. Anti-A antibodies will attach to type A antigens and anti-B antibodies will attach to type B antigens. Therefore, an individual with type A blood can only possess anti-B antibodies (if the individual possessed anti-A antibodies, they would attack the red blood cells of that individual). An individual with type B blood possesses anti-A antibodies. Type AB blood contains both A and B antigens on the red blood cells. Therefore, individuals with this blood type possess neither anti-A nor anti-B antibodies and can receive a transfusion of any blood type. Individuals with type AB blood are referred to as *"universal recipients."*

Type O blood contains no antigens on the cell's surface. In this case, any antibodies that the transfusion recipient may produce (anti-A or anti-B antibodies) have no antigens to attack. Therefore, there is no immune response against this blood. Individuals with type O blood are referred to as *"universal donors"* because this blood is suitable for transfusion in all individuals.

Another type of cell surface antigen found on red blood cells is the *Rh factor*. This factor was named for the rhesus monkey in which the factor was first identified. Red blood cells that contain the Rh factor are referred to as *Rh-positive* and red blood cells without this factor are referred to as *Rh-negative*.

This antigen also stimulates antibody production. Therefore, Rh-negative individuals, who produce anti-Rh antibodies, should receive only Rh-negative blood. Rh-positive individuals, who do not produce anti-Rh antibodies, can receive either Rh-negative or Rh-positive blood. Approximately 85% of whites are Rh-positive and 15% are Rh-negative. Over 99% of Asians, 95% of American blacks, and 100% of African blacks are Rh-positive.

Rh incompatibility may occur when a Rh-negative mother carries an Rh-positive fetus. At the time of delivery, a small amount of the baby's Rh-positive blood may gain access to the maternal circulation. In response, the immune system of the mother produces *anti-Rh antibodies*. During the subsequent pregnancy, the fetus is exposed to these antibodies as they cross the placenta. If this fetus is also Rh-positive, then the anti-Rh antibodies attack the fetal red blood cells and cause *hemolytic disease of the newborn* (*erythroblastosis fetalis*). This may occur in about 3% of second Rh-positive babies and about 10% of third Rh-positive babies. The incidence continues to increase with subsequent pregnancies.

PHARMACY APPLICATION: ERYTHROBLASTOSIS FETALIS

When an Rh-negative mother has been exposed to Rh-positive blood during birth, miscarriage or ectopic pregnancy, she may produce anti-Rh antibodies. As discussed previously, if the fetus in a subsequent pregnancy is also Rh-positive, these maternal antibodies may attack the fetal red blood cells, causing erythroblastosis fetalis. This hemolytic disease is characterized by anemia, jaundice, enlargement of the liver and spleen, and generalized edema.

An important advance in immunopharmacology has been the development of a treatment for preventing erythroblastosis fetalis. This treatment is based on the observation that a primary antibody response to the Rh antigen can be blocked if specific anti-Rh antibodies are administered passively at the time of the exposure to the Rh antigen. This technique is a *passive* form of immunization in which the injected antibodies inactivate the Rh antigens and the mother is prevented from becoming *actively* immunized to these antigens.

Antibody production by the mother may be blocked by treating her with Rh_O (D) immune globulin at the time of exposure to the Rh-positive blood. Commercial forms of Rh_O (D) immune globulin, such as RHOGAM®, contain a high titer of anti-Rh antibodies. When women have received this prophylactic treatment, erythroblastosis fetalis has not been observed in subsequent pregnancies. Rh_O (D) immune globulin is administered intramuscularly. The antibodies have a half-life of approximately 21–29 days.

5.1.3 Leukocytes

There are normally 4,000–11,000 *leukocytes* (*white blood cells*) per microliter of human blood. Unlike red blood cells, white blood cells act primarily within the tissues and are an important component of the immune system. Those found in the blood are in transit. Because of their amoeboid movement, white blood cells can squeeze through pores in the capillary walls and move toward sites of infection. White blood cells are also found in lymphoid tissues, such as the thymus, spleen, and lymph nodes. These cells are referred to as "white" blood cells because they lack hemoglobin and are essentially colorless.

The general *inflammatory and immune functions* of these white blood cells include the following:

- Destruction of invading microorganisms (bacteria and viruses)
- Identification and destruction of cancer cells
- Phagocytosis of tissue debris, including dead and injured cells

The immune system is discussed in detail in Chapter 18. However, many of the functions of the various types of white blood cells are summarized here.

There are five types of white blood cells that are classified as either granulocytes or agranulocytes (possessing cytoplasmic granules or not, respectively):

- Granulocytes
- Neutrophils
- Eosinophils
- Basophils
- Agranulocytes
- Monocytes
- Lymphocytes

Granulocytes are *phagocytic cells*. Their nuclei tend to be segmented into multiple lobes and the cytoplasm of the cells contains numerous granules. These cells are identified by the lobes of the nuclei.

Neutrophils are the most abundant of the white blood cells and account for about 60% of the total number of white blood cells. Mature neutrophils have lobulated nuclei, with two to five lobes connected by thin strands. Because of this unique appearance, neutrophils are also referred to as polymorphonuclear leukocytes (PMNs).

Neutrophils are usually the first to arrive at a site of injury or inflammation. Their primary function is to attack and destroy invading bacteria. In fact, bacterial infection is typically associated with pronounced *neutrophilia* (an increase in the number of circulating neutrophils). These white blood cells are also involved in the removal of tissue debris and, therefore, play a role in the healing process.

Neutrophils eliminate bacteria and tissue debris by way of *phagocytosis*. Small projections of the cell membrane extend outward and engulf the harmful organisms and particles. Ingested materials are then internalized within a cell membrane-bound vesicle. A lysosome, an organelle filled with hydrolytic enzymes, fuses with the vesicle. In this way, the phagocytized material is degraded by these enzymes without any damage to the rest of the cell. Neutrophils have the capacity to phagocytize 5–25 bacteria before they also die.

Eosinophils, which constitute only 1%–4% of the total number of white blood cells, possess a bi-lobed nucleus. These white blood cells are produced in large numbers in individuals with *internal parasitic infections*. The eosinophils attach to the parasites and secrete substances that kill them. These substances include the following:

- Hydrolytic enzymes: released from eosinophil granules (which are modified lysosomes)
- Highly reactive forms of oxygen that are particularly lethal
- Major basic protein: a larvacidal polypeptide also released from granules

Eosinophils also tend to accumulate at the sites of allergic reactions, particularly in the lungs and the skin. The functions of the eosinophils in these areas include the neutralization of inflammatory mediators released from mast cells as well as the phagocytosis of allergen-antibody complexes. In this way, the spread of the inflammatory reaction is limited.

Basophils are the least abundant of the white blood cells and account for less than 1% of the total number of white blood cells. They are similar structurally and functionally to the *mast cells* found in connective tissues, especially in the lungs, skin, and gastrointestinal tract.

Basophils and mast cells play an important role in allergic reactions. The granules of these cells contain various substances including:

- Heparin: which prevents blood coagulation
- Histamine: which promotes bronchoconstriction as well as the vasodilation and increased capillary permeability that leads to inflammation

The white blood cells classified as *agranulocytes* contain very few granules in their cytoplasm. In further contrast to the granulocytes, these cells have a large, nonsegmented nucleus.

Monocytes are the largest of the white blood cells and account for about 5% of the total number of white blood cells in the blood. These white blood cells, which are immature in the blood, leave the vascular compartment and enter the tissues. It is within the tissues that they enlarge, mature, and develop into *macrophages*. Macrophages are large, phagocytic cells that can ingest bacteria, necrotic tissue, and even dead neutrophils. These cells survive much longer than neutrophils and may ingest up to 100 bacteria. The life span of the macrophage may range from months to years, until it is ultimately destroyed as the result of phagocytic activity.

Lymphocytes are typically the second most numerous type of white blood cell and constitute about 30% of the total number of white blood cells. There are two types of lymphocytes:

- B lymphocytes
- T lymphocytes

The primary function of the *B lymphocytes* (also called B cells) is to produce *antibodies*, which are molecules that identify and lead to the destruction of foreign substances, such as bacteria. The B lymphocytes and the antibodies they produce are responsible for *humoral immunity*.

The *T lymphocytes* (also called T cells) provide immunity against viruses and cancer cells. These lymphocytes directly attack and destroy their targets by forming holes in the target cell membrane, causing cell lysis. The T lymphocytes are responsible for *cell-mediated immunity*.

5.1.4 Platelets

The third of the cellular elements within the blood are the *platelets* (*thrombocytes*). Platelets are not cells but small, round or oval *cell fragments*. They are about 2–4 μm in diameter and have no nuclei. Platelets are formed in the red bone marrow as pinched-off portions of very large cells called *megakaryocytes*. Each megakaryocyte, which is confined to the bone marrow, can produce up to 1,000 platelets. Normally, there are approximately 300,000 platelets per microliter of blood. They are replaced about once every 10 days.

Platelets are essential for many aspects of *hemostasis*, or the cessation of blood loss. They play an important role in blood clotting. In fact, they constitute much of the mass of the clot. Several substances are found within the cytoplasm of platelets that contribute to the arrest of bleeding as well as vessel repair:

- Actin and myosin molecules, thrombosthenin: contractile proteins that enable platelets to contract
- Fragments of the endoplasmic reticulum and the Golgi apparatus: produce enzymes and store calcium
- Mitochondria and enzyme systems: form ATP and ADP
- Enzyme systems that produce prostaglandins: substances involved with both the formation of platelet plugs as well as the limitation of clot growth

- Fibrin-stabilizing factor: a protein involved with blood coagulation
- Growth factor: facilitates vascular endothelial cell, vascular smooth muscle cell and fibroblast multiplication and growth, leading to the repair of damaged blood vessels

These substances are discussed more fully in Section 5.2.

5.2   Hemostasis

The prevention of blood loss from a damaged blood vessel is referred to as *hemostasis*. There are three inherent mechanisms that contribute to hemostasis:

- Vascular constriction
- Formation of a platelet plug
- Blood coagulation

Vascular constriction. The first mechanism to occur is *vascular constriction*. Immediately after a blood vessel is cut or severed, the vascular smooth muscle automatically constricts, resulting in a decrease in the flow of blood through the vessel and helping limit blood loss. The vasoconstriction is caused by several factors:

- Sympathetic nerve reflexes in response to pain
- Local myogenic vasospasm in response to the injury
- Locally produced vasoconstrictors released from the damaged tissue and from platelets

When the extent of the trauma to the vessel is increased, then the degree of vascular constriction is increased. Accordingly, a sharply cut blood vessel bleeds far more profusely than a blood vessel damaged by a more crushing injury. The vasoconstriction may last for many minutes or hours. This provides time for the two subsequent mechanisms to develop and get under way.

Formation of a platelet plug. The *formation of a platelet plug* physically blocks small holes in blood vessels. Normally, platelets are unable to adhere to the endothelial lining of the blood vessels; the surface of the platelets contains a coat of glycoproteins that repels the normal endothelium. Interestingly, these same glycoproteins enable the platelets to adhere to damaged vessels.

When platelets contact a damaged vascular surface, in particular, the collagen fibers in the vessel wall, or damaged endothelial cells, the platelets become activated. These platelets become "sticky" and adhere to the damaged tissue. Binding of the platelets to the collagen is facilitated by *von Willebrand factor* (*vWF*). This protein, which is secreted by endothelial cells and platelets, binds to both the exposed collagen and the platelets. In this way, vWF acts as a bridge between the damaged vessel wall and the platelets. The adhered platelets also release ADP and thromboxane A_2, a prostaglandin metabolite, which enhance the stickiness of other platelets. Consequently, more and more platelets adhere to the damaged vessel, ultimately forming a plug. This process is also referred to as *aggregation*. Furthermore, thromboxane A_2, as well as serotonin also released from the platelets, contributes to continued vasoconstriction.

PHARMACY APPLICATION: ANTIPLATELET DRUGS

Platelets play a role in each of the mechanisms of normal hemostasis: vasoconstriction, formation of the platelet plug and blood coagulation. However, they are also involved in pathological processes that lead to atherosclerosis and thrombosis (formation of a blood clot within the vascular system). Antiplatelet drugs interfere with platelet function and are used to prevent the development of atherosclerosis and the formation of arterial thrombi.

The prototype of antiplatelet drugs is aspirin. Aspirin inhibits cyclooxygenase, an enzyme involved in arachidonic acid metabolism. Inhibition of cyclooxygenase blocks the synthesis of thromboxane A_2, the platelet product that promotes both vasoconstriction and platelet aggregation. Because platelets are simply cell fragments, they are incapable of synthesizing new proteins, including enzymes. Therefore, the aspirin-induced inhibition of cyclooxygenase is permanent and lasts for the life of the platelet (7–10 days).

Aspirin is maximally effective as an antithrombotic agent at the comparatively low dose of 160–320 mg per day. (The antipyretic dose of aspirin in adults is 325–650 mg every 4 hours.) Low doses of aspirin cause a steady-state decrease in *platelet* cyclooxygenase activity. Higher doses of aspirin are contraindicated in patients prone to thromboembolism. At higher doses, aspirin also reduces the synthesis of prostacyclin, another arachidonic acid metabolite. Prostacyclin, produced by the *endothelium*, normally inhibits platelet aggregation.

The prophylactic administration of low-dose aspirin has been shown to increase survival following myocardial infarction, decrease the incidence of stroke, and assist in the maintenance of patency of coronary bypass grafts.

Blood coagulation. The third major step in hemostasis is *coagulation,* or the formation of a blood clot. This complex process involves a series of reactions that results in the formation of a protein fiber meshwork that stabilizes the platelet plug.

There are three essential steps that lead to clotting (see Figure 5.1):

- Activation of factor X
- Conversion of prothrombin into thrombin
- Conversion of fibrinogen into fibrin

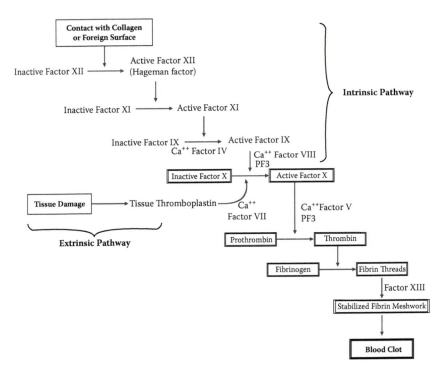

Figure 5.1 The coagulation pathways. Blood coagulation may be elicited by two pathways occurring independently or, more often, concurrently. The intrinsic mechanism begins when blood has contact with the collagen in a damaged vessel wall or with a foreign surface (e.g., test tube). This causes the activation of factor XII, or Hageman Factor, followed by the activation of other clotting factors and, finally, factor X. The extrinsic pathway occurs when damaged tissue releases tissue thromboplastin. This pathway activates factor X directly. The activation of factor X leads to the conversion of prothrombin into thrombin. Thrombin then leads to the conversion of fibrinogen into fibrin threads. It is the fibrin that forms the stabilized meshwork that traps blood cells and forms the blood clot. PF3, platelet factor 3.

The resulting blood clot contains platelets and the physically stabilizing fibrin. In addition, this meshwork usually traps red blood cells, giving the clot its red color.

Altogether, there are 12 *clotting factors* in the plasma. These factors, which are proteins synthesized in the liver, are normally found circulating in the plasma in their inactive forms. The activation of one of these factors leads to the activation of another factor, and so on, resulting in a cascade of reactions culminating in the formation of fibrin. Interestingly, these factors are not numbered for their place in the clotting cascade. Instead, they are numbered in order of their discovery.

Activated *factor X*, along with the Ca^{++} ion, factor V, and platelet factor 3 (collectively, referred to as the *prothrombin activator*) catalyzes the conversion of *prothrombin* into *thrombin*. Thrombin then catalyzes the conversion of *fibrinogen* into *fibrin*, an insoluble, thread-like polymer. The fibrin threads form a meshwork that traps blood cells, platelets and plasma to form the blood clot.

There are two mechanisms by which the clotting cascade may be elicited (see Figure 5.1):

- Extrinsic pathway
- Intrinsic pathway

The *extrinsic pathway* of blood coagulation begins when a blood vessel is ruptured and the surrounding tissues are damaged. The traumatized tissue releases a complex of substances referred to as *tissue thromboplastin*. The tissue thromboplastin further complexes with factor VII and Ca^{++} ions to activate factor X directly.

The *intrinsic pathway* of blood coagulation causes the blood to clot within the vessel itself and is activated when the blood is traumatized or when it contacts the exposed collagen of a damaged vessel wall. This contact activates *factor XII (Hageman Factor)* in the blood. Simultaneously, platelets are activated, such that they begin adhering to the collagen in the vessel wall to form the platelet plug. In addition to ADP and thromboxane A_2, these aggregated platelets also release *platelet factor 3*. This substance plays a role in subsequent clotting reactions. (It is important to note at this point that platelets are involved in all three mechanisms of hemostasis: vascular constriction, formation of the platelet plugs and blood coagulation.)

Activated factor XII leads to the activation of *factor XI*. Activated factor XI, along with Ca^{++} ions and factor IV, leads to the activation of *factor IX*. Activated factor IX, along with Ca^{++} ions, factor VIII and platelet factor 3, leads to the activation of factor X. From the point of factor X activation, the extrinsic and intrinsic mechanisms follow the same common pathway to fibrin formation.

The extrinsic pathway and the intrinsic pathway typically occur simultaneously. The extrinsic mechanism coagulates the blood that has escaped into the tissue prior to the sealing of the vessel, whereas the intrinsic mechanism coagulates the blood within the damaged vessel. Another important difference involves the speed at which these two mechanisms cause coagulation. Because the extrinsic mechanism causes the activation of factor X directly, clotting begins within seconds. The intrinsic mechanism is much slower, usually requiring 1–6 min to form a clot. However, the cascade of reactions characteristic of this mechanism allows for amplification. Each molecule of a given activated clotting factor may activate many molecules of the clotting factor in the next step of the cascade. Therefore, a few molecules of activated Hageman Factor can lead to the activation of hundreds of molecules of factor X and a very powerful coagulation response.

Once the clot is formed, the platelets trapped within it contract, shrinking the fibrin meshwork. This *clot retraction* pulls the edges of the damaged vessel closer together.

Blood coagulation is limited to the site of damage. Once the blood clotting factors have carried out their activities, they are rapidly inactivated by enzymes present in the plasma and in the surrounding tissue.

Positive feedback nature of clot formation. *Thrombin* promotes clot formation at several points in the coagulation cascade through *positive feedback*. Activities of thrombin include the following:

- Acting on prothrombin to make more thrombin, thus facilitating its own formation
- Accelerating the actions of several blood clotting factors (VIII, IX, X, XI and XII)
- Enhancing platelet adhesion and activation
- Activating factor XIII, which strengthens and stabilizes the fibrin meshwork of the clot

Clot dissolution. Once the blood vessel has been repaired, the clot must be removed to prevent permanent obstruction. *Plasmin* is a proteolytic enzyme that digests fibrin (*fibrinolysis*). It is synthesized from its precursor, *plasminogen*. The conversion of plasminogen into plasmin involves several substances, including factor XII (Hageman Factor), which are also involved in the coagulation cascade. Within a few days after the blood has clotted, enough plasmin has been formed to dissolve it. The residue of the clot dissolution is removed by the phagocytic white blood cells: the neutrophils and macrophages.

Prevention of blood clotting and platelet aggregation in the normal vascular system. Several factors contribute to the prevention of blood clotting in the normal vascular system

- *Smoothness* of the endothelial lining: prevents the contact activation of the intrinsic mechanism
- Layer of *glycocalyx* on the endothelium: repels clotting factors and platelets
- *Thrombomodulin*: protein on the endothelium that (1) binds with thrombin, reducing its availability for the clotting process; and (2) activates protein C, which acts as an anticoagulant by inactivating factors V and VIII
- *CD 39*: enzyme on the endothelium that breaks down ADP in the blood to AMP and phosphate (recall that ADP promotes platelet aggregation)
- *Prostacyclin* and *nitric oxide*: secreted by the endothelium, these substances act as vasodilators and inhibitors of platelet aggregation
- *Tissue plasminogen activator*: activates plasmin to dissolve fibrin that is continuously made at low levels

PHARMACY APPLICATION: ANTICOAGULANT DRUGS

Anticoagulant drugs include heparin and warfarin (Coumadin®), dabigatran (Pradaxa®), rivaroxaban (Xarelto®), and apixaban (Eliquis®). These agents are used to prevent deep vein thrombosis. They are also used to prevent the formation of emboli due to atrial fibrillation, valvular heart disease, and other cardiac disorders.

Heparin, which is not absorbed by the gastrointestinal tract, is available only by injection. Its mechanism of action involves the activation of *antithrombin III*. This plasma protein binds with and inactivates thrombin and several other clotting factors. The effect of heparin is immediate.

The most commonly used oral anticoagulant drug in the United States is warfarin. This agent acts by altering vitamin K such that it is unavailable to participate in the synthesis of vitamin K-dependent coagulation factors in the liver (coagulation factors II, VII, IX, and X). Because of the presence of preformed clotting factors in the blood, the full antithrombotic effect of warfarin therapy may require 36–72 hours.

The major adverse effect of warfarin is bleeding. (Ironically, this compound was originally introduced as a very effective rodenticide. As the active ingredient in rodent poison, is causes death due to internal hemorrhaging.) Furthermore, it readily crosses the placenta and can cause a hemorrhagic disorder in the fetus. Therefore, it is contraindicated in pregnant women.

5.3   Alterations in hemostasis

5.3.1   Conditions associated with decreased coagulation

5.3.1.1   Hemophilia

- Caused by a genetic deficiency or lack of certain clotting factors

Three distinct types of hemophilia have been identified:

Type A Hemophilia:
- Most common form (80% or more)
- X-linked recessive disorder
- Results from a deficiency of clotting factor VIII

Type B Hemophilia (Christmas Disease):
- Second most common form of hemophilia (10%–15%)
- X-linked autosomal recessive disorder
- Results from a deficiency of clotting factor IX

Type C Hemophilia (Rosenthal's Disease):
- Least common of all hemophilia cases (<5%)
- Results from a deficiency of clotting factor XI
- Autosomal recessive disorder

Manifestations of Hemophilia:
- Hemophilia may present as a mild, moderate or severe bleeding disorder depending upon the activity of the clotting factors
- Excessive bleeding with trauma or surgery
- Bleeding into soft tissues, muscles and joints
- Excessive menstrual bleeding

Treatment of Hemophilia:
- Avoidance of injury, prevention of bleeding
- Replacement therapy with recombinant clotting factors

There was a significant incidence of HIV and Hepatitis C in patients with hemophilia before the advent of recombinant clotting factors because these factors were previously derived from donor blood.

5.3.1.2   von Willebrand disease

- Most common hereditary bleeding disorder
- Caused by a genetic lack of vWF, a protein produced by the vascular endothelium that is necessary for platelet adhesion
- Causes a reduction in platelet adhesion
- Symptoms may include excessive bruising and bleeding that can be mild to moderate
- Bleeding may occur from gums, nose, and gastrointestinal tract; blood flow during menstruation may be especially heavy

Treatment of von Willebrand disease:
- Infusion of recombinant vWF
- *Desmopressin Acetate*—a vasopressin analog that increases the activity of factor VIII and may stimulate production of vWF by endothelial cells

5.3.1.3   Vitamin K deficiency
- Vitamin K is an essential cofactor for synthesis of factors II, VII, IX, and X by liver enzymes
- It must be obtained from the diet or through bacterial metabolism in the gut
- Conditions that may lead to vitamin K deficiency include intestinal malabsorption or destruction of intestinal flora by antibiotics
- Treatment may include infusion of deficient factors and replacement of parenteral vitamin K

5.3.1.4   Liver disease
Because the clotting factors are synthesized by the liver, any disease or condition that alters liver function may lead to defective production of clotting factors. Diseases that can alter the synthetic function of the liver include:

- Hepatitis
- Cirrhosis
- Liver cancer
- Liver failure

5.3.2   Conditions affecting platelets

5.3.2.1   Thrombocytopenia
Thrombocytopenia is defined as any condition in which the platelet count is abnormally low (<100,000/μL of blood). Decreased platelet production can accompany conditions in which bone marrow function is altered such as:

- Cancer
- Aplastic anemia
- Drug or chemical-induced destruction of platelets
- Radiation exposure
- Infection, HIV
- Deficiency of vitamin B_{12}, folic acid
- Autoimmune destruction

5.3.2.2   Immune thrombocytopenia purpura

- Most commonly occurs in children and adolescents following a viral infection
- Autoimmune disorder in which antibodies bind to platelets in circulation. Antibody-bound platelets are more susceptible to destruction in the spleen. Enlargement of the spleen may result
- Patients may present with abnormal bruising and bleeding
- A chronic, life-long form of the disorder may also occur with lesser incidence
- Treatment may include immune-suppressing drugs like corticosteroids, and possible splenectomy for the chronic form

5.3.2.3   Antiphospholipid syndrome

A hypercoagulability condition caused by the formation of antibodies against negatively charged phospholipids. The mechanism of the disease process is uncertain, but the abnormal antibodies that are produced appear to activate the coagulation cascades. Symptoms include the recurrence of blood clots (deep vein thrombus, peripheral arterial thrombosis) and a significantly increased risk for stroke and miscarriage. A diagnosis of antiphospholipid syndrome is confirmed by the detection of abnormal antibodies in circulation. Treatment focuses mainly on the use of anticoagulant drugs such as warfarin and heparin.

5.3.2.3.1   Drug-induced alterations in hemostasis   A number of pharmacologic agents can impair blood clotting by inhibiting platelet function (see Table 5.1). These agents include the *non-steroidal anti-inflammatories (NSAIDs)*, *ADP receptor inhibitors and gpIIb-IIIa antagonists*. Other drugs can interfere with the action of coagulation cascades and are used therapeutically as *anticoagulants* (see Table 5.1).

5.3.3   Conditions leading to increased blood coagulation (hypercoagulability)

Individuals with hypercoagulability are at increased risk for venous thrombus and emboli. Conditions that can cause hypercoagulability include those that enhance activation of platelets or of the coagulation cascades and include:

1. Inherited disorders of coagulation
   - *Leiden mutation*—genetic defect in clotting factor V that makes it less susceptible to inactivation. Affects 2%–5% of whites
2. Endothelial injury from smoking, diabetes, and atherosclerosis can enhance platelet activation

3. Situations leading to stasis of blood—prolonged bed rest, obesity, pregnancy, prolonged inactivity (long airplane flights)
4. Increased viscosity of blood—polycythemia
5. Trauma or surgery—clotting cascades are activated by tissue or blood vessel injury
6. Cancer—release of pro-coagulation substances. Blood vessel and tissue injury may also accompany growing cancers
7. Drugs:
   * Oral contraceptives
   * Hormone replacement therapy

5.3.4 Disseminated intravascular coagulation (DIC)

DIC is a secondary condition that can occur as a result of overactivation of the intrinsic and extrinsic coagulation pathways. The condition is characterized by the paradoxical effects of both inappropriate activation of the clotting cascades and the destruction of platelets. While over activation of coagulation cascades can lead to widespread thrombosis, the subsequent depletion of platelets and clotting factors due to excessive thrombosis in turn can predispose the patient to excessive bleeding. Excess activation of the fibrinolytic pathways can also occur. Conditions leading to DIC are generally those associated with widespread tissue injury, blood vessel injury and inflammation. Inflammatory mediators such as cytokines appear to play an important role in development of DIC in that they appear to contribute to a pro-coagulation environment (see Figure 5.2). Conditions associated with DIC include:

* Metastatic cancer
* Severe burn injury
* Massive trauma
* Severe bacterial infection, sepsis, septic shock
* Poisonous snake bite

5.3.4.1 Manifestations of DIC
* Excessive bleeding from a number of sites
* Formation of blood clots, deep vein thromboses
* Organ dysfunction due to thrombosis and ischemia

5.3.4.2 Treatment of DIC
* Management of primary disease
* Replacement of clotting factors and platelets
* Cautious use of anticoagulant therapy

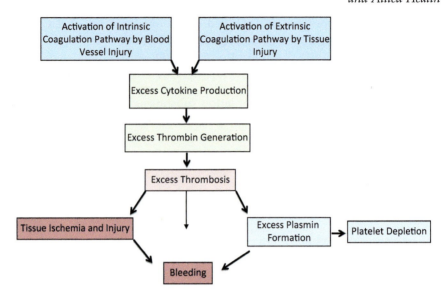

Figure 5.2   Disseminated intravascular coagulation.

5.4   Alterations in hematologic function and oxygen transport

Blood is composed of two main components: a liquid portion called *plasma* and a cellular portion containing red blood cells, white blood cells and platelets. Blood serves a number of important functions in the human body such as transport of oxygen, nutrients, and ions while acting as a buffer between cells and the environment. The total blood volume in a 70-kg man is approximately 5 L.

5.4.1   Hematopoiesis

The process by which blood cells are formed is called *hematopoiesis*. All of the cellular components in blood are derived from a common precursor called a *stem cell*. In the maturing fetus, early production of red blood cells takes place in developing blood vessels. As gestation continues, the production of both red and white blood cells shifts to the fetal liver and spleen and eventually is localized primarily in the bone marrow. Hematopoiesis continues in the bone marrow after birth and is a life-long process. A number of growth factors and cytokines are involved in regulating the process of hematopoiesis. A major regulator of red blood cell production is the hormone *erythropoietin*, which is produced by the adult kidney. Erythropoietin is a glycoprotein released by cells of the kidney in response to the presence of *hypoxia*. The erythropoietin that is produced acts directly on stem cells in the bone marrow to promote the proliferation, maturation and release of new red blood cells. The mature red blood cells that form are biconcave in structure and lack a nucleus. The unique shape of the mature red blood cell maximizes surface area and facilitates diffusion of oxygen across the cell membrane. Since red blood cells do not contain mitochondria, they rely primarily upon glycolysis to meet their metabolic needs. The cell membranes of normal red blood cells must be strong enough to survive transport under high pressure yet be flexible enough to fit though narrow and winding capillaries. A protein *cytoskeleton* provides a framework of support to the red blood cell membrane.

The function of red blood cells is to transport oxygen to tissues. This is accomplished by the intracellular protein *hemoglobin*. The quaternary hemoglobin protein is composed of 2 α and 2 β subunits. Each of the subunits contains a central iron-containing protein called a *heme* protein. It is the iron atom in the heme protein that binds to molecular oxygen. As a result of the four iron-containing heme groups, each molecule of hemoglobin can carry four atoms of oxygen.

5.4.2 Anemia

Anemia is a condition in which there is a reduced number of red blood cells or decreased concentration of hemoglobin in those cells or both. Anemia is often a manifestation of some disease process or abnormality within the body. While there are many causes of anemia, the actual mechanism by which the anemia results is generally due to (1) excess loss or destruction of red blood cells and (2) reduced or defective production of red blood cells. Anemias may be classified according to their cause or effect on red blood cell morphology (see Table 5.2)

5.4.2.1 General manifestations of anemia
A major feature of anemia is a reduced capacity for the transport of oxygen to tissues. This reduced oxygen delivery can result in:

- Ischemia
- Fatigability
- Breathlessness upon exertion
- Exercise intolerance
- Pallor
- Increased susceptibility to infection

5.4.3   Types of anemia

5.4.3.1   Hemolytic anemia

Anemia that results from excess destruction of red blood cells (*hemolysis*). Factors that may cause *hemolysis* include:

- Autoimmune destruction of red blood cells
- Certain drugs (e.g., quinine) or toxins
- Cancers such as lymphoma and leukemia
- Rheumatoid arthritis
- Certain viral infections (e.g., parvovirus)
- Parasitic infections (e.g., malaria)

5.4.3.2   Blood loss anemia

Anemia that results from acute blood loss. With acute loss of large amounts of blood, shock is the major concern. However, with chronic loss of smaller amounts of blood, iron deficiency is a chief concern. Causes of acute and chronic blood loss may include:

- Trauma and hemorrhage
- Malignancy
- Peptic ulcers

1. *Iron-deficiency anemia*
   Iron-deficiency anemia is a major cause of anemia worldwide. It can occur as a result of iron-deficient diets. Vegetarians are at particular risk for iron deficiency, as are menstruating or pregnant women due to their increased requirement for iron. Iron-deficiency anemia may also result from poor absorption of iron from the intestine or persistent blood loss (e.g., ulcers, neoplasia). Because iron is the functional component of hemoglobin, the lack of available iron will result in a decreased hemoglobin synthesis and the subsequent impairment of red blood cell oxygen-carrying capacity.
2. *Cobalamin-deficiency or folate-deficiency anemia*
   Cobalamin (vitamin B_{12}) and folic acid are essential nutrients required for DNA synthesis and red blood cell maturation, respectively. Deficiency of these nutrients will lead to the formation of red blood cells that are of abnormal shape with shortened life spans due to weakened cell membranes. One important cause of vitamin B_{12} deficiency is *pernicious anemia*, which results from a lack of *intrinsic factor* production by the gastric mucosa. Intrinsic factor is required for normal absorption of vitamin B_{12} from the intestine. Any intestinal abnormalities (e.g., neoplasia, inflammation) that interfere with the production of intrinsic factor can lead

Table 5.3   Classification of anemia based on changes in red blood cell (RBC) morphology

1. Size Changes
   Normocytic Anemia—RBC size is unchanged
   E.g., Blood loss anemia
   Macrocytic Anemia—RBC size is increased
   E.g., B_{12}/folic acid deficiency anemia
   Microcytic Anemia—RBC size is reduced
   E.g., Iron-deficiency anemia
2. Color Changes (due to altered hemoglobin content)
   Normochromic—normal hemoglobin concentration
   Hypochromic—reduced hemoglobin concentration
   E.g., Iron-deficiency anemia may be classified as a *microcytic, hypochromic anemia* because both RBC size and hemoglobin content are reduced

to vitamin B_{12} deficiency. Folic acid deficiency most commonly results from poor diet, malnutrition or intestinal malabsorption (see Table 5.3).

5.4.4   Inherited anemia

Anemia may also result from genetic defects in red blood cell structure or function. Two common genetic disorders of red blood cells are *Sickle Cell Anemia* and *Thalassemia*. Both of these disorders result from abnormal or absent genes for the production of hemoglobin.

5.4.4.1   Sickle cell disease

Sickle cell disease is a group of autosomal recessive disorders characterized by abnormal hemoglobin production (see Figure 5.3). In the United States, the highest prevalence of sickle cell disease is in blacks, with a reported incidence of approximately 1 in 500 births. Sickle cell disease is an autosomal recessive disorder that has several patterns of inheritance that determine the severity of the disease in afflicted individual. A normal individual has two genes that code for the beta subunit of hemoglobin. In the *homozygous* form of sickle cell anemia, both genes coding for the beta hemoglobin gene are defective and thus most of the hemoglobin formed (termed *hemoglobin S; HbS*) is defective. As a result, the clinical presentation is most severe in patients with the homozygous form. With the *heterozygous* form (*sickle cell trait*) of the disease, only one of the two genes for the beta subunit of hemoglobin is defective. As a result, less than half of the red blood cell hemoglobin is affected and the clinical presentation is significantly milder.

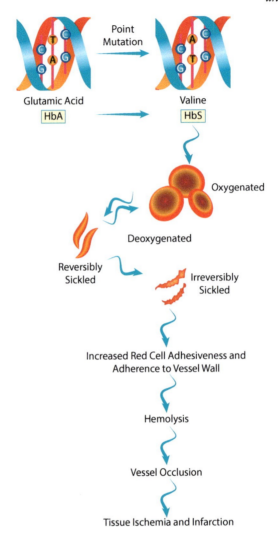

Figure 5.3   Sickle cell anemia.

The mutation observed in sickle cell anemia involves a point mutation in the beta chain of hemoglobin involving the substitution of the amino acid valine for glutamic acid. This amino acid substitution decreases the solubility of hemoglobin when it is deoxygenated. Deoxygenated HgS polymerizes and distorts the flexible red blood cell membrane. The early stages of red blood cell sickling may be reversible if reoxygenation of the HbS occurs. However, if oxygenation is not restored, the polymerization and sickling of affected red blood cell will be irreversible. Sickled red blood cells will block small blood vessels and hemolyze readily, leading to widespread tissue ischemia, injury and possibly infarction (*sickle cell crisis*). This finding high-lights the importance of preventing situations where the blood of patients with sickle cell anemia might become deoxygenated. Factors that may lead to deoxygenation and red blood cell sickling include:

- Strenuous exertion
- Cold exposure
- Acidosis
- High altitudes
- Infections
- Hypoxia

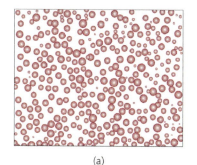

(a)

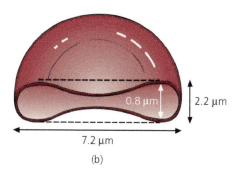

(b)

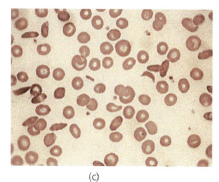

(c)

5.4.4.1.1   Manifestations of sickle cell disease   As a result of their elongated shape and rigidity, affected blood cells do not pass easily through narrow blood vessels and thus may cause blood vessel occlusion. *Hemolysis* of sickled red blood cells is also common. The *spleen* is a major site of red blood cell hemolysis since the blood vessels found within this organ are narrow and convoluted. As a result of the sluggish blood flow, many tissues and organs of the body are eventually affected by this disorder. Specific manifestations may include:

- Impaired oxygen carrying capacity—fatigue, pallor
- Occlusion of blood vessels leading to ischemia, hypoxia, pain
- Organ damage—kidney, lungs, eyes, brain, spleen
- Stasis ulcers of hands and feet due to blood vessel occlusion
- Splenomegaly due to increased destruction of red blood cells in this organ; may necessitate removal of the spleen (*splenectomy*)
- Neurologic complications
- Increased risk of infection and possible septicemia due to stagnation of blood
- Iron overload of tissues such as the heart, spleen, and liver as a result of excess red blood cell hemolysis
- *Acute chest syndrome*—atypical pneumonia that results from pulmonary infarction.

SICKLE CELL ANEMIA AND MALARIA?

The presence of sickle cell genes in the population is increased in regions of Africa where malaria is endemic. It is believed that the presence of this gene mutation offers some protective effect against the malaria parasite that infects red blood cells.

JAUNDICE

Jaundice occurs when there is an excess of bilirubin in the blood. Bilirubin is a breakdown product of hemoglobin that is excreted into the bile. In hemolytic anemia, excess rates of red blood cell destruction lead to the production of bilirubin at rates faster than it can be eliminated from the liver and, as a result, bilirubin backs up into the blood. Bilirubin is pigmented and taints the skin and whites of the eyes with a characteristic yellowish tinge that is indicative of jaundice.

5.4.4.2 Thalassemia

Thalassemia is a genetic disorder characterized by absent or defective production of hemoglobin α or β chains. There are numerous genetic variants of thalassemia since four separate genes encode for the alpha subunit of hemoglobin while two genes code for the beta subunits. Mutation may be point mutations, deletions or insertions. As with sickle cell anemia, afflicted individuals may be *heterozygous* for the trait and have a milder presentation of the disease or *homozygous* and have a more severe form of the disorder. The β form of thalassemia (defective formation of β hemoglobin chains) is most common in individuals from Mediterranean populations, whereas the α form of thalassemia (defective formation of α hemoglobin chains) occurs mostly in Asians. Both the α and β forms of thalassemia are more common in blacks.

5.4.4.2.1 Manifestations of thalassemia In heterozygous individuals, enough normal hemoglobin is usually synthesized to prevent significant anemia. In these individuals, symptoms of anemia may appear only with exercise or physiologic stress. Homozygous individuals are often dependent upon frequent transfusions to treat the resulting severe anemia. Children affected with the homozygous form may be severely growth retarded. The widespread *hypoxia* that can result from impaired oxygen carrying capacity leads to *erythropoietin-induced* increases in hematopoiesis that can eventually affect the structure of the long bones. Severe anemia may also lead to congestive heart failure and marked hepatosplenomegaly. Excessive hemolysis of red blood cells may occur in severe forms of the disease due to overproduction of the normal hemoglobin subunit. Iron deposits from increased absorption and frequent transfusions may injure the liver and heart as well.

5.4.4.2.2 Diagnosis and treatment of sickle cell anemia and thalassemia A simple blood screen for hemoglobin S may detect the presence of sickle cell anemia. If the screening is positive, additional tests will be performed to determine whether one or two sickle cell genes are present. Simple blood tests followed by genetic analysis may also be used to diagnose thalassemia. Testing for sickle cell anemia and thalassemia is part of the newborn screening that is conducted at birth.

Individuals with inherited anemia should avoid physiologic stresses that might exacerbate hypoxia. Infections should be avoided and promptly treated if they occur in order to prevent a possible hypoxic crisis. Proper immunizations and vaccinations should be administered to lessen the chance for infections. Frequent transfusions of normal red blood cells are commonly used in individuals with severe forms of inherited anemia during periods of crisis. These individuals are at risk for iron accumulation as well as contracting blood-borne pathogens such as hepatitis and

HIV from improperly screened blood. Bone marrow transplants may be utilized to effectively cure patients with genetic anemia; however, the procedure carries considerable risk of its own. The drug *hydroxyurea* has been shown to reduce sickling of red blood cells in patients with sickle cell disease and may be helpful for preventing sickle cell crisis. The drug appears to work by stimulating the production of fetal hemoglobin in affected cells.

CASE STUDY

During World War II American soldiers in Southeast Asia were give the drug primaquine in order to prevent malaria. Approximately 10% of African-American soldiers developed a severe hemolytic anemia. A smaller percentage of soldiers from Greek and Italian descent also developed hemolytic anemia.

    The cause of this hemolysis in certain ethnic groups was investigated and later found to be glucose-6-phosphate dehydrogenase (G6PD) deficiency. Explain how primaquine works and why G6PD deficiency lead to hemolysis in soldiers of African-American and Mediterranean descent.

5.4.4.3   *Glucose-6-phosphate dehydrogenase deficiency*

G6PD is an enzyme that helps protect red blood cells against hemolysis during periods of oxidative stress. The gene for G6PD is found on the X-chromosome. A defective gene for G6PD may be fully expressed in homozygous males or partially expressed in heterozygous females. The condition occurs most commonly in patients of Mediterranean or African-American descent. Individuals with defective G6PD production are usually asymptomatic unless exposed to conditions such as fever, infection or hypoxemia that increase oxidative stress or to drugs such as salicylates, sulfonamides or antimalarial drugs that can generate free radicals. *Favism*, an acute hemolytic anemia, may occur in patients of Mediterranean descent following the ingestion of fava beans, which contain the compound DOPA-quinone. During periods of oxidative stress, patients will experience acute hemolysis that can lead to hemoglobinuria, hemoglobinemia, jaundice and, possibly, blood vessel occlusion.

5.4.4.4   *Aplastic anemia*

Aplastic anemia is caused by a lack of red blood cell production by the bone marrow. If erythrocyte stem cells precursors are lacking or destroyed, the process of erythropoiesis will be severely impaired. Aplastic anemia may result from a congenital defect in stem cell production or can be caused

Table 5.4   Possible causes of aplastic anemia

- Radiation exposure
- Chemicals (e.g., organic solvents, heavy metals)
- Chemotherapy drugs
- Certain antibiotics (e.g., chloramphenicol)
- HIV infection
- Toxins

by exposure to agents that damage the bone marrow, such as solvents, radiation, infection, chemotherapeutic drugs, and certain antibiotics (see Table 5.4). Drug-induced aplastic anemia is usually a dose-dependent phenomenon. The clinical manifestations of aplastic anemia will depend upon the extent to which hematopoiesis is impaired. General symptoms of anemia such as pallor, fatigue, lethargy can occur initially. Bleeding in the skin and from the nose, mouth and body orifices may also occur from a lack of platelet production by the abnormal bone marrow. Increased susceptibility to infection is also seen as a result of diminished white blood cell production. The underlying cause of the aplastic anemia needs to be identified and further exposure prevented. Treatment should also include avoidance of physiologic stresses and infection. Transfusions are effective for temporarily improving oxygen carrying capacity. In severe cases, bone marrow transplant may offer a cure.

5.4.4.5   Polycythemia
Polycythemia is a disorder in which the number of red blood cells in circulation is greatly increased. There are two categories of polycythemia, *relative* and *primary*. *Relative polycythemia* results from an increase in the concentration of red blood cells due to a loss of plasma volume. In contrast, *primary polycythemia* (*polycythemia vera*) is caused by excessive proliferation of bone marrow stem cells. Polycythemia vera is a rare neoplastic disorder that occurs in men between the 40 and 60 years of age. A *secondary* form of polycythemia may occur from excess *erythropoietin* production as a physiologic response to hypoxia. Secondary polycythemia may be seen in individuals living at high altitudes, chronic smokers, or individuals with chronic obstructive pulmonary disease.

5.4.4.5.1   *Manifestations of polycythemia*
- Increased blood volume and viscosity
- Increased risk of thrombus
- Occlusion of small blood vessels
- Hepatosplenomegaly from pooling of blood
- Impaired blood flow to tissues (ischemia)

5.4.4.5.2   Treatment of polycythemia
- Increasing fluid volume in relative polycythemia
- Periodic removal of blood to reduce viscosity and volume in primary polycythemia
- Chemotherapy or radiation to suppress activity of bone marrow stem cells in polycythemia vera

Medical terminology

Agglutination(ă-gloo″tĭ-nā′shŭn): Clumping of platelets
Antibody (ăn′tĭ-bŏd″ē): Immunoglobulin molecule produced by B lymphocytes (plasma cells) that destroys or neutralizes antigens
Anticoagulant (ăn″tĭ-kō-ăg′ū-lănt): Agent that prevents coagulation of the blood
Antigen (ăn′tĭ-jĕn): Protein marker on the cell surface that allows the immune system to distinguish between "self" cells and "non-self" cells
Antipyretic (ăn-tĭ-pī-rĕt′ĭk): Agent that reduces fever
Coagulation (kō-ăg″ū-lā′shŭn): Formation of a blood clot
Erythrocyte(ĕ-rĭth′rō-sīt): Mature red blood cell
Erythropoietin(ĕ-rĭth″rō-poy′ĕ-tĭn): Hormone made by the kidney that stimulates red blood cell production in the bone marrow
Fibrinolysis (fī″brĭn-ŏl′ĭ-sĭs): Breakdown of fibrin in a blood clot
Hematopoiesis (hĕm″ă-tō-poy-ē′sĭs): Production of blood cells
Hemolysis (hē-mŏl′ĭ-sĭs): Destruction of red blood cells
Hemostasis (hē″mō-stā′sĭs): Prevention of blood loss
Larvacidal (lăr-vĭ-sī′dăl): Destructive to larva
Leukocyte (loo′kō-sīt): White blood cell
Necrotic (nĕ-krŏt′ĭk): Relating to tissue death or destruction
Neutrophilia (nū″trō-fĭl′ē-ă): Abnormal increase in neutrophils in the blood
Phagocytosis (făg″ō-sī-tō′sĭs): Process by which phagocytes engulf and destroy microorganisms (e.g., bacteria) and cellular debris
Plasma (plăz′mă): Liquid portion of the blood in which the blood cells are suspended
Thrombocyte (thrŏm′bō-sīt): Platelet
Thrombosis (thrŏm-bō′sĭs): Formation of a blood clot within the vascular system

Bibliography

Fox, S. I., *Human Physiology*, 9th ed., McGraw-Hill, New York, 2006.
Ganong, W. F., *Review of Medical Physiology*, 19th ed., Appleton & Lange, Stamford, CT, 1999.
Gaspard, K. J., Composition of blood and formation of blood cells, in *Pathophysiology, Concepts of Altered Health States*, 7th ed., Porth, C. P. Ed., Lippincott, Philadelphia, PA, 2005, chap. 14.

Guyton, A. C., and Hall, J. E., *Textbook of Medical Physiology*, 11th ed., W. B. Saunders, Philadelphia, PA, 2006.

Hambleton, J., and O'Reilly, R. A., Drugs used in disorders of coagulation, in *Basic and Clinical Pharmacology*, 8th ed., Katzung, B. G., Ed., Lange Medical Books/McGraw-Hill, New York, 2001, chap. 34.

Kaushansky, K., and Kipps, T. J., Hematopoietic agents: growth factors, minerals, and vitamins, in *Goodman and Gilman's The Pharmacological Basis of Therapeutics*, 11th ed., Brunton, L. L., Lazo, J. S., and Parker, K. L., Eds., McGraw-Hill, New York, 2006, chap. 53.

Krensky, A. M., Vincenti, F., and Bennett, W. M., Immunosuppresants, tolerogens, and immunostimulants, in *Goodman and Gilman's The Pharmacological Basis of Therapeutics*, 11th ed., Brunton, L. L., Lazo, J. S., and Parker, K. L., Eds., McGraw-Hill, New York, 2006, chap. 52.

Lake, D. F., Akporiaye, E. T., and Hersh, E. M., Immunopharmacology, in *Basic and Clinical Pharmacology*, Katzung, B. G., Ed., Lange Medical Books/McGraw-Hill, New York, 2001, chap. 56.

Majerus, P. W., Broze, G. J., Miletich, J. P. and Tollefsen, D. M., Anticoagulant, thrombolytic, and antiplatelet drugs, in *Goodman and Gilman's: The Pharmacological Basis of Therapeutics*, 9th ed., Hardman, J. G. and Limbird, L. E., Eds., McGraw-Hill, New York, 1996, chap. 54.

Sherwood, L., *Human Physiology from Cells to Systems*, 5th ed., Brooks/Cole, Pacific Grove, CA, 2001.

Silverthorn, D. U., *Human Physiology, an Integrated Approach*, 4th ed., Prentice Hall, Upper Saddle River, NJ, 2007.

Stedman's Medical Dictionary for the Health Professions and Nursing, 5th ed., Lippincott Williams & Wilkins, Baltimore, MD, 2005.

Taber's Cyclopedic Medical Dictionary, 20th ed., F. A. Davis Co., Philadelphia, PA, 2005.

Widmaier, E. P., Raff, H., and Strang, K. T., *Vander's Human Physiology, The Mechanisms of Body Function*, McGraw-Hill, Boston, MA, 2006.

chapter six

The circulatory system

Study objectives

- List the functions of the circulatory system
- Describe how the rate of blood flow to individual tissues differs according to specific tissue function
- Explain the function of each component of the blood vessel wall
- Distinguish between arteries, arterioles, capillaries, and veins in terms of their anatomical characteristics and their functions
- Distinguish between diastolic pressure, systolic pressure, and pulse pressure
- Understand the method by which mean arterial pressure is calculated
- Describe how blood pressure changes as the blood flows through the circulatory system
- Understand Ohm's Law and describe the relationship between blood flow, blood pressure and vascular resistance
- List the factors that affect vascular resistance and explain their physiological significance
- Explain why mean arterial pressure must be closely regulated
- Explain how the autonomic nervous system alters cardiac output, total peripheral resistance and, therefore, mean arterial pressure
- List the sources of input to the vasomotor center
- Describe the mechanism of action and the physiological significance of the baroreceptor reflex, the chemoreceptor reflex, and the low-pressure reflex
- Indicate the source, the factors regulating the release and the physiological significance of the following vasoconstrictors: catecholamines, angiotensin II, vasopressin, endothelin, thromboxane A_2, and serotonin
- Indicate the source, the factors regulating the release or activation, and the physiological significance of the following vasodilators: prostacyclin, nitric oxide, atrial natriuretic peptide, histamine, bradykinin, adenosine, and epinephrine
- Compare and contrast the compliance of systemic arteries and systemic veins
- List the specific blood reservoirs and their common characteristics
- Explain how blood volume, sympathetic stimulation of the veins, skeletal muscle activity and respiratory activity influence venous return
- Describe the effects of gravity on the circulatory system

- Describe the mechanism of active hyperemia
- Define autoregulation of blood flow
- Explain how the myogenic mechanism causes autoregulation of blood flow
- Describe the effects of acute exercise on the circulatory system
- Explain how blood flow through capillaries is regulated by vasomotion
- Describe the physiological significance of the Starling Principle
- Explain how hydrostatic forces and osmotic forces regulate the bulk flow of fluid across the capillary wall
- Describe the four general conditions that can lead to edema formation
- Identify the components of a lipoprotein
- Describe the role of each of the different lipoproteins in lipid transport
- Describe the function of an apolipoprotein
- List risk factors for the development of atherosclerosis
- Discuss the steps involved in the formation of an atherosclerotic plaque
- Compare and contrast the various genetic hyperlipidemias
- What is an aneurysm? Why may it occur? What is a dissecting aneurysm?
- Describe the key feature of the various forms of arteritis
- Compare and contrast Raynaud's disease and Raynaud's phenomenon
- Discuss the etiology of varicose veins. How might they lead to chronic venous insufficiency?
- List factors that would predispose a patient to the formation of a venous thrombus
- Discuss the role of anticoagulant and thrombolytic drug therapy in treatment and prevention of a venous thrombus
- Distinguish primary hypertension from secondary hypertension
- List the risk factors that may contribute to the development of essential hypertension
- Discuss the major consequences of chronic hypertension. What target organs are most affected by hypertension?
- Discuss possible treatment options for essential hypertension
- What are some possible causes of secondary hypertension?
- Describe the various forms of hypertension that are associated with pregnancy
- Define malignant hypertension. Why is it so dangerous?
- What is orthostatic hypotension? What factors might predispose a patient to it?
- Compare and contrast the different types of shock that may occur in a patient based on the cause of the shock
- Describe the physiologic compensatory mechanisms that activate in response to shock
- Explain the statement that "shock not only stops the machine but wrecks the machinery"
- Discuss treatment strategies for each of the various types of shock outlined

The *circulatory system* carries out many important functions that contribute to homeostasis. It obtains oxygen from the lungs, nutrients from the gastrointestinal tract, and hormones from the endocrine glands, and it delivers these substances to the tissues that need them. Furthermore, it removes metabolic waste products, such as carbon dioxide, lactic acid, and urea, from the tissues. Finally, it contributes to the actions of the immune system by transporting antibodies and leukocytes (white blood cells) to areas of infection. Overall, the circulatory system plays a vital role in the maintenance of optimal conditions for cell and tissue function.

Most tissues are *perfused*. In other words, most tissues receive blood flow (epithelial tissue is avascular, as is cartilage). The amount of blood that flows through each tissue, however, depends upon that tissue's function. For example, many organs, such as the heart, the brain, and the skeletal muscles, receive a blood flow that is sufficient to supply their metabolic needs. When metabolic activity increases, as it does during exercise, blood flow to the tissues of these organs increases accordingly. Other organs, however, receive a blood flow that is in significant excess of their metabolic needs. These tissues, including the kidneys, the organs of the digestive system, and the skin, have important homeostatic functions. Among other vital activities, the kidneys filter the blood and remove waste products, and the organs of the digestive system absorb nutrients into the blood. Further, thermoregulation involves the control of blood flow to the body surface where heat is eliminated or conserved. These functions are carried out most effectively and efficiently when the involved tissues receive an abundant blood flow. Under normal resting conditions, the kidneys, which account for only 1% of the body's weight, receive 20% of the *cardiac output (CO)*, the gastrointestinal tract receives approximately 27% of the CO, and the skin receives 6%–15% of the blood pumped by the heart per minute. Because these tissues receive more blood than they need to support metabolic activity, they can easily tolerate a sustained decrease in blood flow. During exercise, when the metabolic demand of the working skeletal muscles and the heart increases substantially, blood flow is directed away from the kidneys and the organs of the digestive system to the skeletal muscles and the heart.

6.1 Blood vessels

The walls of the blood vessels may contain varying amounts of fibrous tissue, elastic tissue, and smooth muscle. All blood vessels are lined with a single layer of endothelial cells, as found forming the endothelium of the heart. The *fibrous connective tissue* provides structural support and stiffens the vessel. The *elastic connective tissue* allows vessels to expand and hold more blood. It also causes the vessels to recoil and exert pressure on the blood within the vessels, which pushes this blood forward. Most blood vessels contain *smooth muscle* that is arranged in either circular or spiral layers. Therefore, contraction of vascular smooth muscle, or *vasoconstriction*, narrows the diameter of the vessel and decreases the flow of blood through it. Relaxation of vascular smooth muscle, or *vasodilation*, widens the diameter of the vessel and increases the flow of blood through it. The smooth muscle of the vessel is innervated by the autonomic nervous system and is, therefore, physiologically regulated. Furthermore, this is where endogenous vasoactive substances and pharmacological agents exert their effects. The *endothelium* has several important physiological functions including contributing to the regulation of blood pressure, blood vessel growth and the exchange of materials between the blood and the interstitial fluid of the tissues (see Table 6.1).

The circulatory system is composed of several anatomically and functionally distinct blood vessels including:

- Arteries
- Arterioles
- Capillaries
- Veins

Arteries carry blood away from the heart (see Figure 6.1). These vessels contain fibrous connective tissue that strengthens them and enables them to withstand the high blood pressures generated by the heart. In general, the arteries function as a system of *conduits*, or pipes, transporting the blood under high pressure toward the tissues. There is little smooth muscle and, therefore, little physiological regulation of vessel diameter in these vessels.

Another noteworthy anatomical feature of the arteries is the presence of elastic connective tissue. When the heart contracts and ejects the blood, a portion of the stroke volume (SV) flows toward the capillaries. However, much of the SV ejected during systole is retained in the distensible arteries. When the heart relaxes, the arteries recoil and exert pressure on the blood within them forcing this "stored" blood to flow forward. In this way, a steady flow of blood toward the capillaries is maintained throughout the entire cardiac cycle.

Table 6.1   Functions of endothelial cells

- Selectively permeable barrier between the vascular compartment and the interstitial fluid of the tissues
- Lining of blood vessels that prevents adherence of blood cells and platelets to the vessel walls
- Production of vasoconstrictor and vasodilator substances that act on underlying vascular smooth muscle
- Role in angiogenesis, or new capillary growth

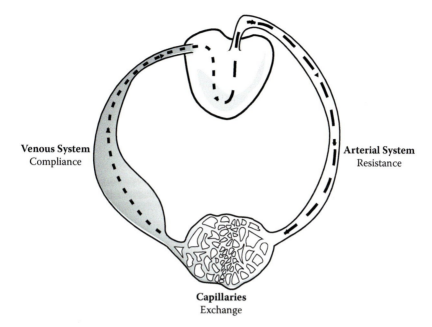

Venous System
Compliance

Arterial System
Resistance

Capillaries
Exchange

Figure 6.1 Schematic diagram of the circulatory system. Arteries carry blood away from the heart. The smallest arterial vessels, the arterioles, are composed mainly of smooth muscle and are the major resistance vessels in the circuit. The capillaries are the site of exchange between the blood and the tissues. Veins carry blood back toward the heart. The small veins are the major compliance vessels in the circuit and, under resting conditions, contain 64% of the blood volume.

As the arteries travel toward the peripheral organs and tissues, they branch and become smaller. Furthermore, the walls of the vessels become less elastic and more muscular. Finally, the smallest arterial vessels, the *arterioles*, are composed almost entirely of smooth muscle with a lining of endothelium. Therefore, depending upon the degree of constriction of the vascular smooth muscle, these vessels may alter their diameter and, consequently, their blood flow, across a very wide range. For this reason, the arterioles are the major *resistance vessels* in the circulatory system. In fact, the primary function of arterioles is to regulate the distribution of the CO and determine which tissues receive more blood and which tissues receive less blood, depending upon the tissue's and the body's needs. In addition, the resistance to blood flow in the arterioles contributes to the regulation of mean arterial pressure, which is discussed in detail in a later section of this chapter.

From the arterioles, blood flows through the *capillaries*, the smallest vessels in the circulatory system. The capillaries are the *site of exchange* between the blood and the interstitial fluid surrounding the cells of the tissues.

The primary mechanism of exchange is simple diffusion as substances move across the capillary walls "down" their concentration gradients, or from an area of high concentration to an area of low concentration. Several important factors influencing the process of diffusion include:

- Surface area of the barrier
- Thickness of the barrier
- Velocity of blood flow

As discussed in Chapter 1, Section B, Fick's Law of Diffusion states that as the surface area of a given barrier increases, so does the degree diffusion. There are approximately 10 billion capillaries in the adult human body with a total exchange surface area of more than 6,300 m²; the equivalent of almost two football fields. Furthermore, most tissue cells are not more than 20 μm away from the nearest capillary.

The capillaries have the thinnest walls of all the blood vessels. They are composed of only a flat layer of endothelium that is one cell thick and is supported by a thin acellular matrix, referred to as the *basement membrane*. The total thickness of this barrier between the blood and the interstitial fluid is only 0.5 μm. As such, the anatomical characteristics of the capillaries that maximize the exchange surface area and minimize the thickness of the barrier, render these vessels ideally suited for the exchange of materials by simple diffusion.

A third factor that influences diffusion across capillary walls is the velocity of blood flow. Although an individual capillary has a diameter of approximately 8–10 μm, the total cross-sectional area of all the systemic capillaries taken together is 2,500–3,000 cm². As the cross-sectional area increases, then the velocity of blood flow decreases. In contrast to the aorta in which blood flows at a rate of 33 cm/s, the capillaries have a velocity of blood flow of 0.33 mm/s. This slow movement of blood facilitates the exchange of materials between the tissues and the vascular compartment.

Following the exchange of substances with the tissues, the blood begins its route back to the heart through the venous system. Blood flows from the capillaries into the *venules*. These small vessels consist mainly of a layer of endothelium and fibrous connective tissue. From the venules, the blood flows into *veins* that become larger as they travel toward the heart. As with the arteries, the walls of these vessels consist of a layer of endothelium, elastic connective tissue, smooth muscle and fibrous connective tissue. However, veins have much thinner walls and wider diameters than the arteries they accompany. These vessels are quite distensible and capable of holding large volumes of blood at a very low pressure. For this reason, the veins are the major *compliance vessels* of the circulatory system (see Figure 6.1). In fact, approximately 64% of the blood volume is contained within the veins under resting conditions. During exercise, the pumping action of the contracting skeletal muscles and the constriction of smooth muscle in the walls of the veins force this blood toward the heart and increase venous return (VR). Therefore, the veins are referred to as *blood reservoirs*. As such, they play an important role in the regulation of VR and, consequently, CO.

Another important anatomical characteristic of the veins is the presence of *valves*. These valves ensure the one-way flow of blood back toward the heart. They are most abundant in the lower limbs where the effects of gravity on the circulatory system are most prevalent and would tend to cause the pooling of blood in the ankles and feet.

Large veins and the *venae cavae* return the blood to the right atrium of the heart. As with the large arteries and the aorta, these vessels function primarily as conduits. There is little smooth muscle and, therefore, little physiological regulation of their diameter.

6.2   Blood pressure

The pressure generated by left ventricular contraction is the driving force for the flow of blood through the entire systemic circulation, from the aorta, through the tissues, and back to the right atrium. The mean pressure in the aorta and the large arteries is typically very high (90–100 mmHg) due to the continual addition of blood to the system by the pumping action of the heart. However, this pressure is *pulsatile*. In other words, it fluctuates due to the alternating contraction and relaxation phases of the cardiac cycle. In a healthy resting adult, *systolic pressure* is approximately 120 mmHg and *diastolic pressure* is approximately 80 mmHg (see Figure 6.2). The *pulse pressure* (PP) is the difference between the systolic and the diastolic pressures:

$$Pulse\ pressure = Systolic\ pressure - Diastolic\ pressure$$

Therefore, using the average values of 120 mmHg (systolic) and 80 mmHg (diastolic), the pulse pressure may be determined:

$$PP = 120\ mmHg - 80\ mmHg = 40\ mmHg$$

The *mean arterial pressure (MAP)* is calculated as follows:

$$MAP = Diastolic\ pressure + 1/3\ (Pulse\ pressure)$$

Therefore, using these same values, the MAP may be determined:

$$MAP = 80\ mmHg + 1/3\ (40\ mmHg) = 93\ mmHg$$

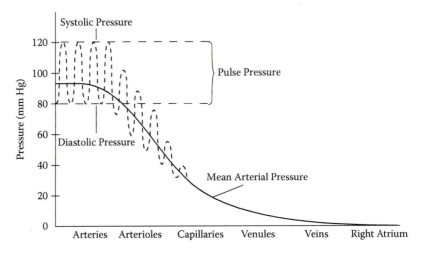

Figure 6.2 Pressures throughout the systemic circulation. At rest, blood pressure in the aorta and the other large arteries fluctuates between a low pressure of 80 mmHg during ventricular diastole and a high pressure of 120 mmHg during ventricular systole. The difference between the diastolic pressure and the systolic pressure is the pulse pressure. Mean arterial pressure in these arteries is approximately 93 mmHg. As the blood continues forward and flows through the arterioles, the pulse pressure is dampened. Because of the high resistance to blood flow in these vessels, the overall pressure drops dramatically. Furthermore, the fluctuations between diastolic pressure and systolic pressure are eliminated so that the blood pressure becomes nonpulsatile. Blood pressure continues to decline, although at a slower rate, as the blood flows through the capillaries and veins back toward the heart.

At rest, the MAP is closer to the diastolic pressure because the diastolic phase of the cardiac cycle lasts almost twice as long as the systolic phase. During exercise when heart rate increases and the length of diastole decreases, the systolic pressure contributes more to the MAP.

As the blood flows through the rest of the system, the pressure continually falls (see Figure 6.2). In addition, the pulsatile nature of the blood pressure is lost as the blood flows through the arterioles. The pulse pressure is damped out by the considerable resistance offered to blood flow by the arterioles. At the arteriolar end of the capillaries, the blood pressure is 30–35 mmHg and at the venular end, the capillary pressure is approximately 10 mmHg. It is important that capillary pressure remains low to avoid the leakage of fluid out of the capillaries into the tissues. Venous pressure is approximately 6–8 mmHg and pressure in the right atrium is close to zero.

6.3   Blood flow

The *flow of blood through a vessel* is determined by two factors:

- Pressure gradient
- Vascular resistance

The relationship between blood flow (Q, milliliters per minute [mL/min]), the pressure gradient (ΔP, millimeters mercury [mmHg]), and vascular resistance (R, millimeters mercury per milliliter per minute [mmHg/mL per min]) is described by *Ohm's Law*:

$$Q = \frac{\Delta P}{R}$$

The *pressure gradient* is the difference between the pressure at the beginning of a blood vessel and the pressure at the end of the blood vessel. The inflow pressure is always greater than the outflow pressure because substances, including blood and air, must flow "down" their pressure gradients; in other words, from an area of higher pressure to an area of lower pressure. The inflow pressure is initially generated by the contraction of the heart. As discussed previously, the blood pressure falls continuously as the blood flows through the circulatory system. This loss of driving pressure is due to the friction generated as the components of the flowing blood that encounter the vessel wall as well as each other. Blood flow through a vessel is directly proportional to the pressure gradient; in other words, the greater the difference between the inflow pressure and the outflow pressure, the greater the flow of blood through the vessel.

The second factor that determines the flow of blood through a vessel is *resistance*. In contrast to the pressure gradient, blood flow through a vessel is indirectly proportional to the resistance. In other words, resistance impedes or opposes blood flow. There are three factors that affect vascular resistance:

- Blood viscosity
- Vessel length
- Vessel radius

Viscosity describes the friction developed between the molecules of a fluid as they interact with each other during flow. More simply put, the "thicker" the fluid, then the greater the viscosity of the fluid. Interestingly, blood is approximately three times more viscous than water.

Viscosity and resistance are directly proportional so that as the viscosity of the fluid increases the resistance to flow increases. In the case of blood flow through the circulatory system, erythrocytes (red blood cells) suspended in the blood are the primary factor determining viscosity. Blood cells exert a frictional drag against each other and against the wall of the blood vessel. *Hematocrit,* the percentage of the blood that consists of red blood cells, is 40%–54% (average = 47%) for an adult male and 37%–47% (average = 43%) for an adult female. Under normal physiological conditions, hematocrit and, therefore, blood viscosity do not vary considerably within an individual. Only pathological conditions, such as chronic hypoxia, sickle cell anemia, and excess blood fibrinogen, may result in hyperviscosity and, consequently, impaired blood flow.

As mentioned previously, friction also develops as blood contacts the vessel wall while flowing through it. Therefore, the greater the vessel surface area in contact with the blood, the greater the amount of friction developed and the greater the resistance to blood flow. Two factors determine the vessel surface area: the length of the vessel and the vessel radius.

The longer the vessel, the more the blood comes into contact with the vessel wall and the greater the resistance. However, *vessel length* in the body remains constant. Therefore, as with blood viscosity, it is not a variable factor causing changes in resistance.

The most important physiological variable determining the resistance to blood flow is *vessel radius*. A given volume of blood comes into less contact with the wall of a vessel with a large radius compared to a vessel with a small radius. Therefore, as the radius of a vessel increases, the resistance to blood flow decreases. In other words, blood flows more readily through a larger vessel than it does through a smaller vessel.

Small changes in vessel radius result in significant changes in vascular resistance and in blood flow. This is because the resistance is inversely proportional to the fourth power of the radius:

$$R \propto 1/r^4$$

If this equation is substituted into Ohm's Law, then blood flow may be calculated as follows:

$$Q = \frac{\Delta P}{1/r^4}$$

Assume two blood vessels of equal length each have a pressure gradient of 1 mmHg. However, blood vessel A has a radius of 1 mm, and blood vessel B has a radius of 2 mm. The flow of blood through vessel A is 1 mL/min, and the flow of blood through vessel B is 16 mL/min. Simply doubling vessel radius causes a 16-fold increase in blood flow.

As mentioned previously, the arterioles are the major resistance vessels in the circulatory system. Because the walls of these vessels contain primarily smooth muscle, they are capable of significant changes in their radius. Therefore, the regulation of blood flow to the tissues is carried out by the arterioles.

Ohm's Law may be rewritten to include the three factors that affect vascular resistance; blood viscosity (η), vessel length (L), and vessel radius (r). The following equation is known as *Poiseuille's Law*:

$$Q = \frac{\pi \, \Delta P \, r^4}{8 \, \eta \, L}$$

6.4   Regulation of arterial pressure

The MAP is the driving force for blood flow through the body's organs and tissues. The MAP must be closely monitored and regulated for several reasons. It must be high enough to provide a force that is sufficient to propel the blood through the entire systemic circuit; from the heart to the top of the head, down to the tips of the toes, and back to the heart again. *Hypotension*, or a fall in blood pressure, may cause insufficient blood flow to the brain, causing dizziness and, perhaps, fainting. However, *hypertension*, or a blood pressure that is too high, may be detrimental to the cardiovascular system. An increase in diastolic pressure increases the afterload on the heart and increases cardiac workload. Furthermore, a chronic elevation in blood pressure increases the risk of various types of vascular damage, such as atherosclerosis and the rupture of small blood vessels. Atherosclerosis will often occur in arteries that supply the heart and the brain, and it impairs the flow of blood to these tissues. The rupture of small blood vessels allows fluid to move from the vascular compartment into the tissues, resulting in edema formation. Several factors that may alter MAP are listed in Table 6.2.

Ohm's Law, which correlates the influence of blood pressure and vascular resistance on blood flow through a vessel (Q = ΔP/R), may also be applied to blood flow through the entire systemic circulation, or CO:

$$\text{Cardiac Output} = \frac{\text{Mean Arterial Pressure}}{\text{Total Peripheral Resistance}}$$

This equation can be reorganized to determine MAP:

$$\text{Mean Arterial Pressure} = \text{Cardiac Output} \times \text{Total Peripheral Resistance}$$

Total peripheral resistance (TPR) is the resistance to blood flow offered by all the systemic vessels taken together, especially by the arterioles, which are the primary resistance vessels. Therefore, MAP is regulated by cardiac activity and vascular smooth muscle tone. Any change in CO or TPR causes a change in MAP. A summary of major cardiovascular principles may be found in Table 6.3.

Table 6.2   Factors that alter blood pressure

Increase in blood pressure
- Decreased blood flow to the brain
- Pain originating in the skin
- Anger, anxiety
- Sexual activity
- Fight-or-flight response
- Exercise
- Collapse of the lungs
- Nicotine
- Caffeine

Decrease in blood pressure
- Pain originating in viscera or joints
- Sleeping
- Happiness
- Inflation of the lungs
- Dehydration
- Shock
  - Cardiogenic
  - Hypovolemic
  - Septic
  - Anaphylactic

Table 6.3   Summary of major cardiovascular principles

$$CO = VR$$

$$CO = HR \times SV$$

$$SV = EDV - ESV$$

$$Q = \frac{\Delta P}{R}$$

$$R \alpha \frac{1}{r^4}$$

$$\text{Pulse Pressure} = P_{systolic} - P_{diastolic}$$

$$MAP = P_{diastolic} + 1/3 \left(\text{Pulse Pressure} \right)$$

$$MAP = CO \times TPR$$

$$VR = \frac{P_V - P_{RA}}{R_V}$$

Notes: CO, cardiac output; VR, venous return; HR, heart rate; SV, stroke volume; EDV, end-diastolic volume; ESV, end-systolic volume; Q, blood flow; ΔP, pressure gradient; R, resistance; r, vessel radius; $P_{systolic}$, systolic pressure; $P_{diastolic}$, diastolic pressure; MAP, mean arterial pressure; TPR, total peripheral resistance, P_V, venous pressure; PRA, right atrial pressure; R_V, venous resistance.

The relationship between CO, TPR and MAP may be considered further. Recall from the earlier discussion that MAP may be calculated from the systolic pressure (SP) and the diastolic pressure (DP):

$$MAP = DP + 1/3(SP - DP)$$

In a healthy individual under normal physiological conditions, systolic pressure is determined primarily by SV. Therefore, any factor that alters SV (and CO) will alter systolic pressure and MAP. Diastolic pressure is determined primarily by TPR. Therefore, any factor that alters TPR will alter diastolic pressure and MAP.

The major factors that affect CO, TPR and, therefore, MAP are summarized in Figure 6.3. These factors may be organized into several categories and will be discussed as such:

- Autonomic nervous systems
- Vasoactive substances
- Venous return
- Local metabolic activity

The effects of the *autonomic nervous system* on MAP are summarized in Figure 6.4. The *parasympathetic system* innervates the SA node and the AV node of the heart. The major cardiovascular effect of parasympathetic stimulation, by way of the vagus nerve, is to decrease HR, which decreases CO and MAP.

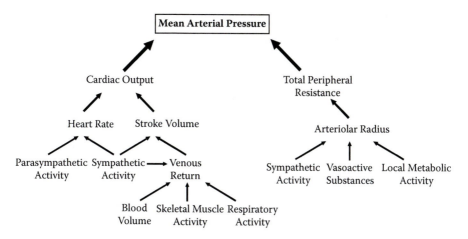

Figure 6.3 Factors that affect mean arterial pressure. Mean arterial pressure is determined by cardiac output (CO) and total peripheral resistance. Important factors that influence these two variables are summarized in this figure.

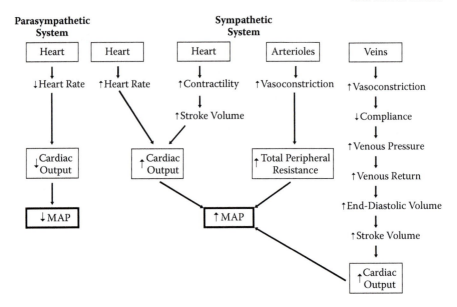

Figure 6.4 Effects of sympathetic and parasympathetic nervous activity on mean arterial pressure. The parasympathetic nervous system innervates the heart and, therefore, influences heart rate and cardiac output (CO). The sympathetic nervous system innervates the heart and the veins and, therefore, influences CO. This system also innervates the arterioles and, therefore, influences total peripheral resistance (TPR). The resulting changes in CO and TPR regulate mean arterial pressure.

The *sympathetic system* innervates most tissues in the heart, including the SA node, the AV node and the ventricular muscle. Sympathetic stimulation causes an increase in HR as well as an increase in ventricular contractility, which enhances SV. The increases in HR and SV cause an increase in CO and, therefore, MAP.

The sympathetic system also innervates vascular smooth muscle and regulates the radius of the blood vessels. All types of blood vessels except capillaries are innervated; however, the most densely innervated vessels include the arterioles and the veins. An increase in sympathetic stimulation of vascular smooth muscle causes vasoconstriction and a decrease in stimulation causes vasodilation. Constriction of arterioles causes an increase in TPR and, therefore, MAP. Constriction of veins causes an increase in VR, which increases end-diastolic volume (EDV), SV (Frank-Starling Law of the Heart), CO and MAP.

Sympathetic nerves are distributed to most vascular beds but are more abundant in the renal, gastrointestinal, splenic, and cutaneous circulations. Recall that these tissues receive an abundant blood flow, more than is necessary to simply maintain metabolism. Therefore, when blood is needed by other parts of the body, such as working skeletal muscles, sympathetic vasoconstrictor activity reduces flow to the tissues receiving excess blood so that it may be redirected to the muscles. Interestingly, there is no sympathetic innervation to cerebral blood vessels. In fact, these vessels do not have α_1-adrenergic receptors so that they cannot be affected by circulating catecholamines. There is no physiological circumstance where blood should be directed away from the brain.

6.4.1   Vasomotor center

Autonomic nervous activity to the cardiovascular system is regulated by the *vasomotor center* (see Figure 6.5). Located in the lower pons and the medulla of the brainstem, the vasomotor center is an integrating center for blood pressure regulation. It receives several sources of input, from the brain as well as the periphery of the body. It processes this information and then adjusts sympathetic and parasympathetic discharge to the heart and the blood vessels accordingly.

Sympathetic nerves going to the arterioles are tonically active. In other words, there is continuous discharge of these nerves, causing *vasomotor tone*. Under resting conditions, this tone results in arterioles being partially constricted. Vasomotor tone is important because it helps to maintain MAP in the range of 90–100 mmHg. Without this partial vasoconstriction of the arterioles, MAP would fall precipitously and blood flow to the vital organs would be compromised. Another physiological advantage of vasomotor tone is that the degree of vasoconstriction can be either increased or decreased. In this way, blood flow to the tissue can be either increased or decreased. Without tone, the vessels could only constrict, and blood flow to the tissue could only decrease.

Other regions of the vasomotor center transmit impulses to the heart via sympathetic nerves or the branches of the vagus nerve. An increase in sympathetic activity to the heart typically occurs concurrently with

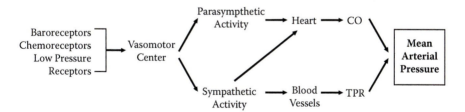

Figure 6.5 The vasomotor center. The baroreceptors, the chemoreceptors and the low-pressure receptors provide nervous input to the vasomotor center in the brainstem. The vasomotor center integrates this input and determines the degree of discharge by the sympathetic nervous system and the parasympathetic nervous system to the cardiovascular system. Cardiac output and total peripheral resistance are adjusted to maintain mean arterial pressure within the normal range.

Table 6.4   Cardiovascular receptors and their stimuli

Receptor	Stimulus
Baroreceptors	Blood pressure
Chemoreceptors	Blood gases ($\downarrow O_2$, $\uparrow CO_2$, $\downarrow pH$)
Low-pressure receptors	Blood volume

an increase in sympathetic activity to the blood vessels and a decrease in vagal stimulation of the heart. Therefore, the resulting increases in CO and TPR work together to elevate MAP more effectively. Conversely, an increase in vagal stimulation of the heart typically occurs concurrently with a decrease in sympathetic activity to both the heart and the blood vessels. Therefore, decreases in both CO and TPR work together to decrease MAP more effectively.

The vasomotor center receives input from multiple sources (summarized in Table 6.4 and Figure 6.5) including:

- Baroreceptors
- Chemoreceptors
- Low-pressure receptors

6.4.2 Baroreceptors

The *baroreceptors* provide the most important source of input to the vasomotor center. These receptors monitor *blood pressure* in the systemic circulatory system. They are found in two locations: the arch of the aorta and the carotid sinuses. As the aorta exits the left ventricle, it curves over the top of the heart, forming an arch, and then descends through the thoracic and abdominal cavities. The coronary arteries, which supply the cardiac muscle, branch off the aorta in this most proximal portion of the aorta. The left and right common carotid arteries also branch off the aortic arch and ascend through the neck toward the head. Each common carotid artery bifurcates, or divides, forming an external carotid artery, which supplies the scalp, and an internal carotid artery, which supplies the brain. The carotid sinus is located at the bifurcation of each common carotid artery. Because blood flow to a tissue is dependent, in large part, upon blood pressure, the baroreceptors are ideally located to monitor blood pressure in regions of the circulatory system responsible for delivering blood to the heart and brain, the two most vital organs in the body.

The baroreceptors respond to stretch or distension of the blood vessel walls. Therefore, they are also referred to as *stretch receptors*. A change in blood pressure will elicit the *baroreceptor reflex*, which involves *negative feedback responses* that return the blood pressure to normal (see Figure 6.6). For example, an increase in blood pressure causes distension of the aorta

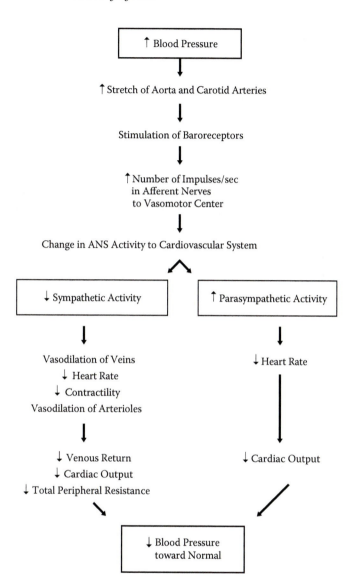

Figure 6.6 The baroreceptor reflex. The baroreceptors are the most important source of input to the vasomotor center. The reflex elicited by these receptors is essential in the maintenance of normal blood pressure.

and the carotid arteries, which stimulates the baroreceptors and there is an increase in the number of afferent nerve impulses transmitted from these receptors to the vasomotor center. The vasomotor center processes this information and adjusts the activity of the autonomic nervous system accordingly. Sympathetic stimulation of vascular smooth muscle and cardiac muscle is decreased. Parasympathetic stimulation of cardiac muscle is increased. Thus, VR, CO, and TPR all decrease so that MAP is decreased back toward its normal value.

On the other hand, a decrease in blood pressure causes less than normal distension or stretch of the aorta and the carotid arteries and a decrease in baroreceptor stimulation. Therefore, fewer afferent nerve impulses are transmitted from these receptors to the vasomotor center. The vasomotor center then alters autonomic nervous system activity such that sympathetic stimulation of vascular smooth muscle and cardiac muscle is increased and parasympathetic stimulation of cardiac muscle is decreased and VR, CO, and TPR increase so that MAP is increased back toward its normal value. The effects of the autonomic nervous system on the cardiovascular system are summarized in Figure 6.5.

It is important to note that the baroreceptor reflex is elicited whether blood pressure increases or decreases. Furthermore, these receptors are most sensitive in the normal range of blood pressures so that even a small change in MAP will alter baroreceptor, vasomotor center, and autonomic nervous system activity. As such, the baroreceptor reflex plays an important role in the short-term regulation of blood pressure. Without this reflex, changes in blood pressure in response to changes in posture, hydration (blood volume), CO, regional vascular resistance, and emotional state would be far more pronounced. The baroreceptor reflex helps to minimize unintentional changes in MAP and maintain adequate blood flow to the tissues.

6.4.3 Chemoreceptors

The *peripheral chemoreceptors* include the *carotid bodies*, located at the bifurcation of the common carotid arteries, and the *aortic bodies*, located in the arch of the aorta. These receptors are stimulated by a decrease in arterial oxygen (*hypoxemia*), an increase in arterial carbon dioxide (*hypercapnia*), and a decrease in arterial pH (*acidosis*). Therefore, as may be expected, the chemoreceptors are primarily concerned with the regulation of ventilation. A secondary function of these receptors is to influence MAP by providing input to the vasomotor center. A decrease in blood pressure causes a decrease in blood flow to the carotid and aortic bodies. Assuming a constant rate of metabolism in these tissues (constant oxygen consumption as well as carbon dioxide and hydrogen ion production), then a decrease in blood flow results in hypoxemia, hypercapnia, and a decrease in local pH. These conditions stimulate the chemoreceptors and cause an increase in the number of nerve impulses transmitted from these receptors to the vasomotor center. The vasomotor center processes this input and adjusts the activity of the autonomic nervous system accordingly. Sympathetic discharge to the cardiovascular system is increased. The predominant effect is an increase in TPR. Because of this negative feedback mechanism, MAP is increased and blood flow to the chemoreceptors is increased back toward its normal value. Interestingly, the chemoreceptor reflex does not affect the cardiovascular system until MAP decreases below 80 mmHg. Therefore, unlike the baroreceptor reflex, this reflex does not help to minimize the daily variations in MAP. Instead, it supplements the activity of the baroreceptor reflex at lower pressures only.

6.4.4   Low-pressure receptors

The *low-pressure receptors* are found within the walls of the atria and the pulmonary arteries. Similar to baroreceptors, low-pressure receptors are also stretch receptors. However, stimulation of these receptors is caused by changes in blood volume in these lower pressure areas. An overall increase in blood volume results in an increase in VR, an increase in the blood volume in the atria and the pulmonary arteries, and stimulation of the low-pressure receptors. Transmission of nerve impulses to the vasomotor center occurs by way of the branches of the vagus nerve. The vasomotor center then elicits reflexes that parallel those of the baroreceptors. An increase in blood volume will initially increase MAP. Therefore, sympathetic discharge decreases and parasympathetic discharge increases so that MAP decreases back toward its normal value. The simultaneous activity of both the baroreceptors and the low-pressure receptors makes the total reflex system more effective in the control of MAP.

The low-pressure receptors may also be referred to as *atrial stretch receptors*. Increased atrial filling and stimulation of these receptors elicit additional compensatory responses including:

- Reflex tachycardia (Bainbridge reflex)
- Reflex vasodilation of renal afferent arterioles
- Decreased secretion of ADH
- Increased secretion of ANP
- Increased urine output (volume reflex)

The net result is a decrease in plasma volume and a decrease in MAP back toward normal.

Vasoactive substances are substances released from many cells and tissues in the body, including the endothelium lining the blood vessels, endocrine glands, and myocytes in the heart, and may all affect vascular smooth muscle tone (see Table 6.5). These substances may either stimulate this muscle to cause vasoconstriction or inhibit this muscle to cause vasodilation. As expected, vasoconstriction will increase TPR and, therefore, MAP. Vasodilation will decrease TPR and, therefore, MAP.

Table 6.5 Vasoactive substances

Vasoconstrictors	Source
Catecholamines	Adrenal medullae
Angiotensin II	Plasma
Vasopressin	Neurohypophysis
Endothelin	Endothelium
Thromboxane A_2	Platelets
Serotonin	Platelets

Vasodilators	Source
Prostacyclin	Endothelium
Nitric oxide	Endothelium
Atrial natriuretic peptide	Atrial myocardial cells
Histamine	Mast cells, basophils
Bradykinin	Plasma, interstitial fluid
Adenosine	Hypoxic cells
Epinephrine	Adrenal medullae

6.4.5 Vasoconstrictors

There are many substances produced in the human body that cause vasoconstriction under physiological and pathophysiological conditions. Important *vasoconstrictors* include:

- Catecholamines
- Angiotensin II
- Vasopressin
- Endothelin
- Thromboxane A_2
- Serotonin

The major circulating hormones that influence vascular smooth muscle tone are the *catecholamines*, epinephrine, and norepinephrine. These hormones are released from the adrenal medulla in response to sympathetic nervous stimulation. In humans, 80% of catecholamine secretion is epinephrine and 20% is norepinephrine. Stimulation of α_1-adrenergic receptors causes vasoconstriction. The selective α_1-adrenergic receptor antagonist, prazosin, is effective in the management of hypertension because it causes the relaxation of both arterial and venous smooth muscle.

Angiotensin II is a circulating peptide with powerful vasoconstrictor properties. The formation of angiotensin II is initiated by the enzyme, renin, which converts the plasma-borne precursor, angiotensinogen, into angiotensin I. Angiotensin-converting enzyme (ACE) then converts angiotensin I into the active molecule, angiotensin II. The location of ACE is ideal for this function because it is found on the surface of endothelial cells in the lungs, which are exposed to the entire CO. The release of renin from specialized cells in the kidneys occurs in response to sympathetic stimulation and when there is a decrease in renal blood flow.

Angiotensin II causes vasoconstriction by the direct stimulation of AT_1 receptors on the vascular smooth muscle. It also enhances the release of the neurotransmitter, norepinephrine, from the sympathetic nerve fibers present in the blood vessels. The vasopressor effects of angiotensin II may be inhibited pharmacologically to decrease TPR and treat hypertension. An important class of orally active drugs is the ACE inhibitors, including captopril and enalapril, which prevent the formation of angiotensin II. More recently, angiotensin receptor antagonists have been developed that act at the vascular smooth muscle. These drugs, including losartan and valsartan, are also orally active.

Vasopressin (anti-diuretic hormone) is a peptide synthesized in the hypothalamus and secreted from the neurohypophysis of the pituitary gland. This substance plays an important role in the long-term regulation of blood pressure through its action on the kidney to increase the reabsorption of water. The major stimulus for the release of vasopressin is an increase in plasma osmolarity. The resulting reabsorption of water dilutes the plasma back toward its normal value of 290 mOsM. This activity is discussed in more detail in Chapter 11, *The Endocrine System* and Chapter 10, *The Renal System*.

Vasopressin also plays an important role in the short-term regulation of blood pressure through its action on vascular smooth muscle. This hormone is one of the most potent known endogenous vasoconstrictors. Two types of vasopressin receptors have been identified: V_1 and V_2 receptors. V_{1A} receptors mediate vasoconstriction and V_2 receptors mediate the antidiuretic effects of this hormone. Specific V_{1A} receptor antagonists of the vasoconstrictor activity of vasopressin are under development.

The vascular endothelium produces several substances that are released basally into the blood vessel wall to alter vascular smooth muscle tone. One such substance is *endothelin*. Endothelin exerts its effects throughout the body causing vasoconstriction as well as positive inotropic and chronotropic effects on the heart. The resulting increases in TPR and CO both contribute to an increase in MAP.

Synthesis of endothelin appears to be enhanced by many stimuli including angiotensin II, vasopressin and the mechanical stress of blood flow on the endothelium. Synthesis is inhibited by vasodilator substances, such as prostacyclin, nitric oxide and atrial natriuretic peptide. There is evidence that endothelin is involved with the pathophysiology of many cardiovascular diseases, including hypertension, heart failure, and myocardial infarction. Endothelin receptor antagonists are currently available for research use only.

Another vasoactive substance produced by the endothelium is *thromboxane A_2 (TxA_2)*. Normally, small amounts of TxA_2 are released continuously; however, increased synthesis appears to be associated with some cardiac diseases.

Synthesized from arachidonic acid, a plasma membrane phospholipid, TxA$_2$ is a potent vasoconstrictor. Furthermore, this substance stimulates platelet aggregation, suggesting that it plays a role in thrombotic events such as myocardial infarction (heart attack). Nonsteroidal anti-inflammatory drugs, such as aspirin and ibuprofen, block the formation of TxA$_2$ and reduce the formation of blood clots.

Serotonin is released from platelets. Along with TxA$_2$, serotonin enhances the vasoconstriction that occurs when a blood vessel is damaged (Table 6.6). The resulting decrease in blood flow contributes to hemostasis, which was discussed in Chapter 5, *Blood and Hemostasis*.

Table 6.6

Drug classification	Generic agents	CO	TPR	PV
Diuretics		↔	↓	↓/↔
Thiazides	Hydrochlorothiazide			
	Chlorthalidone			
	Chlorothiazide			
	Indapamide			
	Metolazone			
Loop diuretics	Furosemide			
	Bumetanide			
	Ethacrynic acid			
	Torsemide			
K$^+$-Sparing diuretics	Amiloride			
	Eplerenone			
	Spironolactone			
Sympatholytics				
Centrally acting	Methyldopa	↓/↔	↓	↔
	Clonidine			
	Guanfacine			
β-Antagonist	Propranolol	↓	↓	↔
α-Antagonist	Prazosin	↔	↓	↔
Vasodilators				
Arterial	Hydralazine	↑	↓	↑
Arterial and venous	Nitroprusside	↔	↓	↔
Ca^{++}-Channel Blockers	Verapamil	↓	↓	↔
	Nifedipine	↔	↓	↔
	Diltiazem	↓	↓	↔
ACE Inhibitors	Captopril	↑	↓	↓
	Enalapril			
Angiotensin II-Antagonists	Losartan	↑	↓	↓
	Valsartan			
	Azilsartan			

PHARMACY APPLICATION: ANTIHYPERTENSIVE DRUGS

Hypertension is the most common cardiovascular disease. In fact, nearly 25% of the adults in the United States are considered hypertensive. Hypertension is defined as a consistent elevation in blood pressure, such that systolic/diastolic pressures are >140/90 mmHg. Over time, chronic hypertension can cause pathological changes in the vasculature and in the heart. Therefore, hypertensive patients are at increased risk for atherosclerosis, aneurysm, stroke, myocardial infarction, heart failure, and kidney failure.

There are several categories of antihypertensive agents:

- Diuretics. Initially, the primary mechanism by which diuretics reduce blood pressure is to decrease plasma volume. Acting at the kidney, diuretics increase sodium loss and, due to the osmotic effects of sodium, increase water loss. The decrease in plasma volume results in a decrease in VR, CO, and MAP. However, the long-term hypotensive effect of the diuretics appears to be due to a decrease in TPR.
- Sympatholytics. Sympathetic stimulation of the cardiovascular system may be altered by several mechanisms.
  - *Centrally acting agents* exert their effects at the vasomotor center in the brainstem and inhibit sympathetic discharge. Reduced sympathetic stimulation of the heart and, especially the vascular smooth muscle, results in some decrease in CO, especially in older patients, and a marked decrease in TPR.
  - *Beta-adrenergic receptor antagonists* reduce myocardial contractility and CO. These agents also reduce the secretion of renin. Therefore, their effects on reducing blood pressure can be explained, in part, by a reduction in the formation of angiotensin II. However, this mechanism does not fully account for the antihypertensive effects of beta blockers. These drugs also reduce peripheral vascular resistance, although, the mechanism of this effect is not known.
  - *Alpha-adrenergic receptor antagonists* reduce peripheral vascular resistance and, therefore, reduce blood pressure.
- Vasodilators. Hydralazine causes direct relaxation of arteriolar smooth muscle. An important consequence of this vasodilation, however, is reflex tachycardia ($\uparrow$CO). It may also cause sodium retention ($\uparrow$plasma volume). The resulting increase in CO tends to offset the effects of the vasodilator. Therefore, these drugs are most effective when administered along with sympathetic agents such as β-adrenergic receptor antagonists that prevent unwanted compensatory responses by the heart.

(Continued)

PHARMACY APPLICATION: ANTIHYPERTENSIVE DRUGS (Continued)

- Ca^{++}-channel blockers. The dihydropyridine agents, such as amlodipine (Norvasc®) and felodipine (Plendil®), are the preferred types of calcium channel blockers used in the treatment of hypertension because they lack inotropic and chronotropic effects on the heart. Therefore, the mechanism of action of these drugs involves a marked decrease in peripheral vascular resistance. Furthermore, they cause less reflex tachycardia than nifedipine.
- ACE inhibitors. ACE inhibitors not only cause vasodilation (↓TPR), they inhibit the aldosterone response to net sodium loss. Normally, aldosterone, which enhances the reabsorption of sodium in the kidney, would oppose diuretic-induced sodium loss. Therefore, the coadministration of ACE inhibitors would enhance the efficacy of diuretic drugs.
- Angiotensin II receptor antagonists. These agents promote vasodilation (↓TPR), increase sodium and water excretion and, therefore, decrease plasma volume. ACE inhibitors and angiotensin II receptor antagonists are the drugs of first choice in patients with heart failure.

6.4.6 Vasodilators

Many substances produced in the human body cause vasodilation under physiological and pathophysiological conditions. *Vasodilators* of particular importance include:

- Prostacyclin
- Nitric oxide
- Atrial natriuretic peptide
- Histamine
- Bradykinin
- Adenosine
- Epinephrine

Another metabolite of arachidonic acid is *prostacyclin* (PGI_2). As with TxA_2, PGI_2 is produced continuously. Synthesized by vascular smooth muscle and endothelial cells, with the endothelium as the predominant source, PGI_2 mediates effects that are opposite to those of TxA_2. Prostacyclin causes vasodilation and inhibits platelet aggregation. Therefore, PGI_2 contributes importantly to the antithrombogenic nature of the vascular wall.

First described in the 1980s as "endothelium-derived relaxing factor," *nitric oxide (NO)* is a vasodilator believed to play a role in the regulation of blood pressure under both physiologic and pathophysiological conditions.

PHARMACY APPLICATION: NITROGLYCERIN AND ANGINA

Angina pectoris (chest pain) is the most common symptom of chronic ischemic heart disease. Angina is caused by an imbalance between the oxygen supply and the oxygen demand of the cardiac muscle. Myocardial oxygen demand increases during exertion, exercise and emotional stress. If coronary blood flow does not increase proportionately to meet this demand, then the affected tissue becomes ischemic and pain develops. This ischemia and pain may be treated pharmacologically with nitroglycerin. This drug causes vasodilation and an increase in blood flow. However, this effect occurs not only in the coronary arteries, but in blood vessels throughout the body. Therefore, in addition to improving coronary blood flow, administration of nitroglycerin may decrease systemic blood pressure. The mechanism of action of nitroglycerin involves the release of NO in the vascular smooth muscle. Most frequently, this drug is administered in the sublingual form and its effects are apparent within 1–3 minutes.

For example, the pharmacologic inhibition of NO synthesis under normal conditions and during septic shock results in a significant elevation of blood pressure. *Atrial natriuretic peptide* (ANP) is produced by specialized myocytes in the atria of the heart. Secretion is stimulated by increased filling and stretch of the atria in response to plasma volume expansion. The effects of ANP include vasodilation, diuresis (increased urine production) and increased sodium excretion. Taken together, these effects decrease blood volume and blood pressure back toward normal.

Histamine and *bradykinin* are important mediators of inflammation. The actions of these substances were discussed in detail in Chapter 3, *The Immune System*.

Adenosine is an important mediator of active hyperemia. This phenomenon is discussed later in this chapter in the section 6.7, *Regulation of blood flow through tissues*.

Epinephrine may cause vasodilation at higher concentrations due to the stimulation of β_2-adrenergic receptors on vascular smooth muscle. These receptors are found primarily on blood vessels in skeletal muscles and in the hepatic and coronary circulations.

6.5 Venous regulation

The vessels of the circulatory system have varying degrees of *distensibility*. This feature allows them to accommodate changes in blood volume. For example, the abrupt addition of the SV to the aorta and large arteries during ventricular systole causes these vessels to expand and "store" a portion of the blood pumped by the heart. The subsequent elastic recoil of the arteries forces the stored blood forward during ventricular diastole. Therefore, the slight distensibility of arteries results in the maintenance of blood flow to the tissues throughout the cardiac cycle.

The most distensible vessels in the circulatory system are the veins. As with the arteries, this feature of the veins also has important physiological implications because it allows them to serve as *blood reservoirs*. The veins are so distensible they can hold large volumes of blood at very low pressures. In fact, under resting conditions, 64% of the blood volume is contained within these vessels.

Compliance (C) in the circulatory system describes the relationship between vascular blood volume (V) and intravascular pressure (P):

$$C = \frac{V}{P}$$

In other words, it is a measure of the inherent distensibility of the blood vessels. The more compliant the vessel, then the greater the volume of blood that it is capable of accommodating.

As mentioned, all blood vessels are compliant. However, the marked difference in distensibility between the arteries and the veins is illustrated by the following:

Compliance of the systemic arteries at rest;

$$C = \frac{13\% \text{ of the blood volume}}{100 \text{ mmHg}}$$

Compliance of the systemic veins at rest;

$$C = \frac{64\% \text{ of the blood volume}}{8 \text{ mmHg}}$$

Due to the significant amount of elastic connective tissue and smooth muscle in their walls, arteries tend to recoil rather powerfully, which keeps the pressure within them high. Of course, this elevated pressure is necessary to drive the blood through the circulatory system. In contrast, veins contain less elastic connective tissue and smooth muscle so the tendency to recoil is significantly less and the pressure remains low.

The venous system, in general, serves as a reservoir for the circulatory system. However, there are some tissues that are particularly important in this respect. These *specific blood reservoirs* include the spleen, the liver, the large abdominal veins and the venous plexus beneath the skin. Common features of the vascular beds within these tissues are that they are very extensive and very compliant. In this way, under normal, resting conditions these vascular beds can accommodate large volumes of blood. In fact, taken together, these tissues may hold up to 1 L of blood, or 20% of the blood volume. Under pathological conditions, such as hemorrhage or dehydration, blood may be mobilized from these tissues, allowing the circulatory system to function relatively normally until the blood volume is restored to normal.

In addition to serving as blood reservoirs, veins help to *regulate* CO by way of changes in VR. VR is defined as the volume of blood that flows from the systemic veins into the right atrium per minute. As will be discussed in Chapter 7, a healthy heart pumps all the blood returned to it. Therefore, CO is equal to VR:

$$CO = VR$$

On the other hand, the heart can only pump whatever blood it receives. Therefore, to increase CO, then VR must also increase.

As with blood flow through a vessel, blood flow through the venous system is determined by Ohm's Law ($Q = \Delta P/R$). In other words, it depends on the pressure gradient in the venous system and venous resistance. Ohm's Law may be rewritten to calculate VR:

$$VR = \frac{P_V - P_{RA}}{R_V}$$

The pressure gradient, or the inflow pressure minus the outflow pressure, is determined by the pressure at the beginning of the venous system (P_V) and right atrial pressure (P_{RA}) at the end of the system. The smaller compliant veins offer very little resistance to blood flow. The slightly stiffer large veins offer a small degree of resistance (R_V).

There are several factors that influence VR including:

- Blood volume
- Sympathetic stimulation of the veins
- Skeletal muscle activity
- Respiratory activity

6.5.1   Blood volume

Blood volume has a direct effect on blood pressure. It also has an important effect on VR. A decrease in blood volume resulting from a hemorrhage or dehydration causes a decrease in venous pressure and a decrease in VR. An increase in blood volume following oral or venous rehydration or a transfusion causes an increase in venous pressure and an increase in VR.

6.5.2   Sympathetic stimulation of the veins

The smaller, more compliant veins, which serve generally as blood reservoirs as well as the specific blood reservoirs, are densely innervated by the *sympathetic system*. Stimulation of the vascular smooth muscle in the walls of these vessels causes vasoconstriction and a decrease in venous compliance. The vasoconstriction increases venous pressure in the veins. The blood is squeezed out of the veins and, due to the presence of the one-way valves, moves toward the heart so that VR increases. A decrease in sympathetic stimulation allows the veins to relax and distend. The vessels become more compliant and capable of holding large volumes of blood at low pressures. In this case, VR decreases.

The effect of sympathetic stimulation on venous resistance is minimal. As previously stated, it is the larger, less flexible veins that provide resistance to blood flow. However, these blood vessels are sparsely innervated. Therefore, there is little change in vessel radius and the physiological effect on blood flow is relatively insignificant.

6.5.3   Skeletal muscle activity

In the extremities (arms and legs), many veins lie between the skeletal muscles. Contraction of these muscles causes compression of the veins and an increase in venous pressure. This external compression squeezes the blood out and forces it back toward the heart causing an increase in VR. This action is referred to as the *skeletal muscle pump*.

The effect of the skeletal muscle pump is essential during exercise. Although there is a mass sympathetic discharge and venous vasoconstriction that enhances VR, this mechanism alone is insufficient to increase VR and, therefore, CO to meet the metabolic demands of strenuous exercise. The skeletal muscle pump mobilizes the blood stored in these tissues and keeps it flowing toward the heart. As the number of muscles involved in the exercise increases, so does the magnitude of the increase in VR and CO.

6.5.4   Respiratory activity

Pressures in the venous system are altered during respiration. *Inspiration* causes a decrease in thoracic pressure and, therefore, a decrease in pressure within the venae cavae and the right atrium. Furthermore, the downward movement of the diaphragm causes an increase in abdominal pressure. Many large veins and specific blood reservoirs are in the abdomen. Compression of these tissues by the diaphragm causes an increase in venous pressure in this region. Therefore, the overall effect of inspiration is to increase the pressure gradient between extrathoracic and intrathoracic veins. This results in an increase in VR.

6.6   Effects of gravity on the circulation

Gravitational forces may have a profound influence on blood flow through the circulatory system. VR and CO may be affected because of these forces. Imagine that the circulatory system is a column of blood that extends from the heart to the feet. As in any column of fluid, the pressure at the surface is equal to zero. Due to the weight of the fluid, the pressure increases incrementally below the surface. This pressure is referred to as the *hydrostatic pressure*.

In an upright adult, the hydrostatic pressure of the blood in the feet may be as high as 90 mmHg. When this pressure is added to the pressure in the veins generated by the pumping activity of the heart, the total pressure in the veins in the feet may be as high as 100 mmHg. The valves in the veins effectively prevent the backward flow of blood toward the feet. However, the valves have no effect on the build-up of pressure in the veins in the lower extremities. The capillaries in the feet are also subjected to the effects of gravity. Pressure in these vessels may be in the range of 135 mmHg.

The increased hydrostatic pressures in the veins and capillaries have two very detrimental effects on the circulatory system:

• Pooling of blood
• Edema formation

Blood tends to pool in the highly distensible veins. Furthermore, excessive filtration of fluid out of the capillaries and into the tissues occurs, causing *edema* or swelling of the ankles and feet, and VR and, therefore, CO are decreased. This leads to a decrease in MAP. The fall in MAP can cause a decrease in cerebral blood flow and, possibly, syncope (fainting).

Compensatory mechanisms in the circulatory system are needed to counteract the effects of gravity. Two important mechanisms include:

• Baroreceptor reflex
• Skeletal muscle activity

Baroreceptors are sensitive to changes in MAP. As VR, CO, and MAP decrease, there is diminished excitation of the baroreceptors. Consequently, the frequency of nerve impulses transmitted from these receptors to the vasomotor center in the brainstem is reduced. This elicits a reflex that will increase HR, increase contractility of the heart and cause vasoconstriction of both arterioles and veins. The increase in CO and TPR effectively increase MAP and, therefore, cerebral blood flow. Constriction of the veins assists in forcing blood back toward the heart and enhances VR.

The *skeletal muscle activity* associated with simply walking decreases venous pressure in the lower extremities significantly. Contraction of the skeletal muscles in the legs compresses the veins and blood is forced toward the heart.

6.7   Regulation of blood flow through tissues

The blood flow to most tissues in the body is determined by the metabolic needs of those tissues. Metabolically active tissues require enhanced delivery of oxygen and nutrients as well as enhanced removal of carbon dioxide and waste products. In general, as the metabolic activity of a tissue increases, its blood flow increases. An important feature of the circulatory system is that each tissue has the intrinsic ability to control its own local blood flow in proportion to its metabolic needs.

6.7.1   Active hyperemia

The increase in blood flow caused by enhanced tissue activity is referred to as *active hyperemia*. Assuming a constant blood pressure, per Ohm's Law ($Q = \Delta P/R$), the increase in blood flow is the result of a decrease in local vascular resistance. Tissue metabolism causes several local chemical changes that can mediate this metabolic vasodilation. These include:

- Decreased oxygen
- Increased carbon dioxide
- Increased hydrogen ions
- Increased potassium ions
- Increased adenosine

As metabolism increases, *oxygen consumption* and *carbon dioxide production* are enhanced. The concentration of *hydrogen ions* is also enhanced as more carbonic acid (formed from carbon dioxide) and lactic acid are produced by the working tissue. Furthermore, the concentration of *potassium ions* in the interstitial fluid is increased. The rate of potassium release from the cells due to repeated action potentials exceeds the rate of potassium return to the cells by way of the Na^+-K^+ pump. Finally, the release of *adenosine* is also believed to play an important role in the regulation of resistance vessels, particularly in the heart and the skeletal muscle.

Each of these chemical changes promotes *vasodilation of arterioles*. In addition, the increase in *tissue temperature* associated with increased metabolism further contributes to metabolic vasodilation. The resulting increase in local blood flow restores these substances to their resting values. More oxygen is delivered and the excess carbon dioxide, hydrogen ions, potassium ions, and adenosine are removed.

It is important to note that local regulatory mechanisms override the effects of extrinsic sympathetic stimulation. For example, during exercise, the mass sympathetic discharge would tend to cause widespread vasoconstriction, even in skeletal muscles. However, local vasodilation in working muscles due to active hyperemia supersedes the effects of the sympathetic nerves. Consequently, these tissues are supplied with the blood that they need.

6.7.2   *Autoregulation*

A different situation arises when the metabolic rate of a tissue remains constant, but the blood pressure changes. Ohm's Law ($Q = \Delta P/R$) states that an increase in blood pressure would tend to increase blood flow to a tissue. However, if there is no change in the metabolic activity of the tissue, then an increase in blood flow is unnecessary. In fact, blood flow to the tissue returns most of the way back to normal rather rapidly. The maintenance of a relatively constant blood flow to a tissue, despite changes in blood pressure, is referred to as *autoregulation*. Once again, resistance changes in the arterioles are involved.

Arteriolar resistance changes that take place to maintain a constant blood flow may be explained by the *myogenic mechanism*—vascular smooth muscle contracts in response to stretch. For example, consider the situation where blood pressure is increased. The increase in pressure causes an initial increase in blood flow to the tissue. However, the increased blood flow is associated with increased stretch of the vessel wall. This leads to the opening of stretch-activated calcium channels in the vascular smooth muscle. The ensuing increase in intracellular calcium results in vasoconstriction and a decrease in the blood flow to the tissue back toward normal.

Another mechanism that may explain autoregulation is the *metabolic theory* described previously as causing active hyperemia. Consider the situation where there is a decrease in blood pressure. The decrease in pressure would cause an initial decrease in blood flow. Assuming a constant rate of metabolism, the decrease in blood flow would lead to a decrease in tissue oxygen and an increase in tissue carbon dioxide, hydrogen ions, potassium ions, and adenosine. Once again, each of these chemical changes promotes vasodilation of the arterioles and an increase in blood flow to the tissue back toward normal.

6.8   *Effects of acute exercise on the circulatory system*

The primary goal of the circulatory system during exercise is to *increase blood flow to the working muscles*. This is accomplished by *increasing MAP* and *decreasing local vascular resistance*:

$$\uparrow\uparrow Q = \frac{\uparrow MAP}{\downarrow R}$$

At the onset of exercise, signals from the cerebral cortex are transmitted to the vasomotor center in the medulla of the brainstem. This *central command* not only inhibits parasympathetic activity, it initiates the *mass sympathetic discharge* that is associated with exercise. Sympathetic activity (including the release of catecholamines from the adrenal medulla) increases proportionally with the intensity of exercise.

Sympathetic stimulation of the heart results in:

- Increased HR and increased myocardial contractility → Increased SV and, therefore,
- *Increased CO*

Sympathetic stimulation of the veins and other blood reservoirs results in:

- Increased P_v → Increased VR → Increased EDV → Increased SV and, therefore,
- *Increased CO*

In other words, the increase in CO occurs by both extrinsic (sympathetic stimulation) and intrinsic (increased VR and the Frank-Starling Law of the Heart) mechanisms. Venous return is also markedly increased by the compression of blood vessels in the working muscles. The increase in CO causes an *increase in MAP*. The increase in MAP contributes to the increase in muscle blood flow.

Sympathetic stimulation of the arterioles results in:

- *Increased TPR*

Most arterioles of the peripheral circulation are strongly constricted by direct sympathetic stimulation. This widespread vasoconstriction serves two purposes. First, it contributes to the increase in MAP. Second, it is an important factor in the *redirection of blood flow* away from the inactive tissues and toward the working muscles. For example, at rest the kidneys and the abdominal organs receive 20% and 27% of the CO, respectively. During exercise, profound vasoconstriction in these vascular beds may reduce the blood flow to each of these circulations to as little as 3% of the CO. On the other hand, the skeletal muscles, which normally receive 20% of the CO at rest, may receive as much as 70%–80% of the CO during exercise.

Resistance in the arterioles of the working muscles is regulated locally. As discussed previously, active hyperemia results in the production of several factors that cause *metabolic vasodilation*. Exercising muscles generate CO_2, H^+ ions, K^+ ions, heat, and adenosine. The vasodilator effect of these locally produced substances overrides the vasoconstrictor effect of the sympathetic system in the muscle and *local vascular resistance is decreased*. The combination of increased driving pressure and decreased local vascular resistance causes an increase in blood flow to the working muscles. Changes in the cardiovascular system during exercise are summarized in Table 6.7.

Table 6.7   Changes in the cardiovascular system during moderate exercise and their mechanisms

- Increased cardiac output (CO): increased heart rate and increased stroke volume (SV)
- Increased heart rate: increased sympathoadrenal input and decreased parasympathetic input to the sinoatrial (SA) node
- Increased SV: increased sympathoadrenal input to the ventricles increases ejection fraction from 60% to as much as 90%; increased venous return (VR) and increased end-diastolic volume (Frank-Starling Law of the Heart)
- Increased VR: increased sympathetic input to the veins; skeletal muscle pumping activity
- Increased total peripheral resistance (TPR): increased sympathetic input to vascular smooth muscle in metabolically inactive tissues (may be partially or entirely offset by vasodilation in working skeletal muscles)
- Increased mean arterial pressure: increased CO and increased TPR (due primarily to increased SV and increased CO)
- Decreased blood flow to kidneys and abdominal organs: increased sympathetic input to vascular smooth muscle (facilitates redirection of blood flow)
- Increased blood flow to skin: decreased sympathetic input to vascular smooth muscle (facilitates thermoregulation)
- Increased blood flow to skeletal muscles and heart: active hyperemia, increased mean arterial pressure

6.9   Capillary exchange

The *capillaries* are the *site of exchange* between the blood and the interstitial fluid surrounding the cells of the tissues. Tissues with a higher metabolic rate have a more extensive capillary network. In other words, there are a greater number of capillaries per unit area. Because of the extensive branching of these vessels, the cells of the body are typically within 20 μm of the nearest capillary. Consequently, the distance that substances must travel between the blood and the cells is minimized. Capillaries are permeable to water and small water-soluble substances, such as glucose, amino acids, lactic acid, and urea. Capillaries are impermeable to proteins.

The *velocity of blood flow* through capillaries is slow compared to the rest of the circulatory system. This is because of the very large *total cross-sectional surface area* of the capillaries. Although each individual capillary has a diameter of only about 8–10 μm, when the cross-sectional areas of all the billions of capillaries are combined, the total is well over 1,000 times larger than that of the aorta. As the total cross-sectional area increases, the velocity of blood flow decreases. The physiological significance of this low velocity of blood flow is that it allows for adequate time for the exchange of materials between the blood and the cells of the tissues.

Blood flow through individual capillaries is *intermittent,* or sporadic. At the beginning of each capillary, where it branches off the arteriole, there is a ring of smooth muscle referred to as the *precapillary sphincter.* This sphincter alternately contracts and relaxes. When contracted, blood flow through the capillary is interrupted. When relaxed, blood flow through the capillary resumes. This process of contraction and relaxation of the precapillary sphincter is referred to as *vasomotion.* It is regulated by the rate of metabolism in the tissue, or the oxygen demand of the tissue. As metabolism in the tissue and its need for oxygen increase, the rate of vasomotion increases and the periods of relaxation are longer. In this way, blood flow through the capillary is markedly increased and the metabolic needs of the tissue are met. At rest, approximately 10%–20% of the body's capillaries are perfused at any given moment. During exercise, these changes in vasomotion allow blood to flow through all the capillaries in the working muscles, contributing significantly to the enhanced perfusion.

There are three primary mechanisms by which substances are exchanged across the capillary wall:

- Diffusion
- Transcytosis
- Bulk flow

The most important mechanism affecting the exchange of substances across the capillary wall is *diffusion.* If a substance is permeable, it moves in or out of the capillary down its concentration gradient. *Lipid-soluble substances* can diffuse through the endothelial cells at any point along the capillary. These molecules, especially oxygen and carbon dioxide, can pass directly through the lipid bilayer. However, *water-soluble substances* move across the membrane only through water-filled pores in the endothelial cells. Small, water-soluble substances, such as glucose, amino acids and ions pass readily through the pores. Water itself may also cross capillary walls through water-selective channels in the endothelial cells referred to as *aquaporins.*

Large, non–lipid-soluble molecules may cross the capillary wall by way of *transcytosis.* This mechanism involves the transport of *vesicles* from one side of the capillary wall to the other. Many hormones, including the catecholamines and those derived from proteins, exit the capillaries and enter their target tissues by way of transcytosis.

The third mechanism of capillary exchange is *bulk flow.* In this case, water and dissolved solutes move across the capillaries because of *hydrostatic pressures* and *osmotic pressures.* When the balance of these two forces causes fluid to move out of the capillary, it is referred to as *filtration.* When these forces cause fluid to move into the capillary, it is referred to as *reabsorption.*

An interesting phenomenon in the circulatory system is that, even though capillaries have numerous pores in their walls, all the fluid does not leak out of them into the interstitial space. If a balloon filled with water had multiple pin-pricks in it, all the water would clearly leak out of it. What prevents this from happening in the capillaries? The *Starling Principle* describes the process by which plasma is held within the vascular compartment.

There are four forces that determine the movement of fluid into or out of the capillary (see Figure 6.7):

- Capillary hydrostatic pressure (P_c)
- Interstitial fluid hydrostatic pressure (P_i)
- Plasma colloid osmotic pressure (π_p)
- Interstitial fluid colloid osmotic pressure (π_i)

Capillary hydrostatic pressure forces fluid out of the capillary. This pressure is higher at the inflow end of the capillary (30 mmHg) than it is at the outflow end (10 mmHg). The *interstitial fluid hydrostatic pressure* would tend to force fluid into the capillary if it were positive. However, this pressure is usually negative and, instead, acts as a suction and pulls fluid out of the capillary. Although it varies depending upon the specific tissue, the average interstitial fluid hydrostatic pressure is about −3 mmHg.

Plasma colloid osmotic pressure is generated by the proteins in the plasma that cannot cross the capillary wall. These proteins exert an osmotic force, pulling fluid into the capillary. In fact, the plasma colloid osmotic pressure, which is about 28 mmHg, is the only force holding the fluid within the capillaries. The *interstitial fluid colloid osmotic pressure* is generated by the small amount of plasma proteins that leak into the interstitial space. Because these

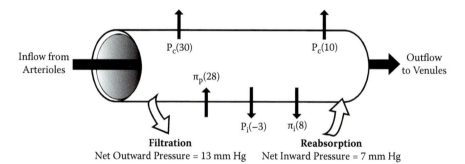

Figure 6.7   The Starling Principle. Illustrated is a summary of the forces determining the bulk flow of fluid across the wall of a capillary. Hydrostatic forces include capillary pressure (P_c) and interstitial fluid pressure (P_i). Capillary pressure pushes fluid out of the capillary. Interstitial fluid pressure is negative and acts as a suction pulling fluid out of the capillary. Osmotic forces include plasma colloid osmotic pressure (π_p) and interstitial fluid colloid osmotic pressure (π_i). These forces are caused by proteins, which pull fluid toward them. The sum of these four forces results in the net filtration of fluid at the arteriolar end of the capillary (where P_c is high) and net reabsorption of fluid at the venular end of the capillary (where P_c is low).

proteins are normally returned to the blood by way of the lymphatic system, the protein concentration in the interstitial fluid is very low. The average interstitial fluid colloid osmotic pressure is 8 mmHg.

Note that, except for the capillary hydrostatic pressure, the magnitude of these forces remains constant throughout the length of the capillary. The capillary hydrostatic pressure decreases steadily as the blood flows from the arteriolar end to the venular end of the capillary. It is the steady decline in this pressure that results in the filtration of fluid at one end and the reabsorption of fluid at the other end of the capillary.

At the *arteriolar end of the capillary*, the pressures forcing fluid out of the capillary include the following:

$$\text{Outward forces} = P_c + P_i + \pi_i$$

$$= 30 \text{ mmHg} + 3 \text{ mmHg} + 8 \text{ mmHg}$$

$$= 41 \text{ mmHg}$$

Although the interstitial fluid hydrostatic pressure is "negative," it causes fluid to be pulled out of the capillary, so this pressure is "added" to the other outward forces. The only force pulling fluid into the capillary is the plasma colloid osmotic pressure:

$$\text{Inward force} = \pi_p$$

$$= 28 \text{ mmHg}$$

The sum of the outward forces (41 mmHg) exceeds that of the inward force (28 mmHg) resulting in a *net filtration pressure* of 13 mmHg. In other words, there is a net movement of fluid out of the capillary at the arteriolar end.

At the *venular end of the capillary*, the sum of the pressures forcing fluid out of the capillary is decreased due to the fall in capillary hydrostatic pressure:

$$\text{Outward forces} = P_c + P_i + \pi_i$$

$$= 10 \text{ mmHg} + 3 \text{ mmHg} + 8 \text{ mmHg}$$

$$= 21 \text{ mmHg}$$

The plasma colloid osmotic pressure remains constant:

$$\text{Inward force} = \pi_p$$

$$= 28 \text{ mmHg}$$

Therefore, at the venular end of the capillary, the inward force (28 mmHg) exceeds the sum of the outward forces (21 mmHg), resulting in a *net reabsorption pressure* of 7 mmHg. In other words, there is a net movement of fluid into the capillary at the venular end.

Bulk flow plays only a minor role in the exchange of specific solutes between the blood and the cells of the tissues. A far more important function of bulk flow is to *regulate the distribution of the extracellular fluid* between the vascular compartment (plasma) and the interstitial space. The maintenance of an appropriate circulating volume of blood is an important factor in the maintenance of blood pressure. For example, dehydration and hemorrhage will cause a decrease in blood pressure. This leads to a decrease in the capillary hydrostatic pressure and net filtration decreases while net reabsorption increases, causing the movement, or bulk flow, of extracellular fluid from the interstitial space into the vascular compartment. This fluid shift expands the plasma volume and compensates for the fall in blood pressure.

Over the course of the day, approximately 20 L of fluid are filtered from the capillaries and about 17 L of fluid are reabsorbed back into the capillaries. The remaining 3 L of fluid is returned to the vascular compartment by way of the *lymphatic system*.

The *lymphatic capillaries* are close-ended vessels that are located near the blood capillaries. As with blood capillaries, the lymphatic capillaries are composed of a single layer of endothelial cells. However, large gaps in between these cells allow not only fluid, but proteins and particulate matter to enter the lymphatic capillaries quite readily. Once the fluid has entered these capillaries, it is referred to as *lymph*. Not surprisingly, the composition of this fluid is similar to interstitial fluid.

Lymphatic capillaries join to form larger *lymphatic vessels*. These vessels have *valves* within them to ensure the one-way flow of lymph. The lymph is moved along by two mechanisms. Automatic, rhythmic waves of contraction of the smooth muscle in the walls of these vessels are the primary mechanism by which lymph is propelled through the system. Second, the contraction of skeletal muscles causes compression of lymphatic vessels. As in the veins, this pumping action of the surrounding skeletal muscles contributes to the movement of the lymph. Ultimately, the lymph is returned to the blood when it empties into the subclavian and jugular veins near the heart.

Four general conditions can lead to *edema* formation, or excess fluid accumulation in the tissue:

- Increased capillary hydrostatic pressure
- Blockage of lymph vessels
- Increased capillary permeability
- Decreased concentration of plasma proteins

Increased capillary hydrostatic pressure promotes filtration and inhibits reabsorption and excess fluid is forced out of the capillary into the interstitial space. An increase in capillary pressure is generally caused by an increase in venous pressure. For example, under conditions of right-sided congestive heart failure, the heart cannot pump all the blood returned to it.

Consequently, the blood becomes backed up in the venous system. This increases the hydrostatic pressure of both the veins and the capillaries, particularly in the lower extremities. Left-sided congestive heart failure may cause pulmonary edema.

Another condition that can impair VR is pregnancy. As the uterus enlarges during gestation, it may cause compression of the veins draining the lower extremities. Once again, venous pressure and capillary pressure are increased. Filtration is enhanced, reabsorption is inhibited, and edema develops in the lower extremities.

Blockage of lymph vessels prevents the return of the excess filtered fluid to the vascular compartment. Instead, this fluid remains within the tissue. Impaired lymph drainage may be caused by local inflammation, cancer, and parasites.

Increased capillary permeability may allow plasma proteins to leak into the interstitial spaces of a tissue. The presence of excess protein in these spaces causes an increase in the interstitial fluid colloid osmotic pressure and pulls more fluid out of the capillaries. Mediators of inflammation, such as histamine and bradykinin, which are active following tissue injury and during allergic reactions, increase capillary permeability and cause swelling.

A *decrease in the concentration of plasma proteins* causes a decrease in the plasma colloid osmotic pressure, resulting in increased filtration, decreased reabsorption, and fluid accumulation within the tissue. Most plasma proteins are made in the liver. Therefore, a decrease in protein synthesis due to liver failure is an important cause of this condition. Malnutrition may also impair protein synthesis. Finally, kidney disease leading to proteinuria (protein loss in the urine) decreases the concentration of plasma proteins.

6.10   Disease of blood vessels

Normal blood flow through arteries and veins requires an intact system of blood vessels and adequate perfusion pressure (CO) to drive the blood through these vessels. A number of disease processes can affect normal function of the arteries and/or veins. Disease-induced changes may impair blood flow through arteries and disrupt delivery of oxygen and nutrients to tissues, whereas disease processes affecting veins will disrupt removal of waste products from tissues and the return of deoxygenated blood back to the heart. Damage to blood vessels can also increase the risk for the development of blood clots in the affected vessel.

6.10.1   Arterial disease

Arteries deliver oxygenated blood to the tissues and organs. Arteries can vary in size from the large aorta that transports blood from the heart, to medium-sized arteries that deliver blood to organs and finally down to small arteries and arterioles that feed blood through capillary beds.

Arterial diseases include conditions such as *atherosclerosis, inflammatory disorders, vasospastic conditions* and *vasospastic disorders.*

6.10.2   Atherosclerosis and dyslipidemia

Atherosclerosis is one of the most common diseases affecting arteries. Atherosclerosis is a complex pathologic process that involves endothelial injury, inflammation, immune cell infiltration, and smooth muscle cell proliferation. Although the formation of atherosclerotic lesions can affect any artery, it is most common in medium- and large-sized arteries, including the aorta, iliac arteries, coronary arteries, and carotid arteries. Table 6.8 lists risk factors that are commonly associated with the development of atherosclerosis.

One of the most significant risk factors for the development of atherosclerosis is high levels of circulating cholesterol. Because dietary lipids and cholesterol are insoluble in the plasma, they are transported as part of complex called a *lipoprotein* (see Figure 6.8). A lipoprotein comprises a

Table 6.8   Risk factors for the development of atherosclerosis

---

- Elevated serum levels of low density lipoprotein (LDL)
- Low serum levels of high density lipoprotein (HDL)
- Family history of dyslipidemia or atherosclerosis
- Smoking
- Hypertension
- Diabetes, insulin resistance
- Age: >45 in men; >55 in women
- Obesity
- Lack of physical activity

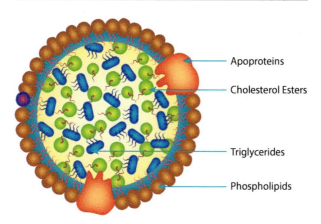

Figure 6.8 Structure of a lipoprotein. (Adapted from *Porth's Pathophysiology: Concepts of Altered Health States* by Grossman, Lippincott Williams and Wilkins, 2013.)

hydrophobic core of cholesterol esters and triglycerides surrounded by a hydrophilic shell of phospholipids. A surface protein called an *apolipoprotein* constitutes the protein portion of the lipoprotein. Apolipoproteins are responsible for determining the metabolic fate of the lipoprotein and they are necessary for the binding of the lipoproteins to cell surface receptors for internalization. There are a number of distinct lipoproteins that are classified according to their density. Table 6.9 describes the various lipoproteins and their functions.

At the tissues, low density lipoprotein (LDL) molecules bind to specific LDL receptors on the cells surface. The receptor-LDL complex is then internalized and the lipids (mainly cholesterol) released for use by the cells. Binding of LDL to cell surface receptors requires the presence of apolipoproteins on the surface on the LDL molecule.

Table 6.10 shows the classification of LDL, total cholesterol, and high density lipoprotein (HDL) levels based on the *Third Report of the National Cholesterol Education Panel*. When serum lipoprotein levels are outside of the recommended range, a *dyslipidemia* is said to be present. The association between elevated levels of serum LDL and low levels of serum HDL with the development of atherosclerosis has been demonstrated in a number of human studies.

Table 6.9   Lipoproteins and their functions

Lipoprotein	Description and function
Chylomicron	Synthesized in the gut wall; mainly composed of triglycerides and some cholesterol; transports dietary lipids from the gut to the liver
Very Low Density Lipoprotein (VLDL)	Synthesized in the liver; primarily composed of triglycerides; delivers triglycerides to fat and muscle; converted in the blood to IDLs
Intermediate Density Lipoprotein (IDL)	Formed from VLDLs in the blood; composed of approximately equal amounts of cholesterol, triglycerides and phospholipids
Low Density Lipoprotein (LDL)	Formed from IDLs in the blood; composed of mainly cholesterol; delivers cholesterol to cells; binds to cell surface receptors and is internalized in tissues; directly involved in the process of atherosclerosis
High Density Lipoprotein (HDL)	Synthesized in the liver; essentially a phospholipid micelle; transports cholesterol from tissues back to the liver; inverse relationship between HDL levels and the development of atherosclerosis

Table 6.10 Classification of LDL, total cholesterol, and HDL (mg/dL)[1]

LDL Cholesterol
- <100   • Optimal
- 100–129   • Near optimal
- 130–159   • Borderline high
- 160–189   • High
- ≥190   • Very high

Total Cholesterol
- <200   • Desirable
- 200–139   • Borderline high
- ≥240   • High

HDL Cholesterol
- <40   • Low
- ≥60   • High

[1] Third Report of the National Cholesterol Education Program (NCEP) Expert Panel on Detection, Evaluation, and Treatment of High Blood Cholesterol in Adults (Adult Treatment Panel III).

The cause of hyperlipidemia is often multifactorial and may include poor diet, sedentary lifestyle, or may be associated with the use of certain drugs such as β-blockers and oral contraceptives. There are also a number of genetic or familial dyslipoproteinemias that can lead to elevated levels of LDL, cholesterol, and triglycerides (see Table 6.11 for a description). Familial dyslipidemias may be difficult to treat and are associated

Table 6.11 Genetic or familial dyslipidemias

Familial Hypercholesterolemia	• Autosomal dominant disorder • Absent or decreased number of LDL receptors to remove cholesterol from circulation
Familial defective Apolipoprotein B-100	• Autosomal dominant disorder • Altered apolipoprotein B reduces affinity of LDL molecules for the LDL receptor
Familial combined Hyperlipidemia	• Uncertain genetic basis • Increased cholesterol, LDL, and triglycerides
Familial Dysbetalipoproteinemia	• Abnormal apolipoprotein E • Increased chylomicrons, VLDL, IDL, and triglycerides
Familial Hypertriglyceridemia	• Uncertain genetic defect • Elevated triglyceride levels • Effect on risk for increased cardiovascular disease is unclear

with a significantly increased risk for atherosclerosis and coronary heart disease. The homozygous form of familial hypercholesterolemia, for example, while rare, is associated with very high levels of LDL cholesterol (800–1,000 mg/dL), which can lead to the formation of cholesterol deposits (xanthomas) in tissues and premature vascular disease in the second or third decade of life.

Steps in the Development of Atherosclerosis

1. The process of atherosclerosis likely begins with endothelial injury in blood vessels. Some factors that can injure the vascular endothelium include hypertension, smoking, diabetes, autoimmune disease, and dyslipidemia.

2. Injury to the vascular endothelium is associated with inflammation, and endothelial dysfunction. Adhesion molecules are expressed on the injured endothelium, allowing circulating monocytes to adhere and infiltrate into the blood vessel wall to become macrophages.

3. The macrophages that have infiltrated into the blood vessel wall now encounter LDL molecules that may have accumulated there are a result of an accompanying dyslipidemia. Activated macrophages release cytolytic enzymes and oxygen radicals that oxidize the LDLs and further damage the blood vessel wall. Macrophages then engulf the oxidized LDL, which fills their cytoplasm. Macrophages that are laden with oxidized LDL molecules are called *foam cells*. These abnormal foam cells produce growth factors that cause excess proliferation of vascular smooth muscle. When they accumulate in significant amounts, these foam cells can form yellowish *fatty streaks* in the blood vessel walls.

4. An atherosclerotic *plaque* can form over time in the blood vessel wall that covers the fatty streak. This plaque comprises collagen fibers, proliferated smooth muscle cells, and a dense extracellular matrix. Fibroblasts infiltrate the area and cause progressive *sclerosis* or hardening of the tissue. *Calcification* of plaques may also occur over time. The formed fibrous plaque can extend into the blood vessel lumen and occlude normal blood flow. Initially, these plaques may be covered by a fibrous cap that helps stabilize the lesion. However, over time this fibrous cap may destabilize and expose the underlying tissue, allowing platelets to attach to the lesion and quickly form a blood clot. When a blood clot forms, it can completely occlude blood flow through the vessel. If the occluded vessel is a coronary artery, a myocardial infarction may result or, if the occlusion affects a carotid artery or a cerebral artery, the result may be a stroke.

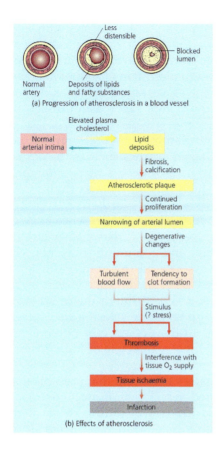

(a) Progression of atherosclerosis in a blood vessel

(b) Effects of atherosclerosis

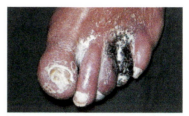

(c) Gangrene as a result of peripheral vascular disease

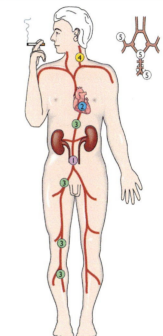

(d) Common sites for the development of peripheral vascular disease. Smoking is a major contributing factor to blood vessel damage and peripheral vascular disease

6.10.3 Inflammatory disease of arteries

Vasculitis refers to inflammation of the blood vessel wall. Several conditions such as *thromboangiitis obliterans*, *giant temporal cell arteritis*, and *polyarteritis nodosa* are inflammatory conditions that can damage arteries of various sizes.

1. *Thromboangiitis obliterans*, also known as *Buerger's Disease*, is an inflammatory disorder that primarily affects medium-sized arteries in the extremities. It occurs most commonly in young men who are heavy tobacco users. Although the exact etiology of this disorder is

uncertain, it manifests with inflammatory lesions of medium-sized arteries in the hands, feet and lower legs that can result in vasospasm, occlusion and thrombus formation. Pain and chronic cyanosis occurs in the affected tissues and can lead to ulceration of tissues and even gangrene. Treatment mainly involves cessation of smoking and attempts to improve blood flow and reduce vasospasm through the use of vasodilator drugs.

2. *Giant Cell Temporal Arteritis* is an inflammatory condition that primarily affects medium- to large-sized arteries such as the temporal, vertebral, and ophthalmic arteries. It occurs most commonly in older patients, with a higher incidence in females than males. It is also more common in individuals from Northern Europe and Scandinavia. The term giant cell comes from the presence of large, multinucleated cells that are observed in the inflammatory lesions. The condition can occur suddenly and commonly presents with headache, swelling and tenderness around the temporal arteries and blurred vision. In severe cases, permanent vision effects might occur as a result of impaired blood flow through the ophthalmic arteries. Nearly 50% of patients with temporal arteritis also present with systemic symptoms related to the presence of polymyalgia rheumatica. Treatment generally involves the use of high doses of corticosteroids.

3. *Polyarteritis Nodosa* is an inflammatory condition that presents with inflammation throughout the blood vessel wall. It most commonly affects small- and medium-sized arteries including those of the kidney, skin, intestine, nerve and muscle. Most cases occur in the fourth or fifth decade of life, and men are two times more likely to be affected than women. Although the exact etiology is uncertain, its occurrence has been associated with active hepatitis B or C infection, as well as intravenous drug abuse. Typical symptoms include weight loss, muscle and joint pain, skin lesions, anorexia, and abdominal pain. Peripheral neuropathies occur in over 50% of affected patients. Organ damage is possible due to alterations in blood flow though the affected arteries. Treatment generally involves the use of high-dose corticosteroids and immunosuppressive agents such as cyclophosphamide.

4. *Vasospastic Conditions Affecting Arteries, Raynaud's disease,* and *Raynaud's phenomenon* are disorders that are characterized by uncontrolled vasospasm of small arteries and arterioles in the fingers and toes. Raynaud's disease is a primary vasospastic disorder of uncertain etiology. It occurs most frequently in otherwise healthy young women and is often precipitated by strong emotions or exposure to cold. Although the etiology is uncertain, Raynaud's disease may be related to excess activity of the sympathetic nerve fibers that

innervate vascular smooth muscle. In contrast, *Raynaud's phenomenon*, is a secondary vasospastic condition that occurs as a result of the presence of other underlying diseases such as scleroderma, malignancy, or from blood vessel injury due to vibrations (e.g., from jackhammers) or prolonged cold exposure (e.g., butchers and time in freezers, frostbite). Localized vasospasm of arterial walls can acutely block blood flow to a particular region of tissue leading to numbness, and discoloration. Raynaud's disease normally follows a more benign course than Raynaud's phenomenon. Severe or prolonged attacks of Raynaud's disease syndrome may result in cyanosis, ulceration and gangrene of fingers or toes. Treatment of Raynaud's involves avoidance of precipitating factors such as cold and strong emotions. Vasodilator drugs or calcium-channel blockers may be used to prevent vasoconstriction. In severe cases, the sympathetic nerves that innervate the local vasculature may be surgically severed.

6.10.4   Aneurysm

An aneurysm is a localized, balloon-like swelling in the wall of an artery caused by weakening of the arterial wall. Although an aneurysm may occur in any artery, the thoracic and abdominal aorta are most susceptible due to their high pressure and significant shear forces on the walls of the vessels. Cerebral aneurysms may also occur and are most frequently located in the *circle of Willis*. Factors that can predispose a patient to the development of an aneurysm include chronic hypertension, the presence of atherosclerotic plaques, vascular infections, blood vessel inflammation and the normal aging process. Patients with *Marfan's syndrome*, a condition that affects the normal production of collagen, may also be predisposed to the development of an aneurysm because the connective tissue support around the arterial walls is reduced.

Aneurysms that involve all three layers of the blood vessel wall are called *true aneurysms* to distinguish them from other types of arterial distention that may occur from external injury or trauma. A *dissecting aneurysm* is a very severe condition in which there is a tear in the inner layers of the blood vessel (tunica intima and tunica media) and, as a result, bleeding occurs in the space below the adventitia of the vessel. Figure 6.9 shows the forms of aneurysm that may occur.

6.10.4.1   Clinical manifestations of aneurysm
- Depending upon size and location, aneurysms may be completely asymptomatic or they may be associated with severe pain.
- Aneurysms in the *thoracic aorta* most commonly present with back or neck pain, cough, difficulty swallowing, or compression of the trachea.

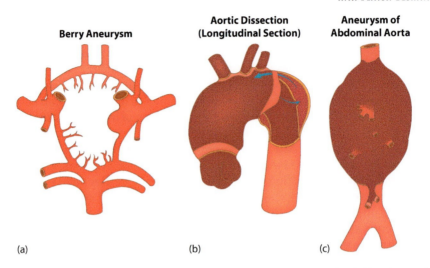

Figure 6.9 Types of aneurysm: (a) Berry aneurysm is a cerebral blood vessel, (b) Dissecting aneurysm of the aorta, (c) Aneurysm of the abdominal aorta. (Adapted from *Porth's Pathophysiology: Concepts of Altered Health States* by Grossman, Lippincott Williams and Wilkins, 2013.)

- Aneurysms in the abdominal aorta are often asymptomatic until they cause pain from compression on spinal nerves or abdominal organs.
- Aneurysm of the *cerebral arteries* often present with symptoms that are characteristic of increased intracranial pressure. Stroke can result if the abnormal blood vessel ruptures and bleeding occurs into the brain tissue.

6.10.4.2   Treatment of aneurysms
- Reduction of blood pressure and blood volume with appropriate drugs.
- Surgical grafting to strengthen arterial walls.
- Dissecting aneurysms are acutely life threatening and require immediate surgical repair.

6.10.5   Disease of the veins

6.10.5.1   Venous thrombosis
A *thrombus* is a blood clot that forms in the lumen of a blood vessel. Although a thrombus may form in an artery as a result of a destabilized atherosclerotic plaque, they are more common in veins due to the lower pressure and reduced blood flow found in the venous circulation. Conditions that may predispose a patient to venous thrombus include those that cause stasis of

blood, overactivation of the clotting cascades or factors that injure blood vessel walls (see Table 6.12).

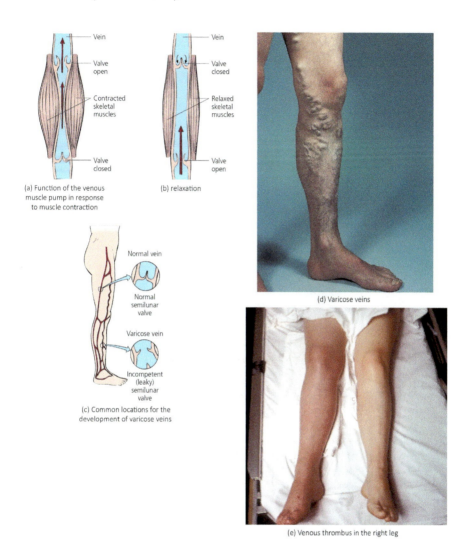

(a) Function of the venous muscle pump in response to muscle contraction

(b) relaxation

(c) Common locations for the development of varicose veins

(d) Varicose veins

(e) Venous thrombus in the right leg

Thrombi may form in superficial vessels of the skin and extremities or in deep veins of circulation or tissues. Most superficial thrombi are benign and self-limiting, whereas *deep vein thrombosus* (DVT) can be much more dangerous. Although a thrombus may present with pain, tenderness and swelling, it is estimated that nearly half of all deep vein thrombi are asymptomatic. Because the majority of deep vein thrombi occur in

Table 6.12   Factors that predispose patients to venous thrombosis

- Hypotension, shock
- Dehydration
- Heart failure, poor cardiac output
- Immobility
- Blood vessel obstruction
- Tissue injury
- Cancer
- Trauma, surgery
- Childbirth
- Infection
- Inflammation

the lower extremities, painful compression or tenderness and swelling of the calf or thigh region might be used to diagnose a DVT in these areas. DVT are associated with significant mortality and morbidity and require intensive treatment.

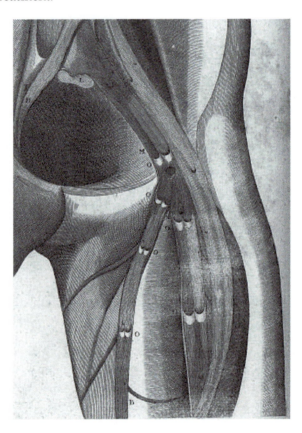

6.10.5.1.1 Treatment and prevention of venous thrombus

- Prevent blood stasis in susceptible patients through ambulation, use of elastic stockings, exercise, or elevation of legs
- Anticoagulation therapy—warfarin, heparin
- Thrombolytic therapy to dissolve clots (e.g., streptokinase, TPA)
- Surgical removal of clots

6.10.5.2 Embolism

An *embolism* is a thrombus that breaks loose and travels through circulation. Unfortunately for many patients with DVT, the first manifestation of the thrombus is a *pulmonary embolism*. A common site for the lodging of emboli is the small pulmonary blood vessels of the lungs. Emboli that lodge in cerebral or coronary blood vessels may also be rapidly fatal. A bolus of fat released by the breakage of long bones, or of air or foreign matter injected into the bloodstream through intravenous or intra-arterial lines can also act as an embolism. Ischemia and possible death of tissues may occur when blood flow is blocked by an embolus.

6.10.5.3 Anticoagulant and thrombolytic drug therapy

Anticoagulant drugs prevent the formation of blood clots by interfering with distinct steps in the blood-clotting cascade. Two of the most commonly used anticoagulants are *warfarin* (administered orally) and *heparin* (administered intravenously). Warfarin prevents the reduction of *vitamin K*, which is a cofactor necessary for activity of a key carboxylase in the clotting cascade. Heparin acts as a cofactor that enhances the activity *antithrombin III*, an enzyme that inactivates clotting factors. Neither warfarin nor heparin has any action against clots that have already formed. A significant potential adverse effect of both warfarin and heparin is unwanted bleeding.

Aspirin is a potent inhibitor of platelet aggregation through its inhibition of the enzyme *cyclooxygenase* in platelets. Inhibition of the cyclooxygenase enzyme reduces the formation of *thromboxane A_2*, a substance that stimulates platelet aggregation and activation. Because platelet aggregation and activation appear to play a major role in thrombus formation, drugs like aspirin may be of significant therapeutic value in preventing their occurrence in at-risk patients.

Thrombolytic drugs are also known as *fibrinolytic* or clot-dissolving drugs. Unlike anticoagulants that prevent the formation of blood clots, thrombolytic drugs can dissolve blood clots once they have formed. A number of thrombolytic drugs are now available for clinical use including *streptokinase, anistreplase, alteplase* (tissue plasminogen activator) and *urokinase*. These agents promote the formation of *plasmin* (from *plasminogen*), an enzyme that degrades the *fibrin* proteins that make up the framework of a thrombus.

The most common unwanted effects of these thrombolytic agents are unwanted bleeding and hemorrhage. Thrombolytic drugs have been shown to be of proven clinical benefit in reducing mortality in patients experiencing a myocardial infarction.

6.10.5.4   Varicose veins

Varicose veins are veins that have become distended over time due to the pooling of blood in the lower extremities. This condition occurs most frequently in individuals who spend long amounts of time standing (pharmacists for example) or who have impaired return of blood from the lower extremities. Pregnancy or obesity can also cause varicose veins due to an increase in intra-abdominal pressure. Veins are thin-walled vessels that are easily distended by the chronic pooling of blood in the lower extremities. Chronic distention of veins can reduce the effectiveness of the one-way venous valves that are present in the lumen to prevent the backflow of blood and lead to a condition termed *valvular incompetence*. Venous valves work in conjunction with skeletal muscle pumps in the legs to move blood back to the heart from the extremities. The most common manifestations of varicose veins are aching and edema. Their appearance through the skin is also unsightly. Treatment involves elevating the legs and the use of support stockings to prevent venous pooling. Surgical interventions may also be used to improve appearances and reduce discomfort.

6.10.5.5   Chronic venous insufficiency

The presence of valvular incompetence or a deep vein thrombus can lead to a condition called *chronic venous insufficiency*. As a result of chronically impaired VR, congestion, edema, poor tissue nutrition, and pathologic changes may occur in the lower extremities. Manifestations of chronic venous insufficiency can include skin atrophy, dermatitis, ulceration, and tissue necrosis. Infection or trauma of the lower extremities in a patient with chronic venous insufficiency can have very serious consequences because poor blood flow will reduce delivery of immune cells and impair wound healing. Treatment for chronic venous insufficiency involves compression of the affected area and possible surgical intervention.

6.11   Disorders of blood pressure

Hypertension (elevated blood pressure) is one of the most common health risks faced by adults. The Centers for Disease Control and Prevention (CDC) estimates that 67 million adults (1 of every 3) have high blood pressure. Another 1 in 3 Americans have prehypertension, which is blood pressure that is higher than normal. Normal blood pressure is 120 systolic/80 diastolic mmHg. Based on current clinical guidelines from the Eighth Joint National Committee (JNC 8), hypertension in patients less than 60 years of age is a blood pressure greater than 140 systolic/90 mmHg diastolic. Prehypertension is considered a blood pressure of 120–139 systolic/80–89 mmHg diastolic. Many patients with hypertension have elevations in both systolic and diastolic blood pressure. A percentage of patients may exhibit *isolated systolic hypertension*, which presents with elevations (>140 mmHg) of only systolic blood pressure. Isolated systolic hypertension is a significant risk factor for ventricular hypertrophy, atherosclerosis, and aneurysm and as such should be managed aggressively.

Chronic untreated hypertension can lead to cardiovascular disease and damage a number of organs such as the heart, kidney, brain, and eyes. Because most patients with hypertension do not exhibit overt symptoms, it is important that patients with hypertension be diagnosed early and treated aggressively to prevent end organ damage. Hypertension is generally categorized as being primary (essential) or secondary in origin.

6.11.1 Primary (Essential) hypertension

Most patients diagnosed with hypertension have the primary or essential form. In these patients, the actual cause of their hypertension in unknown. Although a number of mechanisms have been proposed for the development of primary hypertension (see Table 6.13), the actual cause is likely multifactorial and may involve a combination of genetic and environmental variables.

Although the actual pathogenesis of essential hypertension is uncertain, there are a number of risk factors that have been identified that might predispose patients to its development. Some of these risk factors for hypertension are *non-modifiable* and include:

- Advancing age
- Black race
- Family history of hypertension
- Insulin resistance

Modifiable risk factors for essential hypertension include:

- Obesity
- Cigarette smoking

Table 6.13   Proposed factors in the pathogenesis of primary hypertension

Factor	Effect
Dysfunction of the sympathetic nervous and/or renin-angiotensin-aldosterone systems	Increased peripheral resistance, salt and water retention
Increased dietary sodium intake	Decreased renal sodium excretion, increased fluid volume
Endothelial dysfunction	Increased peripheral resistance
Insulin resistance	Increased peripheral resistance, increased fluid volume
Obesity	Alterations in neurohumoral mediators, insulin resistance, salt and water retention

- High sodium intake
- Excess alcohol consumption
- Low dietary intake of potassium, magnesium, and calcium

Many of the risk factors for essential hypertension are also risk factors for other disorders such as dyslipidemia, atherosclerosis, and type II diabetes. *Metabolic syndrome* is a term used to identify the cluster of condition such as hypertension, elevated blood glucose, dyslipidemia and obesity that often occur together in many patients.

6.11.2   Secondary hypertension

Secondary hypertension is elevated blood pressure that is caused by some identifiable factor. Secondary hypertension likely accounts for less than 10% of all cases of hypertension. Unlike primary hypertension, which requires life-long management, forms of secondary hypertension may be potentially cured if the causative factor is identified and removed. For example, a patient with renal artery stenosis or narrowing may experience secondary hypertension because the reduced renal blood flow will lead to excess activation of the renin-angiotensin-aldosterone system (RAAS). If the stenosis is reversed and renal blood flow restored to normal, it is likely that the secondary hypertension in that patient will resolve. Table 6.14 lists some possible factors that may cause secondary hypertension.

Table 6.14 Examples of secondary hypertension

Factor	Mechanism of hypertension
Endocrine Disorders:	
• Cushing syndrome	• Excess salt and water retention
• Pheochromocytoma	• Excess catecholamine levels
Renal Hypertension:	• Excess activation of the renin-angiotensin-aldosterone system (RAAS)
• Atherosclerosis or stenosis of the renal artery	
Acute Stress	• Excess catecholamines and glucocorticoids
Vascular Disease:	
• Coarcation of the aorta	• Excess activation of the RAAS
• Arteriosclerosis	• Increased peripheral resistance
Drugs:	
• Oral contraceptives	• Excess salt and water retention
• Sympathomimetics	• Increased cardiac output and increased peripheral resistance

6.11.3 Malignant hypertension

A small percentage (approximately 1%) of patients with hypertension may go on to develop a dangerous and rapidly progressing form of hypertension termed *malignant hypertension*. This form of hypertension is associated with sudden and dramatic increases in blood pressure. The condition is more likely to occur in younger adults, particularly those who are of African-American descent. Malignant hypertension has also been associated with renal disease, collagen vascular disorders (e.g., systemic lupus erythematosus) and toxemia of pregnancy. The sudden marked increase in blood pressure can lead to encephalopathy and stroke as well as damage to organs such as the eye, heart and kidney. Treatment of this hypertensive emergency should focus on the rapid reduction of blood pressure through the use of drugs that dilate blood vessels and decrease CO.

6.11.4 Hypertension in pregnancy

Hypertensive disorders complicate 5%–10% of all pregnancies in the United States and remain a significant source of mortality and morbidity both for the mother and fetus. Modest blood pressure and CO variations are normal

Table 6.15   Forms of pregnancy-related hypertension

Gestational Hypertension	High blood pressure develops after 20 weeks of gestation. No proteinuria (protein in the urine). Blood pressure returns to normal postpartum
Preeclampsia	Increased blood pressure that occurs after 20 weeks of pregnancy that is accompanied by proteinuria. Preeclampsia can lead to serious complications in the mother and fetus if untreated. It is most common in first pregnancies or in those with multiple fetuses.
Chronic Hypertension	Blood pressure that was elevated before pregnancy or occurs before the 20th week of gestation. Includes hypertension that first occurs during pregnancy that does not resolve after pregnancy.
Chronic Hypertension with Superimposed Preeclampsia	Worsening of chronic hypertension that was present before pregnancy. Accompanied by proteinuria during pregnancy and increased risk for serious complications.

throughout pregnancy. Blood pressure tends to increase in most pregnant women during the third trimester. Although the exact cause of pregnancy-related hypertension is uncertain, increased activity of the renin angiotensin-aldosterone system is common during pregnancy and hormones such as estrogen, progesterone and prolactin are also elevated. Increased sensitivity to catecholamines and other vasoconstrictor substances may also occur during pregnancy. Table 6.15 describes the common forms of hypertension that can occur during pregnancy.

Appropriate management of hypertension during pregnancy is vital to reduce the risk of fetal and maternal injury. If antihypertensive medications are indicated, the choice of agent must be considered very carefully because some agents can affect blood flow through the placenta and to the fetus. Agents such as ACE inhibitors and angiotensin receptor blocks (ARBs) are contraindicated in pregnancy (pregnancy category X).

6.11.5   Effects of chronic hypertension

Although a small percentage of patients with essential hypertension may present with frequent headaches, most patients are asymptomatic. As a result essential hypertension may go unnoticed and untreated for a number of years. Unless diagnosed early by blood pressure screening and treated appropriately, chronic essential hypertension can progressively damage a number of tissue and organs including:

1. *Blood Vessels*—prolonged high blood pressure in the arteries and arterioles will cause the walls of the blood vessels to thicken to compensate for the excess shear forces. The chronic increased shear forces

can damage the endothelium of blood vessels and predispose them to the development of atherosclerosis. As a result, untreated essential hypertension puts patients at a greater risk of coronary artery disease, cerebrovascular disease, and renal vascular disease. The risk for atherosclerosis is exacerbated in hypertensive patients who have high serum cholesterol, are obese, have diabetes, or who smoke.

2. *Heart*—chronic elevation of arterial pressure means the ventricles of the heart must now pump blood out against a continually elevated afterload (systemic arterial pressure). As compensation for this increased afterload, the left ventricle hypertrophies. Unlike the physiologic hypertrophy that can occur in the hearts of athletes, the ventricular hypertrophy that occurs with hypertension is pathologic. The left ventricle is most affected by hypertension because it is the chamber that must pump blood out to the systemic circulation. Hypertrophied ventricles will require increased blood, oxygen and nutrient supplies and will be at greater risk for arrhythmia. When the ventricular enlargement reaches a certain point, contractile function will no longer be supported and heart failure will ensue.

3. *Kidneys*—chronically elevated pressure can damage the renal vasculature and compromise renal blood flow, oxygen delivery and filtration. As a result, *renal insufficiency* can occur that may eventually progress to *renal failure*. Decreased renal blood flow can lead to activation of the RAAS and contribute to a vicious cycle of increasing blood pressure and decreasing renal function. Hypertension-induced renal injury is exacerbated in diabetic patients.

4. *Eyes*—vision can suffer in patients with chronic hypertension as a result of increased arteriolar pressure in the eyeball or from vascular sclerosis, both of which can damage the retina and the eye as a whole.

6.11.6 Diagnosis and treatment of essential hypertension

Early detection of hypertension in a patient is essential to prevent organ and tissue damage. Comprehensive and frequent blood pressure screening is imperative because it has been shown that 31.6% of patients with hypertension do not realize they have it. Diagnosis of hypertension requires that the patients' blood pressure be measured at least two separate times with the patient seated and the arm elevated to the level of the heart. Stress, caffeine, smoking and exertion can all elevate blood pressure measurements in a patient. Once diagnosed, the treatment of essential hypertension is often multifaceted and will depend upon the severity and responsiveness of the particular patient to various therapies. A brief summary of key recommendations from the JNC 8 report on evidence based guidelines for

Table 6.16 Summary of key recommendations from the Eighth Joint National Committee (JNC) 8 report

Target blood pressure for patients <60 years of age, including those with diabetes and chronic kidney disease, is <140/90 mmHg
Target blood pressure for patients ≥60 years of age is <150/90 mmHg
Initial treatments for non-black patients with hypertension may include thiazide diuretics, calcium channel blockers, angiotensin converting enzyme (ACE) inhibitors or angiotensin receptor blockers (ARBs)
Initial treatments for black patients with hypertension should NOT include ACE inhibitors or ARBs due to decreased responsiveness
All patients with hypertension and chronic kidney disease should receive an ACE inhibitor or ARB for their renal protective effects
No evidence of benefit to treating mild hypertension in low-risk adults

the management of high blood pressure in adults is listed in Table 6.16. Management of the hypertensive patient should always include modification of lifestyle and diet. In the mildly hypertensive patient, these lifestyle modifications alone might reduce blood pressure sufficiently such that pharmacologic interventions are not necessary. In moderate to severely hypertensive patients, pharmacologic interventions should be instituted promptly, in addition to lifestyle changes, to lower blood pressure and prevent the serious consequences of untreated hypertension. Patients who are diagnosed with hypertension at an early stage and who receive effective therapy for their condition will have a significantly lower morbidity and mortality than patients with uncontrolled hypertension. Regular blood pressure screenings are the key to early diagnosis.

6.11.7   Treatment of hypertension

1. *Lifestyle Modifications*
   - Weight loss
   - Exercise
   - Sodium-restricted diet
   - Cessation of smoking
   - Limiting alcohol intake
2. *Pharmacologic*
   a. *Diuretics* (e.g., hydrochlorothiazide)—lower blood pressure by reducing vascular volume. Thiazide diuretics such as hydrochlorothiazide inhibit sodium reabsorption in the distal convoluted tubules of the kidney.
   b. *β-blockers* (e.g., Atenolol)—block β_1 adrenergic receptors in the heart to decrease heart rate and CO.

c. *ACE Inhibitors* (e.g., enalapril)—block the formation of *angiotensin II*, which is a powerful vasoconstrictor; reduce the formation of *aldosterone*, an adrenal hormone that stimulates salt and water retention by the kidney.

d. *Angiotensin Receptor Blockers (ARBs)* (e.g., Valsartan)—Block the actions of angiotensin II at its receptors.

e. *Calcium Channel Blockers* (e.g., nifedipine*)*—reduce blood pressure by relaxing vascular smooth muscle around blood vessels. Certain calcium channel blockers (verapamil) may also reduce CO.

f. *Direct-acting Vasodilators* (e.g., prazosin, hydralazine)—directly relax smooth muscle around peripheral blood vessels.

g. *Centrally Acting Agents* (e.g., methyldopa)—reduce blood pressure by decreasing sympathetic output from the autonomic centers of the brainstem.

6.11.8   Hypotension

Hypotension is an abnormally low blood pressure. One common form of hypotension is *orthostatic hypotension* (also called *postural hypotension*) that occurs upon standing. The act of standing initiates a series of reflex responses in the body that are designed to prevent pooling of blood in the lower extremities and a decrease in blood pressure. These reflexes are initiated by baroreceptors in the aortic arch and carotid arteries and include vasoconstriction in the extremities and increased heart rate. Some possible causes of orthostatic hypotension are listed in Table 6.17.

6.11.8.1   Manifestations of hypotension

- Dizziness (*syncopy*)
- Decreased CO
- Reduced brain blood flow
- Pooling of blood in the extremities
- Falls and injuries are a serious concern, particularly in the elderly

Table 6.17   Causes of orthostatic hypotension

Aging	Associated with reduced baroreceptor response, decreased cardiac output, reduced vascular responsiveness
Decreased Fluid Volume	May be caused by dehydration, diarrhea, vomiting, diuretic use
Autonomic Defects	Impaired ability to vasoconstrict and increase heart rate
Prolonged Bed Rest	Associated with reduced plasma volume and decreased vascular tone
Drug-induced	Vasodilators, centrally acting antihypertensive agents

6.11.8.2   Treatment of hypotension

- Maintain fluid volume
- If lying down, have the patient first sit for several minutes to allow blood pressure to equilibrate than stand slowly
- Elastic support garments and stockings may help prevent pooling of blood in the lower extremities
- Optimize doses of medication that may affect blood pressure, fluid volume or blood vessel tone

---

CASE STUDY

LM is a 79-year-old woman with essential hypertension and angina pectoris. She is currently taking isosorbide dinitrate and hydrochlorothiazide daily. Her children mention that her gait is often unsteady when she gets up, and they are concerned that she may fall and injure herself as a result.

1. What are the likely indications for the each of the drugs she is being prescribed?
2. List factors would put LM at increased risk for orthostatic hypotension.
3. What recommendations might you make to minimize the occurrence of orthostatic hypotension in LM and reduce the risk of her falling?
4. Most hip fractures in the elderly occur as a result of a fall. The outcomes for elderly patients who suffer a hip fracture can be very poor and mortality rates significant. What factors might be responsible for this finding?

6.12   Shock

Shock is a condition that is characterized by inadequate blood flow to organs and tissues. In order to have normal perfusion of tissues, there must be adequate CO, a system of patent blood vessels and adequate blood volume. Shock may occur if one or more of these necessary factors are altered or impaired. Shock may be classified into three main categories based upon the underlying cause. These categories are *hypovolemic shock, distributive (vasogenic) shock,* and *cardiogenic shock.*

6.12.1   Hypovolemic shock

Hypovolemic shock is the most common cause of shock and results from marked decreases in blood volume. Possible causes of hypovolemic shock include:

- Excess blood loss, hemorrhage
- Excess fluid loss from diarrhea, vomiting, severe dehydration, extensive burn injury
- Shifting of fluids from the vasculature to the interstitial spaces (inflammation, ascites)

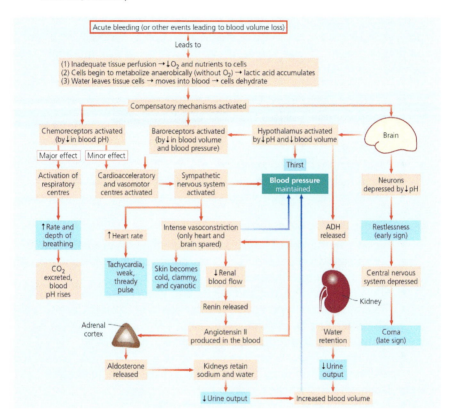

6.12.1.1   *Physiologic responses to hypovolemic shock*

Decreased blood pressure in a patient experiencing shock is detected by *baroreceptors* (pressure sensing neurons) in the aortic arch and carotid arteries. Once activated by a decrease in blood pressure, baroreceptors send impulses to the brain where they elicit a centrally mediated (autonomic) increase in heart rate and CO. Epinephrine is also released by the adrenal medulla to increase peripheral resistance, heart rate and CO. Reduced renal blood flow in a shock patient will also lead to activation of the RAAS, with resulting peripheral vasoconstriction and fluid retention (see chapter 10 for a detailed description of the RAAS). Once activated, these physiologic compensatory mechanisms are able to maintain blood pressure and CO up to a certain point (*compensated shock*);

however, as the loss of blood volume worsens, these compensatory mechanisms are no longer able to maintain blood adequate blood pressure *(decompensated shock)* and, as a result, tissue and organ perfusion will suffer.

6.12.1.2   *Stages of symptoms of hypovolemic shock*

Hypovolemic shock occurs in three stages based on the severity of hypovolemia that is present. These stages are mild (compensated), moderate (progressive) or severe (irreversible).

Stage 1. *Mild or Compensated Shock*
  - Blood volume loss less than 25% of total volume
  - Slight reduction in blood pressure, compensatory mechanisms are effective
  - Mild peripheral vasoconstriction
  - Slight tachycardia (increase in heart rate), cool extremities
  - Thirst centers of the hypothalamus may be activated to increase fluid intake

Stage 2. *Moderate or Progressive Shock*
  - Blood volume loss of approximately of 25%–35% of total volume
  - Significant drop in blood pressure, compensatory mechanisms are inadequate for maintaining CO
  - Significant tachycardia and peripheral vasoconstriction occur
  - Tissues become hypoxic due to poor blood perfusion. *Cyanosis* (bluish tinge) may be evident
  - Urinary output is reduced *(oliguria)* to conserve fluids
  - Symptoms of poor central nervous system (CNS) blood flow such as restlessness, and impaired mental state may become evident

Stage 3. *Severe or Irreversible Shock*
  - Loss of blood volume may approach 50%
  - Marked tachycardia is evident
  - Rapidly falling blood pressure, compensatory mechanisms are ineffective
  - Shallow, rapid breathing
  - Urine output ceases *(anuria)*
  - Unconsciousness
  - Organ and tissue damage from hypoxia
  - Shock is irreversible at this point even if blood volume is restored
  - Death ensues from circulatory collapse

6.12.1.3   *Treatment of hypovolemic shock*

Treatment of hypovolemic shock involves the rapid replacement of fluid and blood. Whole blood plasma or plasma substitutes may be employed.

Saline solutions and solution with plasma volume expanders such as colloidal albumin are useful for replacing fluid volume. Agents such as epinephrine that cause peripheral vasoconstriction will be of limited value in hypovolemic shock unless adequate fluid volume is restored.

6.12.2   Distributive shock

Distributive shock is also termed *vasogenic* shock and occurs as a result of factors that cause marked vasodilation or loss of vascular tone. Specific types of distributive shock are listed Table 6.18.

6.12.2.1   Symptoms of distributive shock

Patients experiencing anaphylactic shock will present with bronchoconstriction, hypotension, itching, urticaria, and angioedema. Compensatory responses will include peripheral vasoconstriction, tachycardia and tachypnea. In contrast, patients experiencing septic shock will often present with warm, flushed extremities as a result of peripheral vasodilation caused by inflammation and increased nitric oxide production. Septic shock is often characterized initially as "warm shock" due to the peripheral vasodilation and flushing that occurs. Symptoms of sepsis such as fever, increased white blood cell numbers, and increased vascular permeability will also be present. "Cold shock" may occur in the latter stages of septic shock as tissue perfusion falls (Figures 6.10 and 6.11).

6.12.2.2   Treatment of distributive shock

In the case of anaphylactic shock, administration of epinephrine will relax bronchial smooth muscle and increase total peripheral resistance (TPR). Antihistamines and corticosteroids may also be of value. Oxygen therapy will help restore normal blood oxygenation. The patient should also be fully

Table 6.18   Types of distributive shock

Neurogenic Shock:
  • Caused by impaired sympathetic input to the blood vessels
  • May result from brain or spinal injury as well as drugs that depress the CNS
     Septic Shock:
  • Most frequently associated with systemic bacterial infection
  • May be triggered by an immune response to bacterial endotoxins
  • Widespread vasodilation occurs in response to the release of inflammatory
     mediators (e.g., histamine, cytokines) and bacterial toxins
     Anaphylactic Shock:
  • Triggered by a systemic allergic reaction to antigens (drugs, food, insect venom)
  • Develops suddenly and manifests with marked vasodilation, bronchospasm,
     and hypotension. May be rapidly fatal if not treated

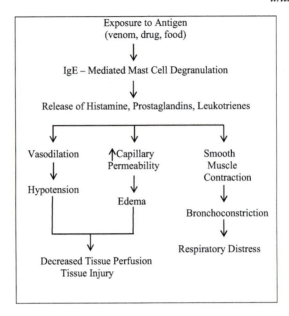

Figure 6.10   Anaphylactic shock.

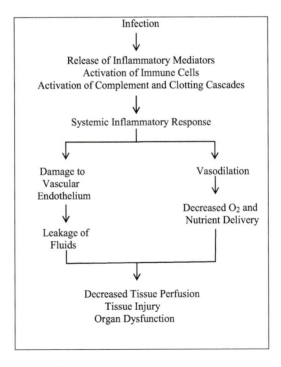

Figure 6.11   Septic shock.

supine to facilitate VR. Treatment of septic shock begins with controlling the agent responsible for the sepsis. Rapid fluid replacement is essential to compensate for fluids lost into tissues as a result of increased vascular permeability. Vasoconstrictor drugs such as norepinephrine would be useful for counteracting the systemic vasodilation that is present.

6.12.3   Cardiogenic shock

Cardiogenic shock occurs when the heart is unable to generate adequate CO (Figure 6.12).
     Possible causes of cardiogenic shock include:

- Heart failure
- Myocardial infarction
- Cardiomyopathy
- Cardiac tamponade
- Pneumothorax
- Cardiac arrhythmia

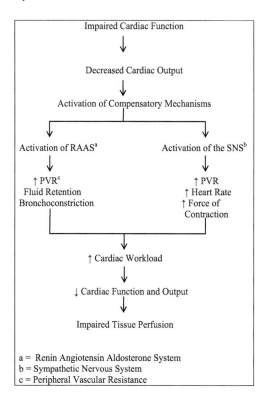

Figure 6.12   Cardiogenic shock.

6.12.3.1 Symptoms of cardiogenic shock

Symptoms of cardiogenic shock are those associated with poor CO and reduced tissue perfusion. They include activation of compensatory mechanisms such as the RAAS, and the sympathetic nervous system.

6.12.3.2 Treatment of cardiogenic shock

Treatment of cardiogenic shock involves interventions designed to improve cardiac function and enhance CO. Vasodilator drugs (organic nitrates) can reduce both preload and afterload on the heart while improving coronary blood flow. Diuretics can be helpful for relieving vascular congestion and edema. Positive inotropic agents such as digoxin and dobutamine may also be employed to increase cardiac contractility.

6.12.4 Complications of shock

During shock, tissues and organs are poorly perfused, if they are perfused at all. The longer the longer the shock persists, the greater the risk for serious complications such as:

- *Altered Tissue Metabolism*: As tissues become hypoxic and are forced to rely on anaerobic metabolism for the production of energy. Lactic acid, a byproduct of anaerobic metabolism, can accumulate in tissues and further impair cellular metabolism and function. Lack of energy production for active ion pumps can lead to electrolyte abnormalities and cellular swelling. Hypoglycemia is also common in patients with shock.
- *Adult Respiratory Distress Syndrome (ARDS, Shock Lung)*: A potentially fatal respiratory failure that accompanies severe shock. The exact cause is uncertain but the condition likely involves diffuse injury to lung tissues as a result of hypoxia, inflammatory mediators, proteolytic enzymes and free radicals. ARDS differs from *respiratory distress syndrome in the newborn*, which results from a lack of surfactant production in premature infants.
- *Disseminated Intravascular Coagulation (DIC)*: Formation of multiple small blood clots that occur throughout the vasculature. May be related to sluggish blood flow and excess activation of platelets and clotting cascades.
- *MODS—Multiple Organ Dysfunction Syndrome*: Occurs when multiple (two or more) organs fail due to poor blood flow. Most commonly seen in patients with severe sepsis or septic shock. Mortality is proportional to the number of organs that fail and may exceed 80% in severe cases. The symptoms will vary depending upon the organs affected.

CASE STUDY

Patient KL is rushed to the emergency room following an automobile accident. Upon examination, the patient was unresponsive and was found to have sustained internal injuries. The patients' blood pressure is 65/45 and at times could not be detected by sphygmomanometer. Heart rate was 165, breathing was shallow and rapid. The patients' extremities exhibited marked pallor and were cold to the touch. Anuria was noted.

  Based on the findings, what stage of shock would KL most likely be experiencing?

  What evidence would you use to support this conclusion?

  Describe any compensatory mechanisms that may be active in KL.

  Are these compensatory mechanisms effective? Why or why not?

Medical terminology

Acidosis (ăs″ĭ-dō′sĭs): Increased acidity or increased hydrogen ion concentration in arterial blood

Baroreceptors (băr′ō-rē-sĕp-tor): In the circulatory system, sensory nerve endings located in the aorta and the carotid arteries that are sensitive to changes in pressure

Chemoreceptors (kē′mō-rē-sĕp-tor): In the circulatory system, sensory nerve endings located in the aorta and the carotid arteries that are sensitive to changes in arterial oxygen, carbon dioxide and pH

Hematocrit (hē-măt′ō-crĭt): Percentage of total blood volume that consists of red blood cells (erythrocytes)

Hypercapnia (hī″pĕr-kăp′nē-ă): Abnormally high level of carbon dioxide in arterial blood

Hypertension (hī″pĕr-tĕn′shŭn): An increase in blood pressure above normal (higher than 140 mmHg systolic and 90 mmHg diastolic)

Hypotension (hī″pō-tĕn′shŭn): A decrease in blood pressure below normal

Hypoxemia (hī″pŏks-ē′mē-ă): Abnormally low level of oxygen in arterial blood

Perfusion (pĕr-fū′zhŭn): Blood flow through a tissue

Proteinuria (prō″tē-ĭn-ū′rē-ă): Loss of proteins in the urine

Pulsatile (pŭsă-tīl): Fluctuating; characterized by a rhythmic beat or throbbing

Resistance (rĭ-zĭs′tăns): In the circulatory system, the opposition to blood flow through a blood vessel

Syncope (sĭn′kō-pē): Loss of consciousness

Vasoactive (văs″ō-ăk′tĭv): Affecting vascular smooth muscle

Vasomotion (văs″ō-mō′shŭn): Change in diameter of a blood vessel

Bibliography

Armstrong, A. W., Myers, C. W., Yeh, D. C., and Rocco, T. P., Integrative cardiovascular pharmacology: Hypertension, ischemic heart disease, and congestive heart failure, in *Principles of Pharmacology, The Pathophysiologic Basis of Drug Therapy*, Golan, D. E., Ed., Lippincott Williams & Wilkins, Philadelphia, PA, 2005, chap. 23.

Benowitz, N. L., Antihypertensive agents, in *Basic and Clinical Pharmacology*, 8th ed., Katzung, B. G., Ed., Lange Medical Books/McGraw-Hill, New York, 2001, chap. 11.

Centers for Disease Control, NCHS Brief. 2013. CDC HTN Hypertension among adults in the United States: National Health and Nutrition Examination Survey, 2011–2012. http://www.cdc.gov/nchs/data/databriefs/db133.htm

Foegh, M. L. and Ramwell, P. W., The Eicosanoids: prostaglandins, thromboxanes, leukotrienes and related compounds, in *Basic and Clinical Pharmacology*, 8th ed., Katzung, B. G., Ed., Lange Medical Books/McGraw-Hill, New York, 2001, chap. 18.

Guyton, A. C., and Hall, J. E., *Textbook of Medical Physiology*, 11th ed., W. B. Saunders, Philadelphia, PA, 2006.

Hoffman, B. B., Adrenoceptor antagonist drugs, in *Basic and Clinical Pharmacology*, 8th ed., Katzung, B. G., Ed., Lange Medical Books/McGraw-Hill, New York, 2001, chap. 10.

Hoffman, B. B., Therapy of hypertension, in *Goodman and Gilman's The Pharmacological Basis of Therapeutics*, 11th ed., Brunton, L. L., Lazo, J. S., and Parker, K. L., Eds., McGraw-Hill, New York, 2006, chap. 32.

Honig, C. R., *Modern Cardiovascular Physiology*, 2nd ed., Little, Brown and Company, Boston, MA, 1988.

Jackson, E. K., Vasopressin and other agents affecting the renal conservation of water, in *Goodman and Gilman's The Pharmacological Basis of Therapeutics*, 11th ed., Brunton, L. L., Lazo, J. S., and Parker, K. L., Eds., McGraw-Hill, New York, 2006, chap. 29.

James, P. A., Oparil, S., Carter, B. L. et al. 2014. Evidence-based guideline for the management of high blood pressure in adults: Report from the Panel members Appointed to the Eight Joint National Committee (JNC 8). *JAMA.* 311:507–520.

Johns Hopkins Vasculitis Center. 2014. http://www.hopkinsvasculitis.org/types-vasculitis/polyarteritis-nodosa/

Johnson, H. M., Thorpe C. T., Bartels, C. M. et al. 2014. Undiagnosed hypertension among young adults with regular primary care use. *J Hypertens.* 32:65–74.

Katzung, B. G. and Chatterjee, K., Vasodilators and the treatment of Angina pectoris, in *Basic and Clinical Pharmacology*, 8th ed., Katzung, B. G., Ed., Lange Medical Books/McGraw-Hill, New York, 2001, chap. 12.

Levy, M. N. and Pappano, A. J., *Cardiovascular Physiology*, 9th ed., Mosby, St. Louis, MO, 2007.

Lo, J. O., Mission, J. F., Caughey, A. B. 2013. Hypertensive disease of pregnancy and maternal mortality. *Curr Opin Obstet Gynecol* 25:124–132.

Marks, R.., Allegrante, J. P., MacKenzie, C. R. et al. 2003. Hip Fractures among the elderly: Causes, consequences and control. *Aging Res Rev.* 2:57–93.

McCulloch, K. M. and McGrath, J. C. Neurohumoral regulation of vascular tone, in *An Introduction to Vascular Biology, From Physiology to Pathophysiology*, Halliday, A., Hunt, B. J., Poston, L., and Schachter, M., Eds., Cambridge University Press, Cambridge, UK, 1998, chap. 5.

Michael, T., Treatment of myocardial ischemia, in *Goodman and Gilman's The Pharmacological Basis of Therapeutics*, 11th ed., Brunton, L. L., Lazo, J. S., and Parker, K. L., Eds., McGraw-Hill, New York, 2006, chap. 31.

National Heart, Lung, and Blood Institute. Third report of the expert panel on detection, evaluation, and treatment of high blood cholesterol in adults (Adult Treatment Panel III). 2004. http://www.nhlbi.nih.gov/health-pro/guidelines/current/cholesterol-guidelines.

Reid, I. A., Vasoactive peptides, in *Basic and Clinical Pharmacology*, 8th ed., Katzung, B. G., Ed., Lange Medical Books/McGraw-Hill, New York, 2001, chap. 17.

Rhoades, R., and Pflanzer, R., *Human Physiology*, Thomson Learning, Pacific Grove, CA, 2003.

Sherwood, L., *Human Physiology from Cells to Systems*, 5th ed., Brooks/Cole, Pacific Grove, CA, 2004.

Silverthorn, D. U., *Human Physiology, an Integrated Approach*, 4th ed., Prentice Hall, Upper Saddle River, NJ, 2007.

Smyth, E. M., Burke, A. and FitzGerald, G. A., Lipid-derived autacoids: Eicosanoids and platelet-activating factor, in *Goodman and Gilman's The Pharmacological Basis of Therapeutics*, 11th ed., Brunton, L. L., Lazo, J. S., and Parker, K. L., Eds., McGraw-Hill, New York, 2006, chap. 26.

Taber's Cyclopedic Medical Dictionary, 20th ed., F. A. Davis Co., Philadelphia, PA, 2005.

Zdanowicz, M. M., *Essentials of Pathophysiology for Pharmacy*, CRC Press, Boca Raton, FL, 2003.

chapter seven

The heart

Study objectives

- Compare the functions of the right side of the heart and the left side of the heart
- Compare the functions of the arterial system and the venous system
- Describe the functions of the three major mechanical components of the heart: atria, ventricles, and valves
- Describe the route of blood flow through the heart
- Discuss the functions of the chordae tendineae and the papillary muscles
- Explain why the thickness of the myocardium varies between the different heart chambers
- Compare and contrast the functional and structural features of cardiac muscle and skeletal muscle
- Discuss the sources of calcium for myocardial contraction
- Explain the mechanism of action of cardiac glycosides in congestive heart failure
- Understand the physiological importance of the myocardial syncytium
- Describe the components of the specialized electrical conduction system of the heart
- Explain how the pacemaker of the heart initiates the heartbeat
- Understand the physiological importance of the AV nodal delay
- Describe the mechanism and the physiological significance of the rapid electrical conduction through the Purkinje fibers
- Compare and contrast the action potentials generated by the SA node and the ventricular muscle cells
- Distinguish between the types of sodium channels and calcium channels involved in the initiation and the conduction of the electrical impulse through the heart
- Discuss the mechanism and the physiological significance of the effective refractory period
- List the types of information obtained from an electrocardiogram
- Describe each of the components of the electrocardiogram
- Define tachycardia and bradycardia
- Understand how arrhythmias may be treated pharmacologically
- Define systole and diastole
- Describe the mechanical events, the status of the valves, and the pressure changes that take place during each phase of the cardiac cycle

- Describe the factors that determine cardiac output
- Distinguish between cardiac output, cardiac reserve, and cardiac index
- Discuss the factors that control heart rate
- Distinguish between the terms chronotropic and inotropic
- Discuss the factors that control stroke volume
- Distinguish between preload and afterload
- Describe the Frank-Starling Law of the Heart
- Understand how the cardiac function curve is generated
- Explain the mechanism of action of diuretics in congestive heart failure and hypertension
- Define ejection fraction
- Describe how cardiac output varies in a sedentary individual versus an endurance-trained athlete
- Compare and contrast diseases of the pericardium. How can they affect cardiac function?
- What is myocarditis, what organisms may cause it? How can it affect the heart muscle?
- Distinguish the different types of cardiomyopathy in terms of their characteristics and hemodynamic consequences
- What is rheumatic fever? How can it affect the heart?
- Compare and contrast the various types of valvular disorders in terms of their causes, manifestations and hemodynamic effects
- Understand the relationship between coronary blood supply and myo-cardial oxygen demand as it relates to myocardial ischemia
- Describe the autoregulation of coronary blood flow
- Distinguish the various forms of angina with regard to their etiology, symptoms and treatment
- Describe the various conditions that compromise acute coronary syndrome
- Provide a rational for pharmacologic and non-pharmacologic therapy in angina and myocardial ischemia
- Understand the etiology of myocardial infarction
- Distinguish the types of myocardial infarction that might occur. How do they differ in terms of their myocardial involvement, location and severity?
- List the major clinical and physiologic manifestations of myocardial infarction. Why does each occur?
- Discuss the role of various compensatory mechanisms in myocardial infarction
- Describe the complications that might arise from a myocardial infarction
- Discuss the rationale for the various treatments used for a patient experiencing a myocardial infarction
- Discuss the possible causes of heart failure

- Distinguish left-heart failure from right-heart failure in terms of etiology and physiologic effects
- Describe how right-heart failure may result from left-heart failure
- Discuss the physiologic mechanisms that become active to compensate for heart failure?
- What are the clinical manifestations of heart failure? Why does each occur?
- Discuss the different approaches that might be used to treat heart failure
- List conditions or factors that might predispose a patient to the development of a cardiac arrhythmia
- Discuss the two mechanisms by which an arrhythmia can arise
- Describe the key features of the various types of atrial and ventricular arrhythmias
- Define heart block and distinguish between first-, second-, and third-degree heart block
- Discuss the rationale and various treatment options for cardiac arrhythmias

The cardiovascular system includes the *heart*, which serves as a pump for the blood, *blood vessels*, which transport the blood throughout the body, and the *blood* itself. Under normal conditions, this system is a continuous, closed circuit, meaning that the blood is found only in the heart and the blood vessels. The heart is discussed in this chapter; the blood vessels and the circulatory system are considered in Chapter 6; and the blood and hemostasis are addressed in Chapter 2.

The heart consists of two separate pumps. The right side of the heart pumps blood to the lungs through the pulmonary circulation to allow gas exchange, the uptake of oxygen, and the elimination of carbon dioxide to take place. The left side of the heart pumps blood to the rest of the tissues of the body through the systemic circulation. In this way, oxygen and nutrients are delivered to the tissues to sustain their activities, and carbon dioxide and other metabolic waste products are removed from the tissues. In both circulations, blood vessels of the *arterial system*, arteries and arterioles, carry blood away from the heart and toward the tissues. The arterioles deliver blood to the *capillaries* where the exchange of substances between the blood and the tissues takes place. From the capillaries, blood flows into the vessels of the *venous system*, veins and venules, which carry blood back to the heart.

The human heart begins pumping approximately 3 weeks after conception and it must continue this activity without interruption all day, every day for an entire lifetime. In a typical individual, this means the heart pumps over 100,000 times per day and propels about 2,000 gallons of blood through almost 65,000 miles of blood vessels. This function of the heart will be discussed in this chapter as well.

7.1   Functional anatomy of the heart

The heart is located in the center of the thoracic cavity. It sits directly above the diaphragm, which separates the thorax from the abdomen, and lies between the lungs and posterior (to the back) of the sternum. The outermost layer of the heart, called the *epicardium*, consists of a thin, fibrous membrane. The heart is enclosed and anchored in place by another fibrous membrane, or sac, referred to as the *pericardium*. The pericardium produces a small amount of *pericardial fluid* that fills the very narrow space between the two membranes. This fluid minimizes the friction produced by the movement of the heart when it beats.

To function mechanically as a pump, the heart must have:

- Receiving chambers
- Delivery chambers
- Valves

The *atria* (sing. *atrium*) are the receiving chambers in that they receive the blood returning to the heart through the veins. The blood then moves to the *ventricles* of the heart, or the delivery chambers. The powerful contractions of the ventricles generate a force sufficient to propel the blood through either the systemic or the pulmonary circulations. *Valves* ensure the one-way, or forward, flow of the blood.

The route of blood flow through the heart begins with the venae cavae, which return blood from the peripheral tissues to the right side of the heart (see Figure 7.1). The *superior vena cava* returns blood from the head and arms to the heart and the *inferior vena cava* returns blood from the truck of the body and the legs to the heart. Blood in the vena cavae has already passed through the tissues of the body and is low in oxygen. This deoxygenated blood first enters the *right atrium* and flows into the *right ventricle*. Contraction of the right ventricle propels this blood to the lungs through the pulmonary circulation by way of the *pulmonary artery*. As it flows through the lungs, the blood becomes enriched with oxygen and eliminates carbon dioxide to the atmosphere. Blood then returns to the heart through the *pulmonary veins*. The oxygenated blood enters the *left atrium* and then the *left ventricle*. Contraction of the left ventricle propels the oxygen-rich blood back to the peripheral tissues through the systemic circulation, passing first through the *aorta*, the largest arterial vessel.

In summary, the heart is a single organ consisting of two pumps: the right heart delivers blood to the lungs and the left heart delivers blood to the rest of the body. Both pumps work simultaneously. The atria fill with blood

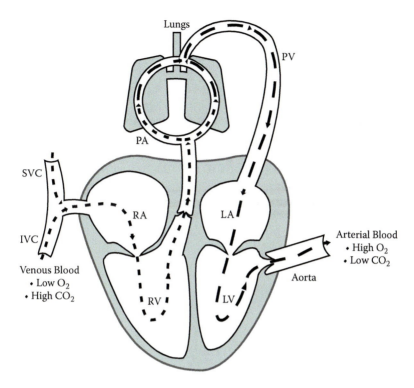

Figure 7.1 Route of blood flow through the heart. Systemic blood returns to the heart by way of the superior (SVC) and inferior (IVC) venae cavae. This blood, which is low in oxygen and high in carbon dioxide, enters the right atrium (RA) and then the right ventricle (RV). The right ventricle pumps the blood through the pulmonary artery (PA) to the pulmonary circulation. It is within the lungs that gas exchange takes place. Next, this blood, which is now high in oxygen and low in carbon dioxide, returns to the heart by way of the pulmonary veins (PV). The blood enters the left atrium (LA) and then the left ventricle (LV). The left ventricle then pumps the blood through the aorta to the systemic circulation and the peripheral tissues.

and then contract at the same time and the ventricles fill with blood and then contract at the same time. To ensure proper filling of the ventricles with blood, contraction of the atria occurs prior to contraction of the ventricles.

There are two sets of valves in the heart to maintain the one-way flow of blood as it passes through the heart chambers:

- Atrioventricular valves
- Semilunar valves

Each of these valves consists of thin flaps of flexible but tough fibrous tissue. Movement of the flaps is passive given that they open and close in response to pressure changes within the heart chambers. The *atrioventricular (AV) valves* are found between the atria and the ventricles. The right AV valve is referred to as the *tricuspid* valve due to its three cusps or leaflets. The left AV valve is called the *bicuspid* valve because it has two cusps. This valve is also referred to as the *mitral valve*. When the ventricles contract, the pressure within them increases substantially, creating a pressure gradient for blood flow from the ventricles back into the atria where the pressure is very low. Closure of the AV valves prevents this potential backward flow of blood. However, what prevents this increased ventricular pressure from causing eversion of the valves, or the opening of the valves in the opposite direction, which would also allow blood to flow backward into the atria? There are strong fibrous ligaments, the *chordae tendineae*, attached to the flaps of the valves (see Figure 7.2). The chordae tendineae arise from cone-shaped

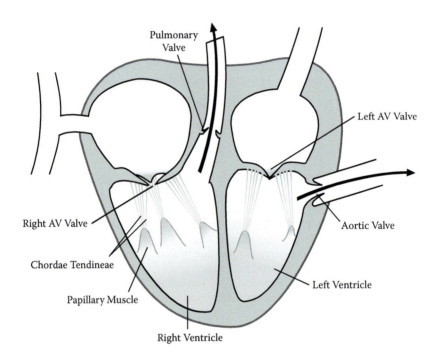

Figure 7.2   Papillary muscles and chordae tendineae. Papillary muscles, which protrude into the ventricles, are continuous with the ventricular muscle. Chordae tendineae extend from the papillary muscles to the flaps of the AV valves. Contraction of the ventricular muscle increases the pressure within the ventricles. This increased pressure closes the AV valves and opens the semilunar valves. In this way, blood is forced out of the semilunar valves to the pulmonary and systemic circulations. Theoretically, this increased pressure could also cause eversion, or the backward opening, of the AV valves into the atria (as indicated by the dotted arrows). However, contraction of the papillary muscles pulls downward on the chordae tendineae. This action opposes eversion and holds the flaps of the AV valves in the closed position.

papillary muscles that protrude into the ventricles. These muscles are continuous with the ventricular muscle. Therefore, when the ventricles are stimulated to contract, the papillary muscles also contract, pulling downward on the chordae tendineae. In this way, the flaps of the valves are not pushed open into the atria (a condition referred to as *prolapse*), but instead are held in place in the closed position. Blood is now forced to continue its forward progression and move from the ventricles into their respective arteries. (It is important to note that the papillary muscles do not open or close the AV valves. Their function is to limit the valves' movement and prevent them from being pushed backward into the atria.)

The *semilunar valves* separate the ventricles from their associated arteries. The *pulmonary valve* is found between the right ventricle and the pulmonary artery, and the *aortic valve* is found between the left ventricle and the aorta. These valves prevent the backward flow of blood from the pulmonary artery or the aorta into their preceding ventricles when the ventricles relax. The semilunar valves also have three cusps. There are no valves between the venae cavae or the pulmonary veins and the atria into which they deliver blood.

It is the closure of the valves that causes the "lub-dub" associated with the heartbeat. The *first heart sound*, or the "lub," occurs when the ventricles contract and the AV valves close. The *second heart sound*, or the "dub," occurs when the ventricles relax and the semilunar valves close.

The heart valves are supported structurally by fibrous connective tissue that forms rings around each valve. These rings are referred to as *annuli fibrosi*.

7.1.1   Myocardial wall

The wall of the heart has three layers:

- Epicardium
- Endocardium
- Myocardium

The outermost layer, the *epicardium*, is the thin, fibrous membrane forming the external surface of the heart. The innermost layer, the *endocardium*, consists of a thin delicate layer of cells lining the chambers of the heart and the valve leaflets. The endocardium is continuous with the *endothelium*, which lines the blood vessels.

The middle layer is the *myocardium*, which is the muscular layer of the heart. This is the thickest layer although the thickness varies from one chamber to the next. Thickness of the myocardium is related to the amount of work that a given chamber must perform when pumping the blood. The atria, which serve primarily as receiving chambers, perform little pumping action.

Under normal resting conditions, most of the blood (75%) moves passively along a pressure gradient (higher pressure to lower pressure) from the veins, into the atria and into the ventricles where the pressure is close to zero. Therefore, it follows that the atria have relatively thin layers of myocardium, as powerful contractions are not necessary. On the other hand, when the ventricles contract, they must develop enough pressure to force open the semilunar valves and propel the blood through the entire pulmonary or systemic circulations. Under normal resting conditions, between heartbeats, the pressure in the pulmonary artery is approximately 8 mmHg and the pressure in the aorta is approximately 80 mmHg. Therefore, to eject blood into the pulmonary artery, the right ventricle must generate a pressure greater than 8 mmHg. However, to eject blood into the aorta, the left ventricle must generate a pressure greater than 80 mmHg. Because the left ventricle performs significantly more work, its wall is much thicker than that of the right ventricle.

Cardiac muscle has many structural and functional similarities with skeletal muscle (Chapter 17) (see Table 7.1). The contractile elements, composed of thin actin filaments and thick myosin filaments, are organized into *sarcomeres*. Therefore, as with skeletal muscle, tension development within the myocardium occurs by way of the *sliding-filament mechanism*. When an action potential travels along the surface of the muscle cell membrane, the impulse also spreads into the interior of the cell along the *transverse (T) tubules*. This stimulates the release of calcium from the *sarcoplasmic reticulum*. Calcium promotes the interaction of actin and myosin resulting in cross-bridge cycling and muscle shortening.

Unlike skeletal muscle, whose only source of calcium is the sarcoplasmic reticulum, cardiac muscle also obtains calcium from the T tubules, which are

Table 7.1   Distinguishing features of cardiac muscle and skeletal muscle

Cardiac muscle	Skeletal muscle
Organized into sarcomeres	Organized into sarcomeres
Sliding-filament mechanism of contraction	Sliding-filament mechanism of contraction
Source of calcium:	Source of calcium:
Sarcoplasmic reticulum	Sarcoplasmic reticulum
Tranverse tubules	
Resting length of sarcomere:	Resting length of sarcomere:
Less than optimal length	Equal to optimal length
Gap junctions provide electrical communication between cells forming a functional syncytium	No gap junctions
Myogenic	Neurogenic
Contraction modified by autonomic nervous system	Contraction elicited by somatic nervous system

filled with extracellular fluid. This calcium, which enters the myocardial cells through L-type Ca^{++} channels, binds to calcium receptors on the external surface of the sarcoplasmic reticulum. Receptor binding then stimulates the release of calcium from the sarcoplasmic reticulum. This mechanism is referred to as *calcium-induced calcium release*. Although most of the calcium utilized in the contractile process is obtained from the sarcoplasmic reticulum (90%), the release is dependent upon the movement of extracellular calcium into the muscle cells.

The amount of calcium that enters the cytoplasm determines the strength of contraction. Any physiological factor or pharmacological agent that increases cytosolic calcium will increase the strength of contraction and, therefore, increase the volume of blood pumped by the heart per minute. Physiological factors that influence cytosolic calcium concentration are discussed later in this chapter.

PHARMACY APPLICATION: CARDIAC GLYCOSIDES AND MYOCARDIAL CONTRACTILITY

A patient is considered to be in heart failure when cardiac output (CO), or the volume of blood pumped by the heart per minute, is insufficient to meet the metabolic demands of the body. One way to improve CO is to enhance myocardial contractility, which will increase stroke volume (SV), or the volume of blood pumped per beat. Contractility may be enhanced by medications that increase cytosolic calcium.

Digoxin is a cardiac glycoside and it may be used in the treatment of severe heart failure. The drug binds to and inactivates the Na^+-K^+-ATPase on the myocardial cell membrane. (Recall that for each ATP expended, three Na^+ ions are pumped out of the cell and two K^+ ions are pumped into the cell.) Inhibition of the Na^+-K^+-ATPase results in the following:

- Decreased extrusion of Na^+ ions from the myocardial cell
- Accumulation of Na^+ ions within the myocardial cell
- Decreased concentration difference for Na^+ ions between the extracellular fluid and the intracellular fluid
- Decreased diffusion of Na^+ ions into the myocardial cell

An important mechanism of calcium removal from the myocardial cell between heartbeats involves the Na^+-Ca^{++} exchangers. The activity of the Na^+-Ca^{++} exchanger relies on the inward diffusion of sodium. As sodium enters the cell by way of the exchanger, calcium leaves the cell, returning to the extracellular fluid. Therefore, inhibition of the Na^+-K^+-ATPase with digoxin ultimately interrupts the activity of the Na^+-Ca^{++} exchangers (resulting in decreased Na^+ ion influx and decreased Ca^{++} ion efflux) and calcium accumulates within the myocardial cell and contractility is increased.

Contraction ends when the calcium is returned to the sarcoplasmic reticulum and the extracellular fluid by way of Ca^{++}-ATPase pumps. Calcium is also returned to the extracellular fluid by way of Na^+-Ca^{++} exchangers.

The arrangement of the myofilaments into sarcomeres renders the cardiac muscle subject to the *length-tension relationship*. When the resting sarcomere length is altered, the amount of tension developed by the myocardium upon stimulation is altered as well. In the heart, the resting sarcomere length is determined by the volume of blood within the ventricle immediately prior to contraction. This length-tension relationship is described by the *Frank-Starling mechanism* and is discussed in more detail in this chapter, Section F.

There are also important differences between skeletal muscle and cardiac muscle. Skeletal muscle cells are elongated and run the length of the entire muscle. Furthermore, there is no electrical communication between these cells. Cardiac muscle cells, on the other hand, are considerably shorter than skeletal muscle fibers, and they branch and interconnect with each other. Intercellular junctions found where adjoining cells meet end-to-end are referred to as *intercalated discs*. There are two types of cell-to-cell junctions within these discs. *Desmosomes* hold the muscle cells together and provide the structural support needed when the heart beats and exerts a mechanical stress that would tend to pull the cells apart. *Gap junctions* are areas of very low electrical resistance (1/400 the resistance of the outside membrane) that allow free diffusion of ions. It is through the gap junctions that the electrical impulse, or heartbeat, spreads rapidly from one cell to another and forms the myocardium into a *syncytium*, where the initiation of a heartbeat in one region of the heart results in the stimulation and contraction of all the cardiac muscle cells at essentially the same time. The heart is composed of two syncytiums: the atrial syncytium and the ventricular syncytium. In each case, but particularly in the ventricles, the simultaneous stimulation of all the muscle cells results in a more powerful contraction, facilitating the pumping of the blood.

Another difference between skeletal muscle and cardiac muscle is that skeletal muscle is neurogenic and requires stimulation from the somatic nervous system to initiate contraction. Because there is no electrical communication between these cells, each muscle fiber is innervated by a branch of an alpha motor neuron. Cardiac muscle, however, is *myogenic*, or self-excitatory—it spontaneously depolarizes to threshold and generates action potentials without external stimulation. The region of the heart with the fastest rate of inherent depolarization initiates the heartbeat and determines the heart rhythm. In normal hearts, this *"pacemaker"* region is the sinoatrial (SA) node.

The heart is richly innervated by the autonomic nervous system (ANS). The sympathetic division, which innervates the entire heart, is excitatory and increases heart rate and contractility. The parasympathetic division, contained in the branches of the vagus nerve, primarily innervates the atria. Vagal activity inhibits the heart and decreases heart rate.

Skeletal muscle contracts only when needed. During intense contractions when oxygen demand is greater than oxygen supply, skeletal muscle may form ATP by way of glycolysis. The drawback to this mechanism of ATP production is the accumulation of lactic acid, which leads to pain and muscle fatigue. In contrast, cardiac muscle must beat all day, every day. Furthermore, it must produce ATP by way of oxidative phosphorylation, which is energetically more efficient and avoids fatigue. To meet this energy demand, the heart must have a substantial blood flow for the delivery of oxygen and nutrients, as well as an abundance of mitochondria where oxidative phosphorylation takes place.

The blood that flows through the chambers of the heart does not supply the heart muscle with oxygen and nutrients. Instead, the myocardium is supplied with blood from the *coronary arteries*. These arteries originate at the very beginning of the aorta and lead to a branching network of vessels (arterioles, capillaries, veins), similar to those found in other tissues. It is when one of these arteries becomes occluded with an atherosclerotic plaque or a thrombus that the patient suffers a *myocardial infarction*, or a "heart attack." On average, under resting conditions, the heart muscle itself receives approximately 5% of the CO, or about 250 mL/min.

Mitochondria occupy approximately 30% of the volume of a cardiac muscle cell. These organelles convert oxygen and nutrients into the ATP needed for muscle contraction. Cardiac muscle consumes, or extracts, 70%–80% of the oxygen delivered to it each minute. This is more than twice the amount consumed by other tissues in the body. Once again, this illustrates the need for a continuous blood flow to the heart muscle as there is very little oxygen reserve. During exercise when cardiac workload is increased, the muscle cannot meet its oxygen needs by extracting more oxygen from the blood. Instead, more blood must be delivered to the myocardium. Blood flow may increase to four to five times the resting rate, or to as much as 1,250 mL/min.

7.2   Electrical activity of the heart

The specialized excitation and electrical conduction system in the heart consists of:

- Sinoatrial node
- Interatrial pathway
- Internodal pathway
- Atrioventricular node
- Bundle of His
- Bundle branches
- Purkinje fibers

The *SA node* is located in the wall of the right atrium near the entrance of the superior vena cava. The specialized cells of the SA node spontaneously depolarize to threshold and generate 70–75 heartbeats/min. Because the SA node has the fastest rate of spontaneous depolarization of any tissue in the heart, it is considered the *pacemaker* of the heart. In other words, it is the SA node that determines the heart rate.

The "resting" membrane potential, or *pacemaker potential*, is different from that of neurons, which were discussed in Chapter 3 (Membrane Potential). First, this potential is approximately –55 mV, which is less negative than that found in neurons (–70 mV) (see Figure 7.3; panel A). Secondly, the pacemaker potential is unstable and slowly depolarizes toward threshold (*Phase 4*). Three important ion currents contribute to this slow depolarization and involve the following types of channels:

- Potassium channels
- F-type sodium channels
- T-type calcium channels

Throughout the pacemaker potential, there is a progressive decrease in the permeability to potassium. As such, positive charges do not diffuse out of the cell.

Pacemaker cells have unique sodium channels referred to as F-type sodium channels (F = funny). They are voltage-gated channels that open when the membrane potential becomes *negative*. The resulting influx of sodium and, therefore, positive charges, contributes to the depolarization of the pacemaker cells during this phase. It is important to note that these F-type sodium channels differ from the fast Na^+ channels, which cause rapid depolarization in other types of excitable cells such as skeletal muscle and neurons. In fact, pacemaker cells are essentially devoid of fast sodium channels.

Toward the end of Phase 4, T-type Ca^{++} channels (T = transient) start to become activated allowing Ca^{++} ion influx. The diffusion of additional positive charges into the pacemaker cells continues to depolarize the membrane toward threshold.

Phase 0 begins when the membrane potential reaches threshold (–40 mV). Recall that the upstroke of the action potential in neurons is due to increased permeability of fast Na^+ channels resulting in a steep, rapid depolarization. However, in the SA node, the action potential develops more slowly because the fast Na^+ channels do not play a role. Whenever the membrane potential is less negative than –60 mV for more than a few milliseconds, these channels become inactivated. With a resting membrane potential of –55 mV, this is clearly the case in the SA node. Instead, when the membrane potential reaches threshold in this tissue, many L-type Ca^{++} channels (L = long-lasting) open, resulting in the depolarization phase of the action potential.

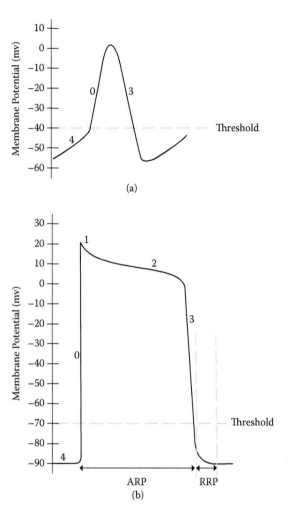

Figure 7.3 Cardiac action potentials. (A) Sino-atrial (SA) Node: During phase 4, the pacemaker potential, the cells of the SA node depolarize toward threshold due to the influx of Na+ ions and Ca++ ions. The upward swing of the action potential, phase 0, results from the influx of calcium through slow Ca++ channels. Repolarization, phase 3, is due to the efflux of K+ ions. (B) Ventricular Muscle: The resting membrane potential, phase 4, is very negative due to the high permeability of the K+ channels. The upward swing of the action potential, phase 0, results from the rapid influx of sodium through fast Na+ channels. The brief repolarization that occurs during phase 1 is due to the abrupt closure of these channels. The plateau of the action potential, phase 2, results from the influx of calcium through slow Ca++ channels. Finally, repolarization, phase 3, is due to the efflux of K+ ions. The absolute, or effective refractory period (ARP) persists until the fast Na+ channels return to their resting state (–70 mV). No new action potentials may be generated during this period. This is followed by the relative refractory period (RRP).

These channels open slowly and, therefore, the slope of this depolarization is less steep than that of neurons.

Phase 3 begins at the peak of the action potential. At this point, the L-type Ca^{++} channels close and K^+ channels open. The resulting efflux of K^+ ions causes the repolarization phase of the action potential.

Because cardiac muscle is myogenic, nervous stimulation is not necessary to elicit the heartbeat. However, the heart rate is modulated by input from the autonomic nervous system. Both the sympathetic and the parasympathetic systems innervate the SA node. Sympathetic stimulation causes an increase in heart rate or an increased number of beats per minute. Norepinephrine, which stimulates β_1-adrenergic receptors, increases the rate of pacemaker depolarization by increasing the permeability to both Na^+ ions and Ca^{++} ions. If the heartbeat is generated more rapidly, then there will be more beats per minute.

Parasympathetic stimulation causes a decrease in heart rate. Acetylcholine, which stimulates muscarinic receptors, increases the permeability to potassium. Enhanced K^+ ion efflux has a two-fold effect. First, the cells become hyperpolarized and, therefore, the membrane potential is farther away from threshold. Second, the rate of pacemaker depolarization is decreased because the outward movement of K^+ ions opposes the effect of the inward movement of Na^+ and Ca^{++} ions. The result of these two effects of potassium efflux is that it takes longer for the SA node to reach threshold and generate an action potential. If the heartbeat is generated more slowly, then there will be fewer beats per minute.

From the SA node, the heartbeat spreads rapidly throughout both atria by way of the gap junctions. As mentioned previously, the atria are stimulated to contract simultaneously. An *interatrial conduction pathway* extends from the SA node in the right atrium across to the left atrium. Its function is to facilitate the conduction of the impulse through the right and left atria simultaneously, creating the atrial syncytium (see Figure 7.4).

An *internodal conduction pathway* (or *Bachmann's bundle*) also extends from the SA node and transmits the impulse directly to the *AV node*. This node is located at the base of the right atrium near the interventricular septum, which is the wall of myocardium separating the two ventricles. The atria and the ventricles are separated from each other by fibrous connective tissue referred to as the *fibrous skeleton* of the heart. Therefore, the electrical impulse cannot spread directly to the ventricles. Instead, the AV node serves as the only pathway through which the impulse can be transmitted to the ventricles. The speed of conduction through the AV node is slowed, resulting in a slight delay (0.1 s). The cause of this *AV nodal delay* is partly due to the smaller fibers of the AV node. More importantly, however, there are fewer gap junctions between the cells of the node, which increases the resistance to current flow. The physiological advantage of the AV nodal delay is that it allows the atria to complete their contraction before ventricular contraction begins. This timing ensures proper filling of the ventricles prior to contraction.

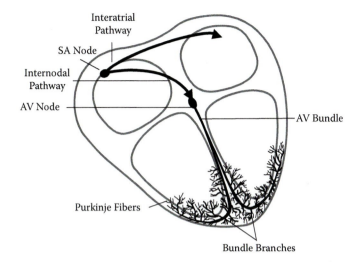

Figure 7.4 Route of excitation and conduction in the heart. The heartbeat is initiated in the sinoatrial (SA) node, or the pacemaker, in the right atrium of the heart. The electrical impulse is transmitted to the left atrium through the interatrial conduction pathway and to the atrioventricular (AV) node through the internodal pathway. From the AV node, the electrical impulse enters the ventricles and is conducted through the AV bundle, the left and right bundle branches and, finally, the Purkinje fibers, which terminate on the true cardiac muscle cells of the ventricles.

From the AV node, the electrical impulse spreads through the *AV bundle* or the *bundle of His* (see Figure 7.4). This portion of the conduction system penetrates the fibrous tissue separating the atria from the ventricles and it enters the interventricular septum, where it divides into the *left and right bundle branches*. The bundle branches travel down the septum toward the apex of the heart and then reverse direction traveling back toward the atria along the outer walls of the ventricles. This route of conduction of the impulse facilitates the ejection of blood from the ventricles. If the impulse were to be conducted directly from the atria to the ventricles, then the ventricular contraction would begin at the top of the chambers and proceed downward toward the apex. This would trap the blood at the bottom of the chambers. Instead, the wave of ventricular electrical stimulation and contraction moves from the apex of the heart toward the top of the chambers where the semilunar valves are located and ejection takes place.

Not surprisingly, the first regions of the ventricles to be stimulated and, therefore, to contract, are the interventricular septum and the papillary muscles. Contraction of the septum makes it more rigid and provides physical support for the subsequent contraction of the rest of the ventricular myocardium. As discussed previously, contraction of the papillary muscles prevents potential eversion of the AV valves during ventricular systole.

The final portion of the specialized conduction system consists of the *Purkinje fibers,* which extend from the bundle branches (see Figure 7.4). These fibers, which spread throughout the myocardium, terminate on the true cardiac muscle cells of the ventricles. The rate of conduction of the impulse through the Purkinje fibers is very rapid, resulting in the functional syncytium of the ventricles discussed earlier. The entire ventricular myocardium is stimulated almost simultaneously, which strengthens its pumping action. The increased rate of conduction (six times the rate of other ventricular muscle cells) is due in part to the large diameter of the Purkinje fibers. Typical myocardial fibers are 10–15 μm in diameter, where Purkinje fibers are 70–80 μm in diameter. Furthermore, there is a very high level of permeability at the gap junctions, which decreases the resistance to current flow. It is estimated that Purkinje fibers conduct impulses at a velocity of 1–4 m/s.

The action potential that is generated in the ventricular muscle is very different from that originating in the SA node (see Figure 7.4). First, the resting membrane potential is not only stable; it is much more negative than that of the SA node. Second, the slope of the depolarization phase of the action potential is much steeper. Finally, there is a lengthy plateau phase of the action potential where the muscle cells remain depolarized for approximately 250–300 ms. The physiological significance of this sustained depolarization is that it leads to sustained contraction (also about 300 ms), which facilitates the ejection of the blood. These disparities in the action potentials are explained by differences in ion channel activity in ventricular muscle compared with the SA node.

At rest, the permeability to K^+ ions in ventricular muscle cells is significantly greater than that of Na^+ ions. Cardiac muscle possesses a unique subtype of potassium channel that is especially leaky at negative membrane potentials, resulting in ventricular muscle cells having a stable resting membrane potential that approaches the equilibrium potential for K^+ of −90 mV (*Phase 4*) (see Figure 7.3, panel B). Upon stimulation by an electrical impulse, the voltage-gated fast Na^+ channels open, causing a marked increase in the permeability to Na^+ ions and a rapid and profound depolarization of the membrane potential to almost +30 mV (*Phase 0*). These voltage-gated Na^+ channels remain open very briefly, and within 1 ms, they are inactivated. The resulting decrease in sodium permeability causes a small repolarization (*Phase 1*).

The ventricular muscle cells do not completely repolarize immediately as do neurons and skeletal muscle cells, however. Instead, there is a plateau phase of the action potential (*Phase 2*). During this phase, there is a decrease in the permeability to K^+ ions and a marked increase in the permeability to Ca^{++} ions. Like the voltage-gated Na^+ channels, the voltage-gated, L-type Ca^{++} channels are also activated by depolarization; however, they open much more slowly. The combination of decreased K^+ ion efflux and increased Ca^{++} ion influx causes the prolonged depolarization.

Repolarization (*Phase 3*) occurs when the Ca^{++} channels close and the K^+ channels open, allowing for the rapid efflux of K^+ ions and a return to the resting membrane potential. These potassium channels, which are involved with repolarization, are similar to those that repolarize neurons and skeletal muscle cells. In other words, they open in response to depolarization and they close in response to a return to a negative membrane potential.

As in neurons, cardiac muscle cells undergo an absolute or *effective refractory period* in which the voltage-gated fast Na^+ channels become inactivated at the peak of the action potential and are incapable of opening regardless of further stimulation. Therefore, the fast Na^+ channels cannot reopen, Na^+ ions cannot enter the cell, and another action potential cannot be generated. These channels do not return to their resting position and become capable of opening in sufficient numbers to generate a new action potential until the cardiac muscle cell has repolarized to approximately -70 mV. The absolute refractory period lasts almost as long as the duration of the associated contraction, about 250–300 ms. The physiological significance of this phenomenon is that it prevents the development of tetanus or spasm of the ventricular myocardium. By the time the cardiac muscle cell can be stimulated to generate another action potential, the contraction from the previous action potential is over. Therefore, the tension from sequential action potentials cannot accumulate and become sustained. This contrasts with skeletal muscle where tetanic contractions readily occur to produce maximal strength (Chapter 12). The pumping action of the heart, however, requires alternating contraction and relaxation so that the chambers can fill with blood. Sustained contraction or tetanus would preclude ventricular filling.

The effective refractory period is followed by a *relative refractory period* that lasts for the remaining 50 ms of the ventricular action potential. During this period, action potentials may be generated; however, the myocardium is more difficult than normal to excite.

7.3   Electrocardiogram

A portion of the electrical current generated by the heartbeat flows away from the heart through the surrounding tissues and reaches the body surface. Using electrodes placed on the skin, this current can be measured and used to produce a recording referred to as the *electrocardiogram* (*ECG*). (The ECG is also referred to as the EKG, which is the abbreviation for the German *elektrokardiogramm*). An important point to remember regarding the ECG is that it represents the sum of all electrical activity throughout the heart at any given moment, not individual action potentials. Therefore, an upward deflection of the recording does not necessarily represent depolarization, nor does a downward deflection represent repolarization. Furthermore, a recording is made only when current is flowing through the heart during the actual process of depolarization or repolarization. No recording is made when the heart is completely depolarized (during the plateau phase of the ventricular action potential) or completely repolarized (between heartbeats). The ECG provides information concerning the following:

- The relative size of the heart chambers
- Various disturbances of rhythm and electrical conduction
- The extent and location of ischemic damage to the myocardium
- The effects of altered electrolyte concentrations
- The influence of certain drugs (e.g., digoxin and anti-arrhythmic drugs)

The ECG provides no information concerning contractility or, in other words, the mechanical performance of the heart as a pump.

The normal ECG is composed of the following (see Figure 7.5):

- *P wave*, caused by atrial depolarization
- *QRS complex*, caused by ventricular depolarization
- *T wave*, caused by ventricular repolarization

There are several noteworthy characteristics of the ECG. First, the firing of the SA node, which initiates the heartbeat, precedes atrial depolarization. Therefore, it should be apparent immediately prior to the P wave. However, due to its small size, it does not generate enough electrical activity to spread to the surface of the body and be detected by the electrodes. Therefore, there is no recording of the depolarization of the SA node.

Second, the area under the curve of the P wave is small compared with that of the QRS complex. This is related to the muscle mass of the chambers. The ventricles have significantly more muscle than the atria and, therefore,

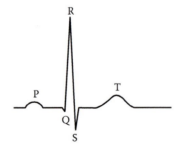

Figure 7.5 Electrocardiogram. The electrocardiogram (ECG) is a measure of the overall electrical activity of the heart. The P wave is caused by atrial depolarization, the QRS complex is caused by ventricular depolarization and the T wave is caused by ventricular repolarization.

generate more electrical activity. Furthermore, although it may not appear to be the case given the spike-like nature of the QRS complex, the areas under the QRS complex and the T wave are approximately the same. This is because these recordings both represent electrical activity of the ventricles even though one is caused by depolarization and the other is caused by repolarization. Either way, the muscle mass involved is the same.

Third, there is no recording during the PR segment. The electrical impulse is being conducted through the AV node and, as with the SA node, there is not enough tissue involved to generate sufficient electrical activity to be detected by the electrodes. The length of the PR segment is determined by the duration of the AV nodal delay.

Finally, there is no recording during the ST segment. This is the period between ventricular depolarization and ventricular repolarization. In other words, the ventricles are completely depolarized and the muscle cells are in the plateau phase of the action potential. As mentioned earlier, unless current is flowing through the myocardium, there is no recording.

Using the ECG, the heart rate may be determined by calculating the time from the beginning of one P wave to the beginning of the next P wave, or from peak to peak of the QRS complexes. A normal resting heart rate in adults is approximately 70 beats/min. A heart rate of less than 60 beats/min is referred to as *bradycardia* and a heart rate of more than 100 beats/min is referred to as *tachycardia*.

PHARMACY APPLICATION: ANTI-ARRHYTHMIC DRUGS

Normal cardiac contraction depends on the conduction of the electrical impulses through the myocardium in a highly coordinated fashion. Any abnormality of the initiation or propagation of the impulse is referred to as an *arrhythmia*. These disorders are the most common clinical problem encountered by a cardiologist. There is a wide range of types of arrhythmias with multiple etiologies and a variety of symptoms. In this section, two types of cardiac tachyarrhythmias are discussed. The most common treatment for these conditions is drug therapy.

Atrial or supraventricular tachycardia is an arrhythmia whose pathophysiology originates above the bifurcation of the bundle of His. Verapamil (a Class IV anti-arrhythmic drug) is an effective agent for this type of arrhythmia. A Ca^{++} channel blocker, it is most potent in tissues where the action potentials depend on calcium currents. These include slow-response tissues such as the SA node and the AV node. The effects of verapamil include a decrease in heart rate and a decrease in the conduction velocity of the electrical impulse through the AV node. The resulting increase in duration of the AV nodal delay, which is

(Continued)

**PHARMACY APPLICATION: ANTI-ARRHYTHMIC
DRUGS (Continued)**

illustrated by a lengthening of the PR segment in the ECG, reduces the number of impulses permitted to penetrate to the ventricles to cause contraction.

Due to the potential for interfering with the pumping action of the heart, ventricular arrhythmias are considered more serious than those occurring in the atria. Ventricular tachycardia is an arrhythmia whose pathophysiology originates distal to the bifurcation of the bundle of His. Procainamide (a Class IA anti-arrhythmic drug) is one of the effective agents used for this type of arrhythmia. Its mechanism of action involves the blockade of the fast Na^+ channels responsible for phase 0 in the fast response tissue of the ventricles. Therefore, its effect is most pronounced in the Purkinje fibers. The effects of this drug's activity include a decrease in the excitability of the myocardial cells and a decrease in conduction velocity. Therefore, a decrease in the rate of the phase 0 upstroke and a prolonged repolarization are observed, resulting in the increased duration of the action potential and the associated refractory period is prolonged and the heart rate is reduced. These effects are illustrated by an increase in the duration of the QRS complex.

7.4   Cardiac cycle

The *cardiac cycle* is the period from the beginning of one heartbeat to the start of the next. As such, it consists of two alternating phases:

- *Systole* is when the chambers contract and eject the blood
- *Diastole* is when the chambers relax, allowing them to fill with blood

Both the atria and the ventricles undergo phases of systole and diastole, however, the duration of each phase in the chambers differs (see Table 7.2). In the

Table 7.2   Systole and diastole in the atria versus the ventricles

	Systole	Diastole	Total
Atria	0.1	0.7	0.8
Ventricles	0.3	0.5	0.8

Note: In a resting adult with a heart rate of 75 beats/min, the cardiac cycle lasts 0.8 seconds. The atria, which are the receiving chambers, have a relatively longer period of diastole (0.7 seconds). The ventricles, which are the delivery chambers, have a relatively longer period of systole (0.3 seconds).

atria, whose primary function is to receive blood returning to the heart from the veins, diastole is the predominant phase and accounts for almost 90% of each cardiac cycle at rest. In the ventricles, where the primary function is to develop enough force to eject the blood into the pulmonary or systemic circulations, systole is much longer lasting and accounts for almost 40% of each cycle at rest.

A discussion of the cardiac cycle requires the relationship of pressure changes, ventricular volume changes, valve activity, and heart sounds. This section will focus on the left side of the heart (see Table 7.3). Identical events occur simultaneously on the right side, although the pressures are lower.

There are four separate events that occur during the cardiac cycle:

- Ventricular filling (diastole)
- Isovolumetric contraction (systole)
- Ejection (systole)
- Isovolumetric relaxation (diastole)

7.4.1   Ventricular filling

This process occurs during ventricular diastole and can be looked at as three phases. When the ventricle has completely relaxed and pressure in the ventricle is lower than the pressure in the atrium, the AV valve opens, because the pressure in the atrium is greater than that of the ventricle due to the continuous return of blood from the veins. The initial phase of filling is rapid. Once the AV valve opens, the blood that had accumulated in the atrium prior to the opening of the AV valve, rushes in. Toward the midpoint of this phase, filling is slower as blood continues to flow from the pulmonary vein into the atrium and then into the ventricle. This phase of filling is referred to as *diastasis*. Up to this point, ventricular filling has occurred *passively* and at rest, approximately 75% of the blood entering the ventricle does so in this manner. The third phase of ventricular filling results from *atrial contraction* when the remaining 25% of the blood is forced into the ventricle. Unlike the first two phases, this is an *active* process. The volume of blood in the ventricles at the end of ventricular filling is referred to as the *end-diastolic volume* (*EDV*) and is approximately 120–130 mL at rest. Note that during the entire diastolic filling period, ventricular pressure is very low (0–10 mmHg) and the aortic (semilunar) valve is closed. The pressure in the aorta during diastole is approximately 80 mmHg, which provides the force needed to close the valve to prevent the backward flow of blood from the aorta into the ventricle during ventricular filling (diastole).

7.4.2   Isovolumetric contraction

This process occurs during ventricular systole. When the ventricular myocardium begins to contract, and squeeze the blood within the chamber, the

Table 7.3 Summary of events occurring during the cardiac cycle

	Filling	Isovolumetric contraction	Ejection	Isovolumetric relaxation
Period	Diastole	Systole	Systole	Diastole
Pressures	$P_A > P_V < P_{aorta}$ $P_A, P_V \approx$ 0–10 mmHg $P_{aorta} \approx$ 80 mmHg	$P_A < P_V < P_{aorta}$ P_V increases toward 80 mmHg	$P_A < P_V > P_{aorta}$ $P_V, P_{aorta} \approx$ 120 mmHg	$P_A < P_V < P_{aorta}$ P_V decreases toward 0 mmHg
AV Valve	Open	Closed	Closed	Closed
Aortic Valve	Closed	Closed	Open	Closed
Ventricular Volume	Increases from 60 mL (end-systolic volume, ESV) to 130 mL (end-diastolic volume, EDV)	No change	Decreases from 130 mL (EDV) to 60 mL (ESV)	No change
ECG	TP segment P Wave PR segment	QRS complex	ST segment	T wave
Heart Sounds	None	First heart sound	None	Second heart sound

pressure increases rapidly as ventricular pressure exceeds atrial pressure, resulting in the closure of the AV valve. The closing of this valve prevents the backward flow of blood from the ventricle into the atrium and results in the first heart sound ("lub"). The ventricle continues its contraction and builds up pressure. There is a period of several milliseconds in which ventricular pressure climbs toward that of the aorta (from less than 10 mmHg up toward 80 mmHg). Until ventricular pressure exceeds aortic pressure, the aortic valve remains closed.

During this point, both valves leading into and out of the ventricle are closed and this period is referred to as *isovolumetric contraction*. During this phase, there is neither filling of the ventricle nor the ejection of blood from the ventricle and, thus, no change in blood volume.

7.4.3   Ejection

Eventually, the buildup of ventricular pressure overtakes the aortic pressure (pressure peaks at 120 mmHg) and the aortic valve is forced open. At this point, *ejection* (systole), or ventricular emptying, takes place. Some blood remains in the ventricle following ejection, approximately 50–60 mL at rest, and is referred to as *end-systolic volume* (*ESV*). Therefore, the volume of blood pumped out of each ventricle per beat, or the *stroke volume* (*SV*), is about 70 mL in a healthy, adult heart at rest.

7.4.4   Isovolumetric relaxation

After systole, the ventricles abruptly relax and the ventricular pressure decreases rapidly. Pressure in the aorta, which has peaked at 120 mmHg during systole, remains above 100 mmHg and the blood in the distended artery is immediately forced back toward the ventricle down a pressure gradient. The backward movement of blood snaps the aortic valve shut. The closure of this valve results in the second heart sound ("dub"). During this portion of ventricular diastole, there is a period of several milliseconds in which ventricular pressure is dissipating and falling back toward zero. Because atrial pressure is close to zero, the AV valve remains closed. Therefore, during this phase of *isovolumetric relaxation*, both valves leading into and out of the chamber are closed. As with isovolumetric contraction, there is no change in the blood volume of the ventricle during this phase of isovolumetric relaxation. When the ventricular pressure falls to a point at which it is once again exceeded by atrial pressure, the AV valve opens, ventricular filling occurs, and the cardiac cycle begins again.

Due to the alternating phases of systole and diastole, the heart pumps blood intermittently. It contracts to pump the blood into the arteries and then it relaxes so it can once again fill with blood. However, capillary blood flow is not interrupted by this cycle and blood flow to the tissues is continuous. This steady blood flow is due to the elastic properties of the arterial walls. When the SV is ejected into the arterial system, some of the blood is pushed forward toward the tissues. The remainder of the SV is retained in the arteries. These large blood vessels are characterized by an abundance of collagen and elastin fibers. These connective tissue fibers allow the arteries to be quite strong, capable of withstanding high pressures, but also reasonably distensible. The rapid addition of the SV causes arterial distension, or stretch, resulting in the "storage" of a portion of this blood in these vessels. During diastole, when the heart relaxes, the arteries recoil and regain their original shape. This recoil squeezes down on the stored blood and pushes it forward toward the tissues. Therefore, blood flow through the circulation is continuous during both ventricular systole and diastole.

7.5   Cardiac output

The primary function of the heart is to deliver a sufficient volume of oxygen-rich blood and nutrients, hormones, and so on to the tissues so that they can effectively carry out their functions. As the metabolic activity of a tissue varies, so will its need for blood. An important factor involved in meeting this demand is CO or the volume of blood pumped into the aorta per minute. Cardiac output is determined by heart rate multiplied by SV:

$$\text{Cardiac output (CO)} = \text{heart rate (HR)} \times \text{stroke volume (SV)}$$

$$CO = HR \times SV$$

An average adult, at rest, may have a heart rate of 70 beats/min and a SV of 70 mL/beat. In this case, the CO would be:

$$CO = 70 \text{ beats/min} \times 70 \text{ mL/beat}$$

$$= 4,900 \text{ mL/min}$$

$$\approx 5 \text{ L/min}$$

This is approximately equal to the total volume of blood in the body. Therefore, the entire blood volume is pumped by the heart each minute.

Many factors are involved in determining a person's CO (see Table 7.4):

- Level of activity
- Size of the body
- Age

Table 7.4   Factors that affect cardiac output

Heart rate
• Autonomic nervous System
• Catecholamines (Epinephrine and Norepinephrine)
• Body temperature

Stroke Volume
• Length of diastole
• Venous return (Preload)
• Contractility of the myocardium
• Afterload
• Heart rate

Miscellaneous
• Level of activity
• Body size
• Age

A primary determinant is the *level of activity* of the body. During intense exercise in an average sedentary person, CO may increase to 18–20 L/min. In a trained athlete, the increase in CO is even greater and may be as much as 30–35 L/min. *Cardiac reserve* is the difference between the CO at rest and the maximum volume of blood that the heart is capable of pumping per minute. The effect of endurance training is to significantly increase cardiac reserve so that a greater volume of blood can be pumped to the working muscles. In this way, exercise performance is maximized and fatigue of the muscles is delayed. On the other hand, patients with heart conditions, such as congestive heart failure or mitral valve stenosis, are not able to increase their CO as much, if at all, during exercise. Therefore, these patients are forced to limit their level of exertion as the disease process progresses.

The *size of the body* is another factor determining CO. Healthy young men have a CO of about 5.5–6.0 L/min, whereas the CO in women averages 4.5–5.0 L/min. This difference does not involve gender in itself, but instead involves the mass of body tissue that must be perfused with blood. The *cardiac index* normalizes CO for body size and is calculated by the CO per square meter of body surface area. An average person of 70 kg has a body surface area of approximately 1.7 m². Therefore:

$$\text{Cardiac index} = 5 \, \text{L/min} \div 1.7 \, \text{m}^2$$

$$= 3 \, \text{L/min/m}^2$$

Cardiac output also varies with *age*. Expressed as cardiac index, it rapidly rises to a peak of more than 4 L/min/m² at 10 years of age and then steadily declines to about 2.4 L/min/m^2 at 80 years of age. This decrease in CO is a function of overall metabolic activity and is, therefore, indicative of declining activity with age.

7.6   Control of heart rate

Heart rate varies considerably depending upon several variables. In normal adults at rest, the typical, average heart rate is about 70 beats/min; however, in children, the resting heart rate is much greater. Heart rate will increase substantially (greater than 100 beats/min) during emotional excitement and exercise, and it will decrease by 10–20 beats/min during sleep. In endurance athletes, the resting heart rate may be 50 beats/min or lower. This condition, referred to as *training-induced bradycardia*, is beneficial because it reduces the workload of the heart.

Mechanisms that alter heart rate have a *chronotropic effect* (*chrono* = time). A factor that increases heart rate is said to have a *positive chronotropic effect*, and a factor that decreases heart rate is said to have a *negative chronotropic effect*. In this section, three factors that control heart rate will be discussed:

- Autonomic nervous system
- Catecholamines
- Body temperature

The *autonomic nervous system* exerts the primary control on heart rate. Because the sympathetic system and the parasympathetic system have antagonistic effects on the heart, the heart rate at any given moment results from the balance or the sum of their inputs. The SA node, which is the pacemaker of the heart, determines the rate of spontaneous depolarization and, along with the AV node, is innervated by both the sympathetic and the parasympathetic systems. The specialized ventricular conduction pathway and ventricular muscle itself are innervated by the sympathetic system only.

Sympathetic stimulation increases heart rate (see Table 7.5). Norepinephrine, the neurotransmitter released from sympathetic nerves, binds to the β-adrenergic receptors in the heart and causes the following effects:

- Increased rate of discharge of the SA node
- Increased rate of conduction through the AV node
- Increased rate of conduction through the bundle of His and the Purkinje fibers

The mechanism of these effects involves the enhanced rate of depolarization of the cells in these tissues due to increased sodium current through the F-type sodium channels. With more Na$^+$ ions entering the cell, the inside

Table 7.5 Effects of autonomic nerves on the heart

Heart tissue	Sympathetic nerves	Parasympathetic nerves
Sinoatrial (SA) Node	↑ Heart rate (primarily via right sympathetic nerves)	↓ Heart rate (primarily via right vagus nerve)
Atrioventricular (AV) Node	↑ Conduction rate	↓ Conduction rate (primarily via left vagus nerve)
Atrial Muscle	↑ Contractility	↓ Contractility
Ventricular Muscle	↑ Contractility (primarily via left sympathetic nerves)	No significant effect

of the cell becomes less negative and approaches threshold more rapidly. In this way, action potentials are generated faster and they travel through the conduction pathway much more quickly so that the heart can generate more heartbeats per minute (see Figure 7.6).

Parasympathetic stimulation decreases heart rate (see Table 7.5). Acetylcholine is the neurotransmitter released from the branches of the vagus nerve, which are the parasympathetic nerves to the heart. Acetylcholine binds to muscarinic receptors and causes the following effects:

- Decreased rate of discharge of the SA node
- Decreased rate of conduction through the AV node

The mechanism of these effects involves the increased permeability to potassium. The enhanced efflux of K^+ ions has two effects on the action potential of the SA node. First, the cells become hyperpolarized so that the membrane potential is farther away from threshold (from a normal resting potential of

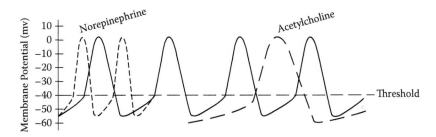

Figure 7.6 Effect of autonomic nervous system stimulation on action potentials of the sinoatrial (SA) node. A normal action potential generated by the SA node under resting conditions is represented by the solid line. The positive chronotropic effect (increased heart rate) of norepinephrine released from sympathetic nerve fibers is illustrated by the short dashed line; and the negative chronotropic effect (decreased heart rate) of acetylcholine released from parasympathetic nerve fibers is illustrated by the long dashed line.

−55 mV down toward −65 mV), and a greater depolarization is now needed to reach threshold and generate an action potential. Second, the rate of depolarization during the pacemaker potential is reduced. The outward movement of positively charged K^+ ions opposes the depolarizing effect of the Na^+ ion and Ca^{++} ion influx. In this way, action potentials are developed more slowly and fewer heartbeats are generated per minute (see Figure 7.6).

At rest, the parasympathetic system exerts the predominant effect on the SA node and, therefore, on heart rate. In a denervated heart, such as a transplanted heart, the resting heart rate is 100 beats/min. This indicates that the SA node, without any input from the autonomic nervous system, has an inherent rate of depolarization of 100 beats/min. However, an intact, or fully innervated heart, generates only 70 beats/min. Therefore, it is evident that the rate of spontaneous discharge by the SA node is suppressed by the influence of the parasympathetic system. In contrast, the sympathetic system dominates during exercise.

It is generally accepted that the maximum heart rate an individual may achieve during exercise can be calculated by the following formula:

$$HR_{max} = 220 - age$$

Therefore, the range of heart rates from 185 to 195 beats/min may be attained in individuals between 25 and 35 years of age. The maximum heart rate that may be attained in an individual 55 years of age is significantly reduced and is about 165 beats/min. Many factors may affect maximum heart rate including level of fitness and various health considerations. Average values for maximum heart rate may be found in Table 7.6.

The activity of the autonomic nerves to the heart is regulated by the vasomotor center in the brainstem. Inputs to the vasomotor center, which subsequently influence autonomic nervous system function, are discussed in detail in Chapter 6.

The second factor that exerts control on heart rate is the release of the *catecholamines*, epinephrine and norepinephrine, from the adrenal medulla.

Table 7.6   Average maximum heart rates and target heart rates

Age (years)	Average maximum heart rate (100%) (beats/min)	Target heart rate zone (50%–70% max) (beats/min)
20	200	100–150
30	190	95–142
40	180	90–135
50	170	85–127
60	160	80–120
70	150	75–113

The circulating catecholamines have the same effect on heart rate as direct sympathetic stimulation, which is to increase heart rate. In fact, in the intact (innervated) heart, the effect of the catecholamines serves to supplement this direct effect. In a denervated heart, the circulating catecholamines serve to replace the effect of direct sympathetic stimulation. In this way, patients who have had a heart transplant may still increase their heart rate during exercise.

Body temperature also affects heart rate by altering the rate of discharge of the SA node. An increase of 1°F in body temperature results in an increase in heart rate of about 10 beats/min. Therefore, the increase in body temperature during a fever, or that which accompanies exercise, serves to increase heart rate and, ultimately, CO. This enhanced pumping action of the heart delivers more blood to the tissues and supports the increased metabolic activity associated with these conditions.

7.7   Control of stroke volume

Many factors contribute to the regulation of SV. Factors discussed in this section include:

- Length of diastole
- Venous return (preload)
- Contractility of the myocardium
- Afterload
- Heart rate

Two important concepts to keep in mind throughout this discussion are the following: "the heart can only pump what it gets" and "a healthy heart pumps all of the blood returned to it." The SA node may generate a heartbeat and cause the ventricles to contract; however, these chambers must be properly filled with blood for this activity to be effective. On the other hand, the volume of blood that returns to the heart per minute may vary considerably. The heart has an intrinsic ability to alter its strength of contraction to accommodate these changes in volume.

Diastole is the period in the cardiac cycle in which relaxation of the myocardium and ventricular filling take place. In an individual with a resting heart rate of 75 beats/min, the length of the cardiac cycle is 0.8 s and the length of ventricular diastole is 0.5 s. As mentioned in the previous chapter, the EDV is approximately 130 mL and the resulting SV is about 70 mL. Consider the case in which the heart rate is increased. Given that CO is determined by heart rate multiplied by SV, an increase in either of these variables should result in an increase in CO. In general, this is quite true. However, the effect of increased heart rate on CO is limited by its effect on the length of diastole. As the heart rate increases, then the length of the cardiac cycle and, therefore, the length of diastole or the time for filling will decrease. At very high heart rates, this may result in a decrease in ventricular filling or EDV, a decrease in SV, and a decrease in CO. Once again, "the heart can only pump what it gets." If there is inadequate time for filling, then despite an increase in heart rate, CO will decrease. This explains why the maximal heart rate during exercise is about 185–195 beats/min in all individuals. Beyond this rate, the ventricles are unable to properly fill with blood and the positive effect of increased heart rate on CO is lost.

Venous return is defined as the volume of blood returned to the right atrium per minute. Assuming a constant heart rate and, therefore, a constant length of diastole, then an increase in venous return, or the rate of blood flow into the heart, will increase ventricular filling, increase EDV, increase SV, and increase CO. Ventricular blood volume prior to contraction is also referred to as *preload*. Once again, "a healthy heart pumps all of the blood returned to it." In fact, the CO is equal to the venous return. The heart has an inherent, self-regulating mechanism by which it can alter its force of contraction based upon the volume of blood that flows into it. This *intrinsic mechanism*, the *Frank-Starling Law of the Heart*, states when ventricular filling is increased, the increased volume of blood stretches the walls of the chambers and the ventricles contract more forcefully. The stronger contraction results in a larger SV. This concept is illustrated by the *cardiac function curve* (see Figure 7.7). As EDV increases, then SV and, therefore, CO increase. This phenomenon is based on the length-tension relationship of cardiac muscle. As will be discussed in Chapter 16, *Muscle*, the resting length of the sarcomere determines the amount of tension generated by the muscle upon stimulation. Due to their attachments to the bones, the resting lengths of the skeletal muscles do not vary greatly. Therefore, the sarcomeres are normally at their optimal length of 2.2 μm, which results in maximal tension development. At this point, the overlap of the actin and myosin filaments in the sarcomere is such that the greatest amount of cross-bridge cycling to generate tension takes place.

The myocardium of the heart, however, is not limited by attachment to any bones. Therefore, the resting length of the sarcomeres of these muscle cells may vary substantially due to changes in ventricular filling. Interestingly, at a normal resting EDV of 130 mL, the amount of ventricular filling and the resting cardiac muscle fiber length is *less than the optimal length*. Therefore, as filling increases, the muscle fibers and their component sarcomeres are stretched and move closer to the optimal length for cross-bridge cycling and tension development. This results in a stronger ventricular contraction and an increase in SV. In other words, a healthy heart operates on the ascending portion of the cardiac function curve, such that an increase in preload results in an increase in SV.

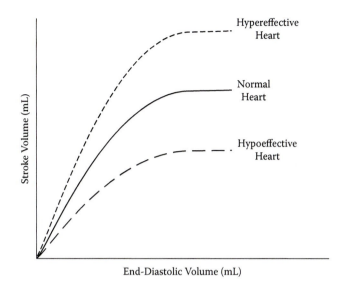

Figure 7.7 Cardiac function curve. This curve illustrates the stroke volume (SV) pumped by the heart for a given end-diastolic volume (EDV) within the ventricle. As ventricular filling (EDV) increases, then SV increases. Factors causing a positive inotropic effect (increased contractility) result in a greater SV for a given amount of filling compared with the normal heart. This "hypereffective" heart is illustrated by the short dashed line that is shifted to the left of that of the normal heart. Sympathetic stimulation, the catecholamines and some medications such as the cardiac glycosides increase contractility. Factors causing a negative inotropic effect (decreased contractility) result in a reduced SV for a given amount of filling. This "hypoeffective" heart is illustrated by the long dashed line that is shifted to the right of that of the normal heart. Damage to the myocardium and some medications, such as β-adrenergic receptor antagonists and calcium channel blockers, decrease contractility.

PHARMACY APPLICATION: DIURETICS AND CARDIAC OUTPUT

Diuretics are a group of therapeutic agents designed to reduce the volume of body fluids. Their mechanism of action is at the level of the kidney and involves an increase in the excretion of Na^+ ions and Cl^- ions and, consequently, an increase in urine production. As discussed in Chapter 2, sodium is the predominant extracellular cation and due to its osmotic effects, it is a primary determinant of extracellular fluid volume. Therefore, if more sodium is excreted in the urine, then more water is also lost, which reduces the volume of the extracellular fluids

(Continued)

PHARMACY APPLICATION: DIURETICS
AND CARDIAC OUTPUT (Continued)

including the plasma. As plasma volume decreases, less blood is available for ventricular filling.

It is this reduction in preload that is, in some cases, beneficial to patients experiencing heart failure. Unlike a healthy heart, a failing heart is unable to pump all the blood returned to it. Instead, the blood dams up and overfills the chambers of the heart. This results in congestion and increased pressures in the heart and the venous system and the formation of peripheral edema. Because the failing heart is operating on the flat portion of a depressed cardiac function curve (see Figure 7.7), treatment with diuretics will relieve the congestion and edema but have little effect on SV and CO.

Stimulation of the ventricular myocardium by the sympathetic system will also increase SV by increasing the *contractility* of the muscle. At any given EDV, norepinephrine released from the sympathetic nerves to the heart will cause a more forceful contraction resulting in the ejection of more blood from the ventricles or an increase in SV and an increase in CO (see Figure 7.7). In other words, the cardiac function curve shifts to the left. Epinephrine released from the adrenal medulla has the same effect on contractility as direct sympathetic stimulation. The mechanism involves the stimulation of β-adrenergic receptors and the subsequent increase in the permeability to calcium. An increase in intracellular calcium results in increased cross-bridge cycling and greater tension development. Sympathetic stimulation, the circulating catecholamines or any other factor that increases contractility has a *positive inotropic effect* on the heart. Therapeutic agents, such as β-adrenergic receptor blockers and calcium channel blockers, which inhibit calcium influx and, therefore, reduce contractility, have a *negative inotropic effect*.

The ventricles are very sparsely innervated by the branches of the vagus nerve. Therefore, parasympathetic stimulation to the heart has little or no significant effect on contractility and SV.

The contractility of the myocardium determines the *ejection fraction* of the heart, which is the ratio of the volume of blood ejected from the left ventricle per beat (SV) to the volume of blood in the left ventricle at the end of diastole (EDV):

$$\text{Ejection fraction} = \frac{SV}{EDV}$$

Under normal resting conditions where the EDV is 120–130 mL and the SV is 70 mL/beat, the ejection fraction is 55%–60%:

$$\text{Ejection fraction} = \frac{70 \text{ mL/beat}}{120 \text{ mL}} = 58\%$$

During exercise when sympathetic stimulation to the heart is increased, the ejection fraction may increase to more than 80%, contributing to a greater SV and a greater CO.

Another factor determining cardiac performance is *afterload* or the diastolic blood pressure in the artery leading from the ventricle. Physiologically, afterload is determined primarily by vascular resistance. Vasoconstriction due to sympathetic nervous stimulation or compression of blood vessels due to skeletal muscle contraction will increase vascular resistance and, therefore, increase afterload.

To push open the semilunar valve and eject the blood, when the ventricle contracts it must develop a pressure that is greater than that in the associated artery. Typically, diastolic blood pressure in the aorta is 80 mmHg. Therefore, the left ventricle must develop a pressure slightly greater than 80 mmHg to open the aortic valve and eject the SV. A dynamic exercise, such as running, may cause only a small increase in diastolic pressure (up to 90 mmHg). However, a resistance exercise, such as weight lifting, has a much greater impact on blood pressure and diastolic pressure may be as high as 150–160 mmHg. A healthy heart can easily contract vigorously enough to overcome any increases in afterload associated with exercise or other types of physical exertion. In contrast, a diseased heart or one weakened by advanced age may not be able to generate enough force to effectively overcome a significantly elevated afterload. In this case, the SV and the CO would be reduced. In addition, a sustained or chronic increase in afterload, as observed in patients with hypertension, will also have a detrimental effect on cardiac workload. Initially, the left ventricle will hypertrophy and the chamber walls will become thicker and stronger to compensate for this excess workload. This form of ventricular enlargement is referred to as *concentric* hypertrophy. However, eventually the balance between the oxygen supply and the oxygen demand of the heart is disrupted, leading to a decreased SV, a decreased CO, and heart failure.

In summary, afterload is determined largely by vascular resistance. An increase in vascular resistance leads to an increase in afterload. Stroke volume is inversely proportional to afterload. An increase in afterload may lead to a decrease in SV.

Changes in *heart rate* also affect the contractility of the heart. As heart rate increases, so does ventricular contractility. The mechanism of this effect involves the gradual increase of intracellular calcium. When the

PHARMACY APPLICATION: CARDIAC GLYCOSIDES AND CARDIAC OUTPUT

Heart failure is defined as when a patient's CO is insufficient to meet the metabolic demands of his/her body. One way to improve CO is to enhance myocardial contractility, which will increase SV. The cardiac glycosides, including digoxin, have been used for many years to treat heart failure due to their positive inotropic effect. Digoxin binds to and inhibits the Na^+-K^+-ATPase in the myocardial cell membrane, which ultimately leads to an increase in the intracellular concentration of calcium. As described previously, this increase in calcium may help to enhance myocardial contractility and, therefore, CO.

electrical impulse stimulates the myocardial cell, the permeability to calcium is increased and calcium enters the cytoplasm from the extracellular fluid, as well as from the sarcoplasmic reticulum, allowing it to contract. Between beats, the calcium is removed from the intracellular fluid and the muscle relaxes. When the heart rate is increased, the periods of calcium influx occur more frequently and the time for calcium removal is reduced. The net effect is an increase in intracellular calcium, an increase in the number of cross bridges cycling, and an increase in tension development.

7.8 Effect of exercise on cardiac output

Endurance training, such as running, alters the baseline or tonic activity of the autonomic nervous system. In the trained athlete, the dominance of the parasympathetic system is even greater than it is in the sedentary individual resulting in a training-induced bradycardia. Whereas the resting heart rate is 70–75 beats/min in a sedentary person, the resting heart rate in the trained athlete may be 50 beats/min or lower. Due to the decrease in heart rate in these individuals, the length of diastole is increased. Assuming a constant rate of venous return, this longer filling period results in a greater EDV and an increased SV (40%–50% greater in the elite athlete compared with the untrained individual). Therefore, at rest when their body's metabolic demands are similar, the CO in the sedentary person and the athlete are also similar (see Table 7.7).

During exercise, the CO increases substantially to meet the increased metabolic demand of the working muscles. However, endurance training results in significantly greater increases in CO, which improves oxygen and nutrient delivery to the working muscles (18–20 L/min in sedentary individuals; 30–35 L/min in trained athletes). Thus, exercise performance is enhanced and fatigue is delayed. To increase CO, both heart rate and SV are increased. The maximum heart rate in all individuals is about 185–195 beats/min.

Table 7.7 Effect of exercise on cardiac output

	Sedentary individual	Endurance-trained athlete
Rest		
Heart rate (beats/min)	71	50
Stroke volume (mL/beat)	70	100
Cardiac output (mL/min)	5,000	5,000
Exercise		
Heart rate (beats/min)	195	195
Stroke volume (mL/beat)	100	160
Cardiac output (mL/min)	19,500	31,200

Therefore, the difference in CO in athletically trained vs. untrained people during exercise involves SV. Stroke volume may increase as much as 50%–60% during exercise. Because the athlete has a much larger SV at rest, the increase in SV during exercise is that much greater (see Table 7.7). In this way, even with a similar maximal heart rate, the endurance-trained athlete pumps a significantly greater volume of blood per minute. To accommodate these larger SVs, the ventricles of these athletes hypertrophy such that the chambers become larger and increase their diameters. This form of ventricular enlargement is referred to as *eccentric hypertrophy*.

7.9   Diseases of the heart

7.9.1   Disorders of the pericardium, myocardium, and endocardium

Cardiovascular disease continues to be a major source of mortality and morbidity in the United States with nearly 50% of yearly deaths attributed to diseases of the heart. Heart disease is a broad term that may include diseases of the *pericardium* (the sac surrounding the heart), *myocardium* (the heart muscle itself), or the *endocardium* lining the heart chambers. Disease processes may also affect the coronary blood vessels that supply oxygenated blood to the heart muscle or the heart valves that help regulate normal blood flow. Infectious agents, the immune system and congenital defects may also be causative factors for a number of specific heart diseases.

7.9.1.1   Disorders of the pericardium

The pericardium is a sac composed of two thin layers of connective tissue that surrounds the heart. A thin layer of lubricating fluid called *serous* fluid separates the individual connective tissue layers. The inside of the pericardium surrounding the heart is filled with approximately 30–40 mL of clear serous fluid that prevents the contracting heart from rubbing against the walls of the pericardium.

7.9.1.1.1   Acute pericarditis
- Pericarditis is inflammation of the pericardium. It may be idiopathic in nature or caused by infection, ischemia, neoplasm, radiation, chemotherapy, or immune activity.

Idiopathic—a disease or condition the cause of which is not known or which arises spontaneously

---

7.9.1.1.1.1   Manifestations
- Pain in the precordial or substernal region that is made worse by deep inspiration, coughing or sneezing
- *"Pericardial friction rub"*—A "sandpaper" sound that may be heard though a stethoscope when inflamed pericardial layers rub together; may be heard through a stethoscope
- Low-grade fever
- *Dyspnea*—shallow breathing to avoid chest pain
- ECG changes are possible

7.9.1.1.2   Pericardial effusion   Pericardial effusion is the collection of fluid that may occur in the pericardial sac.

The type of fluid that accumulates in the pericardial sac will depend upon the condition that is present:

- Serous—heart failure or hypoalbuminemia
- Blood—trauma
- Chylous—condition that impairs lymphatic flow
- Pus, inflammatory exudate—infection

7.9.1.1.2.1   Manifestations   If the volume of fluid in the pericardial sac becomes significant (200–250 mL) it can compress the myocardium and cause or lead to *cardiac tamponade* (Figure 7.8). Compression of the myocardium during cardiac tamponade causes decreased CO and venous return. The right side of the heart is affected first because the right atrium and right ventricle have lower diastolic pressure when compared with the left atrium and left ventricle.

7.9.1.1.2.2   Diagnosis   *Pulsus paradoxus* is a key diagnostic feature of cardiac tamponade. A large fall in systolic blood pressure and SV occurs in patients with cardiac tamponade during inspiration. The presence of pulsus paradoxus may be determined by routine blood pressure measurement. Echocardiography is a rapid and definitive technique for accurately determining the presence and severity of pleural effusion and cardiac tamponade.

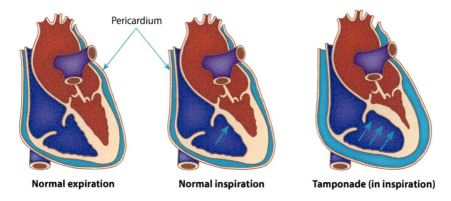

Normal expiration   **Normal inspiration**   **Tamponade (in inspiration)**

Figure 7.8 Cardiac tamponade. Compression of the heart is greater during inspiration due to expansion of the lungs.

7.9.1.1.3 Constrictive (chronic) Carditis Constrictive carditis is a condition in which fibrous scar tissue and even calcifications develop in the pericardium over a period of time. This condition is most commonly associated with chronic inflammation of the pericardium for that persists for months or years. It may be idiopathic or can be caused by infection, uremia, radiation exposure, rheumatic fever, rheumatoid arthritis, or chronic renal failure. The scar tissue that develops in the pericardium may eventually contract and restrict movement of the pericardium. This restriction may compress the myocardium and interfere with ventricular filling and CO.

7.9.1.1.3.1 Rationale for treatment of pericarditis Treatment for pericarditis involves relief of symptoms and elimination of the causative agent(s). Analgesics may be used for relief of pain, whereas anti-inflammatory drugs (e.g., aspirin, salicylates, nonsteroidal anti-inflammatory drugs, corticosteroids) can be employed to reduce inflammation of the pericardial tissues. Antibiotics may be initiated if bacterial infection is the cause of the inflammation. *Pericardiocentesis* or aspiration of accumulated fluid from the pericardial sac is often done to relieve cardiac compression and reduce symptoms.

7.9.2   Diseases of the myocardium

Myocardial diseases are those that originate in the heart muscle.

7.9.2.1   Myocarditis

Inflammation of the heart muscle without a myocardial infarction. It may result from infection with viruses like *Coxsackie B* that replicate in heart muscle or from bacterial or fungal infections.

7.9.2.1.1   Manifestations   Myocarditis may initially be asymptomatic but can present with flu-like symptoms in the acute stages. Many types of myocarditis can resolve with drug therapy and bed rest. However, it can progress to myocardial enlargement or congestive heart failure if chronic inflammation continues.

7.9.2.2   Cardiomyopathies

Cardiomyopathies are a group of diseases affecting the heart muscle. They may be primary in nature with an uncertain etiology or they may be secondary to cardiovascular disease or other identifiable factors. The cardiomyopathies are classified into three distinct types based on their presentation: *dilated, hypertrophic, and constrictive*:

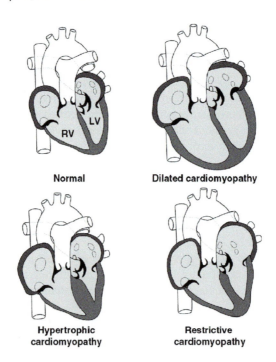

Normal   Dilated cardiomyopathy

Hypertrophic   Restrictive
cardiomyopathy   cardiomyopathy

7.9.2.2.1   Dilated cardiomyopathy   Dilated cardiomyopathy is characterized by gross enlargement of the heart chambers that results in markedly impaired ventricular function. The majority of cases are idiopathic. Secondary causes may include ischemic heart disease, chronic infection, alcoholism, chronic myocarditis, or exposure to chemotherapy agents such as daunorubicin. A genetic cause has been identified in approximately 25%–30% of cases in which the genes coding for contractile proteins may be defective.

7.9.2.2.1.1 Manifestations
- Fatigue due to reduced CO, dyspnea, and pulmonary congestion
- Arrhythmia may occur due to altered conduction in the dilated myocardium

7.9.2.2.2 Hypertrophic cardiomyopathy Hypertrophic cardiomyopathy is characterized by massive enlargement (hypertrophy) of the ventricular muscle and septum that severely limits ventricular filling volume and thus CO. Although some cases may be idiopathic, most primary cases of hypertrophic cardiomyopathy are due to genetic mutations in the genes coding for the cardiac contractile proteins myosin and troponin. The severity of hypertrophic cardiomyopathy can vary greatly. Most patients have a form in which there is significant thickening of the septum. Secondary causes of hypertrophic cardiomyopathy may include chronic hypertension and heart valve disease. Diagnosis is typically made through echocardiogram.

7.9.2.2.2.1 Manifestations
- Fatigue, angina, dyspnea
- Arrhythmia, myocardial infarction and heart failure are all possible outcomes

7.9.2.2.3 Cardiac hypertrophy due to chronic hypertension or heart valve disease Hypertrophy of the myocardium may also occur as a result of chronic hypertension. Generally, the left ventricle is most affected in patients with chronic hypertension. The chronically elevated afterload that accompanies hypertension increases workload on the ventricle and, in turn, leads to hypertrophy. Abnormal heart valve function, possibly due to infection, inflammation or developmental defect, can also lead to cardiac hypertrophy if untreated. Incompetent (leaky) heart valves will allow blood that had been pumped from the ventricle to regurgitate back into the chamber and thus increase filling and workload of that chamber. Stenotic (narrowed) valves can also increase the workload of the ventricles by increasing the resistance to blood flow out of the ventricle. Unlike the physiologic enlargement that can occur in athletes with exercise, the hypertrophy that accompanies hypertension or heart valve disease is pathologic and will lead to eventual impairment of cardiac function and heart failure. Such hypertrophy can also impair normal electrical conduction of the heart muscle and lead to arrhythmia.

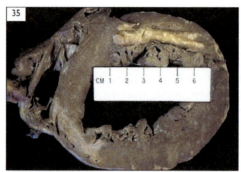

Ventricle affected by hypertrophy

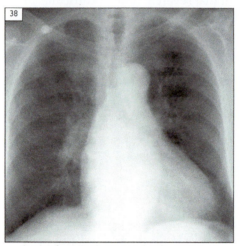

X-ray of cardiac hypertrophy (frontal view)

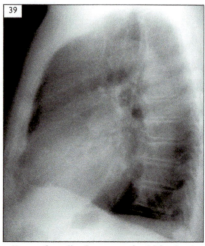

X-ray of cardiac hypertrophy (side view)

7.9.2.2.4   Restrictive cardiomyopathy   Restrictive cardiomyopathy is a disorder characterized by "stiffness" of heart muscle and excessive rigidity of ventricular walls. It is a relatively uncommon disorder that may be caused by systemic diseases such as amyloidosis, glycogen storage disease, or sarcoidosis. Substances such as amyloid or glycogen can infiltrate the heart muscle and impair normal mechanical function. The walls of the ventricle and the ventricular chamber remain relatively normal in terms of thickness and size.

7.9.2.2.4.1   Manifestations
- Excessive rigidity of ventricular walls that limits ventricular filling and markedly diminishes CO
- Fatigue, dyspnea, signs of right-heart failure
- Arrhythmia is common; may lead to congestive heart failure

7.9.2.2.4.2   Treatment of cardiomyopathy   The congestive effects of cardiomyopathy on the pulmonary and systemic circulation may be relieved somewhat by the use of diuretic drugs and with salt and water restriction. Bed rest can reduce workload on the heart, as can vasodilator drugs that cause venous and arterial dilation. Positive inotropes such as digitalis glycosides may be used in dilated cardiomyopathy to enhance contractile function of the heart muscle. Anticoagulant drugs can also be employed to prevent blood clots from forming in pooled blood. In hypertrophic cardiomyopathy, β blockers may be useful to slow heart rate and allow the ventricles a greater time for filling. Prevention of arrhythmias is also important in hypertrophic cardiomyopathy. Surgical removal of a portion of the hypertrophic ventricles may also be carried out to improve overall cardiac function.

7.9.3   Disorders of the endocardium and heart valves

The endocardium is the tissue that lines the chambers of the heart. Disorders of the endocardium often spread to involve the heart valves that are continuous with the endocardium.

7.9.3.1   Infectious endocarditis
- Infection of the endocardium is most often caused by *Streptococcus or Staphylococcus* bacteria. May also be caused by fungi or *Candida* in susceptible patients.
- Predisposing factors include previous damage to the endocardium, intravenous drug use, and systemic bacterial infections (bacteremia). The presence of prosthetic heart valves or heart valve disease has also been shown to increase a patient's risk for infective endocarditis. Organisms generally enter the endocardium from the blood

that enters the heart chambers from the circulation. Blood culture is important for identifying the causative agent. Echocardiography may be used to detect structural changes in the endocardium and heart valves.

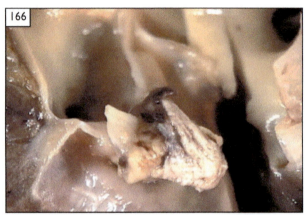

Heart valves affected by infective endocarditis

7.9.3.1.1   Manifestations
- Fever and signs of systemic infection
- Damage to endocardium/myocardium
- Formation of thrombi that can break loose into circulation as emboli
- Damage to the heart valves because they are continuous with the endocardium

7.9.3.1.2   Treatment
- Drug therapy directed at eliminating the causative agent
- Surgical repair of damaged tissue if necessary

7.9.3.2   Rheumatic heart disease
Rheumatic heart disease is a condition that arises as a result of an immune-mediated response to infection with *group A (beta-hemolytic) streptococci* bacteria. The condition is associated with acute, recurrent or chronic inflammation of the heart that may affect the endocardium, myocardium and heart valves. The condition often begins after a respiratory tract infection. It is believed that certain antibodies generated by the immune system against the infecting streptococcal bacteria cross-react with proteins in the human heart that may have similar structure. Tissues of the heart valves are particularly affected. Vegetative lesions and calcifications may

occur in the affected heart valves over time, which, years later, can impair their function and eventually precipitate cardiac hypertrophy and heart failure. Although primarily a disease of school-age children, the long-term effects of rheumatic fever on the heart might not manifest for many years. Joint tissues may also be affected by this immune-mediated process and, as a result, patients with rheumatic fever also present with inflammatory polyarthritis.

7.9.3.2.1   Manifestations
- Low-grade fever
- *Erythema marginatum*—macular lesions that develop on the trunk and abdomen. Often presents as concentric circles that can disappear as the disease progresses
- *Syndenham chorea*—CNS manifestations that include behavioral changes, and *choreiform* (purposeless, jerky) movements. Generally self-limiting
- Polyarthritis that can affect numerous joints
- Subcutaneous nodules that develop over joints of the wrists, elbows and knees
- The most serious manifestation of rheumatic fever endocarditis is chronic disease of the heart valves that may markedly alter cardiac function and lead to heart failure a number of years later

7.9.3.2.2   Treatment
- Antibiotic therapy to eradicate the streptococcal organism. Anti-inflammatory agents may be useful.
- Surgical repair or replacement of damaged heart valves if necessary.

7.9.4   Disorders of the heart valves
Normal heart valves should open fully to allow for the smooth flow of blood between chambers of the heart and out into the large arteries. The valves should also close tightly to prevent any backflow of blood. Damage to heart valves most commonly occurs as a result of inflammation or infection of the endocardium secondary to infective endocarditis or rheumatic fever. Damage may also occur through ischemia or by direct trauma. Congenital defects or abnormalities of the heart valves may also be present at birth. Abnormalities of the *mitral* valve will affect blood flow from the left atrium to the left ventricle, whereas alteration in the *aortic* valve will affect blood flow from the left ventricle into the aorta.

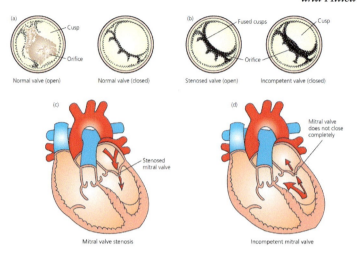

Normal valve (open)   Normal valve (closed)   Stenosed valve (open)   Incompetent valve (closed)

Mitral valve stenosis   Incompetent mitral valve

Two major types of changes are commonly seen with heart valve disease: *stenosis* and *incompetence*. Stenosis is a narrowing of the valve opening due to thickening of the valve cusps. Stenosis may result from scaring of the valves that occurs from rheumatic fever or from a congenital malformation in the valve. The result of stenosis is a turbulent blood flow that leads to decreased efficiency of blood pumping and an increased workload on the chamber that is pumping. *Aortic stenosis* affects the aortic semilunar valve and reduces blood flow from the left ventricle into the aorta. *Mitral stenosis* affects the mitral valve, located between the atria and ventricles, and reduces blood flow between those two chambers. *Incompetent or regurgitant valves* are heart valves that fail to shut completely and therefore allow blood to flow to continue even when closed. Valves may become incompetent after being damaged by rheumatic fever or as a result of congenital mitral valve prolapse (see figure d above). With *aortic regurgitation*, the aortic semilunar valve fails to shut properly and some blood flows back into the left ventricle after contraction. *Mitral regurgitation* is characterized by a backflow of blood from the left ventricle into the left atrium during contraction.

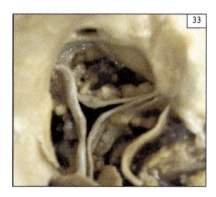

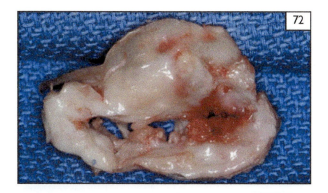

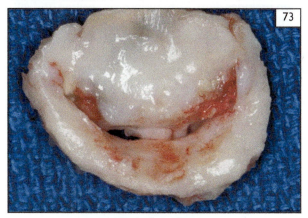

Mitral valve prolapse

7.9.4.1 Mitral valve prolapse

A condition in which the upper edges of the mitral valves protrude into the atrium during contraction. The mitral valves are thickened and enlarged. The actual cause of the disorder is uncertain, but it has a higher incidence in women than men, suggesting a familial basis.

The disorder has also been associated with other diseases of connective tissue such as Marfan syndrome. Although many cases of mitral valve prolapse are completely asymptomatic, some patients may experience fatigue and dizziness as well as atypical chest pain that is not associated with exercise.

7.9.4.1.1 Diagnosis of valvular heart disease

- Auscultation—diagnostic murmur or rumble
- Echocardiography
- ECG changes—reflect chamber enlargement
- Chest X-ray—dilation of heart chambers or aorta
- Hemodynamic changes

7.9.4.1.2   Manifestations

- Decreased CO
- ECG changes, arrhythmia: turbulent blood flow produces a prominent sound or "murmur" that can be heard with a stethoscope
- Dilation of affected atria due to backflow of blood seen with mitral or aortic regurgitation or increased back pressure with mitral valve stenosis
- Hypertrophy of left ventricle due to increased workload associated with aortic stenosis
- Heart failure as a possible long-term consequence of progressive hypertrophy

7.9.4.1.3   Treatment of heart valve disease

Pharmacotherapy of valvular disease often includes *diuretics* to reduce congestion and *anticoagulants* to prevent the formation of an embolism. *Vasodilators* can be of value in reducing afterload in mitral valve disease. *Anti-arrhythmic* drugs may be employed if arrhythmias are present. Positive inotropic agents like *digitalis glycosides* can increase the force of contraction if heart failure occurs. *Antibiotics* may be given prophylactically to prevent endocarditis. A number of techniques have evolved in recent years for surgically treating or correcting valvular defects. *Mitral valvotomy* involves opening of the mitral valve either surgically or with a balloon catheter. *Valvuloplasty* may be performed to surgically repair damaged valves or, if the disease is too advanced, affected valves may be completely replaced with graft valves (porcine, bovine or human) or with mechanical valves.

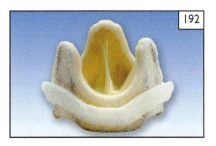

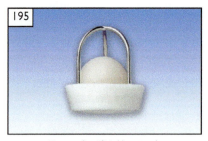

Types of artificial heart valves

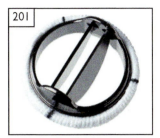

Types of artificial heart valves

7.9.4.2   Congenital heart defects

Congenital defects of the heart are abnormalities that occur during fetal development.

7.9.4.2.1   *Patent ductus arteriosus*   One of the most common congenital abnormalities of the heart is *patent ductus arteriosus* (see Figure 7.9).

During fetal development the lungs are collapsed and blood is shunted around the lungs by a special blood vessel called the *ductus arteriosus* that connects the pulmonary artery with the aorta. When the lungs inflate at

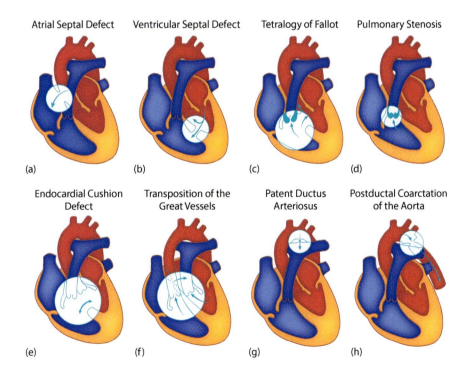

Figure 7.9   Congenital defects of the heart.

birth, blood flows through the pulmonary vessels and the *ductus arteriosus* occludes. In about 1 of every 5,500 births this duct fails to close properly and remains patent. The presence of this duct allows for the backflow of aortic blood into the pulmonary artery. The turbulent blood flow can be detected on auscultation as a murmur. If not corrected, the continued pulmonary congestion places an excess workload on the heart that can result in heart failure years later. Surgical correction of patent ductus arteriosus is relatively simple and essentially involves ligation of the ductus arteriosus.

7.9.4.2.1.1 Atrial or ventricular septal defects Among the most common of congenital heart defects, atrial or ventricular septal defects occur when the septum between the atria or ventricle fails to close during fetal development. Atrial septal defects may be asymptomatic and are often first diagnosed during a routine physical examination. Smaller atrial defects may close spontaneously with aging, whereas larger defects may require surgical correction. Ventricular septal defects are one of the most common congenital heart defects. Shunting of blood will occur from the higher pressure left side of the heart toward the lower pressure right side of the heart. The degree of shunting will depend upon the size of the defect. Large ventricular defects can lead to heart failure and overall failure to thrive. Although many ventricular septal defects will close spontaneously during the first year of life, those that are very large or are causing failure to thrive in the infant should be surgically repaired.

7.10   Myocardial ischemia

The coronary arteries supply oxygenated blood to the myocardium. The coronary arteries fill with oxygenated blood from the aorta during diastole. At rest, the delivery of oxygenated blood and nutrients supplied by the coronary arteries should match the metabolic demands of the heart. Myocardial oxygen demand is increased by factors such as exercise or increased preload and afterload, which increase heart rate and contractility. When the metabolic needs of the heart increase, coronary blood flow should increase accordingly. Coronary blood flow is regulated locally through the accumulation of cardiac metabolites such as lactic acid, CO_2 and adenosine, which cause coronary artery vasodilation and increased blood flow. Increased cardiac workload also results in increased shear forces in the coronary arteries that distends them and triggers the release of nitric oxide from the endothelium that dilates the vascular smooth muscle and increases coronary blood flow.

Myocardial ischemia occurs when the blood flow demands of the heart exceed the supply of oxygenated blood delivered to the myocardium by the coronary arteries. A leading cause of myocardial ischemia is *atherosclerosis* that reduces blood flow through the coronary arteries. Myocardial ischemia can also result from coronary vasospasm, marked hypotension, and anemia.

With age and the progressive occlusion of coronary arteries, smaller *collateral* vessels may begin to carry a greater proportion of blood and provide an alternate means of perfusion for an area of myocardium. These *collateral* blood vessels may run parallel to the larger coronary arteries and be connected to other small coronary vessels by vascular connections called *anastomoses*. Development of collateral circulation may reduce or delay the occurrence of symptoms from myocardial ischemia until the blockage is very progressed. The presence of extensively developed collateral circulation might also explain why many older individuals often survive serious heart attacks when younger individuals, who have not had the chance to develop collateral circulation, often do not.

7.10.1   *Manifestations of myocardial ischemia*

Angina pectoris is the major symptom of myocardial ischemia. Angina pectoris most commonly presents as pain, pressure or a burning sensation in the area of the sternum.

There are three types of angina pectoris:

1. *Classic, exertional, stable angina*
   - Generally caused by a "stable" atherosclerotic plaque.
   - Pain is precipitated by factors that increase workload such as exercise, emotions, stress, and cold exposure. Pain resolves with rest.
   - Symptoms may remain "stable" for a number of years or progress in severity.
   - Treatment is generally symptomatic and designed to reduce myocardial oxygen demand and/or increase coronary artery blood flow.

2. *Unstable angina*
   - Pain that occurs at rest. Coronary blood flow does not meet the metabolic needs of the heart even at rest.
   - Usually associated with extensive blockade of coronary arteries and an unstable atherosclerotic plaque. It is a component of acute coronary syndrome. Also referred to as "pre-infarct" angina because it can lead to an imminent myocardial infarction if not treated.
   - Requires intensive treatment that may include potent antiplatelet/ anticoagulant therapy and surgical interventions such as cardiac catheterization, angioplasty or coronary artery bypass graft.

3. *Variant angina (vasospastic angina, Prinzmetal's angina)*
   - Caused by vasospasm of the coronary arteries. Atherosclerosis may or may not be present.

- May result from excess sympathetic activity.
- Frequently occurs at night or at rest.
- Generally benign but can lead to arrhythmia or infarction if the spasm persists.

Silent ischemia is a particularly dangerous form of myocardial ischemia because of the lack of clinical symptoms, that is, ischemia without angina. It is usually diagnosed by exercise stress testing or Holter monitoring (see Table 7.8).

7.10.2   Acute coronary syndromes

Acute coronary syndromes are a continuum of conditions that includes unstable angina, non-ST elevation myocardial infarction (non-STEMI) and ST elevation myocardial infarction (STEMI). It begins when a previously stable atherosclerotic plaque in a coronary artery destabilizes and loses its protective fibrous cap. When a plaque destabilizes, the necrotic core is exposed, which allows platelets to attach to form a platelet plug. Formation of the platelet plug is accompanied by activation of the clotting cascades, leading to the rapid formation of a blood clot in the coronary artery. This forming clot rapidly occludes blood flow to the myocardium to cause ischemia and angina pain at rest. If the clot resolves or breaks up quickly, no permanent damage will occur to the myocardium. However, if the occlusion of blood flow persists, myocardial injury and necrosis will begin to occur. Initially, the injury will only involve the subendocardial layer of muscle and is characterized by ST depression and T wave inversion without ST elevation (hence the term non-STEMI) on an ECG. Prolonged occlusion of coronary blood flow will result in myocardial injury that involves the full thickness of the heart wall (transumral) and is characterized by marked elevation of the ST segments (STEMI) on the ECG.

7.10.2.1   Rational for treatment of myocardial ischemia
Treatment of myocardial ischemia involves two strategies:

1. Increasing coronary blood flow by dilating coronary arteries
2. Reducing cardiac workload by reducing the heart rate and/or the force of contraction

Table 7.8   Diagnosis of myocardial ischemia

- Electrocardiogram (ECG)—only useful if ischemia is present at time of ECG
- Holter monitoring (24 ambulatory ECG)—can detect episodes of ischemia during a normal day; patient can press a button on the monitor when they experience angina, which can then be correlated with possible ECG changes
- Stress testing with ECG—exercise is used to increase cardiac workload and precipitate ischemia
- Nuclear imaging
- Cardiac catheterization

7.10.2.2   Treatment of myocardial ischemia

The treatment regimen may include both non-pharmacologic and pharma-cologic therapies.

Non-pharmacologic treatment
- Pacing of physical activity
- Avoidance of stress (e.g., emotional, physiologic, cold)
- Reduction of risk factors for ischemic heart disease (e.g., hyperlipid-emia, obesity, hypertension, diabetes, smoking)

Pharmacologic treatment
Organic nitrates—e.g., nitroglycerin
- Dilate coronary arteries and increase myocardial blood flow
- Dilate peripheral arteries and reduce *afterload*
- Dilate peripheral veins and reduce *preload*

β-Adrenergic blockers—e.g., atenolol
- Block myocardial β adrenergic receptors
- Reduce heart rate and CO (resulting in reduced myocardial work-load and oxygen demand)

QUESTION...

Why would the use of β-adrenergic blockers be contraindicated in patients with heart block?

Calcium Channel Blockers—e.g., Nifedipine
- Block calcium channels in vascular smooth muscle
- Dilate coronary arteries and increase myocardial blood flow
- Dilate peripheral arteries and reduce *afterload*

Aspirin, heparin
- Prevent platelet aggregation
- Used for prophylaxis of blood clots particularly in unstable angina

Surgical treatments
Coronary angioplasty
- Uses a balloon catheter to open occluded blood vessels
- Usually performed under local anesthetic
- 5% mortality, high rate of vessel reocclusion
- Placement of drug-treated "stents" in opened vessel reduces rates of occlusion

Coronary artery bypass graft
- Revascularization procedure in which a blood vessel is taken from elsewhere in the body and surgically sutured around a blocked coronary artery
- May involve multiple (1–5) blood vessels
- Reocclusion of transplanted vessel is possible

KEY TERMS

Ischemia—inadequate blood flow to a tissue or part of the body

Hypoxia—deficiency of oxygen in tissues

Preload—the load on the heart at the end of diastole; determined by EDV

Afterload—the force that the contracting heart must generate to eject blood; effected by peripheral vascular resistance and arterial pressure

---

7.11   Myocardial infarction

Myocardial infarction or "heart attack" is a condition in which there is the death of cardiac muscle tissue. Myocardial infarctions are the leading killer of both men and women in the United States. Most infarctions are the direct result of coronary artery occlusions that may occur when atherosclerotic plaque becomes unstable. Emboli from a deep vein thrombosis may also lodge in and occlude a coronary artery. Prolonged vasospasm associated with vasospastic angina might also precipitate a myocardial infarction in certain individuals.

7.11.1   Coronary blood flow and myocardial infarction

The area of the heart affected by a myocardial infarction will be determined by which coronary blood vessel is occluded. The two main coronary arteries supplying the myocardium are the *left coronary artery* (which subdivides into the *left anterior descending* and *circumflex* branches) and the *right coronary artery*. The *left anterior descending* artery supplies blood to the bulk of the anterior left ventricular wall, while the *left circumflex artery* provides blood to the left atrium and the posterior and lateral walls of the left ventricle. The *right coronary artery* mainly provides blood to the right atria and right ventricles. Nearly 50% of all myocardial infarctions involve the *left anterior descending* artery that supplies blood to the main pumping mass of the left ventricle. The next most common site for myocardial infarction is the *right coronary artery*, followed by the *left circumflex*. A myocardial infarction may be *transmural*, meaning it involves the full thickness of the ventricular wall or *subendocardial*, in which the inner one-third to one-half of the ventricular wall is involved. *Transmural infarcts* tend to have a greater effect on cardiac function and pumping ability because a greater mass of ventricular muscle is involved.

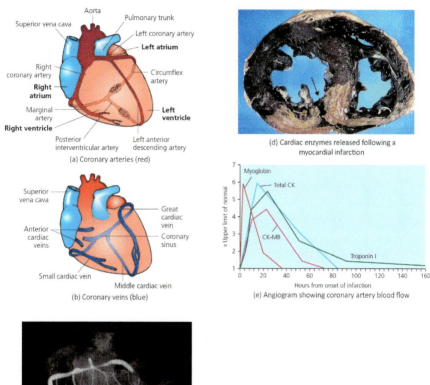

(a) Coronary arteries (red)

(b) Coronary veins (blue)

(c) Massive infarction in the ventricles and septum

(d) Cardiac enzymes released following a myocardial infarction

(e) Angiogram showing coronary artery blood flow

When a myocardial infarction occurs, three zones of affected cardiac muscle may be identified: the *zone of necrosis*, the *zone of injury*, and the *zone of ischemia*. The zone of necrosis refers to the cardiac myocytes that have been killed as a result of prolonged ischemia. These necrotic cells cannot be salvaged and will eventually be replaced by nonfunctional scar tissue. The zone adjacent to the necrotic zone consists of cardiac myocytes that have become injured due to prolonged ischemia. These cells are very important because therapeutic interventions that restore blood flow to the heart muscle could salvage these cells before they become irreversibly injured and go on to necrosis. Salvaging of these injured myocytes by rapid restoration of blood flow will also salvage cardiac muscle function in the patient. Even if they survive the period of ischemia, injured cardiac myocytes may require a period of time before they are able to return to full contractile function. The zone of ischemia contains cardiac myocytes that border the injured myocytes. These ischemic cells will become injured myocytes if the ischemia persists but will likely return to full function once the infarction has passed or blood flow has been reestablished.

7.11.2 Clinical manifestations of myocardial infarction

- Severe chest pain and discomfort: a pressing or crushing sensation often accompanied by nausea, vomiting, sweating, and weakness due to hypotension. Females patients tend to have a greater incidence of atypical presentations with myocardial infarction that often include a preponderance of gastrointestinal symptoms. A small percentage of patients may also experience "silent" myocardial infarctions that have few or none of the common symptoms.
- Irreversible cellular injury generally occurs 20–30 min after the onset of complete ischemia
- Release of myocardial enzymes into circulation from myocardial damaged cells (see Table 7.9)
- Electrocardiogram changes:
  - Myocardial ischemia—inversion of T wave, no S-T elevation (NSTEMI)
  - Myocardial injury—ST elevation (STEMI)
  - Pronounced Q waves—develop several hours after STEMI; do not resolve with time and remain as a lifelong indicator that a patient has suffered a myocardial infarction
- Inflammatory response from the injured myocardium—associated with fever, leukocyte infiltration, increased white blood cell counts, elevated sedimentation rate
- Hyperglycemia

7.11.3 Compensatory mechanisms for myocardial infarction

As a result of the hypotension and hemodynamic changes that accompany a myocardial infarction, the cardiovascular system initiates a number of reflex

Table 7.9   Cardiac biomarkers

Cardiac Troponin T (TnT) Cardiac Troponin I (TnI)	Highly sensitive and specific markers of myocardial injury Serum levels increase 3–6 hours after the onset of chest pain
Myoglobin	Found in both cardiac and skeletal muscle Most sensitive early marker of a myocardial infarction
Creatine Kinase–Muscle/Brain (MB)	Found mainly in heart muscle; not as specific as cardiac troponins; levels increase 3–12 hours after the onset of chest pain

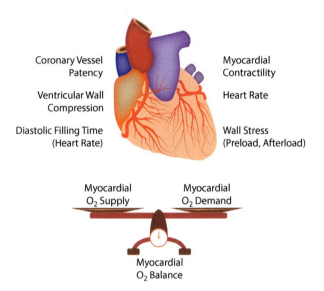

Figure 7.10   Myocardial oxygen balance is a function of supply and demand.

compensatory mechanisms designed to maintain CO and adequate tissue perfusion:

- Catecholamine release—increases heart rate, force of contraction and peripheral resistance. Catecholamines can, however, be arrhythmogenic
- Sodium and water retention
- Activation of renin-angiotensin system leading to peripheral vaso constriction
- Ventricular hypertrophy

Unfortunately, these compensatory changes may increase oxygen demand and workload on the infarcted heart and worsen overall cardiac function.

7.11.4   Complications of myocardial infarction

Once myocardial necrosis occurs, an inflammatory process generally follows for 1–2 days. Dead tissue and debris are then removed in the next 4–10 days by enzymatic digestion and immune cell activity. Scar tissue replacement generally begins 2 weeks after the infarction. During this repair process, the infarcted area is still quite weak and susceptible to rupture. Complete scar tissue replacement of the affected area generally takes 6–8 weeks to complete. Repair of damaged areas occurs by replacement with scar tissue that does not contract or conduct electrical impulses; therefore, alterations in cardiac function are inevitable. Depending upon the extent of the area involved in a myocardial infarction, a number of complications might arise such as:

- Rupture of weakened myocardial wall at the site of the infarction. Rupture of the septum between the ventricles might also occur if the septal wall is involved in the infarction.
- Bleeding into pericardium may cause *cardiac tamponade* and further impair cardiac pumping function. This is most likely to occur with a transmural infarction. Formation of a thromboembolism from pooling of blood in the ventricles.
- Pericarditis—inflammation may result in pericardial friction rub. Often occurs 1–2 days post infarction.
- Arrhythmia—common as a result of hypoxia, acidosis and altered electrical conduction through damaged and necrotic areas of the myocardium. May be life threatening and lead to fibrillation.
- Reduced cardiac function—typically presents with reduced myocardial contractility, reduced wall compliance, decreased SV and increased left ventricular end diastolic volume.
- Congestive heart failure may result if a large enough area of the myocardium has been damaged such that the heart no longer pumps effectively.
- Cardiogenic shock—marked hypotension that can result from extensive damage to the left ventricle. The resulting hypotension will trigger cardiovascular compensatory mechanisms that will further tax the damaged myocardium and exacerbate impaired function. Cardiogenic shock is associated with a mortality rate of 80% or greater.

7.11.5   Rationale for therapy

A main goal of intervention for myocardial infarction is to limit the size of the infracted area and thus preserve cardiac function. Early recognition and intervention in a myocardial infarction has been shown to significantly improve the outcome and reduce mortality in afflicted patients. If employed in the early stages of myocardial infarction, platelet inhibitors

---

KEY TERMS

Cardiac tamponade—excessive pressure that develops from the accumulation of fluid in the pericardium

Pericarditis—inflammation of the pericardium

Stroke volume—volume of blood ejected from each ventricle per beat

End-diastolic volume—volume of blood remaining in the ventricle at the end of systole (contraction)

---

such as aspirin and clot dissolving agents such as tissue plasminogen activator may be very effective in improving myocardial blood flow and limiting damage to the heart muscle. Other drugs such as vasodilators, β adrenergic blockers and angiotensin-converting enzyme (ACE) inhibitors can also improve blood flow and reduce the workload on the injured myocardium and thus reduce the extent of myocardial damage. The development of potentially life-threatening arrhythmias is also common during myocardial infraction as a consequence of hypoxia, acidosis and enhanced autonomic activity and must be treated with appropriate anti-arrhythmia drugs. Supportive therapies such as oxygen, pain management, and sedatives are also utilized.

7.11.5.1 Treatment for myocardial infarction

- Oxygen—used to maintain blood oxygenation as well as tissue and cardiac O_2 levels
- Aspirin and other platelet inhibitors (clopidogrel)—may reduce the overall size of the infarction if administered when a myocardial infarction is first detected
- Thrombolytic agents (tissue plasminogen activator—if employed in the first 1–4 hours following the onset of a myocardial infarction, these drugs may dissolve clots in coronary blood vessels and reestablish blood flow
- Vasodilator drugs—nitroglycerin can increase blood flow to the myocardium and reduce myocardial work by dilating peripheral arteries and veins
- β-Blockers—blunt the effect of catecholamine release on the myocardium and reduce heart rate and myocardial workload
- Pain management—sublingual nitroglycerin, morphine if necessary
- Anti-arrhythmic drugs—to treat and prevent a number of potentially life-threatening arrhythmias that might arise following a myocardial infarction

- ACE Inhibitors—drugs that block activation of the renin-angiotensin system and thus reduce the negative effects of vasoconstriction and salt and water retention on the myocardium
- Surgical reperfusion:
  - Percutaneous coronary intervention (PCI)—may involve placing a balloon catheter in the affected coronary artery to restore blood flow. A spring-loaded metal stent is often placed in the vessel to help keep it open. Stents may be coated with drugs such as sirolimus that release slowly over time to prevent local cellular proliferation and reocclusion of the vessel
  - Coronary artery bypass grafting (CABG)—the procedure involves replacing occluded coronary arteries with graft vessels taken from elsewhere in the body
  - With both PCI and CABG, reocclusion of coronary arteries may still occur over time

7.12 Heart failure

According to statistics, approximately 5.1 million individuals in the United States have heart failure. Nearly half of the individuals who develop heart failure will die within 5 years of diagnosis. Heart failure costs the U.S. nation an estimated $32 billion each year as a result of the cost of health care services, medications to treat heart failure, and missed days of work (Heidenreich 2011). Heart failure is a condition in which the heart is no longer pumping blood effectively. Depending upon the cause, heart failure may be classified as low-output failure or high-output failure. Low-output failure is a reduced pumping efficiency of the heart that is caused by factors that impair cardiac function such as myocardial ischemia, myocardial infarction or cardiomyopathy. With high-output failure, the CO is normal or elevated but still cannot meet the metabolic and oxygen need of the tissues. Common causes of high-output failure can include hyperthyroidism (hypermetabolism) and anemia (reduced oxygen carrying capacity), conditions in which even greatly elevated CO cannot keep up with the increased metabolic requirements of the tissues.

7.12.1 Classification of heart failure

Heart failure may be classified into *systolic failure* or *diastolic failure* based on the ejection fraction, which is the percentage of blood pumped out of the ventricles with each contraction. A normal ejection fraction is between 55% and 70%. Systolic failure occurs when the heart is unable to generate adequate CO as a result of reduced contractility. Left ventricular ejection fraction is significantly decreased with systolic failure. Systolic failure most commonly occurs in patients that have experienced

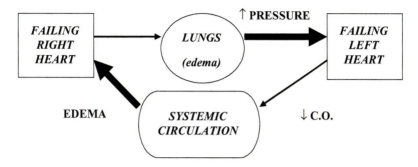

Figure 7.11   Circulatory disturbances in heart failure.

a myocardial infarction. Diastolic failure often accompanies systolic failure and occurs when the ventricles do not relax normally. Cardiac output may be decreased in diastolic failure due a reduced ventricular filling (preload). Diastolic failure may occur in patients with ventricular hypertrophy due to prolonged hypertension or cardiomyopathy or from cardiac tamponade.

From the standpoint of physiologic symptoms, the manifestations of heart failure can be divided into those occurring as a result of *left-heart failure* (left atrium and ventricle) and *right-heart failure* (right atrium and ventricle) (see Figure 7.11).

7.12.2   Left heart failure

The left side of the heart is responsible for pumping oxygenated blood from the lungs out to the peripheral tissues of the body. The most common causes of left-heart failure include myocardial infarction, cardiomyopathy, and chronic hypertension. Left-heart failure is also referred to as *congestive heart failure* due to the pulmonary congestion of blood that accompanies the condition (see Figure 7.12).

7.12.2.1   Manifestations of left-heart failure
- Decreased *SV*, increased *left-ventricular end-diastolic volume (LVEDV)*, increased *preload*.
- Congestion of blood in the pulmonary circulation leading to increased pulmonary pressure and pulmonary edema.
- Dyspnea, cough, frothy sputum. "Rales" or crackling sounds that may be heard through a stethoscope as a result of fluid accumulation in the lungs. *Orthopnea,* the accumulation of fluids and dyspnea are often worse at night or when the patient lies in the supine position because

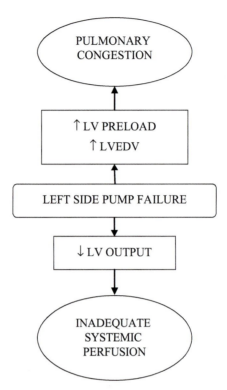

Figure 7.12   Consequences of left-heart failure.

blood and fluids from the lower limbs may redistribute into the pulmonary circulation.

- Poor perfusion of systemic circulation may lead to *cyanosis*.
- Generalized fatigue and muscle weakness.

7.12.3   Right heart failure

Right-heart failure may arise as a consequence of left-heart failure. As a result of the increased pulmonary pressure that accompanies left-heart failure, the resistance to blood flow now faced by the right ventricle is significantly increased as it pumps blood to the lungs. Over time the increased workload on the right ventricle leads to dilation and eventual failure of the

---

KEY TERMS

Stroke volume—the volume of blood pumped by one ventricle during one contraction

LVEDV—"left ventricular end diastolic volume"; the amount of blood that fills the left ventricle during relaxation

Ejection fraction—the fraction of the blood contained in the ventricle at the end of diastole that is expelled during its contraction (the SV divided by EDV)

Preload—the degree to which the myocardium is stretched by venous return. Determined by LVEDV

Afterload—the pressure the heart must overcome to pump blood out into the aorta

Orthopnea—difficulty breathing when lying down

Cyanosis—bluish discoloration of the skin and mucous membranes due to inadequate amounts of oxygen in the blood

---

right heart (see Figure 7.13). Right-heart failure may also result from chronic obstructive pulmonary disease, cystic fibrosis or adult respiratory distress syndrome, which can increase resistance to blood flow through the lungs and thus increase workload on the left heart.

7.12.3.1 Manifestations of right-heart failure
- Increased right ventricular workload
- Venous congestion and distention
- Peripheral edema, ascites
- Swelling of the liver with possible injury and eventual failure
- Gastrointestinal symptoms—anorexia, weight loss, gastrointestinal distress

7.12.4 Physiologic compensation for heart failure

The signs and symptoms of heart failure may not appear in the early stages due to a number of compensatory mechanisms that combine to maintain CO. This early stage of heart failure is termed *compensated heart failure*. The compensatory responses are only effective in the short term and will eventually

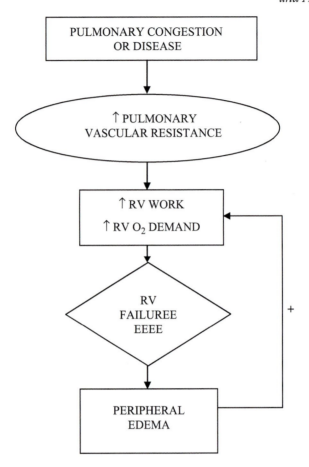

Figure 7.13   Consequences of right-heart failure.

be unable to maintain CO for a long period of time. *Decompensated heart failure* occurs when CO is no longer adequately maintained and overt symptoms of heart failure appear (see Figure 7.14).

Compensatory mechanisms include:

1. *Increased CO*: The normal heart responds to increases in preload or
   LVEDV by increasing SV and CO. The greater the heart is stretched by
   filling, the greater its responsive strength of contraction (*Frank-Starling
   Principle*) (see Figure 7.15). With heart failure there are chronic increases
   in preload that continually distend the ventricular muscle fibers. Over
   time, the compensatory Frank-Starling mechanism becomes ineffective because the cardiac muscle fibers stretch beyond the maximum
   limit for efficient contraction. In addition, the oxygen requirements of

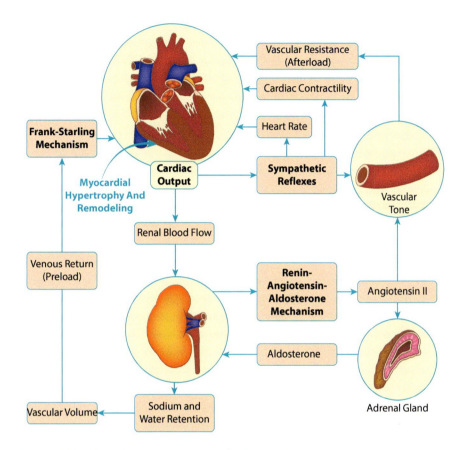

Figure 7.14   Physiologic compensation for heart failure.

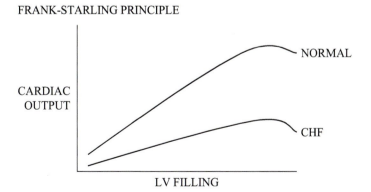

Figure 7.15   Frank-Starling principle graph. Increased filling of the ventricles (venous return) leads to increased force of contraction.

the distended myocardium exceed oxygen delivery. At this point, further increases in preload are not matched by increase in CO.

2. *Increased Sympathetic Activity*: The decrease in CO that accompanies heart failure will lead to decreases in blood flow and blood pressure that activate the sympathetic nervous system. The result of sympathetic activation is an increase in circulating levels of catecholamines, which cause peripheral vasoconstriction as well as increasing heart rate and force of cardiac contraction (positive chronotropic and positive inotropic effects). Unfortunately, the failing myocardium becomes dependent upon circulating levels of catecholamines to help it maintain CO. Over time, the failing myocardium becomes less responsive to the stimulatory effects of these catecholamines and function continues to deteriorate.

3. *Activation of Renin-Angiotensin System*: As a result of decreased CO, blood flow to the kidneys will be significantly reduced. The kidneys respond to this reduction in blood flow by releasing the enzyme *renin*. Renin ultimately leads to the production of *angiotensin II* in the plasma and the release of aldosterone from the adrenal gland. Angiotensin II is a powerful vasoconstrictor that increases systemic blood pressure, whereas aldosterone acts on the kidney tubules to increase salt and water retention, a second factor that will increase systemic blood pressure. Other hormones that appear to be increasingly active during heart failure are *anti-diuretic hormone (ADH)* from the pituitary gland and *atrial natriuretic factor (ANF)*, which is released in response to atrial dilation.

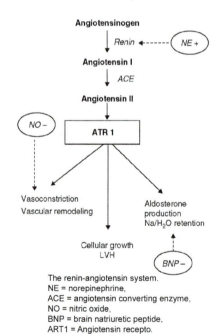

The renin-angiotensin system.
NE = norepinephrine,
ACE = angiotensin converting enzyme,
NO = nitric oxide,
BNP = brain natriuretic peptide,
ART1 = Angiotensin recepto.

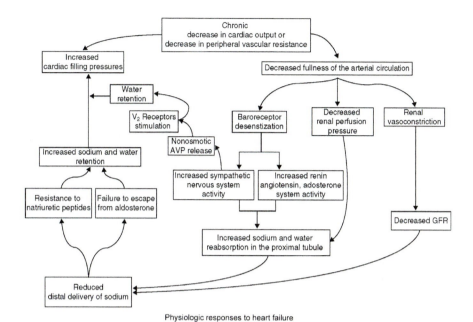

Physiologic responses to heart failure

4. *Ventricular Hypertrophy*: Faced with a chronic increase in workload, the myocardium responds by increasing its muscle mass. While increased muscle mass can increase CO in the short term, contractility eventually suffers as the metabolic demands of the hypertrophied myocardium continue to increase and the efficiency of contraction decreases.

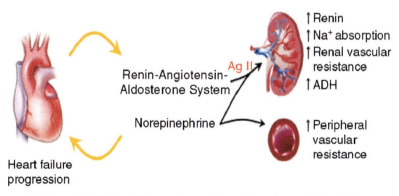

Detrimental effects of the renin-angiotensin system in heart failure

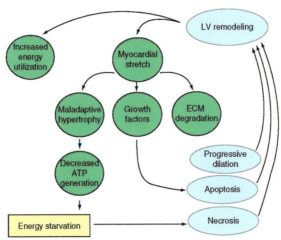

Mechanism of myocardial remodeling in heart failure.
ECM = extracellular matrix

7.12.5 Diagnosis of heart failure

The diagnosis of heart failure is initially based mainly on the patient's history as well as the clinical signs and symptoms. Diagnostic imaging and invasive hemodynamic monitoring may be used for a more detailed assessment of hemodynamic function. Because many patients with heart failure often have underlying cardiovascular disease, radionuclide studies or coronary angiography may be useful for assessing cardiac blood flow. One scale for classifying the severity of heart failure is the New York Heart Association (NYHA) functional classification. In this classification scheme, the severity of heart failure ranges from the least severe (Class I) to the most severe (Class IV) and is based mainly on the severity of symptoms and the impact on daily life functions (see Table 7.10).

Table 7.10   New York Heart Association heart failure classification

Class I	Patients have cardiac disease but ordinary physical activity does not cause undue fatigue, dyspnea or angina
Class II	Patients have cardiac disease that results in a slight limitation of their physical activity; normal activity may cause fatigue, dyspnea, palpitations or angina
Class III	Patients have cardiac disease, which markedly limits their physical activity. Minimal activity causes fatigue, dyspnea, palpitations or angina
Class IV	Patients have debilitating cardiac disease. Symptoms of heart failure may be present at rest

Source: New York Heart Association Functional Classification. http://www.heart.org/en/health-topics/heart-failure/what-is-heart-failure/classes-of-heart-failure.

DIAGNOSIS OF HEART FAILURE

- Dyspnea with exertion, orthopnea, nocturnal dyspnea
- Rales, cough, hemoptysis
- Distention of jugular vein, liver enlargement, ascites
- Peripheral and pulmonary edema
- ECG, chest X-ray for cardiac hypertrophy
- Echocardiography to assess the motion, filling and ejection of the ventricles
- Cardiac catheterization to directly assess hemodynamic function

---

7.12.6   Rationale for treatment of heart failure

The American Heart Association has issued an extensive set of guidelines for treating patients with heart failure (Yancey 2013). Treatments for heart failure can be directed at reducing the workload on the failing heart and/or enhancing cardiac contractility.

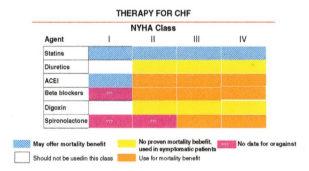

Treatment may include:

- Restriction of physical activity to reduce cardiac workload
- Salt and fluid restriction
- Reduction of preload and afterload through the use of vasodilator drugs such as nitroglycerin
- Potent *diuretic drugs* such as furosemide are used to reduce fluid volume
- The inhibition of angiotensin II formation by *ACE inhibitor drugs or angiotensin receptor blockers (ARBs)*. These agents also counter the compensatory activation of the renin-angiotensin system that can occur with heart failure. Antagonism of aldosterone action may also blunt the progression of cardiac hypertrophy
- Blunting the effects of the catecholamines and sympathetic activation though the use of β-adrenergic receptor antagonists
- Increase cardiac contractility: (positive inotropic agents)

- Digitalis glycosides—digoxin increases the availability of cardiac myocyte calcium, which increases contractility
- Inhibitors of heart-specific phosphodiesterases—drugs such as amrinone increase the cardiac myocyte cAMP level that, in turn, leads to increased contractility

With severe heart failure, the last resort might be a heart transplant, although the current wait for transplant organs can be several years. Mechanical pumps called "left-ventricular assist devices" are currently available and can be used to take over a portion of the heart's pumping function as a temporary measure. However, these mechanical assist devices are not designed as a long-term solution to heart failure. Considerable advances have been recently made in the development and implementation of self-contained mechanical hearts that are designed to be long-term replacements for the failing heart.

7.13 Cardiac arrhythmia

A cardiac arrhythmia or dysrhythmia is any disturbance that occurs to normal heart rhythm. Cardiac arrhythmias can vary in severity from an occasional missed beats to serious abnormalities of rate and rhythm that severely impair the pumping ability of the heart and can be rapidly life threatening. Abnormal cardiac rhythms can arise in tissues of the atria or ventricles as a result of alterations in impulse generation or electrical conduction. Arrhythmias that increase or decrease heart rate will directly affect CO because CO = heart rate × SV. Up to a point, as heart rate increases, CO will also increase. However, at very fast ventricular beating rates, the ventricles may be contracting so quickly that they do not have time to fill properly with blood and as a result CO will fall.

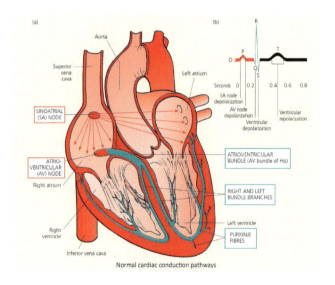

Normal cardiac conduction pathways

7.13.1 Factors that may contribute to the development of a cardiac arrhythmia

A number of different physiologic factors and conditions may alter normal cardiac pacemaker or muscle cell physiology and lead to the development of a cardiac arrhythmia. Some of these factors include:

- Ischemia
- Myocardial infarction
- Electrolyte imbalance
- Altered cellular pH
- Administration of certain drugs
- Congenital defects in the heart

7.13.2 Inherited arrhythmias

A number of genetic variants have been identified that may cause arrhythmia and even sudden death in patients with apparently normal hearts. These genetic variants involve proteins that are found in cardiac ion channels (Na^+, K^+, Cl^-). The presence of these altered proteins can impact the normal opening and closing of these ion channels, thus affecting the depolarization and repolarization of cardiac myocytes and pacemaker cells. Some of these conditions include:

- *Long QT Syndrome (LQTS)*—patients present with prolonged QT intervals on the ECG. This condition is associated with the development of potentially life-threatening ventricular arrhythmias.
- *Brugada Syndrome*—genetic disorder associated with abnormal cardiac sodium channels. The condition typically has an autosomal dominant transmission and presents with ST segment elevations on the ECG. Patients with Brugada syndrome have an increased risk of right bundle branch block, tachyarrhythmia, and sudden cardiac death.

7.13.3 Mechanisms of cardiac arrhythmia

There are two primary mechanisms by which a cardiac arrhythmia might arise: *ectopic pacemakers* and *reentry* impulses.

1. *Ectopic Pacemakers* (see Figure 7.16): The term ectopic refers to the development of abnormal pacemakers in the heart. Under certain conditions, activity of the SA node may be suppressed and other regions of the myocardium that are capable of automaticity take over as the primary pacemaker and assume control over the rate

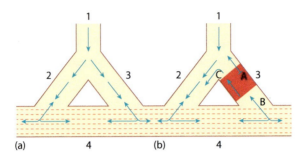

Figure 7.16 Mechanism of cardiac arrhythmia: (a) normal conduction pathway; (b) re-entry current due to the presence of an ischemic region of the myocardium (red).

and rhythm of the heart. In the presence of alterations such as ischemia, hypoxia, electrolyte abnormalities or altered pH, cardiac cells that might not normally function as pacemakers, now become excitable and can act as a secondary or "ectopic" pacemakers. Firing of these ectopic pacemakers can lead to premature cardiac depolarizations that do not follow the normal conduction system of the heart and which are in conflict with those impulses arising from the SA node.

2. *Reentry Impulses* (see Figure 7.16): In a normally functioning myocardium, electrical impulses originating in the SA node follow an orderly progression through the conduction system of the atria and ventricles. These electrical impulses cannot reenter cardiac tissue that has already been depolarized behind them, and they terminate after the ventricles are fully depolarized (Figure 7.16a). In an abnormal myocardium conditions might exist in which there is an area of slowed electrical conduction coupled with a one-way conduction block. Because of the slow rate of depolarization and one-way conduction block, it may be possible for depolarization impulses to travel back upward through the area of one-way conduction block and "reenter" into higher areas of the myocardium which, as a result of the slowed conduction, may have had time to repolarize. Thus, a single wave of depolarization may cause more than one beat (Figure 7.16b). If the timing of reentry is right and the impulse impinges upon the area of myocardium it is entering after the refractory period has occurred, a self-perpetuating "circuitous" type of electrical depolarization might occur.

7.13.4   Types of arrhythmia

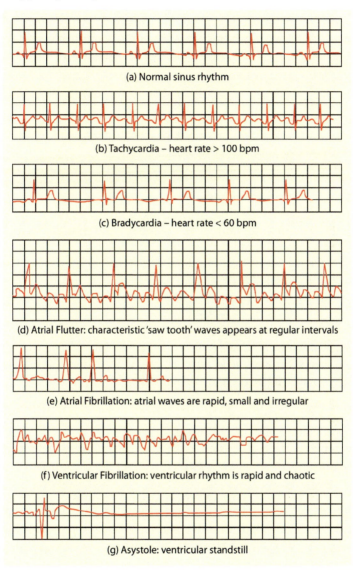

(a) Normal sinus rhythm

(b) Tachycardia – heart rate > 100 bpm

(c) Bradycardia – heart rate < 60 bpm

(d) Atrial Flutter: characteristic 'saw tooth' waves appears at regular intervals

(e) Atrial Fibrillation: atrial waves are rapid, small and irregular

(f) Ventricular Fibrillation: ventricular rhythm is rapid and chaotic

(g) Asystole: ventricular standstill

7.13.4.1   Sinus node arrhythmia

A normally functioning SA node generates 60–100 impulses per minute. Factors such as hyperkalemia, altered sympathetic/parasympathetic input or hypoxia can alter the activity of the SA node. A number of drugs such as digoxin, beta-blockers and sympathomimetics can likewise alter the activity of the SA node.

- *Sinus bradycardia*—excessively slow heart rate (<60 beats/min)
- *Sinus tachycardia*—excessively fast heart rate (>100 beats/min)
- *Sinus arrest*—failure of SA node to discharge, secondary pacemakers may take over (i.e., the AV node)

7.13.4.2   Atrial arrhythmia

7.13.4.2.1   Premature atrial contractions
- Contraction of atrial muscle before the normal contraction that is generated by the SA node
- Most occur from ectopic impulses or reentry impulses
- Also called *premature beats* or *extrasystole*

7.13.4.2.2   Atrial Tachycardia
- Sudden increase in atrial contraction rate to >100 beats/min
- Generally caused by one or more ectopic foci
- The term *paroxysmal atrial tachycardia* is used to describe bouts of atrial tachycardia that begin and end suddenly

7.13.4.2.3   Atrial flutter
- Atrial beating rates of >250 beats/min
- Presents with a classic "saw tooth" pattern of P waves on the ECG
- Often caused by reentry impulses
- The ventricles are protected from the very rapid atrial impulses by the AV node, which is slow to repolarize. As a result of the delay in AV repolarization, the ventricular rate in atrial flutter is generally half that of the atrial rate. However, the ventricles are not protected by the AV node if the arrhythmia arises in the ventricles

7.13.4.2.4   Atrial fibrillation
- Uncoordinated and rapid contraction of the atria
- Often results from multiple reentry currents
- One of the most common chronic arrhythmias. Incidence increases with increasing age
- May occur in patients with ischemic heart disease or mitral valve disease

- Atrial fibrillation puts patients at a significantly increased risk for thrombus formation in the atrium due to stasis of blood. A thrombus formed in the atrium may enter the general circulation to yield an embolism that in turn can lead to a stroke
- Filling of the ventricles during diastole occurs mainly as a passive process, contraction of the atria is necessary only to prime the ventricles or to "top them off" for a full ejection. As a result individuals may survive for months or even years with atrial fibrillation although with a somewhat reduced (by approximately 25%) efficiency of heart pumping

7.13.4.3 Ventricular arrhythmia
7.13.4.3.1 Ventricular premature contractions
- One of the most common types of ventricular arrhythmias
- Can occur occasionally in a normal heart. More common with myocardial ischemia, myocardial hypertrophy or electrolyte imbalances
- Occasional ventricular premature contractions (VPCs) are generally not clinically significant, however, the presence of frequent VPCs may be indicative of an underlying disease process and can progress to ventricular tachycardia or even fibrillation

7.13.4.3.2 Ventricular tachycardia
- Excessive ventricular contraction rates (100–250 beats/min)
- May be caused by and ectopic foci or reentry current that originates in the ventricles
- Tachycardia may be sustained or intermittent
- Can have marked effects on CO due to a reduced time for ventricular filling
- Can predispose a patient to ventricular fibrillation

7.13.4.3.3 Ventricular fibrillation
- The most serious cardiac arrhythmia
- Characterized by a complete loss of ventricular coordination. ECG is completely disorganized
- Cardiac output falls to zero
- Rapid death will ensue if not treated promptly

7.13.4.3.4 Torsades de Pointes Torsades de Points (literally means "twisting of the point) is an unusual form of polymorphic ventricular tachycardia. It is characterized by a prolonged QT interval and gradual twisting of QRS complexes on the ECG. The cause may be congenital or it may be induced by the use of anti-arrhythmic drugs that delay repolarization. Patients may present with palpitations, syncope, and chest pain. The risk of sudden cardiac death is also increased.

7.13.5 Heart block (Figure 7.17)

Heart block is a condition that occurs when abnormalities are present in the conduction pathways of the heart. Such conduction abnormalities may arise from ischemia, hypoxia, electrolyte abnormalities or injury to the myocardium. Excessive vagal (parasympathetic) stimulation or certain drugs might also impair impulse conduction through the AV node and other parts of the conduction pathways.

Heart block may be classified as *first degree, second degree,* or *third degree,* depending upon the severity of the block.

7.13.5.1 First-degree heart block

- All impulses are conducted between atria and ventricles, but at a slowed rate
- Presents on the ECG as a prolonged (>0.20) P-R interval
- Atrial and ventricular rhythms generally remain normal
- May progress over time to a more significant degree of heart block

7.13.5.2 Second-degree heart block

- Some impulses are conducted from the atria to the ventricles, but some are not
- Presents on the ECG as occasional missing QRS complexes
- Subdivided into two specific types:

  - *Mobitz I or Wenckebach*—PR interval progressively prolongs until a QRS complex is dropped
  - *Mobitz II*—P waves are occasionally missing, with subsequent loss of QRS complex for that impulse. PR interval is constant

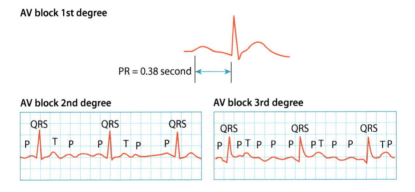

Figure 7.17 Heart block: (a) First degree; (b) Second degree; (c) Third degree.

7.13.5.3   Third-degree heart block

- No impulses are conducted from the atria to the ventricles. Also called "complete AV block"
- The atria and ventricles are being driven by separate pacemakers. Atria may beat at a normal rate if they are being paced by the SA node, whereas the ventricles beat much slower (~30 beats/min) because they are being paced by the Purkinje fibers
- Cardiac output may be significantly reduced due to the slow ventricular rate
- Patients will generally require implantation of a permanent pacemaker

7.13.5.4   Stokes-Adams syndrome

Complete heart block that occurs suddenly and then subsides. Often associated with transient ischemia of the conduction pathways.

7.13.5.5   Bundle branch block

Defective conduction in left or right bundle branches that carry impulses through the ventricular septum. May significantly prolong ventricular depolarization.

QUESTION...

Which cardiac arrhythmias would have the greatest effect on CO and why?

7.13.6   Diagnosis of arrhythmia

A number of techniques may be utilized to diagnose the presence of a cardiac arrhythmia (see Table 7.11). Because the occurrence of an arrhythmia may be episodic, long-term monitoring of cardiac electrophysiology may be necessary in certain patients.

7.13.7   Rationale for the treatment of cardiac arrhythmia

Cardiac arrhythmia may be treated by reducing abnormal automaticity of ectopic pacemakers or by reducing the occurrence of reentry impulses by increasing the duration of the refractory period of the myocardium. In effect, further reducing cardiac conduction may convert a one-way conduction block to a two-way conduction block and thus prevent reentry impulses from initiating a second depolarization. Anti-arrhythmic drugs are generally classified into four distinct classes based upon their mechanism of action.

Table 7.11   Diagnosis of cardiac arrhythmia

1. Resting ECG—done only for a limited time and may miss episodes of arrhythmia
2. Exercise Stress Testing with ECG—exercise may induce changes in the ECG that are indicative of underlying conduction abnormalities or arrhythmia
3. Signal-Averaged ECG—special computerized ECG that averages QRS complexes to detect electrical changes in the heart that predispose a person to arrhythmia and fibrillation
4. Holter Monitoring—ambulatory, portable ECG monitor that can record the electrical activity of the heart for 1–2 days at a time to detect episodes of arrhythmia
5. Cardiac Catheterization—invasive techniques in which electrodes are inserted directly into the heart to measure electrical activity

7.13.8   Treatment of cardiac arrhythmia

7.13.8.1   Pharmacologic

Because of their marked effects on cardiac electrophysiology, *all* of the drugs used to treat cardiac arrhythmias can also cause cardiac arrhythmias.

7.13.8.1.1   Class I anti-arrhythmic drugs
- Block voltage-gated sodium channels, local-anesthetic-like actions on cardiac cells
- Decrease automaticity and reduce conduction velocity
- Used for atrial and ventricular arrhythmias
- E.g., *quinidine, procainamide, lidocaine*

7.13.8.1.2   Class II anti-arrhythmic drugs
- β-adrenoceptor antagonists that block β-adrenergic receptors in the heart
- Blunt the effects of the sympathetic nervous system on the heart
- Increase the refractory period of the AV node
- E.g., *propranolol*

7.13.8.1.3   Class III anti-arrhythmic drugs
- Increase the refractory period and extend overall duration of the cardiac action potential
- E.g., *dofetilide, sotalol*

7.13.8.1.4   Class IV anti-arrhythmic drugs
- Block voltage-gated calcium channels
- Slow depolarization of pacemakers and conduction through AV node
- E.g., *verapamil, diltiazem*

7.13.8.2   Non-pharmacologic treatment of arrhythmia

- Surgical or electrical ablation of accessory conduction pathways that might be involved in conduction of abnormal impulses.
- Implantable cardioverter-defibrillator (ICD)—a device that automatically detects the occurrence of potentially life-threatening arrhythmias and automatically treats them through electrical defibrillation.
- Implantable pacemakers—may be used temporarily or permanently to pace the rate and rhythm of the heart in instances where the normal pacemaker system of the heart has failed.

Medical terminology

Afterload (ăf´tĕr-lōd): Force against which a ventricle of the heart contracts; diastolic pressure in the corresponding artery of a ventricle

Annulus (ăn´ū-lŭs): Ring

Arrhythmia(ā-rĭth´mē-ă): Irregular heartbeat

Atherosclerosis (ăth˝ĕr-ō-sklĕ-rō´sĭs): Common form of arteriosclerosis characterized by cholesterol-lipid-calcium deposits in the walls of arteries causing an occlusion or obstruction to blood flow

Atrium (ā´trē-ŭm): Chamber of the heart that receives venous blood from either the systemic circulation (right atrium) or the pulmonary circulation (left atrium)

Automaticity: Refers to the ability to be self-excitable and generate a heartbeat without nervous stimulation

Bradycardia (brăd˝ē-kăr´dē-ă): Heart rate less than 60 beats/min

Bundle of His (bŭn´dĕl of hĭs): Atrioventricular (AV) bundle; portion of the specialized electrical conduction system found in the interventricular septum

Cardiac index (kăr´dē-ăk ĭn´dĕks): Cardiac output divided by body surface area

Cardiac output (kăr´dē-ăk out´poot): Volume of blood pumped by the heart per minute

Cardiac reserve (kăr´dē-ăk rē-zĕrv´): The difference between the resting cardiac output and the maximal cardiac output

Chordae tendineae (kor´dă tĕnd-ĭn-ē´ă): Tendinous cords that connect the flaps of the atrioventricular valves to the papillary muscles

Chronotropic (krŏn˝ō-trŏp´ĭk): Refers to an agent or factor that influences the heart rate

Contractility (kŏn-trăk-tĭl´ĭ-tē): The force with which ventricular ejection occurs

Cusp (kŭsp): In the heart, a flap of a valve

Desmosome (dĕs´mō-sōm): Intercellular junction that provides attachment and structural support between the cells

Diastasis (dī-ăs´tă-sĭs): Following the period of rapid ventricular filling, the period of slow inflow of blood from the atria to the ventricles

Diastole (dī-ăs´tō-lē): Period of relaxation and filling with blood in the heart

Ejection fraction(ē-jĕk´shŭn frăk´shŭn): The percentage of blood forced out of the ventricle during systole

End-diastolic volume: Volume of blood in the ventricle of the heart just prior to contraction

Endocardium (ĕn˝dō-kăr´dē-ŭm): Endothelial membrane that lines the chambers of the heart

Endothelium (ĕn˝dō-thă´lē-ŭm): Squamous epithelium that lines blood and lymphatic vessels

End-systolic volume: Volume of blood remaining in the ventricle of the heart following ejection

Epicardium (ĕp˝ĭ-kăr´dē-ŭm): Membrane on the surface of the heart

Infarct (ĭn´fărkt): Region of necrosis in a tissue resulting from inadequate blood flow or ischemia

Inotropic (ĭn˝ō-trŏp´ĭk): Refers to an agent or factor that influences the force of muscular contraction

Intercalated disc (ĭn-tĕr´kă-lā-tĕd dĭsk): Occurring at the junction of two myocardial cells; site of transmission of the electrical impulse

Interventricular (ĭn˝tĕr-vĕn-trĭk´ū-lăr): Between the two ventricles

Isovolumetric(ī˝sō-vŏl-yū-mĕt´rĭk): Occurring without a change in volume

Myocardium (mī-ō-kăr´dē-ŭm): Middle layer of the wall of the heart; composed of cardiac muscle

Myogenic (mī´ō-jĕn-ĭk): Originating in muscle; controlled by inherent properties of the muscle instead of nerves; describes the self-excitation of cardiac muscle and single-unit smooth muscle cells

Neurogenic (nū-rō-jĕn´ĭk): Originating in nervous tissue; controlled by nervous factors

Papillary muscle (păp´ĭ-lăr-ē mŭs´ĕl): Cone-shaped muscle arising from the floor of each ventricle and attaching to the chordae tendineae

Pericardium (pĕr˝ĭ-kăr-dē-ŭm): Serous membrane enclosing the heart

Prolapse (prō´lăps): Dropping down of an organ or body part

Preload (prē-lōd): Degree of stretch of the ventricles of the heart just prior to contraction; end-diastolic volume (EDV)

Purkinje fiber (pŭr-kĭn´jē fī´bĕr): Specialized cardiac muscle cell forming the last portion of the electrical conducting system

Septum (sĕp´tŭm): Wall dividing two cavities

Stroke volume: Volume of blood ejected from each ventricle of the heart per beat

Supraventricular (soo˝pră-vĕn-trĭk´ū-lăr): Located above the heart ventricles, specifically, in the atria

Syncytium (sĭn-sĭt´ē-ŭm): Cells of a tissue interconnected electrically by way of gap junctions that function together as a single unit

Systole (sĭs´tō-lē): Period of contraction and ejection of blood from the heart

Tachycardia (tăk˝ē-kăr´dē-ă): Heart rate greater than 100 beats/min

Tetanus (tĕt´ă-nŭs): Smooth, sustained maximal contraction of a muscle

Venous return (vē´nŭs rē-tĕrn´): Volume of blood returning to the right atrium of the heart per minute

Ventricle (vĕn´trĭk-l): Chamber of the heart that delivers blood to either the systemic circulation (left ventricle) or the pulmonary circulation (right ventricle)

Bibliography

American Heart Association, 2002. http://www.justmove.org/fitnessnews/healthf. cfm?Target=hartrates.html.

Du Pont Pharma, *Introduction to Nuclear Cardiology*, 3rd ed., Du Pont Pharma Radiopharmaceuticals, North Billerica, MA, 1993.

Frey, N., Luedde, M., and Katus, H. A., Mechanisms of disease: Hypertrophic cardiomyopathy. *Nat Rev Cardiol.* 2011;9(2):91–100. doi:10.1038/nrcardio.2011.159.

Fox, S. I., *Human Physiology*, 9th ed., McGraw Hill, Boston, MA, 2006.

Go, A. S., Mozaffarian, D., Roger, V. L. et al., Heart disease and stroke statistics—2013 update: A report from the American Heart Association. *Circulation.* 2013;127:e6–e245.

Golan, D. E., Tashjian, A. H., Armstrong, E. J., Galanter, J. M., Armstrong, A. W., Arnout, R. A., and Rose, H., Pharmacology of cardiac rhythm, in *Principles of Pharmacology, The Pathophysiologic Basis of Drug Therapy*, Lippincott Williams & Wilkins, Philadelphia, PA, 2005, chap. 17.

Guyton, A. C., and Hall, J. E., *Textbook of Medical Physiology*, 11th ed., W. B. Saunders, Philadelphia, PA, 2006.

Heidenreich, P. A., Trogdon, J. G., Khavjou, O. A. et al., Forecasting the future of cardiovascular disease in the United States: A policy statement from the American Heart Association. *Circulation.* 2011;123(8):933–944.

Hoffman, B. B., Therapy of hypertension, in *Goodman and Gilman's The Pharmacological Basis of Therapeutics*, 11th ed., Brunton, L. L., Lazo, J. S., and Parker, K. L., Eds., McGraw-Hill, New York, 2006, chap. 32.

Hondeghem, L. M., and Roden, D. M., Agents used in cardiac arrhythmias, in *Basic & Clinical Pharmacology*, 8th ed., Katzung, B. G., Ed., McGraw-Hill, New York, 2001, chap. 14.

Jackson, E. K., Diuretics, in *Goodman and Gilman's The Pharmacological Basis of Therapeutics*, 11th ed., Brunton, L. L., Lazo, J. S., and Parker, K. L., Eds., McGraw-Hill, New York, 2006, chap. 28.

Katzung, B. G., and Parmley, W. W., Cardiac glycosides & other drugs used in congestive heart failure, in *Basic & Clinical Pharmacology*, 8th ed., Katzung, B. G., Ed., McGraw-Hill, New York, 2001, chap. 13.

Levy, M. N., and Pappano, A. J., *Cardiovascular Physiology*, 9th ed., Mosby, St. Louis, MO, 2007.

Lilly, L. S., *Pathophysiology of Heart Disease*, Lea & Febiger, Malvern, PA, 1993, chaps 11 and 17.

McArdle, W. D., Katch, F. I., and Katch, V. L., *Essentials of Exercise Physiology*, 2nd ed., Lippincott Williams & Wilkins, Baltimore, MD, 2000.

Michel, T., Treatment of myocardial ischemia, in *Goodman and Gilman's, The Pharmacological Basis of Therapeutics*, 11th ed., Brunton, L. L., Lazo, J. S., and Parker, K. L., Eds., McGraw-Hill, New York, 2006, chap. 31.

Porth, C. M., *Pathophysiology, Concepts of Altered Health States*, 7th ed., Lippincott Williams & Wilkins, Philadelphia, PA, 2005, chap. 28.

Rhoades, R., and Pflanzer, R., *Human Physiology*, 4th ed., Thomson Learning, Pacific Grove, CA, 2003.

Rocco, T. P., and Fang, J. C., Pharmacotherapy of congestive heart failure, in *Goodman and Gilman's, The Pharmacological Basis of Therapeutics*, 11th ed., Brunton, L. L., Lazo, J. S., and Parker, K. L., Eds., McGraw-Hill, New York, 2006, chap. 33.

Roden, D. M., Antiarrhythmic drugs, in *Goodman and Gilman's, The Pharmacological Basis of Therapeutics*, 11th ed., Brunton, L. L., Lazo, J. S., and Parker, K. L., Eds., McGraw-Hill, New York, 2006, chap. 34.

Rowell, L. B., *Human Cardiovascular Control*, Oxford University Press, New York, 1993.

Sherwood, L., *Human Physiology from Cells to Systems*, 5th ed., Brooks/Cole, Pacific Grove, CA, 2004.

Silverthorn, D., *Human Physiology: An Integrated Approach*, 4th ed., Prentice Hall, Upper Saddle River, NJ, 2007.

Smith, E. R., Pathophysiology of cardiac electrical disturbances, in *Physiopathology of the Cardiovascular System*, Alpert, J. S., Ed., Little, Brown and Company, Boston, MA, 1984, chap. 14.

Stedman's Medical Dictionary for the Health Professions and Nursing, 5th ed., Lippincott Williams & Wilkins, Baltimore, MD, 2005.

Taber's Cyclopedic Medical Dictionary, 20th ed., F. A. Davis Co., Philadelphia, PA, 2005.

White Winters, J. M., Cardiac conduction and rhythm disorders, in *Pathophysiology, Concepts of Altered Health States*, 7th ed., Porth, C. M., Ed., Lippincott Williams & Wilkins, Philadelphia, PA, 2005, chap. 27.

Widmaier, E. P., Raff, H., and Strang, K. T., *Vander's Human Physiology, The Mechanisms of Body Function*, McGraw Hill, Boston, MA, 2006.

Yancey, C., ACCF/AHA Practice Guideline. 2013 ACCF/AHA Guideline for the Management of Heart Failure: A Report of the American College of Cardiology Foundation/American Heart Association Task Force on Practice Guidelines. *Circulation*. 2013;128:e240–e327.

chapter eight

The respiratory system

Study objectives

- Describe the blood-gas interface and explain why the lungs are ideally suited for gas exchange
- List the components and the functions of the conducting airways
- Distinguish between the various types of airways in terms of epithelium and cartilage
- Describe the forces and factors responsible for maintaining inflation of the lungs
- Explain how inspiration and expiration take place
- Distinguish between atmospheric pressure, alveolar pressure, intrapleural pressure and transpulmonary pressure
- Define pulmonary compliance
- Describe the role of elastic connective tissues in the elastic recoil of the lungs as well as in lung compliance
- Explain how surface tension affects the elastic behavior of the lungs
- Describe the functions of pulmonary surfactant
- Explain how interdependence promotes alveolar stability
- Describe the factors that determine airway resistance
- Define tidal volume, residual volume, expiratory reserve volume, and inspiratory reserve volume
- Define functional residual capacity, inspiratory capacity, total lung capacity, and vital capacity
- Distinguish between total ventilation and alveolar ventilation
- Distinguish between anatomical dead space, alveolar dead space, and physiological dead space
- Explain how each factor in Fick's Law of Diffusion influences gas exchange
- List the partial pressures of oxygen (PO_2) and carbon dioxide (PCO_2) in the various regions of the respiratory and cardiovascular systems
- Explain how the PO_2 and the PCO_2 of the alveolar gas are determined
- Explain the effects of airway obstruction and obstructed blood flow on ventilation-perfusion (V:Q) matching
- Describe the local control mechanisms that restore the V:Q ratio to 1
- Explain how oxygen is transported in the blood
- Describe the physiological significance of the steep portion and the plateau portion of the oxyhemoglobin dissociation curve

- Describe the effects of carbon dioxide, pH, temperature, 2,3-bisphosphoglycerate, anemia, and carbon monoxide poisoning on the transport of oxygen
- Explain how carbon dioxide is transported in the blood
- Compare and contrast the functions of the dorsal and the ventral respiratory groups in the medullary respiratory center
- List and describe the sources of input to the medullary respiratory center
- Compare and contrast the function of the peripheral and the central chemoreceptors
- Describe the ventilation response to exercise
- Describe the general symptoms of respiratory disease
- List the major organisms responsible for the common cold
- Discuss the key features of an influenza infection. How do endemics, epidemics, and pandemics differ?
- Describe the drugs that are currently available for treating influenza. How are they similar? How do they differ?
- Compare and contrast typical and atypical pneumonia
- List specific organisms that are associated with hospital-acquired and community-acquired pneumonia
- List populations that are most at risk for pneumonia
- Discuss the etiology and manifestations of tuberculosis. How can we treat it?
- Discuss the possible etiology of bronchial asthma. What are some potential asthma triggers?
- Compare and contrast the "early" and "late" phases of asthma in terms of their etiology, effects on the respiratory passages, and major clinical manifestations
- Describe how asthma attacks are classified based on frequency and severity of attacks
- Describe the various means by which asthma might be treated
- Compare and contrast chronic bronchitis and emphysema in terms of etiology and clinical manifestations
- Describe the different types of pneumothorax that might occur. What might cause each?
- Define atelectasis. What are the various types that might occur? What might cause each?
- Discuss the etiology of cystic fibrosis. What are the major clinical manifestations of cystic fibrosis? Why does each occur?
- What is adult respiratory distress syndrome? How does it differ from respiratory distress syndrome in the newborn?

- List some possible causes of interstitial lung disease. How do interstitial lung diseases differ from diseases such as emphysema and chronic bronchitis?
- List some possible causes of respiratory failure. What are the major clinical manifestations of respiratory failure?

The cells of the body require a continuous supply of oxygen to produce energy and carry out their metabolic functions. Furthermore, these aerobic metabolic processes produce carbon dioxide, which must be continuously eliminated to regulate acid-base balance, or the concentration of H^+ ions in the blood. Therefore, the primary functions of the respiratory system include:

- Obtaining oxygen from the external environment and supplying it to the body's cells
- Eliminating carbon dioxide produced by cellular metabolism from the body

The process by which oxygen is taken up by the lungs and carbon dioxide is eliminated from the lungs is referred to as *gas exchange*.

8.1 Blood-gas interface

Gas exchange takes place at the *blood-gas interface*. This interface exists where the alveoli and the pulmonary capillaries come together. The *alveoli* are the smallest airways in the lungs. The *pulmonary capillaries* are found wrapped around the alveoli. Inspired oxygen moves from the alveoli into the capillaries for eventual transport to the tissues. Carbon dioxide, entering the lungs by way of the pulmonary circulation, moves from the capillaries into the alveoli for elimination by expiration. Both oxygen and carbon dioxide move across the blood-gas interface by way of *simple diffusion*—from an area of high concentration to an area of low concentration.

Fick's Law of Diffusion states the amount of gas that moves across the blood-gas interface is proportional to the surface area of the interface and inversely proportional to the thickness of the interface. In other words, gas exchange in the lungs is promoted when the *surface area* for diffusion is maximized and the *thickness of the barrier* to diffusion is minimized. In fact, anatomically, the lungs are ideally suited for the function of gas exchange. There are 300 million alveoli in the lungs. Furthermore, the walls of each alveolus are surrounded by a network of capillaries. There are as many as 280 billion pulmonary capillaries or almost 1,000 capillaries per alveolus. This results in a vast surface area for gas exchange of approximately 70 m², which is roughly the size of a tennis court.

More specifically, the blood-gas interface consists of the alveolar epithelium, the capillary endothelium, and the interstitium. The alveolar wall is made up of a single layer of flattened *alveolar type I cells*. The capillaries surrounding the alveoli also consist of a single layer of cells, *endothelial cells*. In between the alveolar epithelium and the capillary endothelium is a very small amount of *interstitium*. In some regions, the interstitium may be essentially absent. In this case, the basement membranes of the alveolar epithelial cell and the capillary endothelial cell fuse together. Taken all together, only 0.2–0.5 μm separates the air in the alveoli from the blood in the capillaries. The extreme thinness of the blood-gas interface further facilitates gas exchange by way of diffusion.

8.2 Airways

The airways of the lungs consist of a series of branching tubes. Each level of branching results in another generation of airways. As they branch, the airways become narrower, shorter, and more numerous. A total of *23 generations of airways*, with the alveoli, comprise the twenty-third generation.

8.2.1 Cartilage

The trachea and the primary bronchi contain *C-shaped hyaline cartilage rings* in their walls. The lobar bronchi contain *plates of cartilage* that completely encircle the airways. The cartilage in these large airways provides structural support and prevents the collapse of the airways. As the bronchi continue to branch and move out toward the lung periphery, the cartilage diminishes progressively until it disappears in airways that are about 1 mm in diameter. Airways with no cartilage are referred to as *bronchioles*. As the cartilage becomes sparser, it is replaced by *smooth muscle*. Therefore, the bronchioles, which have no cartilage to support them but do have smooth muscle capable of vigorous constriction, are susceptible to collapse under certain conditions, such as an asthmatic attack.

Air is carried to and from the lungs by the *trachea*, which extends toward the lungs from the larynx. The trachea divides into the *right* and *left primary (main) bronchi*. These *primary bronchi* each supply a lung. The primary bronchi branch and form the *secondary*, or *lobar, bronchi*; one for each lobe of lung. The left lung consists of two lobes and the right lung has three lobes. The lobar bronchi branch and form the *tertiary*, or *segmental, bronchi*; one for each of the functional segments within the lobes. These bronchi continue to branch and move outward toward the periphery of the lungs. The smallest airways without alveoli are the *terminal bronchioles*. Taken all together, the airways from the trachea through and including the terminal bronchioles are referred to as the *conducting airways*. This region, which consists of the first 16 generations of airways, contains no alveoli. Therefore, there is no gas exchange in this area. Consequently, it is also referred to as *anatomical dead space*. The volume of the anatomical dead space is approximately 150 mL (or about 1 mL per pound of ideal body weight).

The conducting airways carry out three major functions:

- Lead inspired air to the more distal gas exchanging regions of the lungs
- Warm and humidify the inspired air as it flows through them
- Defend against microbes, toxic chemicals and foreign matter

The large airways provide a low-resistance pathway for airflow toward the respiratory zone. In other words, they function largely as conduits for the bulk flow of air.

Second, the alveoli are delicate structures and may be damaged by excessive exposure to cold, dry air. The addition of warmth and moisture, particularly in the winter months, protects the alveoli. In fact, this water vapor is visible when one exhales on a cold winter day. The defense against inhaled microbes or foreign particles is discussed in the next section, *Epithelium*. In addition, vagally induced bronchoconstriction in response to irritant receptor stimulation is discussed in the section, *Bronchial Smooth Muscle Tone*.

Branching from the terminal bronchioles are the *respiratory bronchioles*. This is the first generation of airways to have alveoli in their walls. Finally, there are the *alveolar ducts*, which are completely lined with *alveolar sacs*. This region, from the respiratory bronchioles through the alveoli, is referred to as the *respiratory zone*. This zone comprises most of the lungs and has a volume of about 3,000 mL at the end of a normal expiration.

8.2.2   Epithelium

All the conducting airways, the trachea up to the terminal bronchioles, are lined with *pseudostratified ciliated columnar epithelium*. There are approximately 300 cilia per epithelial cell. Interspersed among these epithelial cells are mucus-secreting *goblet cells*. Furthermore, *mucus glands* are found in the larger airways. Consequently, the surface of the conducting airways consists of a mucus-covered ciliated epithelium. The cilia beat upward at frequencies between 600 and 900 beats/min and continuously move the mucus away from the respiratory zone and up toward the pharynx at a rate of 1–2 cm/min. This *mucociliary escalator* provides an important protective mechanism that removes inhaled particles from the lungs and particles larger than about 6 μm are typically stopped from reaching the respiratory zone. Mucus that reaches the pharynx is usually swallowed or expectorated. An additional mechanism by which airway mucus protects the lungs involves the presence of immunoglobulins. These substances, also referred to as antibodies, destroy or neutralize inhaled pathogens. The activity of the immunoglobulins was discussed in detail in Chapter 3, *The Immune System*. Interestingly, the nicotine found in cigarette smoke paralyzes the cilia and impairs their ability to remove the many toxic substances found in smoke.

The respiratory bronchioles are lined with *nonciliated cuboidal epithelial cells* that gradually flatten and become squamous type cells. As mentioned previously, the alveoli are composed of large, flat, *simple squamous epithelium*.

8.3   The pleura

Each lung is enclosed in a double-walled sac referred to as the *pleura*. The *visceral pleura* is the membrane adhered to the external surface of the lungs. The *parietal pleura* lines the walls of the thoracic cavity. The space in between the two layers, the *pleural space*, or *pleural cavity*, is narrow and completely closed.

The pleural space is filled with *pleural fluid*, which lubricates the membranes and reduces friction between the layers as they slide past each other during breathing. The pleural fluid also plays a role in maintaining lung inflation. The cohesion between the molecules of the watery pleural fluid keeps the two layers of the pleura "adhered" to each other. This concept is similar to the effect of water between two glass microscope slides. The two pieces of glass can easily slide over each other; however, the strong attraction of the water molecules for each other opposes the direct separation of the slides. In this way, the lungs are in contact with the thoracic wall, fill the thoracic cavity and remain inflated. In other words, the cohesion of the fluid molecules in the pleural space opposes the tendency of the lungs to collapse.

8.4   Mechanics of breathing

Air will move from an area of high pressure to an area of low pressure. Therefore, a pressure gradient between the atmosphere and the alveoli must be developed. The mechanics of breathing involve volume and pressure changes that take place during ventilation, allowing air to move in and out of the lungs. This section will explain how changes in thoracic volume, lung volume, and pulmonary pressures occur to cause the pressure gradients responsible for inspiration and expiration.

8.4.1   Thoracic volume

The volume of the thoracic cavity increases during inspiration (inhalation) and decreases during expiration (exhalation).

8.4.2   Inspiration

The most important muscle of inspiration is the *diaphragm*. The diaphragm is a thin, dome-shaped skeletal muscle that inserts into the lower ribs and is supplied by the *phrenic nerves*. When the diaphragm contracts, it flattens and pushes downward against the contents of the abdomen. Therefore, contraction of the diaphragm causes an increase in the vertical dimension (top to bottom) of the thoracic cavity and an increase in thoracic volume. In fact, the diaphragm is responsible for 75% of the enlargement of the thoracic cavity during normal, quiet breathing.

Assisting the diaphragm with inspiration are the *external intercostal muscles*. These muscles connect adjacent ribs. When the external intercostal muscles contract, the ribs are lifted upward and outward (much like a handle on a bucket). Therefore, contraction of these muscles causes an increase in the horizontal dimension (front to back) of the thoracic cavity and a further increase in thoracic volume. The external intercostal muscles are supplied by the *intercostal nerves*.

Deeper inspirations are achieved by more forceful contraction of the diaphragm and the external intercostal muscles. Furthermore, *accessory inspiratory muscles*, including the scalenes, the pectoralis minor, and the sternocleidomastoid muscles, contribute to this process. Located mainly in the neck, the scalenes and the sternocleidomastoid muscles raise the sternum and elevate the first two ribs, enlarging the upper portion of the thoracic cavity. The pectoralis minor muscles, located in the upper chest, also pull the rib cage superiorly.

8.4.3 Expiration

Expiration during normal, quiet breathing is *passive*. In other words, no active muscle contraction is required. When the diaphragm is no longer stimulated by the phrenic nerves to contract, it passively returns to its original, preinspiration position under the ribs. Relaxation of the external intercostal muscles allows the rib cage to fall inward and downward, largely due to gravity. These movements cause a decrease in thoracic volume.

During exercise or voluntary hyperventilation, expiration becomes an *active* process. Under these conditions, a larger volume of air must be exhaled more rapidly. Therefore, two muscle groups are recruited to facilitate this process. The most important muscles of expiration are the *muscles of the abdominal wall*. Contraction of these muscles pushes inward on the abdominal contents and increases abdominal pressure. The diaphragm is pushed upward more rapidly and more forcefully toward its preinspiration position.

Assisting the muscles of the abdominal wall are the *internal intercostal muscles*. These muscles are also found between the ribs; however, they are oriented in a direction opposite to that of the external intercostal muscles. Contraction of these muscles pulls the ribs inward and downward.

8.4.4 Lung volume

There are no real physical attachments between the lungs and the thoracic wall. Instead, the lungs literally float in the thoracic cavity, surrounded by pleural fluid. Therefore, the question arises, how does the volume of the lungs increase when the volume of the thoracic cavity increases? The mechanism involves the pleural fluid and the surface tension between the molecules of this fluid. As mentioned previously, the surface tension of the pleural fluid keeps the parietal pleura lining the thoracic cavity and the visceral pleura on the external surface of the lungs "adhered" to each other. In other words, the pleural fluid keeps the lungs in contact with the chest wall. Therefore, as the muscles of inspiration cause the chest wall to expand, increasing the thoracic volume, the lungs are pulled open as well and the lung volume also increases.

8.4.5 Pulmonary pressures

The changes in thoracic volume and lung volume cause the pressures within the airways and the pleural cavity to change. It is these pressure changes that create the pressure gradients responsible for airflow in and out of the lungs. There are four pressures that must be considered (see Figure 8.1):

- Atmospheric pressure
- Intrapleural pressure
- Alveolar pressure
- Transpulmonary pressure

As it does with all objects on the surface of the earth, gravity exerts its effects on the molecules of the atmosphere. The weight generated by these molecules is referred to as *atmospheric*, or *barometric*, *pressure* (P_{atm}). At sea level,

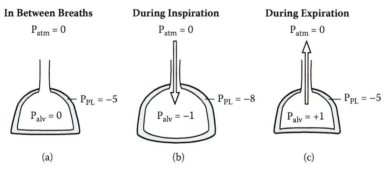

In Between Breaths	During Inspiration	During Expiration
$P_{atm} = 0$	$P_{atm} = 0$	$P_{atm} = 0$
$P_{PL} = -5$	$P_{PL} = -8$	$P_{PL} = -5$
$P_{alv} = 0$	$P_{alv} = -1$	$P_{alv} = +1$
(a)	(b)	(c)

Figure 8.1 Pulmonary pressures. (a) Between breaths. Alveolar pressure (P_{alv}) is equal to atmospheric pressure (P_{atm}), which is 0 mmHg. No air flows in or out of the lungs. (b) During inspiration. As the lung volume increases, the alveolar pressure decreases and becomes subatmospheric (−1 mmHg). The pressure gradient between the atmosphere and the alveoli allows air to flow into the lungs. (c) During expiration. Following inspiration, the lungs recoil and lung volume decreases. Alveolar pressure increases and becomes greater than atmospheric (+1 mmHg). The pressure gradient between the atmosphere and the alveoli forces air to flow out of the lungs.

atmospheric pressure is 760 mmHg. To simplify this discussion, atmospheric pressure will be normalized to 0 mmHg (or 0 mmHg) and all other pressures are referenced to this.

Intrapleural pressure (P_{pl}) is the pressure within the pleural cavity. Under equilibrium conditions, the chest wall tends to pull outward and the elastic recoil of the lungs tends to pull them inward (like a collapsing balloon). These opposing forces create a subatmospheric or negative pressure within the pleural space. In between breaths, intrapleural pressure is −5 mmHg. During inspiration, the lungs follow the chest wall as it expands. However, the lung tissue resists being stretched so that the intrapleural pressure becomes even more negative and is −8 mmHg.

Alveolar pressure (P_{alv}) is the pressure within the alveoli. In between breaths, it is equal to 0 mmHg. Because there is no pressure gradient between the atmosphere and the alveoli, there is no airflow. However, for air to flow into the lungs, the alveolar pressure must fall below atmospheric pressure. In other words, alveolar pressure becomes slightly negative. According to Boyle's Law, at a constant temperature, the volume of a gas and its pressure are inversely related:

$$P \alpha 1/V$$

Therefore, as lung volume increases during inspiration, the pressure within the alveoli decreases. Atmospheric pressure is now greater than alveolar pressure and air enters the lungs. Because the lungs are normally very compliant, or distensible, only a small pressure gradient is necessary for air to flow into the lungs. During a normal inspiration under resting conditions, alveolar pressure is −1 mmHg.

During expiration, the opposite occurs. Lung volume decreases and, therefore, pressure within the alveoli increases. Alveolar pressure is now greater than atmospheric pressure and air flows out of the lungs. Alveolar pressure during a normal expiration under resting conditions is +1 mmHg.

Transpulmonary pressure (P_{tp}) is the pressure difference between the inside and the outside of the lungs. In other words, it is the pressure difference between the alveoli and the pleural space:

$$P_{tp} = P_{alv} - P_{pl}$$

$$= 0 \text{ mmHg} - (-5 \text{ mmHg})$$

$$= +5 \text{ mmHg}$$

In between breaths, the transpulmonary pressure is +5 mmHg. The transpulmonary pressure is also referred to as the *expanding pressure* of the lungs. A force of +5 mmHg expands, or pushes outward on, the lungs so that they fill the thoracic cavity. As might be expected, during inspiration, the transpulmonary pressure increases, causing greater expansion of the lungs:

$$P_{tp} = (-1\,\text{mmHg}) - (-8\,\text{mmHg})$$

$$= +7\,\text{mmHg}$$

The entry of air into the pleural cavity is referred to as a *pneumothorax*. This may occur spontaneously when a "leak" develops on the surface of the lung allowing air to escape from the airways into the pleural space. It may also result from a physical trauma that causes penetration of the chest wall so that air enters the pleural space from the atmosphere. In either case, the pleural cavity is no longer a closed space and the pressure within it equilibrates with the atmospheric pressure (0 mmHg). The transpulmonary pressure is also equal to 0 mmHg and the lung collapses.

In a healthy individual, the lungs are very distensible. In other words, the lungs can be inflated with minimal effort. Furthermore, during normal, quiet breathing, expiration is passive. The lungs inherently recoil to their preinspiratory position. These processes are attributed to the *elastic behavior* of the lungs. The elasticity of the lungs involves the following two interrelated properties:

- Elastic recoil
- Pulmonary compliance

The *elastic recoil* of the lungs refers to their ability to return to their original configuration following inspiration. It may also be used to describe the tendency of the lungs to oppose inflation. Conversely, *pulmonary compliance* describes how easily the lungs inflate. Compliance is defined as the change in lung volume divided by the change in transpulmonary pressure:

$$C = \frac{\Delta V}{\Delta P}$$

A highly compliant lung is one that requires only a small change in pressure for a given degree of inflation. A less compliant lung requires a larger change in pressure for the same degree of inflation. For example, during normal, quiet breathing, human adults inhale a tidal volume of about 500 mL per breath. In an individual with healthy, compliant lungs, the transpulmonary pressure gradient needed to be generated by the inspiratory muscles is very small (approximately 2–3 mmHg). The patient with less compliant, or "stiff," lungs must generate a larger transpulmonary pressure to inflate the lungs with the same 500 mL of air. In other words, more vigorous contraction of the inspiratory muscles is required. Therefore, the *work of breathing* is increased.

The elastic behavior of the lungs is determined by two factors:

- Elastic connective tissue in the lungs
- Alveolar surface tension

The *elastic connective tissue* in the lungs consists of *elastin* and *collagen* fibers. These fibers are found in the alveolar walls and around the blood vessels and bronchi. When the lungs are inflated, the connective tissue fibers are stretched, or distorted. They tend to return to their original shape and cause the elastic recoil of the lungs following inspiration. However, due to the interwoven, mesh-like arrangement of these fibers, the lungs remain very compliant and readily distensible.

The alveoli are lined with fluid. At an air-water interface, the water molecules are much more strongly attracted to each other than to the air at their surface. This attraction produces a force at the surface of the fluid referred to as *surface tension* (ST).

Alveolar surface tension exerts two effects on the elastic behavior of the lungs. First, it decreases the compliance of the lungs. For example, inflation of the lung would increase its surface area and pull the water molecules lining the alveolus apart from each other. However, the attraction between these water molecules, or the surface tension, resists this expansion of the alveolus. Opposition to expansion causes a decrease in compliance. In other words, the alveolus is more difficult to inflate and the work of breathing is increased. The greater the surface tension, the less compliant are the lungs.

The second effect of surface tension is that it causes the alveolus to become as small as possible. As the water molecules pull toward each other, the alveolus forms a sphere, which is the smallest surface area for a given volume. This generates a pressure directed inward on the alveolus, or a *collapsing pressure*. The magnitude of this pressure is determined by the *Law of LaPlace*:

$$P = \frac{2ST}{r}$$

The collapsing pressure (P) is proportional to the alveolar surface tension (ST) and inversely proportional to the radius (r) of the alveolus. In other words, the greater the surface tension and the smaller the radius, the greater the collapsing pressure.

Due to this collapsing pressure, alveoli are inherently unstable. For example, if two alveoli of different sizes have the same surface tension, the smaller alveolus has a greater collapsing pressure and would tend to collapse and empty into the larger alveolus (see Figure 8.2, panel a). As already mentioned, air flows from an area of higher pressure to an area of lower pressure. The air within the smaller alveolus flows into the larger one and

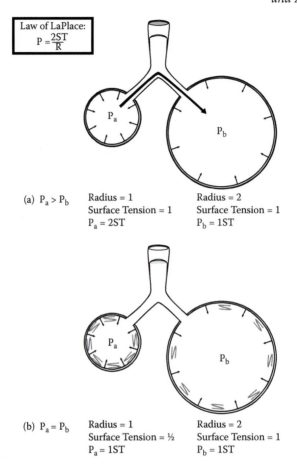

Law of LaPlace:
$$P = \frac{2ST}{R}$$

(a) $P_a > P_b$ Radius = 1   Radius = 2
                     Surface Tension = 1   Surface Tension = 1
                     $P_a = 2ST$ $P_b = 1ST$

(b) $P_a = P_b$ Radius = 1   Radius = 2
                     Surface Tension = ½   Surface Tension = 1
                     $P_a = 1ST$ $P_b = 1ST$

Figure 8.2 Effects of surface tension and surfactant on alveolar stability. (a) Effect of surface tension. According to the *Law of LaPlace* (P = 2ST/r), if two alveoli have the same surface tension (ST), the alveolus with the smaller radius (r) and, therefore, a greater collapsing pressure (P), would tend to empty into the alveolus with the larger radius. (b) Effect of surfactant. Surfactant decreases the surface tension and, therefore, the collapsing pressure, more so in smaller alveoli than it does in larger alveoli. As a result, the collapsing pressures in all alveoli are equal. This prevents alveolar collapse and promotes alveolar stability.

an area of *atelectasis* (airway collapse) develops. Therefore, if alveolar surface tension were to remain the same throughout the lungs, it has the potential to cause widespread alveolar collapse.

Normal lungs, however, produce a chemical substance referred to as *pulmonary surfactant.* Made by *alveolar type II cells* within the alveoli, surfactant is a complex mixture of proteins (10%–15%) and phospholipids (85%–90%), including dipalmitoyl phosphatidyl choline, the predominant constituent.

By interspersing throughout the fluid lining the alveoli, it disrupts the cohesive forces between the water molecules. Pulmonary surfactant has three major functions. Surfactant:

- Decreases surface tension
- Increases alveolar stability
- Prevents transudation of fluid

Pulmonary surfactant *decreases the surface tension* of the alveolar fluid. Reduced surface tension leads to a decrease in the collapsing pressure of the alveoli, an increase in pulmonary compliance (less elastic recoil) and a decrease in the work required to inflate the lungs with each breath. Second, pulmonary surfactant *promotes the stability of the alveoli*. Because the surface tension is reduced, there is a decreased tendency for small alveoli to empty into larger ones (see Figure 8.2, panel b). Third, surfactant *inhibits the transudation of fluid* out of the pulmonary capillaries into the alveoli. Excessive surface tension would tend to reduce the hydrostatic pressure in the tissue outside of the capillaries and capillary filtration is promoted. The movement of water out of the capillaries may result in interstitial edema formation and excess fluid in the alveoli.

Surfactant is more concentrated in the smaller alveoli. Therefore, its effect of lowering surface tension is greater in those alveoli compared with the larger alveoli. In this way, the collapsing pressure is equalized among alveoli of different sizes.

The amount of surfactant produced by alveolar type II cells decreases when breaths are small and constant. On the other hand, the amount of surfactant produced is increased in response to deep breaths due to stretching of the alveolar type II cells. Patients who have had thoracic or abdominal surgery often take small, shallow breaths because of the pain. The patients must be encouraged to regularly take deep breaths. To facilitate this, patients are often provided with an *incentive spirometer*. With a mouthpiece and a piston that rises during inspiration, the patient can visualize how deeply they are breathing.

PHARMACY APPLICATION: INFANT RESPIRATORY DISTRESS SYNDROME

Infant respiratory distress syndrome (IRDS), also known as hyaline membrane disease, is one of the most common causes of respiratory disease in premature infants. In fact, it occurs in 30,000–50,000 newborns per year in the United States; most commonly in neonates born before week 28 of gestation (60%). IRDS is characterized by areas of atelectasis, hemorrhagic edema and the formation of hyaline membranes within the alveoli.

(Continued)

PHARMACY APPLICATION: INFANT RESPIRATORY
DISTRESS SYNDROME (Continued)

IRDS is caused by a deficiency of pulmonary surfactant. Alveolar type II cells, which produce surfactant, do not begin to mature until weeks 25–28 of gestation. Therefore, premature infants may have poorly functioning alveolar type II cells and insufficient surfactant production.

At birth, the first breath taken by the neonate requires high inspiratory pressures to cause the initial expansion of the lungs. Normally, the lungs will retain a portion of this first breath (40% of the residual volume) so that subsequent breaths require much lower inspiratory pressures. In infants lacking surfactant, the lungs collapse between breaths. The airless portions of the lungs become stiff and noncompliant. Therefore, every inspiration is as difficult as the first. In fact, a transpulmonary pressure of 25–30 mmHg is needed to maintain a patent airway (compared with the normal 5 mmHg). This results in a significant increase in the work of breathing and a decrease in ventilation. The inability of the neonate to ventilate adequately leads to progressive atelectasis, hypoxemia, hypercapnia (increased carbon dioxide) and respiratory acidosis. Furthermore, the formation of the hyaline membranes impairs gas exchange, which exacerbates these conditions.

The therapy for IRDS includes mechanical ventilation with continuous positive airway pressure. This maintains adequate ventilation and prevents airway collapse between breaths.

Therapy also includes the administration of exogenous pulmonary surfactant. There are two types of surfactant used to prevent and treat IRDS in the United States. These include surfactants prepared from animal sources as well as synthetic surfactants. Exogenous pulmonary surfactants are administered as a suspension (in saline) through the endotracheal tube used for mechanical ventilation.

Many exogenous pulmonary surfactants are derived from bovine extracts. For example, Infasurf® contains the active ingredient, calfactant, which is an unmodified calf lung extract that includes mostly phospholipids and hydrophobic surfactant-specific proteins. Other exogenous pulmonary surfactants derived from bovine lung extracts include Survanta® (active ingredient, beractant) and Bovactant® (active ingredient, alveofact).

Exosurf® is a synthetic surfactant. It contains colfosceril palmitate, which is a phospholipid and an important constituent of natural and many synthetic pulmonary surfactant compounds.

8.5   Interdependence

Another important factor in maintaining alveolar stability is *interdependence*. Each alveolus in the lungs is surrounded by other alveoli (see Figure 8.3, panel a) and these alveoli are interconnected with each other by connective tissue. Because of these interconnections, any tendency for an alveolus to collapse is opposed by the surrounding alveoli. As the central alveolus collapses, it pulls outward on the surrounding alveoli, stretching them and distorting their shape. In response, the distorted alveoli pull back in the opposite direction to regain their normal shape. In other words, they exert *radial traction* on the central alveolus; the alveolus is pulled open and collapse is prevented.

8.6   Airway resistance

The factors determining the flow of air through the airways are analogous to those determining the flow of blood through the vessels and are described by Ohm's Law:

$$\text{Airflow} = \frac{\Delta P}{R}$$

Airflow through the airways is proportional to the gradient between atmospheric pressure and alveolar pressure (ΔP) and inversely proportional to the *airway resistance* (R).

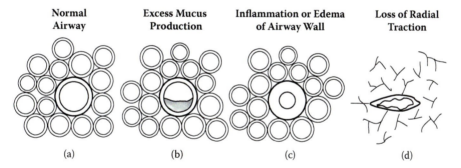

Figure 8.3 Airway obstruction. (a) Normal airway. Illustrated is a normal, patent airway with radial traction offered to it by the surrounding airways. Resistance in this airway is low and air flows through it freely. (b) Excess mucus production. The airway is obstructed by the presence of excess mucus and airway resistance is increased. Airflow is reduced. (c) Inflammation or edema of the airway wall. Thickening of the airway wall due to inflammation or edema narrows the lumen of the airway. The decrease in airway radius increases airway resistance and decreases airflow. (d) Loss of radial traction. Destruction of surrounding airways results in the loss of interdependence, or radial traction. Without the structural support offered by surrounding airways, the central airway collapses and airflow through it is reduced.

The factors determining the resistance to airflow are also analogous to those determining the resistance to blood flow and include viscosity, length of the airway and airway radius. Under normal conditions, the viscosity of the air is fairly constant and the length of the airway is fixed. Therefore, airway radius is the critically important physiological factor determining airway resistance:

$$R \; \alpha \; \frac{1}{r^4}$$

Airway resistance is inversely proportional to the *radius* (r) of the airway to the fourth power. In other words, when the radius is reduced by a factor of two (50%), the airway resistance increases 16-fold.

In normal healthy lungs, the resistance to airflow is so small, that small changes in pulmonary pressure result in large volumes of airflow. As discussed previously, a pressure gradient of 1 mmHg between the atmosphere and the alveolus allows 500 mL of air to enter the lungs. However, there are several factors that may alter airway resistance including:

- Lung volume
- Airway obstruction
- Bronchial smooth muscle tone

8.6.1   Lung volume

As *lung volume* increases, the airway resistance decreases. In other words, as the lungs inflate, the airways expand and become larger. The increase in airway radius decreases airway resistance. Conversely, as lung volume decreases, the airway resistance increases. In fact, at very low lung volumes, the small airways may close completely. This is a problem especially at the base of the lungs where, due to the weight of the lungs, the airways are less well expanded.

8.6.2   Airway obstruction

Airway obstruction may be caused by several factors including:

- Excess mucus production
- Inflammation and edema of the airway wall
- Airway collapse

Both asthma and chronic bronchitis are characterized by the *overproduction of thick, viscous mucus* (see Figure 8.3, panel b). This mucus blocks the airways and, in effect, reduces the radius of the airways and increases airway resistance. A severe asthmatic attack may be accompanied by the formation of mucus plugs, which can completely obstruct airflow.

Asthma and chronic bronchitis, which are considered chronic inflammatory conditions, are also characterized by *inflammation and edema of the airway walls* (see Figure 8.3, panel c). This thickening of the airway wall narrows the lumen of the airway and increases airway resistance. The increase in airway resistance due to excess mucus production and inflammation is reversible pharmacologically.

The pathophysiology of emphysema involves the breakdown, or destruction, of alveoli. This results in the loss of interdependence or the effect of radial traction, on the airways and leads to *airway collapse* (see Figure 8.3, panel d). The increase in airway resistance due to this form of lung obstruction is irreversible.

8.6.3   Bronchial smooth muscle tone

Changes in *bronchial smooth muscle tone* are particularly important in the bronchioles compared with the bronchi. Recall that the walls of the bronchioles consist almost entirely of smooth muscle. Contraction and relaxation of this muscle has a marked effect on the internal radius of the airway. An increase in bronchial smooth muscle tone, or *bronchoconstriction*, narrows the lumen of the airway and increases the resistance to airflow.

The activation of irritant receptors in the trachea and large bronchi by airborne pollutants, smoke and noxious chemicals elicits reflex bronchoconstriction. This reflex is mediated by the *parasympathetic nervous system*, specifically, by the vagus nerve. Acetylcholine released from the vagus nerve stimulates muscarinic receptors on the bronchial smooth muscle to cause bronchoconstriction. This parasympathetic reflex is meant to be a protective response, limiting the penetration of toxic substances deep into the lungs. Parasympathetic stimulation of the lungs also enhances mucus production to trap inhaled particles.

Bronchoconstriction is also elicited by several endogenous chemicals released from mast cells during an allergy or asthmatic attack. These substances, including histamine and the leukotrienes, may also promote the inflammatory response and edema formation.

A decrease in bronchial smooth muscle tone, or *bronchodilation*, widens the lumen of the airway and decreases the resistance to airflow. *Sympathetic nervous stimulation* causes bronchodilation. The adrenergic receptors found on the airway smooth muscle are β_2-adrenergic receptors. Recall that norepinephrine has a very low affinity for these receptors. Therefore, direct sympathetic stimulation of the airways has little effect. Epinephrine, released from the adrenal medulla, causes most of this bronchodilation. Epinephrine has a strong affinity for β_2-adrenergic receptors. Therefore, during a mass sympathetic discharge, as occurs during exercise or the "fight-or flight" response, epinephrine-induced bronchodilation minimizes airway resistance and maximizes airflow.

PHARMACY APPLICATION: PHARMACOLOGICAL
TREATMENT OF ASTHMA

Bronchial asthma is defined as a chronic inflammatory disease of the lungs. It affects an estimated 9–12 million individuals in the United States. Furthermore, its prevalence has been increasing in recent years. Asthma is characterized by reversible airway obstructions such as airway inflammation, increased airway responsiveness to a variety of bronchoactive stimuli, and, in particular, bronchospasm. There are many factors that may induce an asthmatic attack, including allergens, respiratory infections, hyperventilation, cold air, exercise, various drugs and chemicals, emotional upset, and airborne pollutants (e.g., smog, cigarette smoke).

The desired outcome in the pharmacological treatment of asthma is to prevent or relieve the reversible airway obstruction and the airway hyperresponsiveness caused by the inflammatory process. Therefore, categories of medications include bronchodilators and anti-inflammatory drugs.

A commonly prescribed class of bronchodilators is the β_2-adrenergic receptor agonists (e.g., albuterol, metaproterenol). Formoterol fumarate, a long acting, β_2-adrenergic receptor agonist, was approved by the U.S. Food and Drug Administration (FDA) in 2007. These drugs cause relaxation of bronchial smooth muscle and relieve the congestion of the bronchial mucosa. Beta two-adrenergic receptor agonists are useful during an acute asthmatic attack. Furthermore, they are effective when taken prior to exercise in individuals with exercise-induced asthma. These drugs are usually administered by inhalation or by a nebulizer.

Another bronchodilator is ipratropium, an anticholinergic drug that blocks muscarinic receptors on the airway smooth muscle. This results in bronchodilation, particularly in large airways. This agent has no effect on the composition or viscosity of the bronchial mucus and is also used to treat acute asthmatic attacks. Ipratropium is administered by inhalation.

Corticosteroids (e.g., beclomethasone, flunisolide, triamcinolone) have both anti-inflammatory and immunosuppressant actions. These drugs are used prophylactically to prevent the occurrence of asthma in patients with frequent attacks. Because they are not useful during an acute attack, corticosteroids are prescribed along with maintenance bronchodilators. More recently, a combination medication has been developed. Advair® contains the corticosteroid fluticasone propionate as well as the $\beta2$-adrenergic receptor antagonist salmeterol. Each of these drugs is administered by inhalation.

(Continued)

**PHARMACY APPLICATION: PHARMACOLOGICAL
TREATMENT OF ASTHMA (Continued)**

Cromolyn is another anti-inflammatory agent that is used prophylactically to prevent an asthmatic attack. The exact mechanism of action
of cromolyn is not fully understood; however, it is likely to involve the
stabilization of mast cells. This prevents the release of the inflammatory
mast cell mediators involved in inducing an asthmatic attack. Cromolyn
has proven effective in patients with exercise-induced asthma.

A more recent development in the treatment of asthma involves the
leukotriene-receptor antagonists and leukotriene-synthesis inhibitors.
Receptor antagonists include zafirlukast (Accolate®) and montelukast
(Singulair®). Zileuton (Zyflo®) inhibits the enzyme 5-lipoxygenase,
which synthesizes the leukotrienes from arachidonic acid. These drugs
have proven to be effective prophylactic treatment for mild asthma.

8.7   Ventilation

Ventilation is the exchange of air between the external atmosphere and the
alveoli. It is typically defined as the volume of air entering the alveoli per
minute. A complete understanding of ventilation requires the consideration
of lung volumes.

8.7.1   Standard lung volumes

The size of the lungs and, therefore, the lung volumes depend upon an individual's height, weight or body surface area, age and gender. This discussion
will include the typical values for a 70-kg adult male. There are *four standard
lung volumes* (see Figure 8.4 and Table 8.1):

- Tidal volume
- Residual volume
- Expiratory reserve volume
- Inspiratory reserve volume

The *tidal volume* (V_T) is the volume of air that enters the lungs per breath.
During normal, quiet breathing, tidal volume is 500 mL per breath. This volume increases significantly during exercise. The *residual volume* (RV) is the
volume of air remaining in the lungs following a maximal forced expiration.
Dynamic compression of the airways causes collapse and the trapping of air
in the alveoli. Residual volume is normally 1.5 L. It can be much greater in
patients with emphysema because of the increased tendency for airway collapse. *Expiratory reserve volume* (ERV) is the volume of air expelled from the

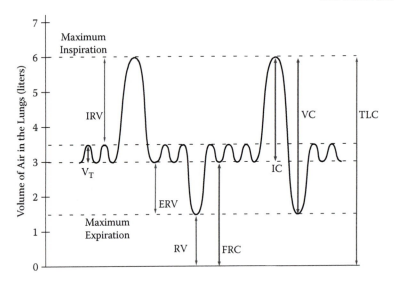

Figure 8.4 Standard lung volumes and lung capacities. Illustrated are the typical values for a 70-kg adult male. Tidal volume (V_T) is 500 mL during normal, quiet breathing. Inspiratory reserve volume (IRV) is obtained with a maximal inspiration and is 2.5 L. Tidal volume and IRV together determine the inspiratory capacity (IC), which is 3.0 L. Expiratory reserve volume (ERV) is obtained with a maximal expiration and is 1.5 L. The volume of air remaining in the lungs following a maximal expiration is the residual volume (RV), which is 1.5 L. The functional residual capacity (FRC) is the volume of air remaining in the lungs following a normal expiration and is 3.0 L. Vital capacity (VC) is obtained with the deepest inspiration and the most forceful expiration and is 4.5 L. The maximum volume to which the lungs can be expanded is the total lung capacity (TLC) and is approximately 6.0 L in adult males and 5.0 L in adult females.

lungs during a maximal forced expiration beginning at the end of a normal expiration. The ERV is normally about 1.5 L. The *inspiratory reserve volume* (IRV) is the volume of air inhaled into the lungs during a maximal forced inspiration beginning at the end of a normal inspiration. The IRV is normally about 2.5 L. It is determined by the strength of contraction of the inspiratory muscles and the inward elastic recoil of the lungs.

There are *four standard lung capacities*, which consist of two or more lung volumes in combination (see Figure 8.4):

- Functional residual capacity
- Inspiratory capacity
- Total lung capacity
- Vital capacity

The *functional residual capacity* (FRC) is the volume of air remaining in the lungs at the end of a normal expiration. The FRC consists of the residual

Table 8.1 Lung volumes and lung capacities in a healthy adult male

Lung volume	Value	Definition
Tidal Volume (V_T)	500 mL	Volume of air that enters the lungs per breath
Residual Volume (RV)	1.5 L	Volume of air remaining in the lungs following a maximal forced expiration
Expiratory Reserve Volume (ERV)	1.5 L	Volume of air expelled from the lungs during a maximal forced expiration (beginning at the end of a normal expiration)
Inspiratory Reserve Volume (IRV)	2.5 L	Volume of air inhaled into the lungs during a maximal forced inspiration (beginning at the end of a normal inspiration)

Lung capacity	Volume	Definition
Functional Residual Capacity (FRC)	3.0 L	Volume of air remaining in the lungs at the end of a normal expiration (RV + ERV)
Inspiratory Capacity (IC)	3.0 L	Volume of air that enters the lungs during a maximal forced inspiration beginning at the end of a normal expiration (V_T + IRV)
Total Lung Capacity (TLC)	6.0 L	Volume of air in the lungs following a maximal forced inspiration (RV + ERV + V_T + IRV)
Vital Capacity (VC)	4.5 L	Volume of air expelled from the lungs during a maximal forced expiration following a maximal forced inspiration (IRV + V_T + ERV)

volume and the expiratory reserve volume and is equal to 3 L. The *inspiratory capacity* (IC) is the volume of air that enters the lungs during a maximal forced inspiration beginning at the end of a normal expiration (FRC). The IC consists of the tidal volume and the inspiratory reserve volume and is equal to 3 L. The *total lung capacity* (TLC) is the volume of air in the lungs following a maximal forced inspiration. In other words, it is the maximum volume to which the lungs can be expanded. It is determined by the strength of contraction of the inspiratory muscles and the inward elastic recoil of the lungs. The TLC consists of all four lung volumes and is equal to about 6 L in a healthy adult male and about 5 L in a healthy adult female. The *vital capacity* (VC) is the volume of air expelled from the lungs during a maximal forced expiration following a maximal forced inspiration. In others words, it consists of the tidal volume as well as the inspiratory and expiratory reserve volumes. Vital capacity is approximately 4.5 L.

These lung volumes and capacities are measured using a spirometer. When the patient inhales, the pen moves upward on the paper affixed to a rotating drum. When the patient exhales, the pen moves downward on the paper. Pulmonary function tests are useful in the diagnosis of pulmonary disease.

8.7.2 Total ventilation

The *total ventilation* (*minute volume*) is the volume of air that enters the lungs per minute. It is determined by tidal volume and breathing frequency:

$$\text{Total ventilation} = \text{tidal volume} \times \text{breathing frequency}$$

$$= 500 \text{ mL/breath} \times 12 \text{ breaths/min}$$

$$= 6,000 \text{ mL/min}$$

With an average tidal volume of 500 mL/breath and breathing frequency of 12 breaths/min, 6,000 mL or 6 L of air moves in and out of the lungs per minute. These values apply to conditions of normal, quiet breathing. Both tidal volume and breathing frequency increase substantially during exercise.

8.7.3 Alveolar ventilation

Alveolar ventilation is less than the total ventilation because the last portion of each tidal volume remains in the conducting airways. Therefore, that air does not participate in gas exchange. As mentioned at the beginning of the chapter, the volume of the conducting airways is referred to as *anatomical dead space*. The calculation of alveolar ventilation includes the tidal volume adjusted for the anatomical dead space and includes only the air that reaches the respiratory zone:

$$\text{Alveolar ventilation} = \left(\text{tidal volume} - \text{anatomical dead space}\right)$$

$$\times \text{ breathing frequency}$$

$$= \left(500 \text{ mL/breath} - 150 \text{ mL dead space}\right)$$

$$\times 12 \text{ breaths/min}$$

$$= 4,200 \text{ mL/min}$$

During exercise, the working muscles need to obtain more oxygen and eliminate more carbon dioxide. Alveolar ventilation is increased accordingly. Interestingly, the increase in tidal volume is greater than the increase in breathing frequency. This is the most efficient mechanism by which to enhance alveolar ventilation. Using the values above, a 2-fold increase in breathing frequency, from 12 to 24 breaths/min, results in an alveolar ventilation of 8,400 mL/min. In other words, alveolar ventilation also increases by a factor of two. However, a 2-fold increase in tidal volume, from 500 mL/breath to 1,000 mL/breath, results in an alveolar ventilation of 10,200 mL/min. Alveolar ventilation is enhanced more in this case because a greater percentage of the tidal volume reaches the alveoli. At a tidal volume of 500 mL/breath and an anatomical dead space of 150 mL, 30% of the inspired air is wasted in that it does not reach the alveoli to participate in gas exchange. However, when the tidal volume is 1,000 mL/breath, only 15% of the inspired air remains in the anatomical dead space (ADS) (see Table 8.2).

8.7.4 Dead space

Anatomical dead space is equal to the volume of the conducting airways. This is determined by the physical characteristics of the lungs because these airways do not contain alveoli to participate in gas exchange.

Alveolar dead space is the volume of air that enters unperfused alveoli. In other words, these alveoli receive airflow but no blood flow. With no blood flow to the alveoli, gas exchange cannot take place. Therefore, alveolar dead space is based on functional considerations rather than anatomical factors. Healthy lungs have little or no alveolar dead space. Various pathological conditions, such as low cardiac output, may result in alveolar dead space.

The anatomical dead space combined with the alveolar dead space is referred to as *physiological dead space*:

Physiological dead space = anatomical dead space + alveolar dead space

Physiological dead space is determined by measuring the amount of carbon dioxide in the expired air. Therefore, it is based on the functional characteristics of the lungs because only perfused alveoli can participate in gas exchange and eliminate carbon dioxide.

Table 8.2 Effect of tidal volume and breathing frequency on alveolar ventilation

Patient	Tidal volume (mL/breath)	Frequency (breaths/min)	Total ventilation (mL/min)	Alveolar ventilation $(V_T - ADS)$ (mL/min)
A	500	12	6,000	4,200
B	500	24	12,000	8,400
C	1,000	12	12,000	10,200

PHARMACY APPLICATION: DRUG-INDUCED HYPOVENTILATION

Hypoventilation is defined as a reduction in the rate and depth of breathing. Inadequate ventilation results in hypoxemia, or a decrease in the oxygen content of the arterial blood. Hypoventilation may be induced inadvertently by various pharmacological agents, including opioid analgesics such as morphine. These medications cause hypoventilation by way of their effects on the respiratory centers in the brainstem. Doses of morphine too small to alter a patient's consciousness may cause discernible respiratory depression. This inhibitory effect on the respiratory drive increases progressively as the dose of morphine is increased. In fact, in humans, death due to morphine poisoning is almost always due to respiratory arrest. Although therapeutic doses of morphine decrease tidal volume, the decrease in breathing frequency is the primary cause of decreased minute volume.

8.8 Diffusion

Oxygen and carbon dioxide cross the blood-gas interface by way of *diffusion*. The factors that determine the rate of diffusion of each gas are described by *Fick's Law of Diffusion*:

$$V_{gas} \; \alpha \; \frac{A \times D \times (\Delta P)}{T}$$

Diffusion is proportional to the surface area of the blood-gas interface (A), the diffusion constant (D) and the partial pressure gradient of the gas (ΔP). Diffusion is inversely proportional to the thickness of the blood-gas interface (T).

The *surface area* of the blood-gas interface is about 70 m^2 in a healthy adult at rest. Specifically, 70 m^2 of the potential surface area for gas exchange in the lungs is both ventilated and perfused. The amount of this surface area may be altered under various conditions. For example, during exercise, an increased number of pulmonary capillaries are perfused (due to increased cardiac output and, therefore, blood flow through the lungs). As a result, a larger percentage of the alveoli are both ventilated and perfused, which increases the surface area for gas exchange. Conversely, a fall in the cardiac output reduces the number of perfused capillaries and, therefore, reduces the surface area for gas exchange. Another pathological condition affecting surface area is emphysema. This pulmonary disease, usually associated with cigarette smoking, causes destruction of alveoli.

The *diffusion constant* for a gas is proportional to the solubility of the gas and inversely proportional to the square root of the molecular weight of the gas:

$$D \alpha \frac{solubility}{\sqrt{MW}}$$

Both oxygen and carbon dioxide are small molecules with low molecular weights. However, carbon dioxide is 20 times more soluble than oxygen. Therefore, the value of the diffusion constant for carbon dioxide is larger than that of oxygen, which facilitates the exchange of carbon dioxide across the blood-gas interface.

The *thickness* of the blood-gas interface is normally less than 0.5 μm. This extremely thin barrier promotes the diffusion of gases. The thickness may increase, however, under conditions of interstitial fibrosis, interstitial edema and pneumonia. Fibrosis involves the excess production of collagen fibers by fibroblasts in the interstitial space. Edema is the movement of fluid from the capillaries into the interstitial space. Pneumonia causes inflammation and alveolar flooding. In each case, the thickness of the barrier between the air and the blood is increased and diffusion is impaired.

The diffusion of oxygen and carbon dioxide also depends on their *partial pressure gradients*. Oxygen diffuses from an area of high partial pressure in the alveoli to an area of low partial pressure in the pulmonary capillary blood. Conversely, carbon dioxide diffuses down its partial pressure gradient from the pulmonary capillary blood into the alveoli.

Dalton's Law states, the partial pressure of a gas (P_{gas}) is equal to its fractional concentration (percentage total gas [% total gas]) multiplied by the total pressure (P_{tot}) of all the gases in a mixture:

$$P_{gas} = \% \text{ total gas} \times P_{tot}$$

The atmosphere is a mixture of gases containing 21% oxygen and 79% nitrogen. Because of gravity, this mixture exerts a total atmospheric pressure (barometric pressure) of 760 mmHg at sea level. Using these values of fractional concentration and total pressure, the partial pressures for oxygen (PO_2) and nitrogen (PN_2) can be calculated:

$$PO_2 = 0.21 \times 760 \text{ mmHg} = 160 \text{ mmHg}$$

$$PN_2 = 0.79 \times 760 \text{ mmHg} = 600 \text{ mmHg}$$

The PO_2 of the atmosphere at sea level is 160 mmHg and the PN_2 is 600 mmHg. The total pressure (760 mmHg) is equal to the sum of the partial pressures.

Under normal, physiological conditions, the partial pressure gradient for oxygen between the alveoli and the pulmonary capillary blood is quite substantial. However, this gradient may be diminished under certain conditions, such as ascent to altitude and hypoventilation. Altitude has no effect on the concentration of oxygen in the atmosphere. However, the effects of gravity on barometric pressure progressively decrease as elevation increases. For example, at an elevation of 17,000 feet, which is the height of Pike's Peak in the Rocky Mountains of Colorado, the barometric pressure is only 380 mmHg. Therefore, the PO_2 of the atmosphere at this altitude is 80 mmHg ($PO_2 = 0.21 \times 380$ mmHg = 80 mmHg). This results in a marked decrease in the partial pressure gradient between the alveoli and the pulmonary capillary blood. Consequently, diffusion is significantly impaired.

Hypoventilation decreases the rate of oxygen uptake into the alveoli. Once again, the partial pressure gradient and the rate of diffusion are reduced. Conditions resulting in impaired diffusion lead to the development of *hypoxemia*, or decreased oxygen in the arterial blood.

8.9   Partial pressures

As explained in the previous section, the PO_2 of the atmosphere is 160 mmHg. The partial pressure of carbon dioxide (PCO_2) is negligible (see Table 8.3 and Figure 8.5).

As air is inspired, it is warmed and humidified as it flows through the conducting airways. Therefore, water vapor is added to the gas mixture. This is accounted for in the calculation of PO_2 in the conducting airways:

$$PO_2 \text{ inspired air} = 0.21 \times (760 \text{ mmHg} - 47 \text{ mmHg})$$

$$= 150 \text{ mmHg}$$

The partial pressure of the water vapor is 47 mmHg. Because of this, the PO_2 in the conducting airways during inspiration is slightly decreased to 150 mmHg. The PCO_2 remains at 0 mmHg.

Table 8.3   Partial pressures of oxygen and carbon dioxide

Location	PO_2 (mmHg)	PCO_2 (mmHg)
Atmosphere	160	0
Conducting Airways (inspired)	150	0
Alveolar Gas	100	40
Arterial Blood	100	40
Tissues	40	45
Mixed Venous Blood	40	45

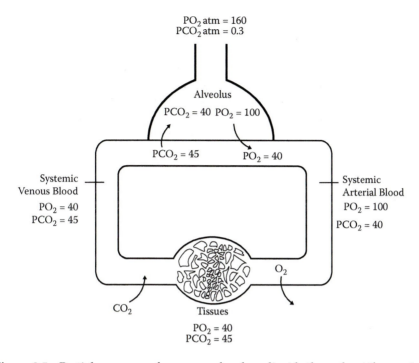

Figure 8.5 Partial pressures of oxygen and carbon dioxide throughout the respiratory and cardiovascular system.

By the time the air reaches the alveoli, the PO_2 has decreased to about 100 mmHg. The PO_2 of the alveolar gas is determined by two processes:

- The rate of replenishment of oxygen by ventilation
- The rate of removal of oxygen by the pulmonary capillary blood

The primary determinant of alveolar PO_2 is the rate of replenishment of oxygen by ventilation. As mentioned previously, hypoventilation causes a decrease in alveolar PO_2. The rate of removal of oxygen by the pulmonary capillary blood is determined largely by the oxygen consumption of the tissues. As metabolic activity and oxygen consumption increase, the PO_2 of the mixed venous blood decreases and the partial pressure gradient for oxygen between the alveoli and the blood is increased and the diffusion of oxygen is enhanced.

The PCO_2 of the alveoli is about 40 mmHg. The alveolar PCO_2 is also determined by two processes:

- The rate of delivery of carbon dioxide to the lungs from the tissues
- The rate of elimination of carbon dioxide by ventilation

As cellular metabolism increases, the rate of production of carbon dioxide also increases. Typically, increased activity is associated with an increase in ventilation so that the increased amounts of carbon dioxide delivered to the lungs are readily eliminated. On the other hand, hypoventilation impairs the elimination of carbon dioxide and causes an increase in alveolar PCO_2.

Assuming oxygen diffuses down its partial pressure gradient from the alveoli into the pulmonary capillary blood until equilibration is reached then, the PO_2 of this blood reaches 100 mmHg. This is the pressure exerted by oxygen molecules in their *gas phase*. In other words, the PO_2 of the blood is determined by the amount of oxygen *dissolved in plasma* as opposed to the amount of oxygen bound to hemoglobin (a concept discussed later in this chapter). This blood flows back to the left side of the heart and into the systemic circulation. Therefore, the PO_2 of the arterial blood is 100 mmHg. Likewise, assuming carbon dioxide diffuses down its partial pressure gradient from the pulmonary capillary blood into the alveoli until equilibration is reached then, the PCO_2 of the blood leaving these capillaries should be 40 mmHg. Therefore, the PCO_2 of the arterial blood is 40 mmHg.

The arterial blood, which is high in oxygen and low in carbon dioxide, is delivered to the tissues. Within the tissues, oxygen is consumed by metabolism and carbon dioxide is produced. Under typical resting conditions, the PO_2 of the tissues is 40 mmHg. Therefore, oxygen diffuses down its concentration gradient from the systemic capillary blood into the cells of the tissues until equilibration is reached. The PO_2 of the venous blood leaving the tissues is also 40 mmHg. The PCO_2 of the tissues is 45 mmHg. Therefore, carbon dioxide diffuses down its concentration gradient from the tissues into the blood until equilibration is reached. The PCO_2 of the venous blood leaving the tissues is 45 mmHg.

The mixed venous blood, which is low in oxygen and high in carbon dioxide, flows back to the lungs to obtain oxygen and eliminate carbon dioxide. Note that the partial pressure gradient for oxygen between the alveoli (100 mmHg) and the mixed venous blood (40 mmHg) is 60 mmHg. The partial pressure gradient for carbon dioxide between the mixed venous blood (45 mmHg) and the alveoli (40 mmHg) is 5 mmHg. According to Fick's Law of Diffusion, the small partial pressure gradient for carbon dioxide would tend to reduce the exchange of this gas. However, the relatively high solubility and diffusion constant of carbon dioxide allows it to diffuse quite readily across the blood-gas interface.

To optimize gas exchange, the uptake of oxygen from the alveolar gas into the pulmonary blood and the elimination of carbon dioxide from the pulmonary blood into the alveolar gas, a given lung unit must be equally well ventilated and perfused. In other words, the air and the blood must be brought together for the exchange of gases to occur efficiently. This is referred to as *ventilation-perfusion (V:Q) matching*. The most effective conditions for gas exchange occur when the V:Q ratio is equal to 1, or when the amount of ventilation in a lung unit is balanced, or matched, by the amount of perfusion. In this region, the mixed venous blood entering the pulmonary capillaries has a PO_2 of 40 mmHg and a PCO_2 of 45 mmHg. The alveolar gas has a PO_2 of 100 mmHg and a PCO_2 of 40 mmHg. Ventilation-perfusion matching results in efficient gas exchange and a PO_2 of 100 mmHg and a PCO_2 of 40 mmHg in the blood leaving the capillaries and returning to the heart (see Figure 8.6, panel a).

Airway obstruction leads to a reduction in the V/Q ratio to a value less than 1. In this lung unit, perfusion is greater than ventilation (see Figure 8.6, panel b). Complete airway obstruction leads to "shunt." Shunt refers to blood that enters the arterial system without passing through a region of ventilated lung. In other words, mixed venous blood travels through the pulmonary circulation without participating in gas exchange. This blood enters the

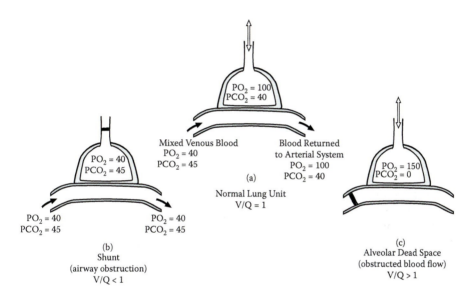

Figure 8.6 Ventilation-perfusion matching. (a) Normal lung unit. Ventilation and perfusion are matched so that the V:Q ratio is equal to 1 and gas exchange is optimized. Mixed venous blood that is low in oxygen and high in carbon dioxide enters the pulmonary capillaries. As the blood flows through these capillaries in the walls of the alveoli, oxygen is obtained and carbon dioxide is eliminated. Blood returning to the heart and the arterial system is high in oxygen and low in carbon dioxide. (b) Shunt. Airway obstruction with normal perfusion can result in a shunt (V:Q < 1). Blood flows through the lungs without obtaining oxygen or eliminating carbon dioxide. This V:Q mismatch causes hypoxemia. (c) Alveolar dead space. Obstructed blood flow with normal ventilation causes the development of alveolar dead space (V:Q > 1). The partial pressures of oxygen and carbon dioxide in the alveoli are similar to those of the conducting airways. This ventilation is wasted because it does not participate in gas exchange.

pulmonary capillaries with a PO_2 of 40 mmHg and a PCO_2 of 45 mmHg. If the lung unit is not ventilated, then this blood exits the capillaries and returns to the heart with the partial pressures of oxygen and carbon dioxide unchanged. The addition of blood that is low in oxygen to the rest of the blood returning from the lungs causes *hypoxemia*. The degree of hypoxemia is determined by the magnitude of the shunt. As airway obstruction increases throughout the lungs, then this widespread decrease in the V:Q ratio results in a greater volume of poorly oxygenated blood returning to the heart and a greater degree of hypoxemia. As discussed, airway obstruction may be caused by many factors including bronchoconstriction, excess mucus production, airway collapse and alveolar flooding.

Obstructed blood flow leads to an increase in the V:Q ratio to a value greater than 1. In this lung unit, ventilation is greater than perfusion (see Figure 8.6, panel c). Complete loss of blood flow leads to *alveolar dead space*. In this lung unit, the air enters the alveoli with partial pressures of oxygen and carbon dioxide equal to those of the conducting airways (PO_2 of 150 mmHg and PCO_2 of 0 mmHg). With no perfusion, oxygen is not taken up from this mixture, nor is carbon dioxide added to the mixture to be eliminated. Alveolar dead space may be caused by pulmonary thromboembolism. This is when a pulmonary blood vessel is occluded by a blood clot. Alveolar dead space may also occur when alveolar pressure is greater than pulmonary capillary pressure. This leads to compression of the capillaries and a loss of perfusion. Alveolar pressure may be increased by positive pressure mechanical ventilation. Pulmonary capillary pressure may be decreased by hemorrhage and a decrease in cardiac output.

Ventilation-perfusion mismatch leads to hypoxemia. Reduced ventilation caused by obstructed airflow or reduced perfusion caused by obstructed blood flow leads to impaired gas exchange. Interestingly, each of these conditions may be minimized by *local control mechanisms* that attempt to match airflow and blood flow in a given lung unit.

Bronchiolar smooth muscle is sensitive to changes in carbon dioxide levels. Excess carbon dioxide causes bronchodilation and reduced carbon dioxide causes bronchoconstriction. Pulmonary vascular smooth muscle is sensitive to changes in oxygen levels. Excess oxygen causes vasodilation and insufficient oxygen (hypoxia) causes vasoconstriction. It is the changes in bronchiolar and vascular smooth muscle tone that alter the amount of ventilation and perfusion in a lung unit to return the V:Q ratio to 1.

In a lung unit with high blood flow and low ventilation (airway obstruction), the level of carbon dioxide is increased and the level of oxygen is decreased. The excess carbon dioxide causes bronchodilation and an increase in ventilation. The reduced oxygen causes vasoconstriction and a decrease in perfusion. In this way, the V:Q ratio is brought closer to 1 and overall pulmonary gas exchange is improved.

In a lung unit with low blood flow and high ventilation (alveolar dead space), the level of carbon dioxide is decreased and the level of oxygen is increased. The reduced carbon dioxide causes bronchoconstriction and a decrease in ventilation. The excess oxygen causes vasodilation and an increase in perfusion. Once again, the V:Q ratio is brought closer to 1 and overall pulmonary gas exchange is improved.

8.10   Gas transport

Once the oxygen has diffused from the alveoli into the pulmonary circulation, it must be carried, or transported, in the blood to the cells and tissues that need it. Furthermore, once the carbon dioxide has diffused from the tissues into the systemic circulation, it must be transported to the lungs where it can be eliminated. This section considers the mechanisms by which these gases are transported.

8.10.1   Transport of oxygen

Oxygen is carried in the blood in two forms:

- Physically dissolved
- Chemically combined with hemoglobin

Oxygen is poorly soluble in plasma. At a PO_2 of 100 mmHg, only 3 mL of oxygen is *physically dissolved* in 1 L of blood. Assuming a blood volume of 5 L, a total of 15 mL of oxygen is in the dissolved form. A normal rate of oxygen consumption at rest is about 250 mL/min. During exercise, oxygen consumption may increase to 3.5–5.5 L/min. Therefore, the amount of dissolved oxygen is clearly insufficient to meet the needs of the tissues.

Most of the oxygen in the blood (98.5%) is transported *chemically combined with hemoglobin*. A large, complex molecule, hemoglobin consists of four polypeptide chains (globin portion), each of which contains a ferrous iron atom (heme portion). Each iron atom can bind reversibly with an oxygen molecule:

$$O_2 + Hb \leftrightarrow HbO_2$$

Therefore, the hemoglobin molecule exists in one of two forms: oxyhemoglobin (HbO_2) or deoxyhemoglobin (Hb). The binding of oxygen to hemoglobin follows the *Law of Mass Action*, such that as the PO_2 increases, as it does in the lungs, more will combine with hemoglobin. When the PO_2 decreases, as it does in the tissues that are consuming it, the reaction moves to the left and the hemoglobin releases the oxygen.

Each gram of hemoglobin can combine with up to 1.34 mL of oxygen. In a healthy individual, there are 15 g of hemoglobin/100 mL of blood. Therefore, the oxygen content of the blood is 20.1 mL O_2/100 mL blood:

$$\frac{15 \text{ g Hb}}{100 \text{ mL blood}} \times \frac{1.34 \text{ mL } O_2}{\text{g Hb}} = \frac{20.1 \text{ mL } O_2}{100 \text{ mL blood}}$$

It is important to note that oxygen bound to hemoglobin has no effect on the PO_2 of the blood. Once again, the *PO_2 of the blood* is determined by the amount of oxygen dissolved in the plasma. The amount of oxygen bound to hemoglobin determines *oxygen content* of the blood. In a normal healthy individual, the percent of hemoglobin saturation directly reflects the number of oxygen molecules present in the blood. However, as will be discussed, under certain pathophysiological conditions, the percent of hemoglobin saturation may not accurately reflect the oxygen content of the blood.

The PO_2 of the blood is the major factor determining the amount of oxygen chemically combined with hemoglobin, or the *percent of hemoglobin saturation*. The relationship between these two variables is illustrated graphically by the *oxyhemoglobin dissociation curve* (see Figure 8.7). As the PO_2 of the blood increases, the combination of oxygen and hemoglobin also increases. However, this relationship is not linear. The amount of oxygen carried by hemoglobin increases steeply up to a PO_2 of about 60 mmHg. Beyond this point, the curve becomes much flatter, such that there is little change in the percent of hemoglobin saturation as PO_2 continues to increase. At a PO_2 of 100 mmHg, which is the normal PO_2 of the alveoli and, therefore, the arterial blood, the hemoglobin is 97.5% saturated with oxygen.

Each region of the curve, the steep portion and the flat plateau portion, has important physiological significance. The *steep portion of the curve*, between 0 and 60 mmHg, is the PO_2 range found in the cells and tissues. This region of the curve is ideal for *unloading* oxygen to the tissues. On average, the PO_2 of the tissues and, therefore the mixed venous blood is about 40 mmHg at rest. At a PO_2 of 40 mmHg, the hemoglobin is 75% saturated with oxygen. In other words, as the blood flows through the systemic capillaries, the hemoglobin releases 22.5% of its oxygen to the tissues. An increase in the metabolic activity of a tissue and, therefore, an increase in oxygen consumption, will decrease the PO_2 in that tissue. The fall in PO_2 in this region of the oxyhemoglobin dissociation curve has a profound effect on the percent of hemoglobin saturation. At a PO_2 of 15 mmHg, the hemoglobin is only 25% saturated with oxygen. In this case, the hemoglobin has released 72.5% of its oxygen to the tissue. Therefore, relatively a small drop in PO_2 (from 40 mmHg down to 15 mmHg) results in a marked increase in the unloading of oxygen (more than three times as much oxygen has been released to the tissue that needs it).

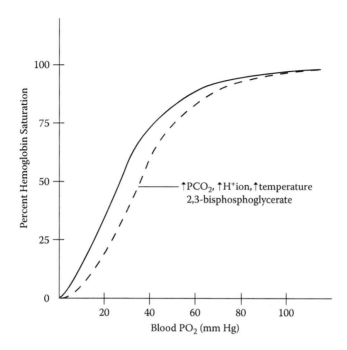

Figure 8.7 Oxyhemoglobin dissociation curve. The percent hemoglobin saturation depends upon the PO_2 of the blood. The PO_2 of the blood in the pulmonary
capillaries is 100 mmHg. Consequently, in the lungs, the hemoglobin loads up with
oxygen and becomes 97.5% saturated. The average PO_2 of the blood in the systemic capillaries is 40 mmHg. Therefore, at the level of the tissues, hemoglobin
releases oxygen and the saturation falls to 75%. Increased PCO_2, H^+ ion concentration, temperature, and 2,3-bisphosphoglycerate shifts the oxyhemoglobin dissociation curve to the right. Therefore, at any given PO_2, the hemoglobin releases more
oxygen to the tissue.

The *plateau portion of the curve*, between 60 and 100 mmHg, is the PO_2
range found in the alveoli. As the mixed venous blood flows through the
pulmonary capillaries in the walls of the alveoli, the hemoglobin loads up
with oxygen. As mentioned above, at a normal alveolar PO_2 of 100 mmHg,
the hemoglobin becomes almost fully saturated with oxygen (97.5%). At a
PO_2 of 60 mmHg, the hemoglobin still becomes 90% saturated with oxygen. In other words, the hemoglobin remains quite saturated with oxygen
even with a marked fall in PO_2 (40 mmHg). This provides a good mar-
gin of safety for the oxygen carrying capacity of the blood. Therefore, if
an individual ascends to some altitude above sea level or has pulmonary
disease such that the alveolar PO_2 falls, the oxygen content of the blood
remains high.

8.10.2   Factors affecting the transport of oxygen

There are several factors that affect the transport of oxygen including:

- PCO_2, pH and temperature
- 2,3-bisphosphoglycerate
- Anemia
- Carbon monoxide

An *increase in the PCO₂*, a *decrease in pH* and an *increase in temperature* all shift the oxyhemoglobin dissociation curve to the right so at any given PO_2, the hemoglobin releases more oxygen to the tissue (see Figure 8.7). Both carbon dioxide and hydrogen ion can bind to hemoglobin. The binding of these substances changes the conformation of the hemoglobin and reduces its affinity for oxygen. This phenomenon is referred to as the *Bohr effect*. An increase in temperature also reduces the affinity of hemoglobin for oxygen. This effect is of benefit to a metabolically active tissue. As the rate of metabolism increases, as it does during exercise, oxygen consumption and, therefore, the demand for oxygen, increases. In addition, the carbon dioxide, the hydrogen ions and the heat produced by the tissue are all increased. These products of metabolism facilitate the release of oxygen from the hemoglobin to the tissue that needs it.

2,3-bisphosphoglycerate (2,3-BPG) is produced by red blood cells. This substance also binds to hemoglobin, shifting the oxyhemoglobin dissociation curve to the right. Once again, the rightward shift of the curve reduces the affinity of hemoglobin for oxygen so that more oxygen is released to the tissues. Levels of 2,3-BPG are increased when the hemoglobin in the arterial blood is chronically undersaturated or, in other words, during *hypoxemia*. Decreased arterial PO_2 may occur at altitude or as the result of various cardiovascular or pulmonary diseases. The rightward shift of the curve is beneficial at the level of the tissues because more of the oxygen that is bound to the hemoglobin is released to the tissues. However, the shift of the curve may be detrimental in the lungs because the loading of hemoglobin may be impaired.

Levels of 2,3-BPG may be decreased in blood stored in a blood bank for as little as 1 week. A decrease in 2,3-BPG shifts the oxyhemoglobin dissociation curve to the left. In this case, at any given PO_2, the unloading of oxygen to the tissues is decreased. The progressive depletion of 2,3-BPG can be minimized by storing the blood with citrate-phosphate-dextrose.

Anemia causes a decrease in the oxygen content of the blood and, therefore, a decrease in the supply of oxygen to the tissues. It is characterized by a low hematocrit that may be caused by several pathological conditions, such as a decreased rate of erythropoiesis (red blood cell production), excessive loss of erythrocytes or a deficiency of normal hemoglobin in the erythrocytes. Although there is a decrease in the oxygen content of the blood, it is important to note that anemia has no effect on the PO_2 of the blood or on the

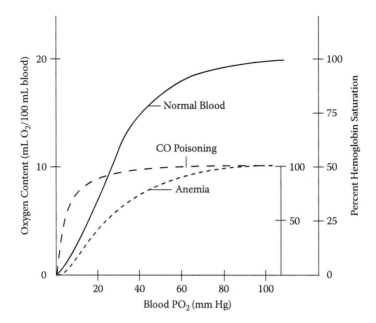

Figure 8.8 Effect of anemia and carbon monoxide poisoning on oxygen transport. Anemia results from a deficiency of normal hemoglobin. The PO_2 of the blood and the percent hemoglobin saturation remain normal. However, because there is less hemoglobin present to transport oxygen, the oxygen content of the blood is decreased. Carbon monoxide (CO) impairs the transport of oxygen to the tissues by two mechanisms. First, it binds preferentially with hemoglobin and prevents the hemoglobin from binding with oxygen, resulting in the hemoglobin remaining fully saturated (although with carbon monoxide instead of oxygen) and the oxygen content of the blood being decreased. Second, CO shifts the oxyhemoglobin dissociation curve to the left and inhibits the release of oxygen from the hemoglobin. As with anemia, the PO_2 of the blood is unaffected.

oxyhemoglobin dissociation curve (see Figure 8.8). Arterial PO_2 is determined only by the amount of oxygen dissolved in the blood, which is unaffected. Furthermore, the affinity of hemoglobin for oxygen has not changed. What has changed is the amount of hemoglobin in the blood. If there is less hemoglobin available to bind with oxygen, then there is less oxygen in the blood.

Anemia does not stimulate ventilation. As will be discussed in a subsequent section, the peripheral chemoreceptors are sensitive to decreases in PO_2, not oxygen content.

Carbon monoxide is a by-product of the combustion of hydrocarbons such as gasoline. It may cause sickness and death due to poisoning because it interferes with the transport of oxygen to the tissues by way of two mechanisms:

- Formation of carboxyhemoglobin
- Leftward shift of the oxyhemoglobin dissociation curve

Carbon monoxide has a much greater affinity (240 times) for hemoglobin than does oxygen so that *carboxyhemoglobin* is readily formed. Therefore, even small amounts of carbon monoxide can tie up the hemoglobin and prevent the loading of oxygen. Furthermore, the formation of carboxyhemoglobin causes a *leftward shift of the oxyhemoglobin dissociation curve* (see Figure 8.8) so, at any given PO_2, the unloading of oxygen to the tissues is impaired. Therefore, not only does the hemoglobin carry less oxygen, it does not release this oxygen to the tissues that need it. The concentration of hemoglobin in the blood and the PO_2 of the blood are normal.

Carbon monoxide poisoning is particularly insidious. An individual exposed to carbon monoxide is usually unaware of it as this gas is odorless, colorless and tasteless. Furthermore, it does not elicit any irritant reflexes resulting in sneezing, coughing or feelings of dyspnea (difficulty in breathing). Finally, as with anemia, carbon monoxide does not stimulate ventilation.

8.10.3   Transport of carbon dioxide

Carbon dioxide is carried in the blood in three forms:

- Physically dissolved
- Carbaminohemoglobin
- Bicarbonate ions

As with oxygen, the amount of carbon dioxide *physically dissolved* in the plasma is proportional to its partial pressure. However, carbon dioxide is 20 times more soluble in the plasma than is oxygen. Therefore, approximately 10% of the carbon dioxide in the blood is transported in the dissolved form.

Carbon dioxide can combine chemically with the terminal amine groups (NH_2) in blood proteins. The most important of these proteins for this process is hemoglobin. The combination of carbon dioxide and hemoglobin forms *carbaminohemoglobin*:

$$Hb \cdot NH_2 + CO_2 \leftrightarrow Hb \cdot NH \cdot COOH$$

Deoxyhemoglobin can bind more carbon dioxide than oxygenated hemoglobin. Therefore, the unloading of the oxygen in the tissues facilitates the loading of carbon dioxide for transport to the lungs. Approximately 30% of the carbon dioxide in the blood is transported in this form.

The remaining 60% of the carbon dioxide is transported in the blood in the form of *bicarbonate ions*. This mechanism is made possible by the following reaction:

$$H_2O + CO_2 \xleftrightarrow{\quad CA \quad} H_2CO_3 \leftrightarrow H^+ + HCO_3^-$$

The carbon dioxide produced during cellular metabolism diffuses out of the cells and into the plasma. It then continues to diffuse down its concentration gradient into the red blood cells. Within the red blood cells, the enzyme, *carbonic anhydrase* (CA), facilitates the combination of carbon dioxide and water to form *carbonic acid* (H_2CO_3). The carbonic acid then dissociates into hydrogen ion (H^+) and bicarbonate ion (HCO_3^-). As the bicarbonate ions are formed, they diffuse down their concentration gradient out of the red blood cell and into the plasma. This process is beneficial because bicarbonate ion is far more soluble in the plasma than carbon dioxide. As the negatively charged bicarbonate ions exit the red blood cell, chloride ions, the most abundant anions in the plasma, enter the cells by way of HCO_3^--Cl^- carrier proteins. This process, referred to as the *chloride shift*, maintains electrical neutrality. Many of the hydrogen ions bind with hemoglobin. As with carbon dioxide, deoxyhemoglobin can bind more readily with hydrogen ions than oxygenated hemoglobin.

This entire reaction is reversed when the blood reaches the lungs. Because carbon dioxide is eliminated by ventilation, the reaction is pulled to the left. Bicarbonate ions diffuse back into the red blood cells. The hemoglobin releases the hydrogen ions and is now available to load up with oxygen. The bicarbonate ions combine with the hydrogen ions to form carbonic acid. The carbonic acid then dissociates into carbon dioxide and water. The carbon dioxide diffuses down its concentration gradient from the blood into the alveoli and is exhaled. A summary of the three mechanisms by which carbon dioxide is transported in the blood is illustrated in Figure 8.9.

8.11   Regulation of ventilation

The rate and depth of breathing are perfectly adjusted to meet the metabolic needs of the tissues and to maintain a PO_2 of 100 mmHg, a PCO_2 of 40 mmHg and a pH of 7.4 in the arterial blood. Breathing is initiated spontaneously by the central nervous system. It occurs in a continuous, cyclical pattern of inspiration and expiration. There are three major components of the regulatory system for ventilation:

- Medullary respiratory center
- Receptors and other sources of input
- Effector tissues (respiratory muscles)

Aggregates of cell bodies within the medulla of the brainstem comprise the *medullary respiratory center*. There are two distinct functional areas:

- Dorsal respiratory group
- Ventral respiratory group

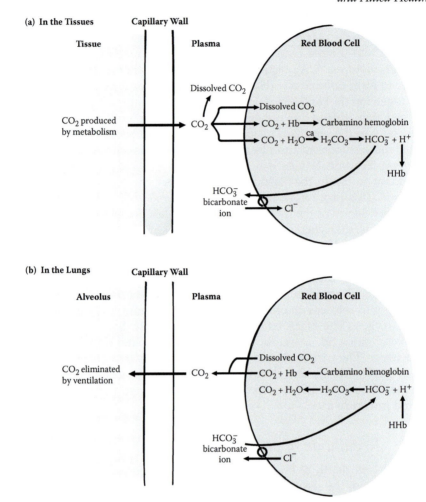

Figure 8.9 Transport of carbon dioxide in the blood. Carbon dioxide (CO_2) is transported in the blood in three forms: dissolved, bound with hemoglobin and as bicarbonate ion (HCO_3^-). The carbon dioxide produced by the tissues diffuses down its concentration gradient into the plasma and into red blood cells. A small amount of carbon dioxide remains in the blood in the dissolved form. Within the red blood cell, carbon dioxide can bind with reduced hemoglobin to form carbaminohemoglobin. In addition, due to the presence of the enzyme, CA, carbon dioxide can combine with water to form carbonic acid (H_2CO_3). Carbonic acid then dissociates into bicarbonate ion and hydrogen ion (H^+). The hydrogen ion is picked up by the reduced hemoglobin (HHb). The bicarbonate ion diffuses down its concentration gradient from the red blood cell into the plasma. To maintain electrical neutrality, as the bicarbonate ion exits the cell, a chloride ion (Cl^-) enters the cell. This is referred to as the chloride shift. In the lungs, these reactions reverse direction and the carbon dioxide is eliminated by ventilation.

The aggregate of cell bodies in the dorsal region of the medulla is the *dorsal respiratory group* (DRG). The DRG consists primarily of *inspiratory neurons*. These neurons are self-excitable and repetitively generate action potentials to cause inspiration. The inspiratory neurons descend to the spinal cord where they stimulate neurons that supply the inspiratory muscles, including those of the phrenic nerves and the intercostal nerves. These nerves then stimulate the diaphragm and the external intercostal muscles to contract and cause inspiration. When the inspiratory neurons are electrically inactive, expiration takes place. Therefore, this cyclical electrical activity of the DRG is responsible for the basic rhythm of breathing. Furthermore, the DRG is likely the site of integration of the various sources of input that alter the spontaneous pattern of inspiration and expiration.

The aggregate of cell bodies in the ventral region of the medulla is the *ventral respiratory group* (VRG). The VRG consists of both expiratory and inspiratory neurons. This region is inactive during normal, quiet breathing. (Recall that expiration, at this time, is a passive process.) However, the VRG is active when the demands for ventilation are increased, such as during exercise. Under these conditions, action potentials in the *expiratory neurons* cause forced, or active, expiration. These neurons descend to the spinal cord where they stimulate the neurons that supply the expiratory muscles, including those that innervate the muscles of the abdominal wall and the internal intercostal muscles. Contractions of these muscles cause a more rapid and more forceful expiration.

Inspiratory neurons of the VRG augment inspiratory activity. These neurons descend to the spinal cord where they stimulate the neurons that supply the accessory muscles of inspiration including those that innervate the scalene muscles and the sternocleidomastoid muscles. Contractions of these muscles cause a more forceful inspiration.

In summary, the regulation of ventilation by the medullary respiratory center determines the:

- Interval between the successive groups of action potentials of the inspiratory neurons, which determines the rate or *frequency of breathing* (as the interval shortens, the breathing rate increases)
- Frequency of action potential generation and the duration of this electrical activity to the motor neurons and, therefore, the muscles of inspiration and expiration, which determine the depth of breathing, or the *tidal volume* (as the frequency and duration of stimulation increases, the tidal volume increases)

The medullary respiratory center receives excitatory and inhibitory inputs from many areas of the brain and the peripheral nervous system including:

- Lung receptors
- Proprioceptors

- Pain receptors
- Limbic system
- Chemoreceptors

Pulmonary stretch receptors are responsible for initiating the *Hering-Breuer Reflex*. These stretch receptors are located within the smooth muscle of both large and small airways. They are stimulated when the tidal volume exceeds 1 L. Nerve impulses are transmitted by the vagus nerve to the medullary respiratory center and inhibit the inspiratory neurons. The primary function of these receptors and the *Hering-Breuer Reflex* is to prevent overinflation of the lungs.

Irritant receptors are located throughout the respiratory system in the nasal mucosa, the upper airways, the tracheobronchial tree and possibly the alveoli. Mechanical or chemical stimulation of these receptors can cause a reflex cough or sneeze. In either case, a deep inspiration is followed by a forced expiration against a closed glottis, which causes a marked increase in intrapulmonary pressure. The glottis then opens suddenly, resulting in an explosive expiration. The ensuing high airflow rate is meant to eliminate the irritant from the respiratory tract. In a cough, expiration occurs by way of the mouth, and in a sneeze, expiration is through the nose. Stimulation of irritant receptors also causes hyperpnea (increased ventilation) and bronchoconstriction.

Proprioceptors are located in muscles, tendons, and joints. Stimulation of these receptors causes an increase in ventilation. Proprioceptors are believed to play a role in initiating and maintaining the elevated ventilation associated with exercise.

Pain receptors also influence the medullary respiratory center. Pain may cause a reflex increase in ventilation in the form of a "gasp." Somatic pain typically causes hyperpnea and visceral pain typically causes apnea, or decreased ventilation.

Breathing is modified during the expression of various emotional states. For example, the normal cyclical pattern of breathing is interrupted during laughing, crying, sighing or moaning. The modifications in ventilation associated with these activities are elicited by input from the *limbic system* to the medullary respiratory center.

Chemoreceptors provide the most important input to the medullary respiratory center in terms of regulating ventilation to meet the metabolic requirements of the body. Chemoreceptors are sensitive to changes in PO_2, PCO_2 and pH. There are two types of chemoreceptors:

- Peripheral chemoreceptors
- Central chemoreceptors

The *peripheral chemoreceptors* include the carotid bodies and the aortic bodies. The *carotid bodies*, which are more important in humans, are located near the bifurcation of the common carotid arteries. The *aortic bodies* are found in the arch of the aorta. The peripheral chemoreceptors respond to a decrease in PO_2, an increase in PCO_2 and a decrease in pH (increase in H^+ ion concentration) in the arterial blood.

The *central chemoreceptors* are located near the ventral surface of the medulla, in close proximity to the respiratory center. These receptors are surrounded by the extracellular fluid (ECF) of the brain. They respond to changes in H^+ ion concentration. The composition of the ECF surrounding the central chemoreceptors is determined by the cerebrospinal fluid (CSF), local blood flow and local metabolism.

A summary of the responses of the peripheral and the central chemoreceptors to reduced arterial oxygen, increased arterial carbon dioxide and increased arterial hydrogen ion concentration is found in Table 8.4.

8.11.1   Chemoreceptor response to decreased arterial PO_2

Hypoxia has a direct depressant effect on the central chemoreceptors as well as the medullary respiratory center. In fact, hypoxia tends to inhibit activity in all regions of the brain. Therefore, the ventilatory response to hypoxemia is elicited only by the peripheral chemoreceptors.

A decrease in arterial PO_2 causes stimulation of the peripheral chemoreceptors. The ensuing elevation in ventilation increases the uptake of oxygen and returns PO_2 back to its normal value of 100 mmHg. However, this stimulatory effect does not occur until the arterial PO_2 falls below 60 mmHg. The physiological explanation for this delayed response to hypoxemia is provided by the shape of the oxyhemoglobin dissociation curve (see Figure 8.7). The plateau portion of the curve illustrates that hemoglobin remains quite saturated (90%) at a PO_2 of 60 mmHg. Therefore, when the PO_2 of the arterial blood is between 60 and 100 mmHg, the oxygen content of the blood is still very high. An increase in ventilation at this point is not critical. However, below a PO_2 of 60 mmHg, the saturation of hemoglobin and, therefore, the oxygen content of the blood decrease rapidly. Stimulation of the peripheral chemoreceptors, to increase ventilation and enhance the uptake of oxygen, is now essential to meet the metabolic needs of the body. Let it be clear, however, that this ventilatory response to hypoxemia is due to the change in PO_2, not oxygen content. For example,

Table 8.4   Chemoreceptor responses to changes in arterial PO_2, PCO_2, and H^+ ion concentration

Change in arterial blood	Effect on peripheral chemoreceptors	Effect on central chemoreceptors
↓ Arterial PO_2	Stimulates (PO_2 < 60 mmHg)	Depresses
↑ Arterial PCO_2	Weakly stimulates	Strongly stimulates
↑ Arterial H^+ ion	Stimulates	No effect

as discussed previously, anemia and carbon monoxide poisoning, which decrease oxygen content but not PO_2, do not cause an increase in ventilation.

It is important to note that a decrease in PO_2 is not the primary factor in the minute-to-minute regulation of ventilation. This is because the peripheral chemoreceptors are not stimulated until the PO_2 falls to life-threatening levels. A decrease of this magnitude would likely be associated with abnormal conditions, such as pulmonary disease, hypoventilation or ascent to extreme altitude.

8.11.2   *Chemoreceptor response to increased arterial PCO_2*

An increase in arterial PCO_2 causes weak stimulation of the peripheral chemoreceptors. The ensuing mild increase in ventilation contributes to the elimination of carbon dioxide and the decrease in PCO_2 back toward its normal value of 40 mmHg. The response of the peripheral chemoreceptors to changes in arterial PCO_2 is much less important than that of the central chemoreceptors. In fact, less than 20% of the ventilatory response to an increase in arterial PCO_2 is elicited by the peripheral chemoreceptors.

An increase in arterial PCO_2 results in the marked stimulation of the central chemoreceptors. In fact, this is the most important factor in the regulation of ventilation. As we are all aware, it is impossible to hold one's breath indefinitely. As the carbon dioxide accumulates in the arterial blood, the excitatory input to the respiratory center from the central chemoreceptors overrides the voluntary inhibitory input and breathing resumes. Furthermore, this occurs well before the arterial PO_2 falls low enough to stimulate the peripheral chemoreceptors.

Interestingly, the central chemoreceptors are insensitive to carbon dioxide itself. However, they are very sensitive to changes in the H^+ ion concentration in the ECF surrounding them. How does an increase in arterial PCO_2 cause an increase in H^+ ion concentration in the brain? Carbon dioxide readily crosses the blood-brain barrier. As the arterial PCO_2 increases, carbon dioxide diffuses down its concentration gradient into the ECF of the brain from the cerebral blood vessels. Due to the presence of the enzyme, CA, the following reaction takes place in the ECF of the brain:

$$CO_2 + H_2O \xleftrightarrow{\text{CA}} H_2CO_3 \leftrightarrow H^+ + HCO_3^-$$

CA facilitates the formation of carbonic acid (H_2CO_3) from carbon dioxide and water. The carbonic acid then dissociates to liberate hydrogen ion (H^+) and bicarbonate ion (HCO_3^-). The hydrogen ions strongly stimulate the central chemoreceptors to increase ventilation. The ensuing elimination of the excess carbon dioxide from the arterial blood returns the PCO_2 back to its normal value.

Conversely, a decrease in the arterial PCO_2 due to hyperventilation, results in a decrease in the H^+ ion concentration in the ECF of the brain. Decreased stimulation of the central chemoreceptors and, therefore, a decrease in the excitatory input to the medullary respiratory center, causes a decrease in ventilation. Continued metabolism allows the carbon dioxide to accumulate in the blood such that the PCO_2 returns to its normal value.

8.11.2.1   *Chemoreceptor response to increased arterial hydrogen ion concentration*

An increase in arterial hydrogen ion concentration, or a decrease in arterial pH, stimulates the peripheral chemoreceptors and enhances ventilation. This response is important in maintaining acid-base balance. For example, under conditions of *metabolic acidosis,* caused by the accumulation of acids in the blood, the enhanced ventilation eliminates carbon dioxide and, thereby, reduces the concentration of the H^+ ions in the blood. Metabolic acidosis may occur in patients with uncontrolled diabetes mellitus or when tissues become hypoxic and produce lactic acid.

An increase in arterial hydrogen ion concentration has no effect on the central chemoreceptors. Hydrogen ions are unable to cross the blood-brain barrier.

8.12   *Ventilatory response to exercise*

Exercise results in an increase in oxygen consumption and an increase in carbon dioxide production by the working muscles. To meet the metabolic demands of these tissues, ventilation increases accordingly. Minute ventilation increases linearly in response to oxygen consumption and carbon dioxide production up to the level of approximately 60% of an individual's work capacity. During this period of mild-to-moderate exercise, mean arterial PO_2 and PCO_2 remain relatively constant at their normal values. In fact, the partial pressures of these gases may even improve (arterial PO_2 is increased, arterial PCO_2 is decreased). Therefore, it does not appear that hypoxic or hypercapnic stimulation of the peripheral chemoreceptors plays a role in the ventilatory response to mild-to-moderate exercise.

Beyond this point, during more severe exercise associated with anaerobic metabolism, the minute ventilation increases faster than the rate of oxygen consumption, but proportionally to the increase in carbon dioxide production. The mechanism of the ventilatory response to severe exercise involves the *metabolic acidosis* caused by anaerobic metabolism. The lactic acid produced under these conditions liberates H^+ ions, which effectively stimulate the peripheral chemoreceptors to increase ventilation.

During exercise, the increase in minute ventilation results from increases in both tidal volume and breathing frequency. Initially, the increase in tidal volume is greater than the increase in breathing frequency. As discussed earlier in this chapter, increases in tidal volume increase alveolar ventilation more effectively. Subsequently, however, as metabolic acidosis develops, the increase in breathing frequency predominates.

The mechanisms involved with the ventilatory response to exercise remain quite unclear. No single factor, or combination of factors, can fully account for the increase in ventilation during exercise. Therefore, much of this response remains unexplained. Factors that appear to play a role include the following:

- Impulses from the cerebral cortex
- Impulses from proprioceptors
- Body temperature
- Epinephrine

At the beginning of exercise, there is an immediate increase in ventilation. This increase is thought to be caused by two mechanisms involving the cerebral cortex. Neurons of the primary motor cortex stimulate alpha motor neurons in the spinal cord to cause skeletal muscle contraction. In addition, *impulses from the motor cortex*, transmitted through collateral interconnections to the medullary respiratory center, stimulate ventilation. The motor cortex is also involved in the stimulation of the cardiovascular system during exercise. These adjustments, which occur before any homeostatic factors (e.g., blood gases) have changed, are referred to as *anticipatory adjustments*. The immediate increase in ventilation may account for as much as 50% of the total ventilatory response to exercise. A *conditioned reflex*, or a learned response to exercise, may also be involved. Once again, impulses from the cerebral cortex provide input to the medullary respiratory center.

Proprioceptors originating in muscles and joints of the exercising limbs provide substantial input to the medullary respiratory center. In fact, even passive movement of the limbs causes an increase in ventilation. Therefore, the mechanical aspects of exercise also contribute to the ventilatory response.

The increased metabolism associated with exercise increases *body temperature*. The increase in body temperature further contributes to the increase in ventilation during exercise. (Not surprisingly, ventilation is also enhanced in response to a fever.)

Exercise is associated with a mass sympathetic discharge and *epinephrine*, which is believed to stimulate ventilation, release from the adrenal medulla is markedly increased.

8.13   *Disorders of the respiratory system*

Respiratory disease and illness is a major cause of mortality and morbidity in the United States. Respiratory structures such as the airways, alveoli and pleural membranes may all be affected by various disease processes. These respiratory diseases include infections such as pneumonia and tuberculosis, as well as *obstructive* disorders such as asthma, bronchitis, and emphysema that obstruct airflow into and out of the lungs. Other conditions such as pneumothorax, atelectasis, respiratory distress syndrome and cystic fibrosis are classified as *restrictive* disorders because they limit normal expansion of the lungs. Pulmonary function may also be affected by exposure to inhaled particles or by the growth of cancers. General symptoms of respiratory disease are listed in Table 8.5.

Table 8.5   General symptoms of respiratory disease

- *Cough*—acute or chronic
- *Hypoxia*—decreased levels of oxygen in the tissues
- *Hypoxemia*—decreased levels of oxygen in arterial blood
- *Hypercapnia*—increased levels of CO_2 in the blood
- *Hypocapnia*—decreased levels of CO_2 in the blood
- *Clubbing*—of distal fingers or toes can occur with conditions of low oxygenation
- *Dyspnea*—difficulty breathing
- *Tachypnea*—rapid rate of breathing
- *Cyanosis*—bluish discoloration of skin and mucus membranes due to poor oxygenation of the blood
- *Hemoptysis*—blood in the sputum
- *Pain*—pleural pain from infection or inflammation; chest wall or rib pain from cough

8.13.1   Respiratory infections

Infections of the respiratory tract can occur in the upper or lower respiratory tract or both. Organisms capable of infecting respiratory structures include bacteria, viruses, and fungi. The manifestations of respiratory infections can range from mild to severe and even life threatening, depending upon the organism involved and extent of infection. A healthy respiratory tract has a number of defenses that are designed to protect against infectious organisms (see Table 8.6). Cigarette smoking and airway inflammation can impair these protective mechanisms and allow infectious organisms to reach the bronchi and lungs where they can cause pneumonia. The presence of an upper respiratory tract infection can likewise predispose a patient to a lower respiratory tract infection.

8.13.1.1   Infections of the upper respiratory tract

8.13.1.1.1   The common cold and rhinosinusitis   The majority of upper respiratory tract infections are caused by viruses. The most common viral pathogens for the "common cold" are *rhinovirus, parainfluenza virus, respiratory syncytial virus, adenovirus, and coronavirus.* Common cold viruses replicate best in the cooler tissues of the upper airways. These viruses tend to have seasonal

Table 8.6   Defenses of the respiratory system

1. Moist, mucus-covered surfaces—trap particles and organisms
2. IgA, lysosomes found on respiratory surfaces
3. Ciliated Epithelium—clears trapped particles and organisms from airway passages
4. Cough Reflex and Epiglottis—prevents aspiration of particles and irritants into lower airways
5. Pulmonary Macrophages—phagocytize foreign particles and organisms in the alveolar spaces

variations in their peak incidence. They are readily spread from person to person via respiratory secretions, and gain entry to the body through the nasal mucosa, and surfaces of the eye. Common colds are normally self-limiting with symptoms generally lasting less than 1 week. Rhinosinusitis is inflammation of the nasal passages and sinuses. It may be caused by viral or bacterial (most commonly *H. influenza*, *S. pneumoniae*). Treatment of rhinosinusitis is mainly symptomatic, but antibiotics may be indicated with serious bacterial infections.

8.13.1.1.1.1 *Manifestations of the common cold and rhinosinusitis*

- *Rhinitis*—inflammation of the nasal mucosa
- *Sinusitis*—inflammation of the sinus mucosa
- *Pharyngitis*—inflammation of the pharynx and throat
- Headache
- Nasal discharge and congestion
- Common cold viruses are also a leading source of ear infections (*otitis media*) in children

8.13.1.1.2 *Influenza*

Influenza is one of the most significant human respiratory infections. It is caused by viruses that belong to the *Orthomyxoviridae* family. Three distinct forms of Influenza virus have been identified, A, B and C. Of these three variants, type A is the most common and causes the most serious illness in humans. Two identifying proteins on the surface of the virus, namely hemagglutinin (H) and neuraminidase (N), are also used to further subtype influenza viruses (see Figure 8.10). The hemagglutinin protein is used by the flu virus to attach to cells of the respiratory epithelium, whereas the neuraminidase protein acts as an enzyme that facilitates budding of new flu viruses from host cells. The influenza virus is a highly transmissible respiratory pathogen. The incubation period for influenza infection is typically 1–4 days. Influenza viruses are RNA viruses with "segmented" genomes, meaning that the RNA is found in multiple fragments instead on one long unit. A segmented genome may contribute to high rates of genetic diversity by facilitating the exchange of genetic information across the various segments of RNA. Because the organism has a high tendency for genetic mutation, new variants of the virus are constantly arising in different places around the world. Influenza viruses undergo a gradual process of minor genetic changes over time termed *antigenic* drift. Over the course of years, the accumulated effect of these minor genetic changes eventually result in an influenza virus that has undergone so many antigenic changes that it essentially becomes a new strain of flu virus. At this point an *antigenic shift* is said to have occurred. Historically, serious *pandemics* of influenza were generally seen every 8–10 years as a result of these antigenic shifts. Although most cases of influenza in healthy adults are self-limiting, the incidence of serious illness mortality rates from influenza is significantly higher in elderly patients and children.

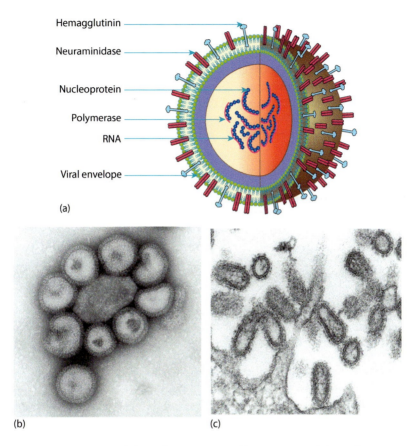

Hemagglutinin
Neuraminidase
Nucleoprotein
Polymerase
RNA
Viral envelope

(a)

(b)   (c)

Figure 8.10 Structure of the influenza virus. (a) Structure of the influenza virus; (b) negative-stained transmission electron micrograph (TEM) of influenza viral particle; TEM of 1918 influenza pandemic virus virons. (Adapted from *Porth's Pathophysiology: Concepts of Altered Health States* by Grossman, Lippincott Williams and Wilkins, 2013.)

8.13.1.1.2.1 Symptoms of influenza infection
- Headache
- Fever, chills, malaise
- Muscle aches
- Nasal discharge
- Unproductive cough
- Rhinotracheitis—inflammation of the nose and throat

Influenza infection can cause marked inflammation of the respiratory epithelium leading to acute tissue damage and a loss of ciliated cells that protect the respiratory passages from other organisms. As a result, influenza infection may predispose the respiratory passages to infection by bacteria. It is also possible for the influenza virus to infect the tissues of the lower respiratory passages (*influenza* pneumonia) in susceptible individuals. Influenza pneumonia is most likely to occur in elderly patients and those who are immunocompromised. It can progress rapidly and lead to tachypnea, hypotension, hypoxemia and death.

8.13.1.1.2.2   Treatment of influenza

- Bed rest, fluids
- Analgesics, cough medicine
- Keeping the patient warm can help
- Antiviral drugs (see Table 8.7)
- Influenza vaccine—provides protection against certain A and B influenza strains that are expected to be prevalent in a certain year. The vaccine must be updated and administered yearly to be effective. The influenza vaccine is particularly indicated in the elderly, individuals weakened by other disease and health care workers.

8.13.1.2   Infections of the lower respiratory tract

The respiratory tract is protected by a number of very effective defense mechanisms designed to keep infectious organisms and particulates from reaching the lungs (see Table 8.6). In order for an organism to reach the lower respiratory tract the organism must be particularly virulent, present in very large number or there is a weakening of the host defense barriers. One factor that might weaken the respiratory defense barriers is cigarette smoking, which can paralyze the cilia lining the cells of the respiratory passages, and impair removal of secretions, particles and microorganisms. The presence of a respiratory pathogen such as the cold or influenza virus may also cause an inflammatory reaction that impairs the defense barriers of the respiratory passages and open an individual up to infection by other respiratory pathogens.

Table 8.7   Drugs for treating influenza

Amantadine, Rimantadine:
- Used orally or by aerosol administration
- Effective only against type A influenza
- Inhibits viral uncoating in infected host cells
- High rates of resistance have developed to these agents, their use is not recommended

Neuraminidase Inhibitors (Zanamavir, Oseltamivir):
- Can be used by inhalation (Zanamavir) or orally (Oseltamivir)
- Effective against both types A and B influenza
- Inhibits the activity of viral *neuraminidase* enzyme that is necessary for the budding and spread of the newly made influenza viruses

8.13.1.2.1   Pneumonia   Pneumonia is a condition that involves inflammation of lower lung structures such as the alveoli or interstitial spaces. It may be caused by bacteria, viruses, protozoa or by fungi such as *Pneumocystis jiroveci*. Despite advances in drug therapy, pneumonia is still the sixth leading cause of death in the United States. The prevalence and severity of pneumonia has been heightened in recent years due to the emergence of HIV as well as antibiotic resistance. A number of specific patient populations are at increased risk for developing pneumonia (see Table 8.8). Pneumonia may be classified according to the pathogen that is responsible for the infection. There tend to be distinct organisms that cause pneumonia in the hospital setting versus the community setting.

8.13.1.2.1.1   Classification of pneumonia
Hospital or Healthcare Acquired (nosocomial)
- Infection occurs in a hospital, clinical setting or nursing home
- Most commonly enteric gram-negative organisms (*Escherichia coli, Pseudomonas aeruginosa, Staphlococcus aureus*)

Community Acquired
- Infection occurs in a community setting such as the workplace or school
- Common organisms include *Streptococcus pneumoniae, Haemophilus pneumoniae,* and *mycoplasma pneumoniae* as well as the *influenza viruses*

A second classification scheme for pneumonia is based upon the specific organisms that are infecting the lungs and includes *typical* and *atypical* pneumonia.

Typical Pneumonia
- Usually bacterial in origin and may include organisms such as:
  - *S. pneumoniae*—gram-positive aerobic bacteria
  - *Legionella   pneumophilia*—gram-negative   rod   responsible   for Legionnaires disease
- Organisms are replicating in the spaces of the alveoli

Table 8.8   Individuals most at risk for pneumonia

- Elderly
- Those with viral infection
- Chronically ill
- Immunosuppressed patients
- Smokers
- Patients with cardiopulmonary disease or chronic respiratory disease

Manifestations of Typical Pneumonia
- Inflammation and fluid accumulation is seen in the alveoli
- White blood cell infiltration and exudation that can been seen on chest X-ray
- Manifests with high fever, chest pain, chills, malaise
- Purulent sputum, may be bloody or rust colored
- Pleuritic pain with inspiration
- Varying degrees of hypoxemia may be present

Atypical Pneumonia
- May be caused by organisms such as *Mycoplasma pneumoniae* and viruses such as the influenza viruses and the respiratory syncytial virus
- Organisms are replicating in the spaces around the alveoli including the alveolar septum and interstitum

Manifestations of Atypical Pneumonia
- Generally milder symptoms than typical pneumonia
- Lack of white blood cell infiltration in alveoli
- Lack of fluid accumulation in the alveoli, no purulent sputum
- Generally less effects on alveolar gas exchange
- Not usually evident on X-ray
- The presence of atypical pneumonia may make the patient susceptible to bacterial (typical) pneumonia

8.13.1.2.1.2   *Pneumonia in immunocompromised patients*   A variety of organisms can cause severe respiratory infections and pneumonia in patients who are immunocompromised. A number of these organisms are opportunistic and not typically associated with respiratory disease in healthy, immunocompetent individuals. These organisms include:

- Bacteria—*Mycobacterium tuberculosis, Mycobacterium avium*
- Fungi—*Pneumocystis jirovecii, Aspergillus fumigatus, Histoplasma capsulatum, Candida*
- Viruses—Cytomegalovirus, influenza, herpes Simplex virus, varicella-zoster virus

Pneumonia in immunocompromised individuals can be particularly dangerous given the weakened immune status of the host and the virulent nature of many of these organisms.

8.13.1.2.1.3   Treatment of pneumonia

- Appropriate antibiotics if bacterial in origin. The health care provider should consider the possibility of antibiotic-resistant organisms being present. Growing rates of antibiotic resistance are a major concern with *S. pneumoniae*. The presence of bacteria should be confirmed to avoid unnecessary use of antibiotics.
- Supportive therapy
- A vaccine for *pneumococcal* pneumonia is currently available and highly effective. This vaccine is recommended for children over 5 years of age and adults over 65 years of age.

8.13.1.2.2   Tuberculosis   Tuberculosis (TB) is an infectious disease caused by the organism *Mycobacterium tuberculosis*. According to the World Health Organization (WHO) in 2013, 9 million people fell ill with TB and 1.5 million died from the disease. TB is second only to HIV/AIDS as the greatest killer worldwide due to a single infectious agent. Over 95% of TB deaths occur in low- and middle-income countries, and it is among the top 5 causes of death for women 15–44 years of age.

Unlike most other bacteria, *M. tuberculosis* is surrounded by an outer capsule that makes the organism very resistant to destruction. *M. tuberculosis* is primarily transmitted via the airborne route through respiratory aspirates and secretions. Being an aerobic organism, the tuberculosis mycobacterium prefers to replicate in the oxygen-rich tissues of the lungs. Once in the lung tissues, the organism causes an extensive inflammatory reaction as it is attacked first by polymorphonuclear leukocytes and later by macrophages. The primary inflammatory lesion that forms in the lungs from tuberculosis infection is called a *Ghon focus*. If the lesion also spreads to involve regional lymph nodes it is now termed a *Ghon's complex* (see Figure 8.11). Necrosis of infected lung tissues may result in a cheesy appearance to the tissue that is referred to as a *caseous necrosis*. *Liquefecation* of the necrotic lesions might also occur over time.

In an otherwise healthy individual, the immune system is usually able to contain the organism and over time will encapsulate it through *calcification* of the lesions. These calcified Ghon's complexes are readily visualized by chest X-ray for the remainder of the patient's life (see Table 8.9). Because live *M. tuberculosis* are often found within these encapsulations, impairment of immune function in the infected individual may lead to *reactivation* of the primary infection.

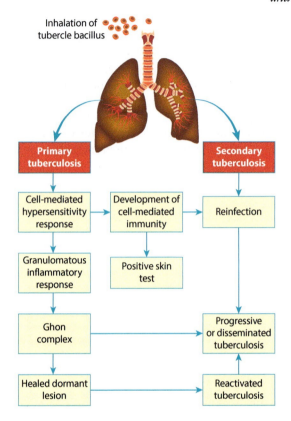

Figure 8.11 Primary and secondary tuberculosis. (Adapted from *Porth's Pathophysiology: Concepts of Altered Health States* by Grossman, Lippincott Williams and Wilkins, 2013.)

Table 8.9   Testing for tuberculosis

- Mantoux Test—skin test for reaction against the tuberculin purified protein derivative standard (PPDS)
- Acid-fast staining of sputum cultures to visualize *M. tuberculosis*
- Chest radiograph to identify Ghon's complex

8.13.1.2.2.1   Manifestations of primary tuberculosis
- Productive, prolonged cough
- Chest pain, *hemoptysis*
- Chill, fever, night sweats
- Anorexia, weight loss

8.13.1.2.2.2   Treatment of tuberculosis   Although a number of potential vaccines against tuberculosis are undergoing clinical testing, an effective vaccine is not currently available in the United States. Management of tuberculosis often requires prolonged treatment with powerful antimyco-bacterial drugs such as isoniazid, rifampin, and ethambutol. Unfortunately in recent years, the treatment of tuberculosis has been complicated by the rise of TB organisms that are resistant to one or more of the commonly used anti-tubercular agents. According to the WHO, globally in 2013, an estimated 480,000 people developed multidrug-resistant TB (MDR-TB). In cases of MDR-TB, mortality can be on the order of 70%–90%. Factors that affect immune function such as proper nutrition and management of other diseases are also essential for successful treatment of tuberculosis.

QUESTION...

What are some factors that might contribute to tuberculosis drug resistance?

8.13.2   Cancers of the respiratory tract

8.13.2.1   Laryngeal cancer

- Accounts for approximately 2%–3% of all cancers
- Incidence is increased with smoking and particularly in smokers who also consume alcohol
- Squamous cell carcinomas are most common
- Symptoms may include hoarseness, cough and pain with swallowing
- Outcomes depend upon timing of detection

8.13.2.2   Lung cancer

- Lung cancer is the most common cancer worldwide, accounting for 1.8 million new cases and 1.6 million deaths in 2012 (CDC 2015). Lung cancer is the leading cancer killer in both men and women in the United States (American Cancer Society 2015). An estimated 158,040 Americans are expected to die from lung cancer in 2015
- The vast majority of lung cancers are carcinomas of lung tissue. There are two main types of lung cancers, *non-small cell and small cell:*

1. *Non-Small Cell Lung Cancer:*
   - 85% of all lung cancers
   - Includes *adenocarcinoma, squamous cell carcinoma, and large cell carcinoma:*
     - *Adenocarcinoma*—40% of lung cancers. Arises from secretory cells such as those that produce respiratory mucus. Occurs mainly in former or current smokers, but may occur in nonsmokers. More common in women than men. It tends to be slower growing than other forms of lung cancer

- *Squamous Cell Carcinoma*—25%–30% of all lung cancers. Epidermal in origin. Strong association with smoking history and as a result they tend to arise near bronchi
- *Large Cell Lung Carcinoma*—10%–15% of all lung cancers. Highly undifferentiated cells that grow and spread quickly

2. *Small Cell Lung Cancer:*
   - 10%–15% of all lung cancers
   - May arise from neuroendocrine cells in the bronchi
   - Strongest association with smoking
   - Highly aggressive cancer cells that spread rapidly and early in the course of the disease

8.13.2.2.1   Manifestations of lung cancer

- Localized lung effects may include dyspnea, cough and wheezing. Bloody sputum (hemoptysis) may occur along with a dull, nonlocalized pain
- Systemic symptoms may occur as the cancer grows and metastasizes. These symptoms may include anorexia, weight loss, and fatigue
- *Paraneoplastic syndrome*—a complex set of physiologic effects caused by substances produced by growing cancer cells. Substances produced by tumor cells may include hormones such as ACTH, ADH that can lead to *Cushing syndrome* or the syndrome of inappropriate antidiuretic hormone secretion (*SIADH*). Tumor cells may also produce antigenic substances that can trigger and antibody attack on the nervous system and lead to a variety of neurologic symptoms. The presence of a paraneoplastic syndrome often precedes the detection of cancer by a number of months.

8.13.2.2.2   Treatment of lung cancer   Diagnosis of lung cancer may be made through chest X-ray, CT scanning, PET scanning, bronchoscopy or biopsy. Once the presence of a lung cancer is verified it is "staged" using the TNM system where T represents the size of the primary tumor, N represents the extent of lymph node involvement, and M represents the presence or absence of metastasis. Primary therapy for lung cancer includes chemotherapy, and radiation. Targeted therapies based on the physical, metabolic and genetic characteristics of specific types of lung cancer cells have shown significant promise. Such targeted therapies include drugs that inhibit angiogenesis, block growth factor receptors, and antagonize proteins involved in cancer cells growth and spread.

8.13.3   Obstructive and restrictive pulmonary disorders

Obstructive pulmonary disorders are those that are associated with obstruction of the airways and include asthma, chronic bronchitis, and emphysema. *Restrictive* pulmonary disorders are those that reduce or impair lung compliance (the ability of the lung tissues to stretch) and include atelectasis, pulmonary fibrosis, pulmonary edema, and acute respiratory distress syndrome (ARDS).

8.13.4 Obstructive pulmonary disorders

8.13.4.1 Asthma

The incidence of asthma has been steadily increasing in recent years. Approximately 259 million American suffer from asthma. Nearly 7.1 million asthma sufferers are under the age of 18. Asthma accounts for nearly 2 million emergency room visits each year and costs $56 billion dollars annually. A key component of the asthmatic response is airway "hyperreactivity." In susceptible individuals, exposure to certain "triggers" (see Table 8.10) can induce marked bronchospasm and airway inflammation in susceptible patients. Patients who respond to asthma triggers likely have an underlying genetic susceptibility to these triggers. A number of asthma-related genes have been identified in patients who exhibit airway hyperactivity when exposed to asthma triggers. Although the function of these genes is not clear, they appear to be involved in mast cell degranulation, cytokine production, antigenic recognition, mucus production, and protection of the respiratory epithelium (WHO 2015).

Asthma may be classified as *atopic* or *intrinsic*. Atopic asthma is caused by extrinsic or allergic factors and is the most common form of asthma. In contrast, intrinsic asthma is caused by factors such as cold air, exercise, drugs, and strong emotions.

8.13.4.1.1 Atopic asthma Atopic asthma occurs as a result of exposure to an exogenous allergen or antigen. Individuals with atopic asthma produce large amounts of the IgE antibody that attaches to *mast cells* that are present in many tissues. With subsequent exposure, the atopic trigger binds to IgE on the surface of mast cells that in turn causes their degranulation and the release of inflammatory mediators such as *histamine, leukotrienes,* and *eosinophilic chemotactic factor.* The response of a certain Helper-T cell subset (T_2H) appears to be upregulated in patients with asthma. This particular subset of Helper T-cells is responsible for stimulating the differentiation of activated B-lymphocytes (B-cells) into IgE-producing plasma cells instead of IgG and IgM producing plasma cells. The reason for an increased expression of the T_2H subset of Helper T-cells in asthmatic patients is unclear (Figure 8.12).

Table 8.10 Asthma triggers

Atopic triggers
Allergens—pollen, pet dander, fungi, dust mites
Pollutants
Cigarette smoke

Intrinsic triggers
Cold air
Strong emotions
Exercise
Respiratory tract infections

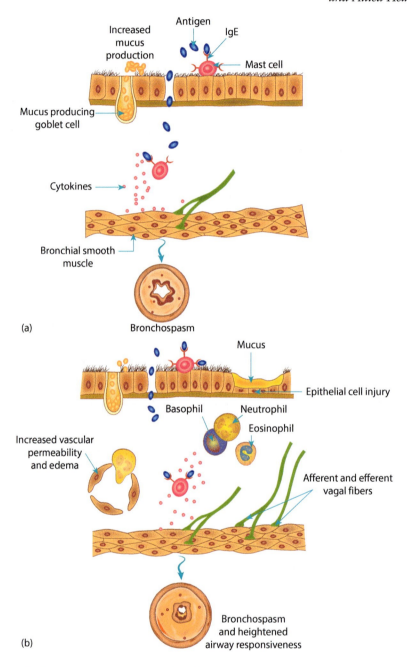

Figure 8.12   Airway changes associated with respiratory disease. (a) Early phase of asthma; (b) Late phase of asthma. (Adapted from *Porth's Pathophysiology: Concepts of Altered Health States* by Grossman, Lippincott Williams and Wilkins, 2013.)

QUESTION?

What are some of the factors that might be responsible for the increased occur-rence of asthma in recent years?

The typical response of a patient with atopic asthma can be divided into an "early" phase and a "late phase."

1. *Early Phase of Asthma*
   Occurs rapidly (less than 30 min) after exposure to an asthmatic trig-ger. The early phase of asthma is characterized by marked constriction and spasm of bronchial airways that is accompanied by airway edema and the production of excess mucus. Activation of parasympathetic nervous system may also occur and can exacerbate bronchospasm and further increase mucus production.

2. *Late Phase of Asthma*
   The late phase of asthma can occur several hours after the initial onset of symptoms and manifests mainly as an inflammatory response. Infiltration of immune cells such as neutrophils, eosinophils and baso-phils further enhance the inflammatory response. Cytokines such as tumor necrosis factor (TNF-α) and interleukins (IL-4, -5, and -13) have also been shown to play an important role in the airway inflammation associated with atopic asthma.

   8.13.4.1.2   Manifestations of asthma
   - Coughing, wheezing
   - Difficulty breathing
   - Rapid, shallow breathing
   - Increased respiratory rate
   - Excess mucus production
   - Barrel chest due to trapping of air in the lungs
   - Significant anxiety

   8.13.4.1.3   Complications of asthma   The chronic inflammation of the airways that can accompany persistent asthma attacks may result in remodeling of the airways. Remodeling changes may be irreversible and include fibrosis, neovascularization, smooth muscle hypertrophy and epithelial changes. Such remodeling can lead to a thickening of the airways that further impairs the flow of air. Possible complications of asthma can also include the occurrence of *status asthmaticus*, which is a life-threatening condition of prolonged bronchospasm that is often not responsive to drug therapy. *Pneumothorax* is also a possible consequence as a result of lung pressure increases that can result from the extreme difficulty involved in expiration during a prolonged asthma attack. Marked hypoxemia and acidosis might also occur and can result in overall respiratory failure.

8.13.4.1.4 Treatment of asthma The appropriate drug treatment regimen for asthma is based upon the frequency and severity of the asthma attacks (see Tables 8.11 and 8.12) and may include:

- Avoidance of triggers, and allergens. Improved ventilation of the living spaces, use of air conditioning.
- *Bronchodilators* (e.g., albuterol, terbutaline)—short acting or long acting *beta-adrenergic* receptor activators. May be administered as needed in the form of a nebulizer solution using a metered dispenser or they may be given subcutaneously. These drugs block bronchoconstriction but do not prevent the inflammatory

Table 8.11 Clinical classification of asthma

- Mild intermittent—attacks occur two times per week or less
- Mild persistent—attacks occur more than two times per week
- Moderate persistent—attacks that occur daily or almost daily and are severe enough to effect activity
- Severe persistent—attacks are very frequent and persist for a long period of time. Attacks severely limit activity

Table 8.12 Staging of the severity of an acute asthma attack

Stage I (mild):
- Mild dyspnea
- Diffuse wheezing
- Adequate air exchange

Stage II (moderate):
- Respiratory distress at rest
- Marked wheezing

Stage III (severe):
- Marked respiratory distress
- Cyanosis
- Marked wheezing or absence of breath sounds

Stage IV (respiratory failure):
- Severe respiratory distress, lethargy, confusion, prominent pulsus paradoxus

response. Long-acting beta agonists should always be given in conjunction with an inhaled corticosteroid

- *Xanthine drugs* (e.g., Theophylline)—cause bronchodilation but may also inhibit the late phase of asthma. These drugs are often used orally as second line agents in combination with other asthma therapies such as steroids. Drugs such as theophylline can have significant central nervous system, cardiovascular and gastrointestinal side effects that limit their overall usefulness.
- *Anti-inflammatory drugs* (corticosteroids)—current mainstays for asthma therapy. Used orally or by inhalation to blunt the inflammatory response of asthma. Inhaled corticosteroids have significantly less risk for serious side effects. The most significant unwanted effects occur with long-term oral use of corticosteroids and may include immunosuppression, increased susceptibility to infection, osteoporosis, and effects on other hormones such as the glucocorticoids.
- *Cromolyn sodium*—anti-inflammatory agent that blocks both the early and late phase of asthma. The mechanism of action is unclear but may involve mast cell function or responsiveness to allergens.
- *Leukotriene modifiers* (e.g., Zafirlukast)—new class of agents that blocks the synthesis of the key inflammatory mediators leukotrienes.

8.13.5   Chronic obstructive pulmonary disease (COPD)

The WHO defines COPD as lung disease characterized by chronic obstruction of lung airflow that interferes with normal breathing and is not fully reversible. COPD includes both chronic bronchitis and emphysema.

8.13.5.1   Bronchitis
Bronchitis refers to a condition in which there is inflammation of the bronchial passages. Bronchitis may occur in both acute and chronic forms.

1. *Acute Bronchitis*: Inflammation of the bronchial passages most commonly caused by infection with bacteria or viruses. Acute bronchitis is generally a self-limiting condition in healthy individuals but can have much more severe consequences in individuals who are weakened with other illness or who are immunocompromised. Symptoms of acute bronchitis often include productive cough, dyspnea, and possible fever.
2. *Chronic Bronchitis*: Chronic bronchitis is an obstructive pulmonary disease that is most frequently associated with chronic cigarette smoking (approximately 90% of cases). Chronic bronchitis may

also be caused by prolonged exposure to inhaled particulates such as coal dust or other pollutants. The disease is characterized by chronic inflammation of the airways and excess mucus production in the lower respiratory tract. This mucus accumulation can impair function of the ciliated epithelium and lining the respiratory tract and prevent the clearing out of debris and organisms. As a result, patients with chronic bronchitis often suffer repeated bouts of respiratory infection.

8.13.5.1.1 Manifestations of chronic bronchitis (see Figure 8.12)
- Chronic inflammation of bronchial passages
- Productive, chronic cough
- Production of excessive respiratory mucus
- Purulent sputum; frequent respiratory infections
- Hypertrophy of bronchial smooth muscle
- Airway obstruction, dyspnea—markedly reduced FEV
- Hypoxia, hypoxemia, cyanosis—may lead to a compensatory *polycythemia*
- Air trapping due to mucus plugs and hypertrophied airway smooth muscle
- *Cor pulmonale*—symptoms of right heart failure caused by pulmonary disease. Increased resistance to pulmonary blood flow can increase workload on the right heart and cause symptoms of right-side heart failure such as peripheral edema and venous congestion

8.13.5.1.2 Treatment of chronic bronchitis
- Cessation of smoking or exposure to irritants
- Bronchodilators to open airway passages
- Expectorants to loosen mucus
- Anti-inflammatories to relieve airway inflammation and reduce mucus secretion
- Prophylactic antibiotics for respiratory infections
- Oxygen therapy

8.13.5.2 Emphysema
Emphysema is a respiratory disease that is characterized by destruction and permanent dilation of the terminal bronchioles and alveolar air sacs (see Figure 8.13). The vast majority (>95%) of all patients with emphysema were chronic cigarette smokers. Although the exact etiology of emphysema is complex and multifactorial, it appears that chronic exposure to cigarette smoke causes chronic inflammation of the alveolar airways that results in infiltration by lymphocytes and

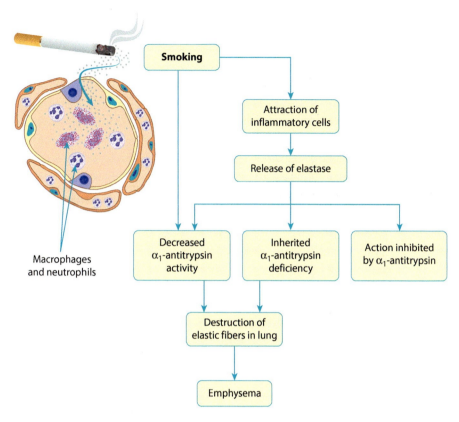

Figure 8.13 Structural changes in the alveolar sacs with emphysema. (Adapted from *Porth's Pathophysiology: Concepts of Altered Health States* by Grossman, Lippincott Williams and Wilkins, 2013.)

macrophages. Excess release of inflammatory cytokines and protease enzymes (such as trypsin) from immune cells can damage and destroy the elastic proteins (i.e., *elastin*) that are found in walls of the alveoli. As a result, alveolar air sacs become enlarged and distended as their structure is affected and their elasticity lost. Levels of the protective anti-protease enzyme α_1-*antitrypsin* are also decreased over time in individuals who are chronic cigarette smokers. The endogenous α_1-antitrypsin enzyme inactivates destructive protease enzymes in lung tissue. A rare form of genetic emphysema occurs in individuals who are not cigarette smokers but who do have a defect in the gene that produces α_1-antitrypsin.

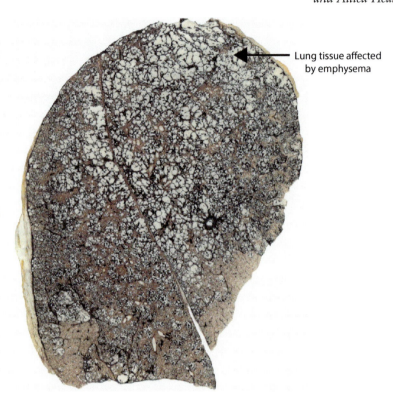

Lung tissue affected by emphysema

The presentation of emphysema may be *centriacinar* or *panacinar* (see Figure 8.14). With centriacinar emphysema the destruction of the alveolar walls occurs mainly in the respiratory bronchioles and regions of the alveoli in closest proximity to the airways. This form of emphysema is most common in cigarette smokers because these areas of the respiratory passages and alveoli receive the highest concentrations of cigarette smoke. In contrast, panacinar emphysema involves destruction of the alveolar walls throughout alveolar clusters. Panacinar emphysema is typically seen in patients with emphysema caused by a genetic lack of α_1-antitrypsin.

8.13.5.2.1 Manifestations of emphysema The major physiologic changes seen in emphysema are a loss of alveolar elasticity and a decrease in the overall surface area for gas exchange within the lungs. Note that chronic bronchitis and emphysema are a continuum of disease processes effecting both the airways and alveoli. As a result many long-term smokers may exhibit symptoms of both chronic bronchitis and emphysema at the same time.

Manifestations may include:

- Tachypnea with prolonged expirations. Because a compensatory increase in respiratory rate in patients with emphysema is often

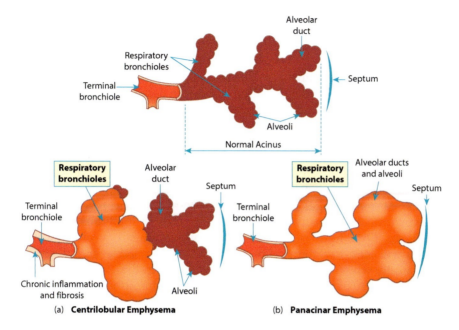

Figure 8.14   Types of emphysema. (a) Centrilobular; (b) Panacinar. (Adapted from *Porth's Pathophysiology: Concepts of Altered Health States* by Grossman, Lippincott Williams and Wilkins, 2013.)

effective in maintaining arterial blood gases, one does not usually see hypoxia or cyanosis until the end stages of the disease. Patients with emphysema often exhale through "pursed lips," which increases the resistance to expired air and generates a backpressure that helps keep the airways inflated. Patients may also sit in a "tripod" posture to enhance the efficiency of the respiratory muscles (see Table 8.13)

- Dyspnea may occur at rest, worsened with exertion
- Barrel chest from prolonged expiration and air trapping
- Decreased breath sounds

Table 8.13   Comparison of symptoms for chronic bronchitis and emphysema

Chronic bronchitis	Emphysema
• Mild dyspnea possible	• Dyspnea is common
• Productive cough with purulent sputum	• Barrel chest
• Frequent respiratory infections	• Tachypnea
• Cyanosis is common	• Decreased breath sounds
• Polycythemia	• Cyanosis is rare
• Cor pulmonale	

8.13.6   Cystic fibrosis

Cystic fibrosis is a genetic disorder that affects function of exocrine glands of the respiratory, gastrointestinal and reproductive tracts. Approximately 30,000 American are currently living with cystic fibrosis. The disease is more prevalent in whites of Northern European descent. The disorder is an autosomal recessive condition caused mutations in a single gene on chromosome 7. The defective gene codes for a protein called the *cystic fibrosis transmembrane conductance regulator protein* (*CFTCR*). This protein is a cAMP-regulated chloride channel found in secretory cells that line the airways, pancreas, and reproductive tract. Abnormal activity of this protein results in the production of overly thick mucus that cannot be cleared from the respiratory passages and accumulates to form *mucus plugs*. The accumulated mucus also becomes a breeding ground for numerous respiratory pathogens. Over time, chronic infection and inflammation of respiratory tissues will lead to deterioration of lung function and eventual respiratory failure, which is the leading cause of death in these patients. Excess mucus may also be produced by cells of the gastrointestinal tract leading to possible gastrointestinal blockage and impairment of digestion. Exocrine function of the pancreas is also affected by this disorder and can result in impaired digestion of nutrients as well as possible destruction of the pancreas. Homozygous patients present with marked clinical symptoms, whereas those who are heterozygous are carriers of the disease often present with mild symptoms (although some may not present with clinical symptoms at all).

8.13.6.1   Manifestations of cystic fibrosis

- Thick, viscous mucus in the respiratory and gastrointestinal tract
- Frequent, serious respiratory infections
- Obstruction of respiratory passages
- Progressive deterioration of respiratory function
- Dyspnea, hypoxemia
- Respiratory failure
- Pancreatic destruction, diabetes
- Gastrointestinal blockage
- Poor nutrient digestion

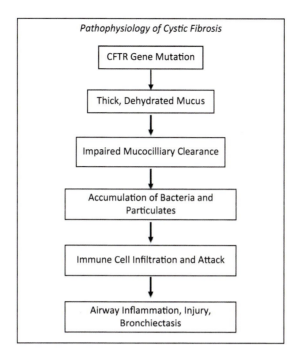

Pathophysiology of Cystic Fibrosis

CFTR Gene Mutation

↓

Thick, Dehydrated Mucus

↓

Impaired Mucocilliary Clearance

↓

Accumulation of Bacteria and Particulates

↓

Immune Cell Infiltration and Attack

↓

Airway Inflammation, Injury, Bronchiectasis

8.13.6.2 Diagnosis of cystic fibrosis

A standard method for diagnosis of cystic fibrosis is the sweat chloride test. In this test sweat production is stimulated through a small electric current and content of chloride in the sweat analyzed. Normal sweat chloride values are 10–35 milliequivalents per liter (mEq/L). Patients with cystic fibrosis usually have a sweat chloride value greater than 60 mEq/L. The presence of cystic fibrosis may be confirmed by DNA tests for the mutated fibrosis transmembrane conductance regulator (CFTR) gene. Screening of newborns for cystic fibrosis is currently mandated in all 50 U.S. states.

8.13.6.3 Treatment of cystic fibrosis

- Use of prophylactic antibiotics to prevent respiratory infections
- Frequent manual drainage of respiratory secretions
- Mucolytic agents

- Bronchodilators
- Pancreatic enzyme replacement, supplementation with vitamins and minerals
- *Ivacaftor* is a new drug approved for the treatment of CF in patients with specific mutations. The drug works by increasing activity of the abnormal chloride channels in these patients. Unfortunately, the mutations treated by ivacaftor only occur in approximately 5% of patients with cystic fibrosis. Combinations of new drugs that can be used along with ivacaftor to treat the most common forms of cystic fibrosis are currently underway
- Lung transplantation is a viable option for patient with end-stage disease

8.13.7   Restrictive pulmonary disorders

8.13.7.1   Pleuritis, pleural effusion

The pleura is a thin, double-walled membrane that surrounds the lungs. The space between the two layers of the pleura is called the pleural cavity and contains a lubricating fluid called *serous fluid*. *Pleuritis* (also known as *pleurisy*) is a condition that occurs when there is inflammation of the pleura. Pleuritis is most commonly caused by bacterial (pneumonia) or viral infections that originate in the respiratory tract. It may also be caused by rheumatoid disease and lung cancer metastases. Symptoms of pleuritis include chest pain that is worsened with inspiration. This may in turn lead to the patient taking shorter breaths to minimize expiration and subsequent pain.

Pleural Effusion is a condition that occurs when fluid accumulates in the pleural cavity. Fluids may be bloody in the case of trauma, clear (serous) in the case of heart or renal failure, or purulent in the case of infection. Accumulation of fluid in the pleura can limit expansion of the lungs during inspiration and may lead to dyspnea. For both pleuritis and pleural effusion, the goal of therapy is to treat the underlying cause of the condition.

8.13.7.2   Pneumothorax (see Figure 8.15)

The pleural cavity is the space in which the lungs reside. Pneumothorax is the entry of air into the pleural cavity. In order for normal lung expansion to occur, there must be a negative pressure within the pleural cavity with respect to atmospheric pressure outside the pleural cavity. The inside of the pleural cavity is essentially a vacuum and when air enters the pleural cavity the negative pressure is lost and the delicate lungs collapse. Because each lung sits in a separate pleural cavity, pneumothorax of one plural cavity will not cause collapse of the other lung.

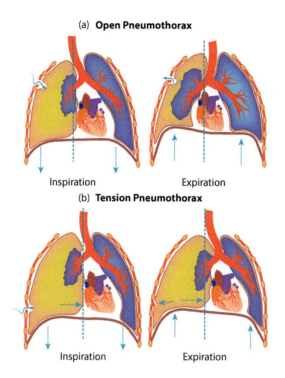

Figure 8.15   Types of pneumothorax. (a) Traumatic (open); (b) Tension (closed). (Adapted from *Porth's Pathophysiology: Concepts of Altered Health States* by Grossman, Lippincott Williams and Wilkins, 2013.)

8.13.7.2.1   Types of Pneumothorax

1. *Open or Communicating Pneumothorax*
   - Often results from a traumatic chest wound
   - Air enters the pleural cavity from the atmosphere and as a result the lung collapses due to equilibration of pressure within the pleural cavity with atmospheric pressure

2. *Tension Pneumothorax*
   - Occurs when air "leaks" from the lungs into the pleural cavity
   - May be caused by factors such as lung cancer, extreme air trapping, or pulmonary diseases such as COPD
   - The increased plural pressure prevents lung expansion during inspiration and the lung remains collapsed

3. *Closed or Spontaneous Pneumothorax*
   - A condition in which there is a one-way movement of air into but not out of the pleural cavity
   - May involve a hole or wound to the pleural cavity that forms a flap and allows air to enter and the lung to collapse. Upon expiration the hole or opening closes and prevent the movement of air back out of the pleural cavity
   - Tension pneumothorax can be life-threatening because the pressure in the pleural cavity will continue to increase with each breath and may result in further compress the heart, the large blood vessels in the thorax or the opposite lung

8.13.7.2.2   Manifestations of pneumothorax
- Tachypnea, dyspnea
- Chest pain
- Possible compression of thoracic blood vessels and heart, with tension pneumothorax

8.13.7.2.3   Treatment of pneumothorax
- Removal of air from the pleural cavity with a needle or chest tube
- Repair of trauma and closure of opening into pleural cavity

8.13.7.3   Atelectasis
Atelectasis is a condition in which there is incomplete expansion of lungs. It may be caused by blockage of the airways or compression of the lung tissue.

8.13.7.3.1   Types of atelectasis
1. *Absorption atelectasis*
   - Occurs when the bronchial passages are blocked by mucus, tumors or edema
   - May result from conditions such as chronic bronchitis, or cystic fibrosis in which there is the accumulation of excess mucus in the respiratory passages

2. *Compressions atelectasis*
   - Occurs when air, blood, fluids or a tumor compresses lung tissues externally

8.13.7.3.2   Manifestations of atelectasis
- Dyspnea, cough
- Reduced gas exchange. The effects of atelectasis on gas exchange will depend upon the amount of lung tissue that is prevented from expanding
- Shunting of blood to areas of the lungs that are inflated. The *ventilation-perfusion coupling* ability of the lungs will help ensure that blood is directed to areas of the lungs where gas exchange can still occur

8.13.7.3.3 Treatment of atelectasis
- Removal of airway blockage
- Removal of, for example, air, blood, fluids, or tumors that are compressing lung tissues

8.13.7.4 Bronchiectasis (see Figure 8.16)

Bronchiectasis is a condition that results from prolonged injury or inflammation of respiratory airways and bronchioles. It is characterized by

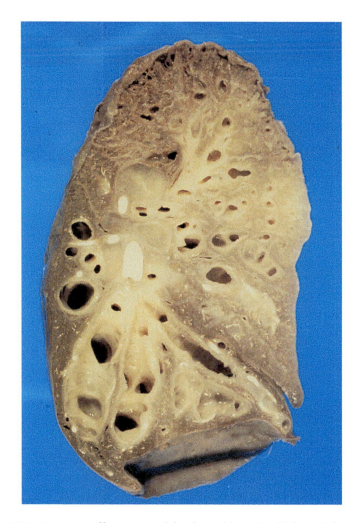

Figure 8.16 Airways affects caused by bronchiectasis. (Adapted from *Porth's Pathophysiology: Concepts of Altered Health States* by Grossman, Lippincott Williams and Wilkins, 2013.)

abnormal dilation of the bronchus or bronchi caused by destruction of the elastic tissues in the airway walls. Airway defenses and the ability to clear respiratory secretions is likewise impaired. It is most frequently associated with mucus blockage, infections such as tuberculosis, cystic fibrosis, and prolonged exposure to respiratory toxins. The major manifestations of bronchiectasis are chronic cough, excess mucus accumulation, and frequent respiratory infections. The condition cannot be reversed and is treated with antibiotics, bronchodilators, and physical (respiratory) therapy.

8.13.8   Acute respiratory distress syndrome

ARDS is a syndrome associated with destruction of alveolar membranes and their related capillaries. It may occur as a result of direct injury to the lungs or as a result of dramatic decreases in blood flow to the lung ("shock lung"). It is also more likely to occur in patients who are critically ill. Mortality for ARDS can be on the order of 40%–50%. Patients who survive ARDS are likely to experience lasting injury to their lungs. Possible causes of ARDS are listed in Table 8.14.

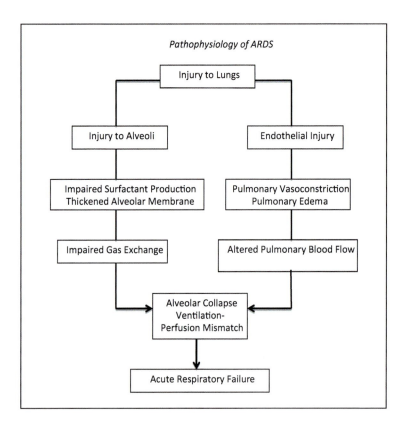

Table 8.14   Possible causes of ARDS

- Septicemia, uremia
- Trauma
- Near drowning
- Inhalation of toxic gases or agents
- Aspiration of gastric contents
- Widespread pneumonia
- Drug overdose
- Systemic shock

8.13.8.1   *Manifestations of ARDS*

- Dyspnea
- Endothelial damage—infiltration by immune cells with subsequent release of inflammatory mediators, proteolytic enzymes and free radicals
- Decreased surfactant production, atelectasis
- Hypoxemia—CO_2 is significantly more water-soluble than O_2 and can still be eliminated from the lungs via diffusion, as a result blood levels of oxygen are more affected by ARDS than CO_2. Hypoxemia leads to hyperventilation, which in turn can cause respiratory alkalosis
- Increased permeability and accumulation of fluids in alveoli and around alveolar spaces
- Pulmonary fibrosis
- Respiratory failure

8.13.8.2   *Treatment of ARDS*

Treatment of ARDS is mainly supportive with the goal of keeping the patient alive until the lung tissues can heal.

- Oxygen therapy
- Anti-inflammatory drugs are controversial
- Careful fluid management
- Correction of acid-base imbalances
- Prevent infections

8.13.9   *Respiratory distress syndrome of the newborn*

The etiology of newborn respiratory distress syndrome differs considerably from that of the adult. Respiratory distress in the newborn is most commonly caused by a lack of surfactant by the lungs. Pulmonary surfactant is a mixture of lipids and proteins and is produced by type II cells of the alveoli. A thin layer of surfactant covers the surface of the alveoli and provides surface tension that keeps the thin-walled alveoli from collapsing. Surfactant also moistens the alveolar surfaces to facilitate gas exchange. Respiratory distress syndrome of the newborn occurs most commonly in infants who are born premature and whose lungs have not developed to the point where they are producing adequate surfactant. Clinical manifestations become evident immediately at birth and can be rapidly fatal if not treated.

8.13.9.1 Manifestations of respiratory distress syndrome in the newborn

- Rapid, shallow breathing
- Atelectasis and lung collapse
- Lung inflammation and damage
- Hypoxemia and dyspnea
- Nasal flaring, grunting upon inspiration

8.13.9.2 Treatment of respiratory distress syndrome in the newborn

- Delay or prevent premature delivery of infant if possible
- Treatment of premature newborn with synthetic surfactant delivered directly into the lower respiratory tract. Exogenous surfactant will need to be supplied until the infant's lungs have matured to the point at which they are producing their own surfactant
- Injection of cortisol in the mother prior to delivery may significantly reduce the incidence of respiratory distress syndrome in premature infants. Cortisol has also been shown to stimulate activity of type II cells
- Mechanical ventilation

8.13.10 Interstitial lung diseases

Interstitial lung diseases represent a number of restrictive disorders whose main characteristic is scaring and fibrosis of lung tissue. The result of extensive lung scarring is reduced lung compliance and overall decreased lung volumes. Many causes of interstitial lung disease involve occupational exposure to injurious substances such as coal dust ("black lung"), asbestos (asbestosis), silicone dust (silicosis), radiation, drugs or toxins (see Table 8.15). Chronic lung infections, pulmonary edema or tumors might also lead to scaring and fibrosis of lung tissue. However, the etiology of a significant percentage of interstitial lung disease remains unknown.

8.13.10.1 Manifestations of interstitial lung disease

- Dyspnea, tachypnea
- Cough

Table 8.15 Possible causes of interstitial lung diseases

Exposure to Injurious Substances:
- Coal dust
- Asbestos
- Silicone dust
- Talc
- Organic dusts—e.g., hay, cotton
- Noxious gases
- Radiation
- Anticancer drugs
- Infectious agents

Other Causes:
- Sarcoidosis—an immune disorder characterized by the formation of granulomas that affect the lungs, skin and eyes
- Immunologic disorders—e.g., rheumatoid arthritis, systemic lupus erythematosus

---

- Hypoxemia
- Clubbing of fingers due to chronic hypoxia
- Progressive deterioration of pulmonary function and possible respiratory failure

8.13.10.2   Treatment of interstitial lung diseases

Treatment options for these disorders are limited and mainly focus on removal of the injurious substances. Anti-inflammatory drugs may be of use in limiting damage from chronic inflammation. Oxygen therapy may be instituted in severe cases.

8.13.11   Respiratory failure

Respiratory failure is a condition that results when the lungs are no longer able to sufficiently oxygenate the blood or remove CO_2 from it. It may occur as the end result of chronic respiratory diseases or it may be an acute event caused by factors such as pneumothorax or opioid drug overdose (see Table 8.16). Respiratory failure may be classified as being mainly *hypercapnic* or *hypoxemic* in terms of presentation. Hypercapnic failure is associated with excess levels of CO_2 and occurs when there is inadequate alveolar ventilation (e.g., depression of the respiratory centers). Hypoxemic failure occurs when there is inadequate exchange of oxygen between the alveoli and their associated capillaries (e.g., severe COPD). However, most patients with respiratory failure exhibit a combined presentation of hypercapnia and hypoxemia.

8.13.11.1   Manifestations of respiratory failure
- Hypoxemia
- Hypercapnia

Table 8.16   Causes of respiratory failure

Acute:
- Pneumothorax
- Drug overdose (e.g., opioids, sedatives)
- Pleural effusion—accumulation of fluids in the pleural cavity
- Airway obstruction
- Status asthmaticus
- Inhalation of toxins or noxious gases

Chronic:
- Emphysema
- Interstitial lung diseases
- Cystic fibrosis
- Spinal cord or brain injury
- Congestive heart failure
- Neuromuscular disorders—e.g., muscular dystrophy, myasthenia gravis. amyotrophic lateral sclerosis
- Pulmonary emboli
- Diffuse pneumonia
- Pulmonary edema

- Ventilation-perfusion mismatch—areas of the lungs are ventilated but nor perfused with blood
- Cyanosis, possible but not always present
- Central nervous system symptoms—slurred speech, confusion, impaired motor function
- Altered blood pH
- Initial tachycardia and increased cardiac output followed by bradycardia and decreased cardiac output

8.13.11.2   Treatment of respiratory failure
- Treatment of underlying cause or disease
- Bronchodilators
- Correction of blood pH
- Oxygen therapy
- Mechanical ventilation

Medical terminology

Aerobic (ĕr-ō′bĭk): Requiring oxygen

Alveolar dead space (ăl-vē′ō-lăr dĕd spās): Volume of the poorly perfused alveoli; the resulting lack of gas exchange contributes to physiological dead space

Anatomical dead space (ăn″ă-tŏm′ĭk-ăl dĕd spās): Volume of the conducting airways where there is no gas exchange

Anemia (ă-nē´mē-ă): Condition resulting from a decrease in the number of circulating red blood cells or a decrease in hemoglobin

Apnea (ăp-nē´ă): Temporary cessation of breathing

Atelectasis (ăt˝ē-lĕk´tă-sĭs): Collapse of the airways

Bohr effect (bor ē-fĕkt´): Hydrogen ions or an acid environment changes the structure of hemoglobin causing it to release more oxygen in the tissues

Chemoreceptor (kē˝mō-rē-sĕp´tor): In the respiratory system, a receptor that is stimulated by a decrease in oxygen, an increase in carbon dioxide, or an increase in hydrogen ion resulting in an increase in ventilation

Compliance (kŏm-plī´ăns): In the respiratory system, the distensibility of the lungs

Dyspnea (dĭsp-nē´ă): Difficulty breathing

Exogenous (ĕks-ŏj´ē-nŭs): Originating outside of the body or an organ

Hering-Breuer reflex (hĕr´ĭng-broo´ĕr rē´flĕks): Reflex inhibition of inspiration due to stimulation of stretch receptors in the lungs

Hypercapnia (hī˝pĕr-kăp´nē-ă): Increased carbon dioxide in the blood

Hyperpnea (hī˝pĕrp´nē-ă): Increased ventilation due to an increase in tidal volume, an increase in breathing frequency, or both

Hypoxemia (hī-pŏks-ē´mē-ă): Decreased oxygen in the arterial blood

Insidious (ĭn-sĭd´ē-ŭs): Gradual, subtle, or indistinct in onset

Intrapleural (ĭn˝tră-ploo´răl): Within the pleural cavity surrounding the lungs

Nebulizer (nĕb´ū-lī˝zĕr): Apparatus that produces a fine mist for inhalation

Neonate (nē´ō-nāt): Newborn infant up to 1 month of age

Noncompliant (nŏn-kŏm-plī´ănt): In the respiratory system, stiff, poorly distensible lungs that are difficult to inflate

Phrenic nerve (frĕn´ĭk nĕrv): Portion of the somatic motor nervous system that innervates the diaphragm

Physiological dead space (fĭz˝ē-ō-lŏj´ĭ-kăl dĕd spās): Sum of the anatomical dead space and the alveolar dead space; represents all of the regions of the lungs that do not participate in gas exchange and do not eliminate carbon dioxide

Pleura (ploo´ră): Double-walled membrane that encloses each lung

Pneumothorax (nū-mō-thō´răks): Entry of air into the pleural cavity causing collapse of the lung

Proprioceptor (prō˝prē-ō-sĕp´tors): Receptors in muscles and joints that provide an awareness of body position and movement

Recoil (rē´koyl): Spring back; in the respiratory system, the return of the lungs to their preinspiratory volume

Shunt (shŭnt): In the respiratory system, blood that perfuses unventilated alveoli

Surfactant (sŭr-făk´tănt): In the respiratory system, a substance secreted by alveolar type II cells that decreases the surface tension of the fluid lining the alveoli

Transpulmonary (trănz˝pŭl´mō-nĕ-rē): Across the surface of the lungs
Transudation (trănz˝-ū-dā´shŭn): Movement of fluid across the wall of the
capillary and into the interstitial space

Bibliography

American Cancer Society. 2015. Cancer Facts and Figures. http://www.cancer.org/
research/cancerfactsstatistics/cancerfactsfigures2015/index.
Centers for Disease Control and Prevention. 2015. National Center for Health
Statistics. https://www.google.com/search?client=safari&rls=en&q=cdc+center+
for+national+health+statistics&ie=UTF-8&oe=UTF-8.
Fox, S. I., *Human Physiology*, 9th ed., McGraw Hill, Boston, MA, 2006.
Gutstein, H. B., and Akil, H., Opioid analgesics, in *Goodman and Gilman's, The
Pharmacological Basis of Therapeutics*, 9th ed., Brunton, L. L., Lazo, J. S., and
Parker, K. L., Eds., McGraw-Hill, New York, 2006, chap. 21.
http://www.healthinfotranslations.com/incentive_spirometer_441477.php.
Levitsky, M. G., *Pulmonary Physiology*, 5th ed., McGraw-Hill, New York, 1999.
Marieb, E. N., and Hoehn, K., *Anatomy & Physiology*, 3rd ed., Pearson Benjamin
Cummings, San Francisco, CA, 2008.
Porth, C. M., *Pathophysiology, Concepts of Altered Health States*, 7th ed., J. B. Lippincott
Company, Philadelphia, PA, 2005.
Robergs, R. A., and Roberts, S. O., *Exercise Physiology, Exercise, Performance, and
Clinical Applications*, Mosby, St. Louis, MO, 1997.
Schmann, L., Obstructive pulmonary disorders, in *Perspectives on Pathophysiology*,
Copstead, L.-E. C., Ed., W. B. Saunders Company, Philadelphia, PA, 1995, chap. 20.
Schmann, L., Ventilation and respiratory failure, in *Perspectives on Pathophysiology*,
Copstead, L-E. C., Ed., W. B. Saunders Company, Philadelphia, PA, 1995, chap. 22.
Schwartzstein, R. M., and Parker, M. J., *Respiratory Physiology, A Clinical Approach*,
Lippincott Williams & Wilkins, Philadelphia, PA, 2006.
Sherwood, L., *Human Physiology, From Cells to Systems*, 5th ed., Brooks/Cole, Pacific
Grove, CA, 2004.
Silverthorn, D. U., *Human Physiology, An Integrated Approach*, 4th ed., Prentice Hall,
Upper Saddle River, NJ, 2007.
Stedman's Medical Dictionary for the Health Professions and Nursing, 5th ed., Lippincott
Williams & Wilkins, Baltimore, MD, 2005.
Taber's Cyclopedic Medical Dictionary, 20th ed., F. A. Davis Co., Philadelphia, PA, 2005.
Ward, J. P. T., Ward, J., Wiener, C. M., and Leach, R. M., *The Respiratory System at a
Glance*, Blackwell Science Ltd., Oxford, UK, 2002.
West, J. B., *Pulmonary Physiology and Pathophysiology, An Integrated, Case-Based
Approach*, Lippincott Williams & Wilkins, Philadelphia, PA, 2001.
West, J. B., *Respiratory Physiology, The Essentials*, 7th ed., Lippincott Williams &
Wilkins, Philadelphia, PA, 2005.
Widmaier, E. P., Raff, H., and Strang, K. T., *Vander's Human Physiology, The Mechanisms
of Body Function*, McGraw-Hill, Boston, MA, 2006.
World Health Organization. 2015a. Genetics and Asthma. http://www.who.int/
genomics/about/Asthma.pdf.
World Health Organization. 2015b. Tuberculosis Factsheet. http://www.who.int/
mediacentre/factsheets/fs104/en/.

chapter nine

The digestive system

Study objectives

- Describe the anatomical and functional characteristics of each of the four layers of the digestive tract wall: mucosa, submucosa, muscularis externa and serosa
- Distinguish between the two types of gastrointestinal motility: segmentation and peristalsis
- Explain how each of the three types of sensory receptors within the digestive tract are stimulated: chemoreceptors, osmoreceptors and mechanoreceptors
- Explain how the following mechanisms regulate the activity of the digestive system: intrinsic nerve plexuses, extrinsic autonomic nerves and gastrointestinal hormones
- List the components of saliva and their functions
- Describe how salivary secretion is regulated
- Explain how swallowing takes place
- For each of the following organs: esophagus, stomach, small intestine and large intestine, describe:
    - Specialized anatomical modifications
    - The type of motility and how it is regulated
    - The types of secretions and how they are regulated
    - The digestive processes that take place
    - The absorptive processes that take place
    - Other functions
- List general symptoms of gastrointestinal disease
- Describe the various disorders that can affect the esophagus
- Discuss peptic ulcer disease in terms of its cause(s), effects and treatment
- What are the main features of irritable bowel syndrome? Why might it occur? How does it differ from inflammatory bowel disease?
- Compare and contrast Crohn's disease and ulcerative colitis in terms of their clinical similarities and differences. How might each be treated?
- Explain how various conditions can alter intestinal motility or the absorption of nutrients
- How might one detect colorectal cancer? What are some factors that might predispose an individual to it? Discuss the relationship between gastrointestinal polyps and adenocarcinoma?

- What is diverticular disease? Why might it occur? Define diverticulitis
- List the major functions of the liver
- Discuss the key features of the hepatitis viruses in terms of their epidemiology, effects on the liver and possible long-term consequences
- Describe the three stages of alcoholic liver disease
- Define liver cirrhosis. List the major manifestations of cirrhosis. Explain why each of these manifestations occurs
- Define jaundice, why might it occur?
- How does cholelithiasis differ from cholecystitis? List factors that may predispose an individual to cholelithiasis
- Discuss acute and chronic pancreatitis. What might cause each? What are some of the possible effects of each on the body?

The overall function of the digestive system is to make ingested food available to the cells of the body. Most ingested food is in the form of large molecules (macromolecules) that must be broken down by mechanical and biochemical processes into their smaller components (see Table 9.1). These smaller units are then absorbed across the wall of the digestive tract and distributed throughout the body, although not all ingested materials are completely digested and absorbed by the human gastrointestinal tract. For example, cellulose, the fibrous form of plant carbohydrates, is indigestible by humans. Normally, about 95% of ingested food materials are made available for use by the body. Interestingly, as long as food remains within the digestive tract itself, it is technically outside of the body. Not until the materials have crossed the epithelium that lines the tract, is it considered to have "entered" the body.

The digestive system consists of the following:

- The gastrointestinal tract
- Accessory digestive organs

Table 9.1 Ingested and absorbable molecules for the three major categories of nutrients

Carbohydrates	Monosaccharides
• Polysaccharides (Starch)	• Glucose
• Disaccharides	• Galactose
• Sucrose (Table Sugar)	• Fructose
• Lactose (Milk Sugar)	
Proteins	Amino acids
Fats	Monoglycerides
• Triglycerides	Free fatty acids

The *gastrointestinal tract* is essentially a tube that runs through the center of the body from the mouth to the anus. This tube consists of the following organs:

- Mouth
- Pharynx
- Esophagus
- Stomach
- Small intestine
- Large intestine

Although these organs are continuous with one other, each has important anatomical modifications that allow them to carry out their specific functions.

The *accessory digestive organs* exist outside of the gastrointestinal tract itself; however, each of these organs empty secretions into the tract that contribute to the process of digestion. These accessory digestive organs include the following:

- Salivary glands
- Liver
- Gallbladder
- Pancreas

9.1   Digestive tract wall

The digestive tract wall has the same basic structure from the esophagus through the colon. There are four major layers within the wall:

- Mucosa
- Submucosa
- Muscularis externa
- Serosa

9.1.1   Mucosa

The innermost layer of the digestive tract wall, the *mucosa*, is composed of three layers: the mucous membrane, the lamina propria, and the muscularis mucosa. The *mucus membrane* provides important protective, absorptive, and secretory functions for the digestive tract. The nature of the epithelial cells lining the tract varies from one region to the next. The average life span of these epithelial cells is only a few days, so rapidly dividing stem cells continually produce new cells to replace worn-out epithelial cells. Mucus-secreting goblet cells are found in the mucosa throughout much of the gastrointestinal tract. The *lamina propria* is a thin, middle layer of connective tissue that contains the capillaries and small lymphatic vessels positioned to collect digested nutrient molecules. It also contains numerous lymph nodules that provide protection against infectious agents. The outer *muscularis mucosa* is a thin layer of smooth muscle. Contraction of this muscle may alter the effective surface area for absorption in the lumen.

9.1.2   Submucosa

The *submucosa* of the digestive tract wall is a thick middle layer of connective tissue that provides the wall with its distensibility and elasticity as nutrient materials move through the system.

9.1.3   Muscularis externa

The outer layer of the wall is the *muscularis externa*. In most regions of the tract, it consists of two layers of muscle: an inner circular layer and an outer longitudinal layer. Contraction of the circular layer narrows the lumen of the tube, whereas contraction of the longitudinal layer causes the tube to shorten.

The muscle tissue of the digestive tract consists of *single-unit smooth muscle*. Within each layer, the muscle cells are connected by gap junctions forming a syncytium. In this way, action potentials generated at a given site may travel along the muscle layer. The smooth muscle undergoes slow but continuous electrical activity, producing rhythmic contractions of the digestive tract wall. The cycles of depolarization and repolarization in the smooth muscle are referred to as *slow-wave potentials*. Interestingly, recent studies have suggested that the generation of the slow waves in gastrointestinal smooth muscle involves specialized cells referred to as *interstitial cells of Cajal* (ICC). These cells have long cellular processes as well as gap junctions, which allow the ICCs to communicate with each other as well as smooth muscle cells, permitting the spread of depolarization from one cell to the next.

Slow-wave potentials do not reach threshold during each cycle, so contraction does not necessarily occur with each depolarization. Smooth muscle contraction will take place only when the slow wave depolarizes all the way to threshold. At this point, voltage-gated Ca^{++} channels open, Ca^{++} ions enter the muscle cells and one or more action potentials are generated. The influx of Ca^{++} ions contributes to both the depolarization phase of the action potential as well as the muscle contraction itself. These action potentials result in *phasic contractions*. The force and duration of muscle contraction is determined by the number of action potentials generated. Typically, phasic contractions last only a few seconds. Tissues that exhibit phasic contractions include the body of the esophagus, the gastric antrum, and the small intestine. Other tissues, including the lower esophageal sphincter (LES), the upper region of the stomach, and many sphincters located throughout the gastrointestinal tract, exhibit *tonic contractions*. These contractions are slow and sustained and may last minutes to hours.

Muscular activity, or *gastrointestinal motility*, is enhanced by stretching the muscle, as occurs when food materials distends the digestive tract wall. It is also enhanced by parasympathetic nervous stimulation and by several specific gastrointestinal hormones. Motility is inhibited by sympathetic nervous stimulation and by blood-circulating epinephrine.

The two basic types of gastrointestinal motility are:

- Segmentation
- Peristalsis

The contents of the digestive tract must be constantly churned and mixed. In this way, the materials are exposed to digestive enzymes and they meet the wall of the tract for absorption. This mixing is carried out by *segmentation*, or stationary muscular contractions. This form of motility divides a portion of the tract into alternating constricted regions and unconstricted regions. Segmentation contractions move back and forth as a previously constricted region relaxes and a previously relaxed region contracts. This activity results in the thorough mixing of the contents with digestive enzymes and other secretions. This is the more important form of motility in the small intestine, where most digestion and absorption takes place.

The contents of the tract must also be continually moved forward so it can be acted upon by the sequential regions of the tract. *Peristalsis* is a muscular contraction that produces a ring of contraction that moves along the length of the tract. This wave-like contraction causes propulsion and forces the contents forward. Peristalsis is more important in the pharynx, the esophagus and the stomach.

Gastrointestinal sphincters are formed where the circular layer of smooth muscle is thickened. Sphincters occur at several points along the tract. Their function is to limit the movement of food materials from one region to another. For example, the pyloric sphincter is found between the stomach and the duodenum of the small intestine. This sphincter plays an important role in limiting the rate of gastric emptying. Sphincters undergo *tonic contractions*, which may be sustained for minutes or hours.

9.1.4   Serosa

The connective tissue membrane that surrounds the wall of the digestive tract is the *serosa*. This membrane secretes a watery fluid that provides lubrication and prevents friction between the digestive organs as they move about in the abdomen. The serosa is continuous with the *peritoneum*, which is the serous membrane lining the abdominal cavity. The peritoneum also forms sheets of tissue, or *mesentery*, which suspend the digestive organs from the wall of the abdomen. The mesentery acts as a sling which, while offering structural support for the organs, also provides for the range of movement needed during the digestive process.

9.2   Regulation of gastrointestinal function

The digestive tract contains three types of sensory receptors that are sensitive to chemical or mechanical changes within the system. These include:

- Chemoreceptors
- Osmoreceptors
- Mechanoreceptors

Chemoreceptors respond to various chemical components within the gastrointestinal lumen. For example, chemoreceptors in the duodenum of the small intestine are stimulated by excessive amounts of hydrogen ions secreted by the stomach. *Osmoreceptors* are sensitive to the osmolarity of the contents within the lumen of the tract. As the digestive process progresses, large nutrient molecules are split into their smaller components. This increases the number of molecules and, therefore, increases the osmolarity of the material being processed. Excessive osmolarity may suggest that absorption is not keeping pace with digestion. *Mechanoreceptors* respond to stretch or distension of the gastrointestinal tract wall.

Receptor stimulation may lead to the activation of any or all the following regulatory mechanisms within the tract:

- Enteric nervous system
- Intrinsic nerve plexuses
- Extrinsic autonomic nerves
- Gastrointestinal hormones

The *enteric nervous system* consists of submucosal (Meissner's) and myenteric (Auerbach's) plexuses. These plexuses within the wall of the intestine contain 100 million neurons (about the same number of neurons as found in the spinal cord). The enteric nervous system includes both intrinsic neurons and extrinsic neurons.

9.2.1   Intrinsic nerve plexuses

The *intrinsic nerve plexuses* are interconnecting networks of nerve cells located entirely within the gastrointestinal tract. These plexuses are responsible for *intratract reflexes*. The stimulation of a receptor in one region of the tract neurally influences the activity of another region of the tract.

These reflexes occur directly, independent of the central nervous system. Intratract reflexes provide a mechanism for self-regulation of the tract and help to coordinate the activity of the organs within it. Examples of such reflexes include:

- *Enterogastric reflex*: where receptor stimulation in the duodenum of the small intestine elicits neural activity that regulates both muscle contraction and glandular secretion in the stomach
- *Gastroileal reflex*: where increased gastric activity causes increased activity in the ileum and increased movement of chyme through the ileocecal sphincter
- *Ileogastric reflex*: where distension of the ileum causes a decrease in gastric motility
- *Intestino-intestinal reflex*: where overdistension of a given segment of the intestine causes relaxation throughout the rest of the intestine

9.2.2   Extrinsic autonomic nerves

Gastrointestinal activity is also modified by *extrinsic autonomic nerves*. The tract is innervated by both the parasympathetic and the sympathetic divisions of the autonomic nervous system. Parasympathetic innervation is provided primarily by the vagus nerves (esophagus, stomach, pancreas, gallbladder, small intestine, and upper large intestine) and the pelvic nerves (rest of the large intestine). Sympathetic innervation is provided by pathways that pass through the celiac, inferior mesenteric, and superior mesenteric ganglia. The effects of these two divisions tend to oppose each other. The parasympathetic system stimulates most digestive activities, whereas the sympathetic system inhibits them. Interestingly, the autonomic nerves to the digestive system, especially the vagus nerve of the parasympathetic system, can be discretely activated. In this way, digestive activity can be modified without affecting tissue function in other regions of the body.

9.2.3   Gastrointestinal hormones

A third factor contributing to the regulation of digestive activity is the secretion of *gastrointestinal hormones*. These hormones may be released in one region of the tract, travel in the circulatory system to other regions of the tract and influence the activity of effector cells in that region. A summary of the source, the stimulus for release, and the actions of several important hormones is found in Table 9.2.

   A summary of these three mechanisms that regulate the activity of the digestive system is illustrated in Figure 9.1. A local change in the tract may lead to the stimulation of one or more of the three types of receptors present

Table 9.2   Digestive hormones

Hormone	Source	Stimulus for release	Actions of hormone
Gastrin	G cells in pyloric region of the stomach	Protein in stomach; vagal stimulation	Stimulates parietal cells (HCl) and chief cells (pepsinogen) in the stomach; enhances gastric motility
Secretin	Endocrine cells in mucosa of duodenum	Acid in duodenum	Inhibits gastric emptying; inhibits gastric secretion; stimulates secretion of bicarbonate from the pancreas; stimulates secretion of bicarbonate-rich bile from the liver
Cholecystokinin	Endocrine cells in mucosa of duodenum	Breakdown products of lipid and, to a small extent, protein digestion in duodenum	Inhibits gastric emptying Inhibits gastric secretion; stimulates contraction of the gallbladder; stimulates secretion of digestive enzymes from the pancreas
Glucose-dependent Insulinotropic Peptide (GIP); formerly referred to as gastric inhibitory peptide	Endocrine cells in mucosa of duodenum	Glucose, lipids, acid, and hyperosmotic chyme in duodenum; distension of duodenum	Inhibits gastric emptying; inhibits gastric secretion; stimulates secretion of insulin from pancreas

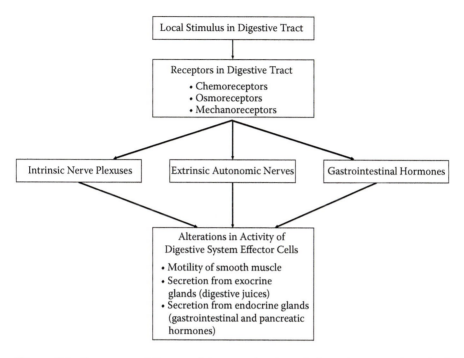

Figure 9.1 Summary of the regulatory mechanisms influencing gastrointestinal function.

in the tract wall. Receptor stimulation may then activate any or all three regulatory mechanisms. These mechanisms then alter the activity of the effector tissues within the digestive system including smooth muscle, exocrine glands, and endocrine glands.

The following sections will discuss each region of the digestive system separately. Where appropriate, the basic digestive processes will be considered: motility, secretion, digestion, and absorption.

9.3 Mouth

The *mouth* is the region from the lips to the pharynx. The first step in the digestive process is chewing or *mastication*. This initial mechanical breakdown of the food facilitates its movement to the stomach. The mouth is lined with *stratified squamous epithelium*, which provides extra protection from injury by coarse food materials.

Three pairs of salivary glands secrete saliva into the oral cavity:

- Parotid glands: located between the angle of the jaw and the ear
- Sublingual glands: located below the tongue
- Submandibular glands: located below the jaw

Saliva contains:

- Water
- Mucus
- Lysozyme
- Salivary amylase
- Lingual lipase

Approximately 99.5% of saliva is *water*. Swallowing is facilitated by the moistening of food materials. Furthermore, water serves as a solvent for molecules that stimulate the taste buds. The presence of *mucus*, which is thick and slippery, lubricates the mouth and the food and assists in swallowing. *Lysozyme* is an enzyme that lyses or kills many types of bacteria that may be ingested with the food.

Saliva begins the process of chemical digestion with *salivary amylase*. This enzyme splits starch molecules (amylose) into fragments. Specifically, polysaccharides, or starches, are broken down into maltose, a disaccharide consisting of two glucose molecules. Salivary amylase may account for up to 75% of starch digestion before it is denatured by hydrochloric acid in the stomach.

A small amount of *lingual lipase* is also present, predominately in infants, and plays a role in the breakdown of dietary lipid. This enzyme is optimally active at an acidic pH and, therefore, remains active through the stomach and into the intestine.

Due to parasympathetic stimulation of the salivary glands, saliva is secreted continuously at a basal rate of approximately 0.5 mL/min. Secretion may be enhanced by two types of reflexes:

- Simple or unconditioned salivary reflex
- Acquired or conditioned salivary reflex

The *simple or unconditioned salivary reflex* occurs when food is present within the oral cavity causing stimulation of chemoreceptors and pressure receptors. These receptors then transmit impulses to the *salivary center* in the medulla of the brainstem. Parasympathetic efferent impulses are transmitted back to the salivary glands and secretion is enhanced.

The *acquired or conditioned salivary reflex* is elicited in response to the thought, sight, smell or sound of food. As demonstrated with Pavlov's dog, these stimuli result in a learned response. Another stimulus that enhances salivation is nausea. Salivary secretion is inhibited by fatigue, sleep, fear and dehydration. Overall, 1–2 L of saliva may be produced per day.

PHARMACY APPLICATION: EFFECTS OF ANTICHOLINERGIC DRUGS ON THE DIGESTIVE SYSTEM

In addition to their therapeutic actions, many drugs have undesirable side effects that may influence the digestive system. An example of such a drug is scopolamine, one of the most effective agents used for the prevention of motion sickness. This drug may be administered transdermally in a multilayered adhesive unit, or "patch." Its mechanism of action likely involves the inhibition of muscarinic receptors in the vestibular apparatus of the inner ear. This interrupts the transmission of nerve impulses from the inner ear to the emetic center in the medulla of the brainstem and vomiting in response to motion is inhibited. However, the salivary glands are also quite sensitive to the activity of muscarinic receptor antagonists. In fact, scopolamine and other anticholinergic agents may severely inhibit the copious, watery secretion of the salivary glands. In this case, the mouth becomes dry and swallowing and speaking may become difficult. Other anticholinergic agents may be used to (1) reduce muscle rigidity and muscle tremor in Parkinson's disease (benztropine mesylate); (2) reduce bronchospasm and airway mucus secretion in asthma and chronic obstructive pulmonary disease (COPD) (ipratropium); and (3) reduce the accumulation of secretions in the trachea and the possibility of laryngospasm prior to the administration of general anesthesia. In each case, these medications also inhibit salivary secretion and cause "dry mouth."

9.4   Pharynx

The *pharynx* is the cavity at the rear of the throat and links the mouth with the esophagus. It serves as a common passageway for both the respiratory and the digestive systems. The *swallowing reflex* takes place largely in the pharynx. This is an example of an all-or-none reflex in which, once the process has begun, it cannot be stopped. Swallowing may be initiated voluntarily when the tongue pushes a bolus of food toward the back of the mouth and into the pharynx. The stimulation of pressure receptors in the pharynx results in the transmission of nerve impulses to the *swallowing center* in the medulla of the brainstem. This elicits a coordinated, involuntary reflex that involves the contraction of muscles in the appropriate sequence. A wave of contraction sweeps down the constrictor muscles of the pharynx. The epiglottis moves downward over the larynx to seal off the trachea and the upper esophageal sphincter (UES) relaxes, allowing the bolus of food to enter the esophagus. Once the food bolus enters the esophagus, the UES closes to prevent the swallowing of air. This phase of the swallowing reflex is referred to as the *pharyngeal stage* and lasts approximately 1 s.

9.5   Esophagus

The *esophagus*, located behind the trachea, is a muscular tube connecting the pharynx and the stomach. It is lined with *stratified squamous epithelium*. The only substance secreted by the esophagus is *mucus*. The protective mucus provides lubrication for the passage of food and it helps to prevent damage to the esophageal wall by coarse food materials. The esophagus is sealed off by two sphincters, one at either end of the tube: the *UES* and the *LES*. Each of these sphincters is normally closed except during the process of swallowing. The normal function of the respiratory system creates a subatmospheric pressure in the thoracic cavity. If, indeed, the esophagus were open to the atmosphere, this pressure gradient would pull air into the esophagus and stomach during each inspiration. Therefore, the closure of these sphincters prevents large volumes of air from entering the digestive tract. In addition, the LES prevents the reflux of the corrosive gastric contents into the esophagus.

The *esophageal stage* of the swallowing reflex involves a *primary peristaltic wave* of contraction that is initiated by the swallowing center and mediated by the vagus nerve. This wave, which begins at the UES, moves slowly down the esophagus at a rate of 2–6 cm/s until it reaches the LES. Therefore, it may take a bolus of food 10 s to pass through the esophagus. Some food particles that are particularly large or sticky may remain in the esophagus after the primary peristaltic wave. The distension of the esophagus by the presence of these particles elicits *secondary peristaltic waves* that do not involve the swallowing center. The smooth muscle of the LES relaxes immediately prior to the arrival of the peristaltic contraction to allow for the movement of the food into the stomach.

9.6   Stomach

The *stomach*, located on the left side of the abdominal cavity just below the diaphragm, lies between the esophagus and the small intestine. It is the most distensible portion of the gastrointestinal tract. As with the esophagus, it has a sphincter at either end; the previously mentioned LES is located at the entrance to the stomach and the *pyloric sphincter* is located at the exit of the stomach leading to the duodenum of the small intestine. The LES is normally closed except during swallowing. The pyloric sphincter is subject to tonic contraction, which keeps it almost, but not completely, closed. In this way, fluids may easily pass through it. The movement of food materials through this sphincter requires strong gastric contractions. Even then, only a few milliliters are pushed through at a time. Gastric contractions mash the food materials and thoroughly mix them with the gastric secretions. This produces a thick, semifluid mixture referred to as *chyme*.

The stomach is divided into three regions:

- *Fundus*: uppermost region of the stomach located above the junction with the esophagus

- *Body*: middle or main portion of the stomach
- *Antrum*: terminal region of the stomach leading to the gastroduodenal junction

The stomach performs several important functions:

- Holds ingested food until it can be processed by the remainder of the digestive tract
- Mechanically mashes ingested food and mixes it with gastric secretions
- Begins the process of protein digestion

Food is held in the body of the stomach, which may expand to hold as much as 1 L of chyme. As food enters the stomach, it undergoes reflex relaxation. This reflex is referred to as *receptive relaxation*. It enhances the ability of the stomach to accommodate a marked increase in volume with only a small increase in stomach pressure. The fundus does not typically store food given that it is located above the esophageal opening into the stomach. Instead, it usually contains a pocket of gas.

9.6.1 Gastric motility

In addition to the circular and longitudinal layers of smooth muscle, there is an extra layer of smooth muscle in the stomach. The *oblique layer* of smooth muscle begins at the UES and fans out across the anterior and posterior surfaces of the stomach. It fuses with the circular layer in the lower region of the stomach. This extra layer of muscle enhances gastric motility and, therefore, the mixing and mashing of the food.

Contraction of gastric smooth muscle occurs in the form of *peristalsis*. Peristaltic contractions begin in the body of the stomach and proceed in a wave-like fashion toward the duodenum. These contractions are weak in the upper portion of the stomach where the muscle layers are relatively thin. The contractions become much stronger in the lower portion of the stomach as the muscle layers become thicker. As the wave of contraction sweeps through the antrum, a small amount of chyme is pushed through the partially open pyloric sphincter. When the peristaltic contraction reaches the pyloric sphincter, the sphincter closes and the rest of the chyme in this region is forced back toward the body of the stomach where more mixing and mashing takes place. This propulsion of chyme back into the stomach is referred to as *retropropulsion*.

It may take many hours for the contents of the stomach to be processed and moved into the small intestine. Several factors influence gastric motility and, therefore, the rate of gastric emptying. These include:

- Volume of chyme in the stomach
- Fluidity of the chyme
- Volume and chemical composition of the chyme in the duodenum

The major gastric factor that affects motility and the rate of emptying is the *volume of chyme in the stomach*. As the volume of chyme increases, the wall of the stomach becomes distended and mechanoreceptors are stimulated. This elicits reflexes that enhance gastric motility by way of the intrinsic nerves and the vagus nerve. The release of the hormone, gastrin, from the antral region of the stomach further contributes to enhanced motility.

The degree of *fluidity of the chyme* also affects the rate of gastric emptying. Ingested liquids move through the pyloric sphincter and begin to empty almost immediately. Ingested solids must first be converted into a semifluid mixture of uniformly small particles. Only particles about 1 mm³ or smaller move readily into the duodenum. The faster the necessary degree of fluidity is achieved, the more rapidly the contents of the stomach may empty into the duodenum.

The most important factors that regulate gastric motility and the rate of emptying of the stomach involve the *volume and chemical composition of the chyme in the duodenum*. Receptors in the duodenum are sensitive to:

- Distension
- Lipids
- Acid
- Osmolarity of the chyme

The goal of these duodenal factors is to maintain a rate of gastric emptying that is consistent with the proper digestion and absorption of nutrient molecules in the small intestine. In other words, emptying must be regulated so that the duodenum has adequate opportunity to process the chyme that it already contains before it receives more from the stomach. Regulation occurs by way of the *enterogastric reflex*, which inhibits gastric motility, increases contraction of the pyloric sphincter and, therefore, decreases the rate of gastric emptying. This reflex is mediated through the intrinsic nerves and the vagus nerve. Regulation also occurs by way of a *hormonal response* that involves the release of the *enterogastrones* from the duodenum. These hormones include *secretin, cholecystokinin,* and *glucose-dependent insulinotropic peptide* (GIP).

As the volume of the chyme in the duodenum increases, it causes *distension* of the duodenal wall and the stimulation of *mechanoreceptors*. This receptor stimulation elicits reflex inhibition of gastric motility mediated through the intrinsic nerves and the vagus nerve. Distension also causes the release of GIP from the duodenum, which contributes to the inhibition of gastric contractions.

Duodenal receptors are also sensitive to the chemical composition of the chyme and detect the presence of lipids, excess hydrogen ions, and hyperosmotic chyme, as well. These conditions also elicit the enterogastric reflex and the release of the enterogastrones to decrease the rate of gastric emptying.

Of the three major categories of nutrients, *lipids* are the slowest to be digested and absorbed. Furthermore, these processes take place only in the small intestine. Therefore, to ensure complete lipid digestion and absorption, the rate of movement of lipid from the stomach to the duodenum must be carefully regulated. The presence of lipid in the duodenum stimulates intestinal chemoreceptors. This receptor stimulation elicits reflex inhibition of gastric motility and slows the addition of more lipids from the stomach. Lipid also causes the release of cholecystokinin from the duodenum. This hormone contributes to the inhibition of gastric contractions. The significance of the inhibitory effect of lipid is illustrated by the comparison between a high-fat meal (up to 6 hours for gastric emptying) and a meal consisting of carbohydrates and protein (3 hours for gastric emptying). Therefore, a fatty meal is "more filling" than a low-fat meal due its effect on gastric motility.

An important gastric secretion is *hydrochloric acid*, which performs several functions in the stomach. This acid from the stomach is neutralized by pancreatic bicarbonate ions in the duodenum. Excess acid in the chyme stimulates chemoreceptors in the duodenum. This receptor stimulation elicits reflex inhibition of gastric motility. Excess acid also causes the release of secretin from the duodenum. This hormone contributes to the inhibition of gastric contractions. In this way, the neutralization process may be completed before additional acid arrives in the chyme from the stomach.

Chyme within the duodenum has, by this point, undergone some degree of carbohydrate and protein digestion. Salivary amylase has fragmented starch molecules and, as will be discussed, pepsin from the stomach has fragmented proteins. Therefore, the number of disaccharides and small peptides has increased, which leads to an increase in the *osmolarity of the chyme*. The rate of absorption of these smaller molecules must keep pace with the rate of digestion of the larger molecules. If not, the stimulation of *osmoreceptors* in the duodenum by the hyperosmotic chyme will inhibit gastric motility and gastric emptying. This effect is mediated through reflex inhibition.

9.6.2 Gastric secretion

The human stomach secretes 2–4 L of gastric juice per day. The gastric mucosa, which produces these secretions, is divided into two functional regions:

- Oxyntic gland area
- Pyloric gland area

The *oxyntic gland area* is located in the proximal 80% of the stomach. These glands consist of three types of cells:

- Mucus neck cells
- Parietal cells
- Chief cells

The pyloric gland area is located in the remaining distal 20% of the stomach.

In addition to a large amount of water, secretions of the stomach include the following:

- Hydrochloric acid
- Pepsinogen
- Mucus
- Intrinsic factor
- Gastrin

Hydrochloric acid (*HCl*) is produced by the *parietal cells*. This is a strong acid that dissociates into H^+ ions and Cl^- ions. These ions are actively transported into the lumen of the stomach by the *proton pump* (*H^+-K^+-ATPase*). These pumps transport H^+ ions uphill against a million-to-one concentration gradient into the lumen of the stomach while they transport K^+ ions in the opposite direction. Functions of HCl include:

- Activating pepsinogen, the precursor for the enzyme, pepsin
- Assisting in the breakdown of connective tissue and muscle fibers within the ingested food
- Killing of most types of microorganisms ingested with the food

Pepsinogen is produced by the *chief cells*. Within the lumen of the stomach, this precursor molecule is split by HCl to form the active enzyme, *pepsin*. Optimally active at an acidic pH (pH = 2), pepsin begins protein digestion by fragmenting the proteins into smaller peptide chains.

Mucus is produced by the *mucus neck cells* and by the *surface epithelial cells* of the stomach wall. A thick layer of mucus adheres to the wall of the stomach forming the *gastric mucosal barrier*. The function of this barrier is to protect the gastric mucosa from injury, specifically, from the corrosive actions of HCl and pepsin. Together with bicarbonate ions released into the lumen of the stomach, mucus neutralizes the acid and maintains the mucosal surface at a nearly neutral pH.

PHARMACY APPLICATION: DRUG-INDUCED GASTRIC DISEASE

In addition to their beneficial effects, some medications may cause cellular injury and disease. An example of this phenomenon involves nonsteroidal, anti-inflammatory drugs (NSAIDS). These drugs include aspirin (a derivative of salicylic acid), ibuprofen (arylpropionic acid; Advil®), and acetaminophen (para-aminophenol derivative; Tylenol®). Because of their beneficial pharmacological effects, the consumption of these agents has increased significantly in recent years. The NSAIDS

(Continued)

PHARMACY APPLICATION: DRUG-INDUCED GASTRIC DISEASE (Continued)

are used to treat fever, pain, acute inflammation, and chronic inflammatory diseases, such as arthritis. They are also used prophylactically to prevent heart disease, stroke, and colon cancer.

Unfortunately, frequent exposure to NSAIDS may also cause two detrimental effects. These agents inhibit the activity of cyclooxygenase, an important enzyme in the synthesis of gastroprotective prostaglandins. More importantly, NSAIDS may cause breaks in the gastric mucosal barrier. The normal gastric mucosa is relatively impermeable to H^+ ions. When the gastric mucosal barrier is weakened or damaged, H^+ ions leak into the mucosa in exchange for Na^+ ions. As H^+ ions accumulate in the mucosa, intracellular buffer systems become saturated, the pH decreases, and cell injury and cell death occur. These damaged cells then secrete more HCl, which causes more injury, and so on, resulting in a positive feedback cycle. An ulcer may form when injury from the gastric secretions, HCl and pepsin, overwhelms the ability of the mucosa to protect itself and replace damaged cells. Local capillaries are also damaged, causing bleeding or hemorrhage into the gastric lumen.

Intrinsic factor is produced by the *parietal cells*. Within the stomach, it combines with *vitamin B_{12}*, forming a complex required for the absorption of this B_{12} in the ileum of the small intestine. Vitamin B_{12} is an essential factor in the formation of red blood cells. Individuals unable to produce intrinsic factor cannot absorb vitamin B_{12} and, therefore, red blood cell production is impaired. This condition, referred to as *pernicious anemia*, occurs as the result of an autoimmune disorder that involves the destruction of parietal cells.

Gastrin is a hormone produced by gastric endocrine tissue, specifically, the G *cells* in the pyloric gland area. It is released into the blood and carried back to the stomach. The major function of gastrin is to enhance acid secretion by directly stimulating both parietal cells (HCl) and chief cells (pepsinogen). Gastrin also stimulates the local release of histamine from *enterochromaffin-like cells* in the wall of the stomach. *Histamine* stimulates parietal cells to release HCl.

There are three major phases of gastric secretion:

- Cephalic phase: 20%–30% of the gastric secretory response to a meal
- Gastric phase: 60%–70% of the gastric secretory response to a meal
- Intestinal phase: approximately 10% of the gastric secretory response to a meal

The *cephalic phase* of gastric secretion occurs before food even enters the stomach. Thoughts of food; sensory stimuli, such as the smell, sight or taste of food; and activities, such as chewing and swallowing, all enhance gastric secretion. The cephalic phase is mediated by the vagus nerve and gastrin, which is released in response to vagal stimulation. These mechanisms promote the secretion of HCl and pepsinogen.

The *gastric phase* is elicited by the presence of food in the stomach. Distension of the stomach wall as well as the presence of protein, caffeine and alcohol all enhance gastric secretion. This phase is mediated by the intrinsic nerves, the vagus nerve and gastrin. Each of these mechanisms promotes the secretion of HCl and pepsinogen. Other factors that influence gastric acid secretion include histamine (enhances) and somatostatin (inhibits).

PHARMACY APPLICATION: PHARMACOLOGICAL TREATMENT OF GASTRIC ULCERS

The pharmacological treatment of ulcers involves the inhibition of gastric acid secretion. However, more than one approach may be used to accomplish this goal: H_2-receptor antagonists and proton-pump inhibitors.

Histamine does not play a role in normal acid production. However, histamine may stimulate the release of HCl under pathological conditions. In the case of an ulcer, when H^+ ions enter the gastric mucosa, they stimulate the release of histamine from enterochromaffin-like cells. The histamine then stimulates H_2-receptors on the parietal cells to release more HCl. Therefore, excess acid release may be prevented with the administration of H_2-receptor antagonists, such as cimetidine (Tagamet®) and famotidine (Pepcid®). However, the inhibition of histamine-induced acid secretion is not adequate in all patients. More recently, proton-pump inhibitors, such as omeprazole (Prilosec®) and lansoprazole (Prevacid®), pantoprazole (Protonix®), and rabeprazole (Aciphex®) have been used in the treatment of ulcers and gastroesophageal reflux disease (GERD). These drugs bind irreversibly to the proton pump (H^+-K^+-ATPase), which is found only in the parietal cell. This causes permanent inhibition of enzyme activity. Thus, the secretion of H^+ ions into the lumen of the stomach is inhibited. The secretion of acid resumes only after new molecules of H^+-K^+-ATPase are inserted into the gastric mucosa.

The *intestinal phase* has two components that influence gastric secretion:

* Excitatory component
* Inhibitory component

The *excitatory component* involves the release of *intestinal gastrin*. This occurs in response to the presence of the products of protein digestion in the duodenum. Intestinal gastrin travels in the blood to the stomach, where it enhances the secretion of HCl and pepsinogen. The magnitude of this effect is very small, however, and accounts for approximately 10% of the acid secretory response to a meal.

In contrast to the excitatory component, the *inhibitory component* of the intestinal phase has a very strong influence on gastric secretion. As with gastric motility, the volume and composition of the chyme in the duodenum affect gastric secretion. Distension of the duodenal wall as well as the presence of lipids, acid and hyperosmotic chyme all inhibit secretion by way of the enterogastric reflex and the release of the enterogastrones.

9.7 Liver

The *liver* is the largest internal organ, weighing more than 1.5 kg (3.5–4.0 lbs.) in an adult. The blood flow to the liver is 1,350 mL/min (27% of the cardiac output) on average and comes from two sources:

- Hepatic artery
- Hepatic portal vein

The *hepatic artery* supplies the liver with 300 mL/min of oxygenated blood from the aorta. The remaining 1,050 mL/min of blood flow is delivered by the *hepatic portal vein*, a vessel that brings blood directly from the digestive tract. Although this blood is low in oxygen, it contains a high concentration of nutrients absorbed from the intestines.

The liver performs many important functions, including:

- Storage of blood
- Filtration of blood
- Storage of vitamins and iron
- Formation of blood coagulation factors
- Metabolism and excretion of certain drugs, bilirubin and hormones
- Metabolism of carbohydrates, proteins, and lipids
- Formation of bile

The liver is a large and distensible organ. As such, large quantities of blood may be stored in its blood vessels providing a *blood reservoir* function. Under normal physiological conditions, the hepatic veins and hepatic sinuses contain approximately 450 mL of blood, or almost 10% of the blood volume. When needed, a significant portion of this blood may be mobilized to increase venous return and cardiac output.

Blood flowing from the intestines to the liver through the hepatic portal vein often contains bacteria. *Filtration of this blood* is a protective function provided by the liver. Large phagocytic macrophages, referred to as *Kupffer cells*, line the hepatic venous sinuses. As the blood flows through these sinuses, bacteria are rapidly taken up and digested by the Kupffer cells. This system is very efficient and it removes more than 99% of the bacteria from the hepatic portal blood.

The liver serves as an important *storage site for vitamins and iron*. Sufficient quantities of several vitamins may be stored to prevent vitamin deficiency for some period:

- Vitamin A: up to 10 months
- Vitamin D: 3–4 months
- Vitamin B_{12}: at least 1 year

Iron is stored in the liver in the form of *ferritin*. When the level of circulating iron becomes low, ferritin releases iron into the blood.

Several substances that contribute to the *blood coagulation* process are formed in the liver. These include fibrinogen, prothrombin, and several of the blood clotting factors (II, VII, IX and X). Deficiency in any of these substances leads to impaired blood coagulation.

The liver is capable of *detoxifying or excreting into the bile many drugs,* such as sulfonamides (antibacterial drugs), penicillin, ampicillin, and erythromycin. *Bilirubin,* the major end-product of hemoglobin degradation, is also excreted in the bile. In addition, several *hormones* are metabolized by the liver including thyroid hormone and all the steroid hormones, such as estrogen, cortisol, and aldosterone.

In terms of nutrients, the liver is the most important metabolic organ in the body. It receives a large volume of nutrient-rich blood directly from the digestive tract that provides an abundant amount of substrates for metabolism. *Metabolic processes involving carbohydrates* include the following:

- Storage of a significant amount of glycogen
- Conversion of galactose and fructose into glucose
- Gluconeogenesis

Metabolic processes involving proteins include the following:

- Deamination of amino acids
- Formation of urea (for removal of ammonia from the body fluids)
- Formation of plasma proteins
- Conversion of amino acids into other amino acids and other essential compounds

Most cells in the body metabolize lipids; however, some processes of *fat metabolism* occur mainly in the liver. These include:

- Oxidation of fatty acids to supply energy for other body functions
- Synthesis of cholesterol, phospholipids and lipoproteins
- Synthesis of fat from proteins and carbohydrates

Another important product of liver metabolism is *bile*, which is necessary for the digestion and absorption of dietary lipids. Bile is an aqueous, alkaline fluid consisting of a complex mixture of organic and inorganic components. The major organic constituents of bile are the *bile salts*, which account for approximately 50% of the solid components. Derived from cholesterol, bile salts are *amphipathic molecules*. In other words, these molecules have a hydrophilic region and a hydrophobic region. Inorganic ions are also present in the bile and include Na^+, K^+, Ca^{++}, Cl^-, and HCO_3^- ions. The total number of cations exceeds the total number of anions.

Bile is produced continuously by the liver. The bile salts are secreted by the hepatocytes and the water, sodium bicarbonate, and other inorganic salts are added by the cells of the bile ducts within the liver. The bile is then transported by way of the *common bile duct* to the duodenum. Bile facilitates fat digestion and absorption throughout the length of the small intestine. In the terminal region of the ileum, the final segment of the small intestine, the bile salts are actively reabsorbed into the blood. They are then returned to the liver by way of the hepatic portal system and resecreted into the bile. This recycling of the bile salts from the small intestine back to the liver is referred to as the *enterohepatic circulation*.

Bile secretion by the liver is stimulated by the following:

• Bile salts
• Secretin
• Parasympathetic stimulation

The return of the *bile salts* to the liver from the small intestine is the most potent stimulus of bile secretion. In fact, these bile salts may cycle two to five times during each meal. The intestinal hormone, *secretin*, which is released in response to acid in the duodenum, enhances the aqueous alkaline secretion by the liver. Secretin has no effect on the secretion of bile salts. During the cephalic phase of digestion, before food even reaches the stomach or intestine, *parasympathetic stimulation*, by way of the vagus nerve, promotes bile secretion from the liver.

9.8 Gallbladder

The gallbladder is attached to the inferior surface of the liver. This pear-shaped organ is about 7–10 cm long. During a meal, bile enters the duodenum from the common bile duct through the *Sphincter of Oddi*. Between meals, this sphincter is closed to prevent the bile from entering the small intestine. Most of the bile secreted from the liver is backed up the common bile duct into the *cystic duct* and into the gallbladder. Because the gallbladder is a small organ, it can accommodate only 35–100 mL of bile when full.

Within the gallbladder, sodium is actively removed from the bile. Chloride follows the sodium down its electrical gradient and water follows osmotically and, therefore, the organic constituents of the bile are concentrated 5- to 20-fold. During a meal, when the bile is needed for digestion, the gallbladder contracts and the bile is squeezed out and into the duodenum. Contraction is elicited by *cholecystokinin*, an intestinal hormone released in response to the presence of chyme, especially lipids, in the duodenum.

9.9   Pancreas

The pancreas, which is about 12–15 cm long, is located behind the stomach along the posterior abdominal wall. Exocrine glands within the pancreas secrete an aqueous fluid referred to as pancreatic juice. The pancreas secretes approximately 1 L of this fluid per day. Pancreatic juice is alkaline and contains a high concentration of bicarbonate ions. It is transported to the duodenum by the pancreatic duct. Pancreatic juice neutralizes the acidic chyme entering the duodenum from the stomach. Neutralization not only prevents damage to the duodenal mucosa; it creates a neutral or slightly alkaline environment that is optimal for the function of pancreatic enzymes. The pancreas also secretes several enzymes that are involved in the digestion of carbohydrates, proteins and lipids.

There are three major phases of pancreatic secretion:

- Cephalic phase: approximately 20% of the pancreatic secretory response to a meal
- Gastric phase: 5%–10% of the pancreatic secretory response to a meal
- Intestinal phase: approximately 70%–80% of the pancreatic secretory response to a meal

As with gastric secretion, both nervous stimulation and hormones regulate secretion from the pancreas. During the *cephalic phase* and the *gastric phase*, the pancreas secretes a low-volume, enzyme-rich fluid. This secretion is mediated by the vagus nerve.

Most pancreatic secretion takes place during the *intestinal phase*. The intestinal hormone, *secretin*, stimulates the release of a large volume of pancreatic juice with a high concentration of bicarbonate ions. Secretin, "nature's antacid," is released in response to acidic chyme in the duodenum (maximal release at pH < 3.0). The intestinal hormone, *cholecystokinin*, is released in response to the presence of the products of protein and lipid digestion. Cholecystokinin then stimulates the release of digestive enzymes from the pancreas.

9.10   Transport of bile and pancreatic juice

Bile is secreted by the liver, stored in the gallbladder and used in the small intestine. It is transported toward the small intestine by the *hepatic duct* (from the liver) and the *cystic duct* (from the gallbladder), which join to form the *common bile duct*. Pancreatic juice is transported toward the small intestine by the *pancreatic duct.* The common bile duct and the pancreatic duct join to form the *hepatopancreatic ampulla,* which empties into the duodenum. The entrance to the duodenum is surrounded by the *Sphincter of Oddi.* This sphincter is closed between meals to prevent bile and pancreatic juice from entering the small intestine. The Sphincter of Oddi relaxes in response to the intestinal hormone, cholecystokinin, thus allowing biliary and pancreatic secretions to flow into the duodenum.

9.11   Small intestine

The small intestine is the longest (>3 m in a living human) and most convoluted organ in the digestive system. It is divided into three segments:

* Duodenum: first 20–30 cm
* Jejunum: next approximately two-fifths of the small intestine
* Ileum: remaining three-fifths of the small intestine

The small intestine is the region where most digestion and absorption take place. As such, the mucosa of the small intestine is well adapted for these functions with the following anatomical modifications:

* Plicae circulares
* Villi
* Microvilli

The *plicae circulares,* or circular folds, form internal rings around the circumference of the small intestine. These rings are found along the length of the small intestine. They are formed from inward foldings of the mucosal and submucosal layers of the intestinal wall. The plicae circulares are particularly well developed in the duodenum and jejunum and increase the absorptive surface area of the mucosa about three-fold.

Each plica is covered with millions of smaller projections of mucosa referred to as *villi.* Two types of epithelial cells cover the villi:

* Goblet cells
* Absorptive cells

The *goblet cells* produce mucus. The *absorptive cells,* found in a single layer covering the villi, are far more abundant. Taken together, the villi increase the absorptive surface area another 10-fold.

Microvilli are microscopic projections found on the luminal surface of the absorptive cells. Each absorptive cell may have literally thousands of microvilli forming the *brush border.* These structures increase the surface area for absorption another 20-fold. All together, these three anatomical adaptations of the intestinal mucosa, plicae circulares, villi, and microvilli, increase the surface area as much as 600-fold, which has a profound positive effect on the absorptive process.

9.11.1   Motility of the small intestine

Both segmentation and peristalsis take place in the small intestine. *Segmentation* mixes the chyme with the digestive juices and exposes the chyme to the intestinal mucosa for absorption. This form of motility causes only a small degree of forward movement of the chyme along the small intestine. *Peristalsis*, a wave-like form of muscle contraction, primarily moves chyme along the intestine and causes only a small amount of mixing. These contractions are weak and slow in the small intestine. In this way, there is sufficient time for complete digestion and absorption of the chyme as it moves forward. Intestinal peristaltic contractions are normally limited to short distances (1–4 cm).

Segmentation contractions occur as the result of the *basic electrical rhythm* (*BER*) of the pacemaker cells in the small intestine. This form of muscular activity is slight or absent between meals. The motility of the small intestine may be enhanced during a meal by the following:

- Distension of the small intestine
- Gastrin
- Extrinsic nerve stimulation

During a meal, segmentation occurs initially in the duodenum and the ileum. The movement of chyme into the intestine and the *distension of the duodenum* elicit segmentation contractions in this segment of the small intestine. Segmentation of the empty ileum is caused by *gastrin* released in response to distension of the stomach. This mechanism is referred to as the *gastroileal reflex*. *Parasympathetic stimulation*, by way of the vagus nerve, further enhances segmentation. *Sympathetic stimulation* inhibits this activity.

9.11.2   Digestion and absorption in the small intestine

Most digestion and absorption of carbohydrates, proteins, and lipids occurs in the small intestine. A summary of the digestive enzymes involved in these processes is found in Table 9.3.

9.11.3   Carbohydrates

Approximately 50% of the human diet is composed of starch. Other major dietary carbohydrates include the disaccharides, sucrose (30%, table sugar, composed of glucose and fructose) and lactose (6%, milk sugar, composed of glucose and galactose). Starch is initially acted upon by amylase. *Salivary amylase* starts the breakdown of starch molecules in the mouth and within

Table 9.3 Digestive enzymes

Nutrient molecule	Enzyme	Action of enzyme	Source of enzyme	Site of action
		Carbohydrate		
Polysaccharide (Starch)	Amylase	Fragment polysaccharides into disaccharides (maltose)	Salivary glands, pancreas	Mouth, stomach, small intestine
Disaccharides	Disaccharidases (maltase, lactase, sucrase)	Hydrolyze disaccharides into monosaccharides (glucose, galactose, fructose)	Absorptive cells of small intestine	Brush border of absorptive cells
		Protein		
Protein (Long Peptide Chain)	Pepsin	Fragment proteins into smaller peptides	Stomach chief cells	Stomach
Peptides	Trypsin, chymotrypsin, carboxypeptidase	Hydrolyze peptides into di- and tripeptides	Pancreas	Small intestine
Di- and Tripeptides	Aminopeptidases	Hydrolyze di- and tripeptides into amino acids	Absorptive cells of small intestine	Brush border of absorptive cells
		Lipid		
Triglyceride	Lingual lipase[a]	Hydrolyze triglycerides into monoglycerides and free fatty acids	Salivary glands	Mouth, stomach
	Pancreatic lipase	Hydrolyze triglycerides into monoglycerides and free fatty acids	Pancreas	Small intestine

[a] The role of lingual lipase in the digestion of dietary lipids is minor: It accounts for less than 10% of the enzymatic breakdown of triglycerides.

the stomach, until HCl denatures the enzyme. *Pancreatic amylase* carries on this activity in the small intestine. Amylase fragments polysaccharides into disaccharides (maltose, composed of two glucose molecules).

The disaccharide molecules, primarily maltose, are presented to the brush border of the absorptive cells. As the disaccharides are absorbed, *disaccharidases* (maltase, sucrase, and lactase) split these nutrient molecules into monosaccharides (glucose, fructose and galactose).

Glucose and galactose enter the absorptive cells by way of *secondary active transport.* Cotransport carrier molecules associated with the disaccharidases in the brush border transport both the monosaccharide and a Na^+ ion from the lumen of the small intestine into the absorptive cell. This process is referred to as "secondary" because the cotransport carriers, themselves, operate passively and do not require energy. However, they do require a concentration gradient for the transport of Na^+ ions into the cell. This gradient is established by the active transport of Na^+ ions out of the absorptive cell at the basolateral surface.

Fructose enters the absorptive cells by way of facilitated diffusion. All monosaccharide molecules exit the absorptive cells by way of facilitated diffusion and enter the blood capillaries.

The ability of the human small intestine to absorb free sugars is quite remarkable. It has been estimated that hexoses equivalent to 22 pounds of sucrose can be absorbed daily. There appears to be little physiologic regulation of sugar absorption.

9.11.4   Proteins

Protein digestion begins in the stomach by the action of the gastric enzyme, *pepsin*. This enzyme fragments large protein molecules into smaller peptide chains. Digestion is continued in the small intestine by the pancreatic enzymes, *trypsin, chymotrypsin,* and *carboxypeptidase.* Similar to pepsin (pepsinogen), these enzymes are secreted as inactive precursors (trypsinogen, chymotrypsinogen and procarboxypeptidase). The intestinal enzyme *enterokinase* activates trypsin at the brush border. Trypsin then activates chymotrypsin and carboxypeptidase. These pancreatic enzymes hydrolyze the peptide chains into amino acids (40%), as well as dipeptides and tripeptides (60% combined).

As seen with glucose and galactose, the amino acids enter the absorptive cells by way of secondary active transport. Once again, energy is expended to pump Na^+ ions out of the absorptive cells, creating a concentration gradient for the cotransport of amino acids and Na^+ ions into the cell.

Dipeptides and tripeptides are also presented to the brush border of the absorptive cells. As the nutrient molecules are absorbed, aminopeptidases split them into their constituent amino acids. The activity of the *aminopeptidases* accounts for approximately 60% of protein digestion. The amino acid molecules then exit the absorptive cells by way of facilitated diffusion and enter the blood capillaries.

9.11.5   Lipids

Dietary fat consists primarily of triglycerides. Fat digestion begins in the mouth and stomach by the action of the salivary enzyme, lingual lipase. However, the role of this enzyme is minor given that it accounts for less than 10% of the enzymatic breakdown of triglycerides. *Gastric lipase* is also responsible for a very small degree of lipid digestion.

Lipids are digested primarily in the small intestine. The first step in this process involves the action of the *bile salts* contained in the bile. Bile salts cause *emulsification*, which is the dispersal of large fat droplets into a suspension of smaller droplets (<1 μm). This process creates a significantly increased surface area upon which fat-digesting enzymes can act.

Intact triglycerides are too large to be absorbed. Therefore, *pancreatic lipase* acts on the lipid droplets to hydrolyze the triglyceride molecules into *monoglycerides* and *free fatty acids*. These constituent molecules are water-insoluble and would tend to float on the surface of the aqueous chyme. Therefore, they must be transported to the absorptive surface. This process is carried out by *micelles*, which are sphere-like structures formed by the amphipathic bile salts. The bile salts associate with each other such that the polar region of the molecules orient outward, making them water-soluble. The nonpolar region faces inward, away from the surrounding water. The monoglycerides and free fatty acids are carried in this interior region of the micelle. Upon reaching the brush border of the absorptive cells, the monoglycerides and free fatty acids leave the micelles and enter the cells by simple diffusion. Because they are nonpolar, these molecules move passively through the lipid bilayer of the cell membrane. This process takes place primarily in the jejunum and proximal ileum. The bile salts are absorbed in the distal ileum by way of either passive diffusion or secondary active transport.

Within the absorptive cells, the monoglycerides and free fatty acids are transported to the endoplasmic reticulum, which contains the necessary enzymes to resynthesize these substances into triglycerides. The newly synthesized triglycerides then move to the Golgi apparatus. Within this organelle, they are packaged in a lipoprotein coat consisting of phospholipids, cholesterol, and apoproteins. These protein-coated lipid globules, referred to as *chylomicrons*, are now water-soluble. Approximately 90% of the chylomicron consists of triglycerides.

Chylomicrons leave the absorptive cell by way of exocytosis. Because they are unable to cross the basement membrane of the blood capillaries, the chylomicrons enter the *lacteals*, which are part of the lymphatic system. The vessels of the lymphatic system converge to form the thoracic duct, which drains into the venous system near the heart. Therefore, unlike the products of carbohydrate and protein digestion that are transported directly to the liver by way of the hepatic portal vein, absorbed lipids are diluted in the blood of the circulatory system before they reach the liver. This dilution of the lipids prevents the liver from being overwhelmed with more fat than it can process at one time.

9.11.6　Water and electrolytes

Each day in an average adult, about 5.5 L of food and fluids move from the stomach to the small intestine as chyme. An additional 3.5 L of pancreatic and intestinal secretions produce a total of 9 L of material in the lumen. Most of this ($\geq$7.5 L) is absorbed from the small intestine. The absorption of nutrient molecules, which takes place primarily in the duodenum and jejunum, creates an osmotic gradient for the passive absorption of water.

Sodium may be absorbed either passively or actively. Passive absorption occurs when the electrochemical gradient favors the movement of Na^+ between the absorptive cells through "leaky" tight junctions. Sodium is actively absorbed by way of transporters in the absorptive cell membrane. One type of transporter carries a Na^+ ion and a Cl^- ion into the cell. Another carries a Na^+ ion, a K^+ ion, and two Cl^- ions into the cell.

9.12　Large intestine

The *large intestine* is the region of the digestive tract from the ileocecal valve to the anus. Approximately 1.5 m in length, this organ has a larger diameter than the small intestine. The mucosa of the large intestine is composed of absorptive cells and mucus-secreting goblet cells. The mucosal layer of the large intestine imitates the small intestine in that it contains lymphatic nodules to protect against microbial infection. In contrast to the small intestine, the mucosa in this organ does not form villi.

The large intestine consists of the following structures:

- Cecum
- Appendix
- Colon
- Rectum

The *cecum*, which is the most proximal portion of the large intestine, receives chyme from the ileum of the small intestine through the *ileocecal valve*. The *appendix*, the small projection at the bottom of the cecum, is a lymphoid tissue. This tissue contains lymphocytes and assists in the defense against bacteria that enter the body through the digestive system.

The largest portion of the large intestine is the *colon*. It consists of four regions: ascending colon (travels upward toward the diaphragm on the right side of the abdomen), transverse colon (crosses the abdomen under the diaphragm), descending colon (travels downward through the abdomen on the left side), and the sigmoid colon (S-shaped region found in the lower abdomen). The sigmoid colon is continuous with the *rectum*, which leads to the external surface of the body through the *anus*.

The large intestine typically receives 500–1500 mL of chyme from the small intestine per day. As discussed, most digestion and absorption has already taken place in the small intestine. In fact, there are no digestive enzymes produced by the large intestine. At this point in the human digestive tract, the chyme consists of indigestible food residues (e.g., cellulose), unabsorbed biliary components, and any remaining fluid. Therefore, the two major functions of the large intestine are:

- Drying
- Storage

The colon absorbs most of the water and salt from the chyme resulting in this *"drying"* or concentrating process. The absorption of water occurs passively down its osmotic gradient, following the active transport of ions, resulting in only about 100 mL of water being lost through this route daily. The remaining contents, now referred to as *feces*, are *"stored"* in the large intestine until they can be eliminated by way of defecation.

In addition to water, the large intestine also absorbs electrolytes, several B complex vitamins and vitamin K. The normally occurring bacteria, also referred to as *microflora*, that reside in the large intestine produce vitamin K and folic acid, which are then absorbed.

9.12.1   Motility of the large intestine

The longitudinal layer of smooth muscle in the small intestine is continuous. In the large intestine, this layer of muscle is concentrated into three flat bands referred to as *taniae coli*. Furthermore, the large intestine appears to be subdivided into a chain of pouches or sacs referred to as *haustra*. The haustra are formed because the bands of *taniae coli* are shorter than the underlying circular layer of smooth muscle and causes the colon to bunch up.

Movements through the large intestine are typically quite sluggish. It will often take 18–24 hours for materials to pass through its entire length. The primary form of motility in the large intestine is *haustral contractions*, or *haustrations*. These contractions are produced by the inherent rhythmicity of smooth muscle cells in the colon. Haustrations, which result in the pronounced appearance of the haustra, replicate the segmentation contractions seen within the small intestine. Haustrations are *nonpropulsive* and serve primarily to slowly move the contents back and forth, exposing them to the absorptive surface.

In contrast to segmentation contractions in the small intestine (9–12 per min), haustral contractions occur much less frequently (up to 30 min between contractions). These very slow movements allow for the growth of *bacteria* in the large intestine. Normally, the bacterial flora in this region is harmless, unless it enters the bloodstream, such as would result from eating tainted food due to unsanitary processing and preparation.

A second form of motility in the large intestine is the *mass movement*. Three or four times per day, typically after a meal, a strong propulsive contraction occurs that moves a substantial bolus of chyme forward toward the distal portion of the colon. Mass movements may result in the sudden distension of the rectum that elicits the defecation reflex.

9.12.2   Secretion of the large intestine

The large intestine produces an *alkaline mucus secretion*. The function of this secretion is to protect the mucosa from mechanical or chemical injury. *Mucus* provides lubrication to facilitate the movement of the contents of the lumen. *Bicarbonate ions* neutralize the irritating acids produced by the local bacterial fermentation. Colonic secretion increases in response to mechanical or chemical stimuli. The mechanism of the enhanced secretion involves both intrinsic nerve and vagal nerve reflexes.

9.13   Gastrointestinal disorders

Gastrointestinal diseases include a diverse range of disorders that may be localized to a particular structure or gastrointestinal organ or may be generalized throughout the gastrointestinal tract. Gastroesophageal reflux disease (GERD) is the most common gastrointestinal disorder, while colorectal cancer accounts for more than half of all gastrointestinal cancers and is the leading cause of gastrointestinal-related mortality (Peery et al., 2012). Many gastrointestinal disorders share a number of general symptoms that are listed in Table 9.4.

9.13.1   Abnormalities of the esophagus

The esophagus is a flexible muscular tube that conveys food from the throat to the stomach.

9.13.1.1   Swallowing disorders—dysphagia
- Difficulty swallowing that may be caused by obstruction of the esophagus or impaired motility of the esophageal walls
- Obstruction may be caused by neck tumors, congenital narrowing or esophageal diverticula (see below)
- Neuromuscular disorders such as stroke or brain injury may impair the cranial nerves that are involved in swallowing

Table 9.4   General symptoms of gastrointestinal disease

- Anorexia—loss of appetite
- Nausea
- Vomiting
- Diarrhea, constipation
- Bleeding—obvious or "occult"

1. *Achalasia*
   - A condition caused by failure of the LES (cardiac sphincter) to relax and allow food to enter the stomach. It may be related to defects in neural input to the esophagus.
   - Achalasia is a chronic condition that causes distention of the lower esophagus that may lead to chronic inflammation and eventual ulceration of the esophagus.
   - The condition presents with dysphagia, vomiting, and chest pain that is often exacerbated by eating.
   - Aspiration of trapped esophageal contents into the lungs is a significant concern when the patient is lying down.

2. *Esophageal Diverticula*
   - Diverticula are small pockets that form in the esophageal walls. They occur most frequently from congenital weakness of the esophagus walls.
   - Food can easily become trapped in a diverticulum, leading to inflammation and infection of the esophagus with possible ulceration.

3. *Mallory-Weiss Syndrome*
   - A condition in which longitudinal tears occur in the walls of the lower esophagus.
   - Most commonly occurs after an episode of severe vomiting (i.e., alcoholism, acute illness).
   - May be associated with acute bleeding and esophageal injury

9.13.1.1.1   *Gastroesophageal reflux disease (GERD)*
- Gastroesophageal reflux is a condition caused by the backflow of stomach contents into the lower esophagus.
- It results from weakness or incompetence of the LES that normally blocks reflux of stomach contents into the esophagus.
- Because of their high acid content (low pH), reflux of stomach contents will cause irritation and inflammation of the esophagus (*esophagitis*) that can lead to ulceration of the esophagus.
- A *hiatal hernia* may also cause gastroesophageal reflux. A hiatal hernia is a condition in which the top of the stomach protrudes up through the opening of the diaphragm.

9.13.1.2   *Manifestations of GERD*
- Burning pain in the epigastric region ("heartburn") that may be worsened by alcohol consumption, caffeine, smoking, exercise, and obesity; lying down may exacerbate reflux

- Esophagitis, possible ulceration of esophagus
- *Barrett's esophagus*—strictures and scaring that can result from chronic inflammation of the esophageal walls; can lead to narrowing of the esophagus with subsequent dysphagia (see Figure 9.2)

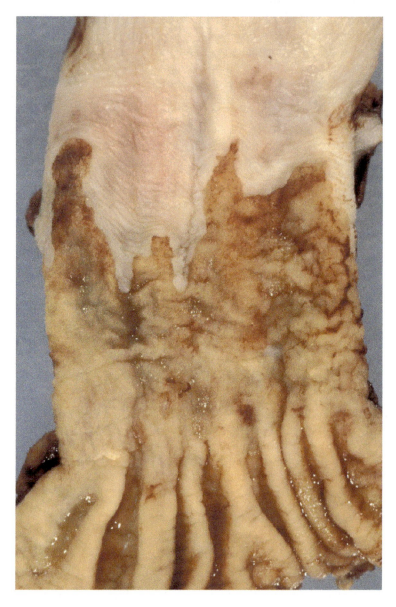

Figure 9.2 Barrett's esophagus image. (Adapted from *Porth's Pathophysiology: Concepts of Altered Health States* by Grossman, Lippincott Williams and Wilkins, 2013.)

- Dysphagia, poor nutrition
- Possible increased risk of esophageal cancer with chronic esophagitis and Barrett's esophagus

9.13.1.3   Treatment of GERD
- Consumption of frequent small meals rather than large ones
- Sleep with head elevated
- Avoid fatty meals, chocolate and caffeine, all of which may affect gastric emptying
- Consumption of fluids with meals to wash food out of esophagus
- Use of antacids or proton-pump inhibitors (see Table 9.5) to reduce pH of stomach contents
- Surgery if a hiatal hernia is present

9.13.2   Disorders of the stomach

9.13.2.1   Gastritis
- Gastritis is a condition in which there is inflammation of the gastric mucosa (stomach lining)
- It may present as an acute or chronic disorder

9.13.2.1.1   Acute gastritis
- Transient irritation and inflammation of the stomach lining
- May be caused by factors such as alcohol consumption, aspirin or NSAID use, and stress

Table 9.5   Drugs for treatment of peptic ulcer disease

Antibiotics for eradication of *H. pylori*:
- Three-drug combination that may include two antibiotics such as clarithromycin, amoxicillin or metronidazole plus a proton-pump inhibitor

Antacids (e.g., *magnesium hydroxide, aluminum hydroxide*):
- Act by neutralizing gastric acid and raising gastric pH
- Possible unwanted effects may include diarrhea or constipation

H_2 Receptor Antagonists (e.g., *Ranitidine, Cimetidine*):
- Inhibit the action of histamine at H_2 receptors to inhibit gastric acid secretion
- Unwanted effects may include diarrhea, muscle pain and rashes

Proton-Pump Inhibitors (e.g., *Omeprazole*):
- Block the intestinal H^+-K^+-ATPase pump to inhibit gastric acid secretion
- Unwanted effects may include headache, diarrhea and rashes

Mucosal Protective Agents (e.g., *Bismuth, Sucralfate*):
- Enhance the mucosal protective barriers or provide an additional physical barrier over the surface of the gastrointestinal tract
- Few side effects but may include constipation

- The inflammation associated with acute gastritis is a self-limiting process that does not usually result in long-term injury to the gastric mucosa

9.13.2.1.2 Chronic gastritis
- Chronic irritation and inflammation of the stomach lining
- May be cause by bacterial infection with *H. pylori*, alcohol abuse, or long-term aspirin and NSAID use
- Can lead to atrophy and ulceration of the gastric mucosa

9.13.2.2 Peptic ulcers (Figure 9.3)

The term *peptic ulcer* refers to erosion of the mucosa lining of any portion of the gastrointestinal tract. If the ulcer occurs in the stomach lining, it is specifically referred to as a *gastric ulcer*. In the United States, most ulcers occur in the duodenum and in elderly patients. *Causes of peptic ulcer disease include*:

- Infection with the bacteria *H. pylori*, which occurs in 80%–95% of patients with peptic ulcer disease. The mechanism by which *H. pylori* infection leads to peptic ulcers is shown in the figure below.
- Injury or death of mucus-producing cells.
- Excess acid production in the stomach. The hormone *gastrin* stimulates the production of acid in the stomach; therefore, any factors that increase gastrin production will in turn increase the production of stomach acid. See box on *Zollinger-Ellison syndrome*.
- Chronic use of aspirin and NSAIDs. Prostaglandins produced in the gut have a protective effect in that they increase mucus and bicarbonate production and increase blood flow to the gastric mucosa. Both aspirin and NSAIDs inhibit the production of prostaglandins in the gut. Aspirin and NSAIDs are also chemically corrosive to the gastric mucosa.

9.13.2.2.1 Stress ulcers   Prolonged physiologic stress can also lead to the formation of ulcers in the gastrointestinal tract. These *"stress ulcers"* may

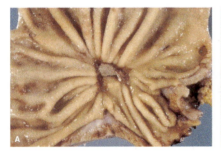
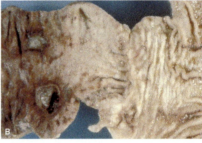

Figure 9.3 Section of the intestine affected by ulcerative colitis. (a) Gastric ulcer; (b) Duodenal ulcer (Adapted from *Porth's Pathophysiology: Concepts of Altered Health States* by Grossman, Lippincott Williams and Wilkins, 2013.)

result from altered gastrointestinal blood flow and increased acid secretion. Patients at risk for the development of stress ulcers include those with severe trauma, sepsis, burn injury or respiratory distress syndrome. *Cushing ulcers* are a specific form of peptic ulcer seen in patients with brain injury. They are likely caused by excessive stimulation of the vagal nerve that enhances acid production and decreased blood flow to the gastric mucosa.

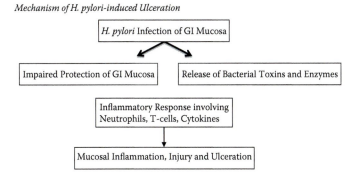

Mechanism of H. pylori-induced Ulceration

ZOLLINGER-ELLISON SYNDROME

- Tumors of the gastrin-secreting endocrine cells of the pancreas or less frequently the duodenal wall
- Because gastrin stimulates acid production in the gut, high gastrin levels lead to excessive acid production, which can lead to GERD and peptic ulceration
- Complications may include gastrointestinal perforation, hemorrhage, and obstruction
- The gastrin-producing tumors are malignant in nearly half of the cases diagnosed and can metastasize

---

9.13.2.2.1.1 Manifestations of Peptic Ulcer Disease
- Episodes of remission and exacerbation
- Pain that is often worse on an empty stomach and often relieved by food or antacids

9.13.2.2.1.2 Complications of Peptic Ulcers
- Complications of peptic ulcer disease may include gastrointestinal bleeding and possible hemorrhage (20%–25% of patients). Bleeding may be occult or may present as melena or hematemesis
- Perforation of ulcers is possible and can lead to peritonitis due to the leakage of gastrointestinal contents into the abdomen. Mortality rates associated with ulcer perforation are very significant

9.13.2.2.1.3   Diagnosis of Peptic Ulcers

- Presentation of clinical symptoms
- Endoscopy to visualize ulcers and biopsy for the presence of *H. pylori*
- X-ray with barium contrast
- Breath test for CO_2 production: patients swallow a urea capsule and the amount of CO_2 produced by bacterial activity is measured in the exhaled air

9.13.2.2.1.4   Treatment of Peptic Ulcer Disease

- Avoidance of alcohol, smoking and NSAIDs
- Antibiotic therapy has been shown to be highly effective in eradicating *H. pylori* in the vast majority of patients. The current standard for the treatment of *H. pylori*-related ulcers is administration of antibiotics to eradicate the organism in conjunction with a proton-pump inhibitor to reduce the production of acid. This treatment regimen can lead to complete healing of the ulcers
- Antacids, H_2 antagonists, proton-pump inhibitors
- Mucosal protectants

9.13.3   Disorders of the intestines

9.13.3.1   Irritable bowel syndrome (IBS)

- IBS may be one of the most common gastrointestinal disorders. It is most common in young and middle-aged women
- Patients present with symptoms of gastrointestinal pain, gas, bloating, and altered bowel function (diarrhea-predominate or constipation-predominate). Symptoms may be localized to the lower intestine and colon and are often relieved by defecation
- No underlying pathophysiologic processes have yet to be identified in these patients. Bowel hyperreactivity and excessive motility of the bowels may be contributing factors
- Emotional factors, stress and certain foods may exacerbate the symptoms
- Treatment may include psychological counseling, dietary changes such as increased fiber consumption. Agents that affect various serotonin receptors in the gastrointestinal tract have been used in more severe cases of IBS. Anti-diarrheal, anticholinergic, and antispasmodic agents might also be of value

9.13.3.2   Inflammatory bowel disease

The term inflammatory bowel disease (IBD) includes the conditions *Crohn's disease (CD)* and *ulcerative colitis (UC)*. Both of these diseases are characterized

Table 9.6   Comparison of key characteristics in crohn's disease and ulcerative colitis

Characteristic	Crohn's disease	Ulcerative colitis
Peak Age of Onset	20–30 years of age	15–25 years of age
Areas Affected	Colon and rectum	Large and small intestine
Inflammation	Skin lesions	Continuous
Involvement	Mainly mucosa	Mainly submucosa
Bloody Stool	Rarely evident	Common
Diarrhea	Common	Common
Malabsorption	Common	Rare
Abdominal Pain	Common	Common
Fistulae, Abscesses	Common	Rare
Clinical Course	Exacerbation and remission	Exacerbation and remission
Cancer Risk	Uncertain?	Increased

by chronic inflammation of various regions of the gastrointestinal tract (see Table 9.6). In the United States, it is currently estimated that approximately 1–1.3 million people suffer from IBD (CDC Website, CDC.gov).

9.13.3.2.1   Crohn's disease (CD)

- Although the exact etiology of Crohn's disease in unknown, there appears to be a significant genetic component. Several gene mutations such as *CARD15/NOD2, IBD3, IBD5, and IBD10* have been linked to the development of CD. Much recent interest has focused on the possible role of pro-inflammatory *cytokines* in the pathogenesis of this disorder.
- Distribution of Crohn's disease shows a distinct predisposition to certain populations including Jews and individuals from the United States, Western Europe and Scandinavia. The disease often presents in the late teens to early twenties and is present for the life of the patient with intermittent periods of remission and exacerbation.
- The disease may affect any region of the gastrointestinal tract but is most commonly seen in the distal ileum and colon.
- Although CD affects all layers of the bowel, the inflammation is particularly evident in the *submucosal* layer of the intestine. The pattern of inflammation seen is a *granulomatous inflammation* with distinct "cobblestone" appearance to the mucosa. The inflammatory lesions are not constant along the length of the intestine but rather present with a "skip" pattern that intersperses areas of inflammation with normal looking, non-inflamed tissue (see Figure 9.4).

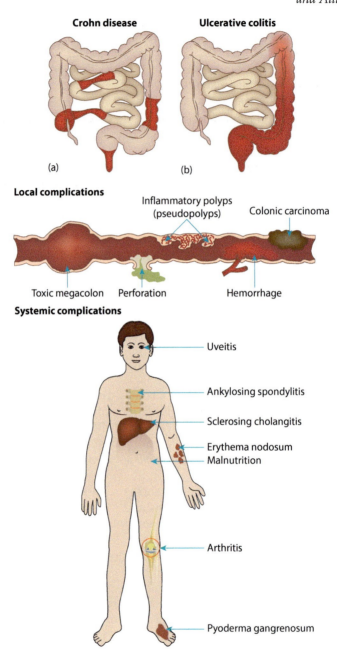

Figure 9.4   Local and systemic complications of Crohn's disease. (a) Crohn disease can affect both the large and small intestine; (b) Ulcerative colitis affects the distal colon. (Adapted from *Porth's Pathophysiology: Concepts of Altered Health States* by Grossman, Lippincott Williams and Wilkins, 2013.)

9.13.3.2.1.1   Manifestations of Crohn's disease

- Periods of exacerbation and remission
- Diarrhea, blood is usually not evident in the stool but may be occult (i.e., detected by clinical assay)
- Intestinal pain similar to indigestion
- Fever
- Weight loss and nutritional deficiency that may be related to impaired nutrient absorption from the small intestine
- Nausea, anorexia, vomiting
- Complications may include intestinal obstruction, abscess formation and the development of *fistulas* (abnormal connections between the intestines and possibly other abdominal organs). Radiographic contrast studies may be used to determine if fistulae are present

9.13.3.2.1.2   Treatment of Crohn's disease

- Nutritional supplementation to offset the poor nutrition that can result from anorexia and intestinal malabsorption. Total parenteral nutrition may be indicated in severe cases
- Anti-inflammatory (e.g., sulfasalazine) and immunomodulatory drugs (e.g., corticosteroids, azathioprine, methotrexate). Monoclonal antibody drugs such as infliximab that block inflammatory cytokines such as TNF-α have also been shown to be effective in treating IBD

9.13.3.2.2   Ulcerative colitis (see Figure 9.5)

- Inflammatory disease that affects the colon and rectum

Ulcerative colitis

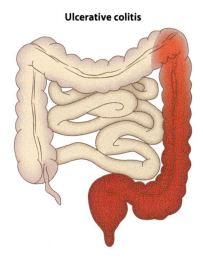

Figure 9.5   Ulcerative colitis.

- Although the exact etiology of UC is unknown, genetic and immunological factors are likely contributors to the disease. Abnormal T-cell activity, excess cytokine production and the formation of antibodies against colonic epithelial cells have been documented in patients with UC. Individuals between 20 and 40 years of age are most susceptible, particularly those with a family history of UC or those of Jewish descent
- The disease primarily affects the *mucosal* layer of the large intestine
- Unlike Crohn's disease the pattern of inflammation is continuous throughout the affected area
- UC, similar to Crohn's disease, also presents with periods or remission and exacerbation

9.13.3.2.2.1   *Manifestations of ulcerative colitis*
- Chronic, bloody diarrhea
- Fever, pain, anorexia, weakness
- Possible iron deficiency anemia from chronic blood loss
- Possible complications may include *toxic megacolon* (see Box), perforation of the intestine, significant blood loss. An increased incidence of colon cancer has also been documented in patients with UC

TOXIC MEGACOLON

- Life-threatening distention of the colon
- May lead to perforation of the colon, septicemia, and peritonitis
- Mortality associated with a perforated colon is on the order of 40% or more

---

9.13.3.2.2.2   *Treatment of ulcerative colitis*
- Anti-inflammatory (e.g., sulfasalazine) and immunomodulatory drugs (e.g., corticosteroids, azathioprine, methotrexate). Monoclonal antibody drugs such as infliximab that block inflammatory cytokines such as TNF-α have also been shown to be effective in treating UC
- Nicotine appears to exert a protective effect in UC but not Crohn's disease
- Surgical resection of diseased bowel may be required

9.13.3.2.3   *Diagnosis of IBD*
- Patient history and physical examination
- Sigmoidoscopy, colonoscopy, biopsy

9.13.3.2.4   Systemic manifestations of IBD   A significant percentage of patients with Crohn's disease or UC may present with systemic symptoms such as polyarthritis, cutaneous lesions, hepatobiliary effects and uveitis.

The cause of these systemic manifestations is uncertain but may be related to excess inflammation or immune activity.

     9.13.3.2.4.1 Diverticular disease (see Figure 9.6) A condition characterized by the presence of *diverticula*, which are multiple saclike protrusions of the colonic mucosa. *True diverticulum* involves all layers of the intestinal wall, whereas *false diverticulum* only involves the muscularis layer. Diverticular disease occurs with increased frequency in patients over 60 years of age and may be related to age-related changes in the bowel as well as diet. Individuals who consume a low-fiber, low-bulk diet also appear at greater risk for the formation of diverticula formation.

   9.13.3.2.5 Manifestations of diverticular disease
- Many instances are asymptotic. Most cases of diverticula are first identified during routine diagnostic testing such as colonoscopy
- Changes in bowel habits
- Excess flatulence
- A possible serious complication of diverticular disease might be infection or inflammation of the diverticula (*diverticulitis*) due to trapping of intestinal contents and accumulation of intestinal contents in the diverticula. This may lead to eventual perforation of the intestinal wall and sepsis

   9.13.3.2.6 Treatment of diverticular disease
- Increase bulk and fiber in the diet
- Antibiotics if diverticulitis is present

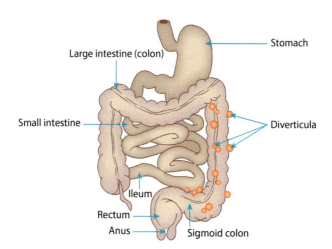

Figure 9.6   Diverticula disease. (Adapted from *Porth's Pathophysiology: Concepts of Altered Health States* by Grossman, Lippincott Williams and Wilkins, 2013.)

9.13.4   Disorders of intestinal motility and absorption

Peristalsis is the wave-like contraction of smooth muscle that is responsible for propelling contents through the gastrointestinal tract. Gastrointestinal motility is regulated by the enteric nervous systems as well as by a number of local acting gastrointestinal hormones such as gastrin, secretin, glucagon-like peptide-1 and motilin. Changes in intestinal motility as well alterations in colonic absorption of fluids and electrolytes may result in *diarrhea* or *constipation*. Although many individuals may experience normal fluctuations in bowel activity, prolonged episodes of diarrhea or constipation may be indicative of a more serious underlying disorder.

9.13.4.1   Diarrhea

Diarrhea is the excessive passage of stools and may be an acute or chronic condition. Acute diarrhea is most commonly caused by infectious organisms such as bacteria and viruses. Bacterial toxins can stimulate the secretion of fluids into the intestines and cause a *secretory diarrhea*. Overload of the intestine with nonabsorbable substances such as sorbitol or lactose in lactase-deficient individuals can lead to *osmotic diarrhea*. Chronic diarrhea may occur in patients with IBD or malabsorption disorders.

9.13.4.1.1   Manifestations of diarrhea
- Cramping pain
- Dehydration
- Bloody stools may be observed if inflammation is present
- Electrolyte imbalance
- Metabolic acidosis due to intestinal bicarbonate losses
- Impaired digestion and intestinal absorption

9.13.4.1.2   Treatment of diarrhea
- Restoration of fluids and electrolytes
- Antibiotics if the cause is bacterial in origin
- Drugs such as loperamide or diphenoxylate can be used to decrease intestinal secretions and motility

9.13.4.2   Constipation

Constipation is a condition that is characterized by difficult or infrequent defecation. A number of factors such as low-fiber diet, low fluid intake, and inactivity can cause acute episodes of constipation. Chronic forms of constipation may occur in patients with neurologic disease or spinal cord injury. *Hirschsprung disease* is a condition in which the ganglion cells in the large intestine do not develop properly during gestation. Patients with this condition suffer from very poor colonic motility and severe constipation. Drugs such as opioids and anticholinergic agents can also cause significant constipation. Treatment of constipation focuses mainly on increasing fluid and fiber intake as well as increasing activity. Laxative drugs may also be used with care to treat acute constipation.

9.13.4.3 Intestinal malabsorption

The absorption of most nutrients (fats, carbohydrates, amino acids) and a number of vitamins occurs primarily in the small intestine. Malabsorption occurs when the absorption of these nutrients from the gut is defective. Intestinal malabsorption may be caused by pancreatic disorders because pancreatic enzymes released into the intestine are important for converting nutrients into forms that are readily absorbed by the intestine. Other conditions that can cause intestinal malabsorption include:

9.13.4.3.1 Lactase deficiency

- Congenital lack of *lactase* enzyme in the intestinal brush border leads to lactose intolerance. Ingested lactose, which is normally metabolized to monosaccharides by lactase, is not absorbed from the gut and remains there to be acted upon by bacteria. The result is flatuance, intestinal irritation and osmotic diarrhea. Avoidance of dietary lactose will prevent the symptoms.

9.13.4.3.1.1 Celiac disease

- An immune-mediated disorder caused by the ingestion of gluten-containing grains. Clinical manifestations include marked intestinal inflammation, intestinal malabsorption, abdominal pain, and diarrhea. A gluten-free diet is indicated for patients diagnosed with celiac disease.

9.13.4.3.1.2 Bile salt deficiency

- Bile salts are produced by the liver from cholesterol and stored in the gallbladder. They are released into the duodenum in response to food intake. Their main action is to emulsify dietary fats so they may easily cross the brush border of the intestine. Conditions such as liver disease or obstruction of the bile ducts can affect the production and release of bile salts, respectively. The resulting malabsorption of fats can lead to *steatorrhea*. Because the absorption of fat-soluble vitamins such as A, D, K, and E may also be affected; patients may also suffer from the effects of deficiency of one or more of these vitamins. Lack of vitamin A has been associated with the development of night blindness. Because vitamin D is involved in the absorption of calcium from the gut, deficiency of this vitamin can lead to bone demineralization. Vitamin K is important for the synthesis of clotting factors by the liver and deficiency of this vitamin impair clotting function.

9.13.5   Gastrointestinal cancers

9.13.5.1   Esophageal cancer

Esophageal cancers most commonly arise as adenocarcinomas associated with Barrett's esophagus of chronic GERD. The risk of developing esophageal adenocarcinoma is also increased by tobacco use. The first clinical manifestation of esophageal cancer is often dysphagia that occurs after significant tumor growth and spread. Long-term prognosis is often poor given the fact that the cancer has often already grown significantly and metastasized when first diagnosed.

9.13.5.2   Stomach cancer

The incidence of stomach cancer in the United States has decreased steadily in recent decades. Risk factors for the development of stomach cancer include chronic gastritis, ingestion of carcinogens such as nitrates and nitrosamines, family history, and chronic *H. pylori* infection. Most stomach cancers develop in the antrum region and are asymptomatic until well progressed. This late detection leads to a poor prognosis. Symptoms at the time of detection may include anorexia, pain, indigestion, vomiting and weight loss.

9.13.5.3   Colorectal cancer

Colorectal cancer is the second leading cause of cancer deaths in the United States after lung cancer. Most cases of colorectal cancer are carcinomas that arise from preexisting colorectal benign *adenomatous polyps*. A number of factors may contribute to the development of colorectal cancer including high-fat diet, low-fiber diet, age over 50 years, and genetic predisposition. Colorectal cancer may be detected though proctoscopy, by the presence of occult blood in the stool, or by blood tests for the presence of several tumor-specific antigens.

9.13.5.3.1   Manifestations of colorectal cancer
- Diarrhea or constipation
- Blood in the stool (obvious or occult)
- Pain is rare
- Weakness, malaise, anorexia, weight loss
- Bowel obstruction
- Common sites of metastasis for colorectal cancer are the brain, lungs, and bone
- Long-term prognosis depends upon how early the cancer is detected and the extent to which it has spread

9.14   Hepatobiliary disorders

The liver is a large glandular organ composed of a two main lobes. The large left and right lobes of the human liver are further subdivided into a number of smaller lobules, which are the functional units of the liver. The

Table 9.7 Functions of the liver

- Carbohydrate, fat, and protein metabolism
- Metabolism of steroid and sex hormones
- Production of bile
- Elimination of bilirubin
- Drug metabolism
- Synthesis of plasma proteins and clotting factors
- Storage of glycogen, minerals, and vitamins

liver is responsible for performing a number of crucial functions that are essential for normal life (see Table 9.7). Alteration of liver function may result from exposure to a number of factors such as viruses, alcohol, toxins, and drugs and can result in conditions such as *hepatitis* and *cirrhosis*. In light of the many key functions of the liver, factors that affect liver function will often have profound effects on normal physiology and function.

9.14.1 Tests of liver function

Elevated serum levels of liver enzymes such as *alanine aminotransferase (ALT)* and *aspartate aminotransferase (AST)* can be used to assess injury to liver cells. The excretory function of the liver may be assessed by measurement of serum bilirubin or γ-glutamyltransferase (GGT). The synthetic function of the liver may be assessed by the measurement of serum albumin or prothrombin time (a measurement of clotting factor activity). Imaging techniques such as ultrasonography and CT (computed tomography) scanning can provide information about liver architecture, structural abnormalities and flows.

9.14.2 Infectious disease of the liver

9.14.2.1 Viral hepatitis

The term "hepatitis" refers to inflammation and injury of the liver. Hepatitis may be caused by a number of injurious agents such as viruses, alcohol, toxins and drugs. When the liver is inflamed and injured as a result of viral infection, it is termed a *viral hepatitis*. Alcoholic hepatitis will be discussed under the topic of cirrhosis. In the United States there are three main *hepatitis viruses* designated hepatitis A, B, and C. Two other variants, hepatitis D and E are also present in certain populations. All of the hepatitis viruses target the hepatocytes of the liver for their site of infection and replication. The main features of the various hepatitis viruses are shown in Table 9.8.

Table 9.8   Characteristics of common hepatitis viruses

Characteristic	Hepatitis A	Hepatitis B	Hepatitis C
Viral Genome	ssRNA	dsDNA	ssRNA
Incubation Period (Days)	15–50	45–160	14–180
Route of Transmission	Fecal/oral, sexual	Blood and body fluids	Blood and body fluids
Potential for Chronic Infection	None	15%–20% of infected patients develop chronic liver disease	75%–85% of infected patients develop chronic liver disease

9.14.2.1.1   Epidemiology of viral hepatitis
Hepatitis A Virus (HAV)
- Transmitted via the fecal-oral route, usually through fecal-contaminated food, water, or shellfish. Numerous outbreaks have been traced to infected food handlers and poor sanitation. May also be transmitted through sexual contact. The highest incidence occurs in children and adolescents and, in the United States, outbreaks are sometimes seen in day-care centers
- The virus replicates in the liver but is shed in the stools
- HAV infection is generally self-limiting and does not lead to chronic liver disease

Hepatitis B Virus (HBV)
- Blood-borne pathogen
- Major routes of transmission include intravenous drug use, unprotected sexual contact, and exposure to contaminated blood products
- Can produce chronic hepatitis and lead to liver failure and liver carcinoma

Hepatitis C Virus (HCV)
- Blood-borne pathogen
- Major route of transmission is through contaminated blood and body fluids
- Accounts for most cases of transfusion-related viral hepatitis
- HCV is the most common cause of chronic hepatitis, cirrhosis, and liver cancer

Hepatitis D Virus (HDV)
- Blood-borne pathogen
- Can only coinfect individuals with active hepatitis B infection
- Transmitted through contaminated blood and body fluids. Higher incidence in i.v. drug abusers
- Clinical course is similar to HBV

Hepatitis E Virus (HEV)
- Fecal-oral route of transmission similar to HAV
- Outbreaks are more common in developing nations and refugee camps because of poor sanitation and fecal contamination of water supplies
- Young children are most frequently affected
- The effects of hepatitis E infection are particularly severe in pregnant women

9.14.2.1.2   Manifestations of viral hepatitis
- Manifestations may range from asymptomatic to severe
- Fatigue, malaise, anorexia, nausea occur with acute infection
- *Jaundice* (see box)
- Liver inflammation and abdominal pain
- Abnormal liver function and enzyme levels
- Chronic active infection can lead to liver cirrhosis

JAUNDICE

- A yellowing of the skin and whites of the eyes due to excess levels of circulating bilirubin.
- Bilirubin is formed from hemoglobin during the normal and abnormal breakdown of red blood cells. Free bilirubin formed in the blood is conjugated by the liver and eliminated into the intestinal tract along with bile.
- Conditions that impair the ability of the liver to conjugate and eliminate bilirubin will result in the accumulation of bilirubin in the blood with accompanying jaundice.
- Causes of Jaundice may be:
    - *Prehepatic*—excess RBC hemolysis, hemolytic anemia
    - *Intrahepatic*—hepatitis, cirrhosis, liver cancer
    - *Posthepatic*—obstruction of bile outflow, cholelithiasis

9.14.2.1.3   Chronic complications of viral hepatitis

- Chronic active or persistent hepatitis can lead to progressive liver injury, liver failure and death. The chronic form of hepatitis is most common with hepatitis B, C, D, but rare with hepatitis A and E.
- Chronic active hepatitis is also associated with an increased incidence of hepatocellular carcinoma.

9.14.2.1.4   Treatment of viral hepatitis

- Many hepatitis infections will resolve within 4–8 weeks without treatment. Hepatitis A rarely becomes chronic and seldom requires treatment other than supportive measures. The long-term course of hepatitis B and C is less predictable.
- Effective vaccines are currently available against hepatitis A and B.
- Drug therapy for HBV is currently designed to suppress viral replication and includes the use of pegylated-interferon and agents such as lamivudine and adefovir that inhibit viral DNA polymerase. New triple drug therapy for HCV may be curative.

9.14.3   Alcoholic liver disease

The incidence of alcoholism in the United States is estimated at 7% of the population, with approximately 2 million individuals suffering from alcoholic liver disease. After ingestion, alcohol (ethanol) is converted by the alcohol dehydrogenase enzyme in hepatocytes to acetaldehyde. It is believed that the accumulation of acetaldehyde is responsible for many of the toxic effects that are observed with ethanol ingestion. Alcoholic liver disease presents in three progressive stages:

- *Alcoholic Steatosis*—"Fatty Liver." Accumulation of fat in the hepatocytes. May occur as a result of altered fat metabolism by the liver. Changes associated with steatosis include increased synthesis of fatty acids and triglycerides. Enlargement of the liver is accompanied by symptoms that may include anorexia, nausea, and jaundice. At this point, the fatty changes are generally reversible if alcohol consumption ceases.

- *Alcoholic Hepatitis*—inflammation, degeneration and necrosis of hepatocytes with continued alcohol intake. Symptoms can range from mild to severe and can include anorexia, and weight loss. Jaundice is often a hallmark sign associated with the presence of alcoholic hepatitis. Although structural changes in alcoholic hepatitis are also reversible to a large extent if alcohol consumption ceases, patients who continue to drink general progress to cirrhosis within 1–2 years.
- *Alcoholic Cirrhosis*—diffuse scarring and fibrosis of the liver that occurs after many years of alcohol abuse. Because the liver plays such an important role in many normal physiologic processes, alcoholic cirrhosis is a multi-system disease.

9.14.4 Cirrhosis

Cirrhosis is characterized by diffuse scarring and fibrosis of the liver in response to chronic inflammation and injury. One of the major features of cirrhosis is the replacement of functional liver tissue by nonfunctional scar tissue. Alcoholic liver disease and viral hepatitis are leading causes of cirrhosis; however, there may be additional causes (see Table 9.9). As functional hepatocytes are lost, so is normal liver function. Cirrhosis will eventually result in liver failure. Given the great reserve capacity of the liver, 80%–90% of functional hepatocytes must be lost before overt liver failure ensues.

9.14.4.1 Manifestations of cirrhosis and liver failure

- *Hepatosplenomegaly*—swelling of spleen and liver. Swelling of the liver can increase portal pressure, whereas swelling of the spleen can lead to increased destruction of red blood cells (anemia) white blood cells (leukopenia) and platelets (thrombocytopenia).
- *Ascites*—accumulation of fluid in the peritoneal cavity. Results from portal hypertension and decreased plasma protein production by the liver. Presents with massive fluid-filled distention of the abdomen.
- *Portal Hypertension* (see box)

Table 9.9   Types of cirrhosis

- *Alcoholic Cirrhosis* (portal cirrhosis, Laennec's cirrhosis)—caused by excess ethanol intake likely due to acetaldehyde toxicity (a metabolite of ethanol)
- *Biliary Cirrhosis*—damage that begins in the bile ducts and bile canaliculi that leads to cirrhosis. Presents in two forms:
  - *Primary*—autoimmune disease of uncertain origin. Usually develops slowly and can be treated if detected early
  - *Secondary*—caused by bile duct obstruction (intrahepatic or extrahepatic). E.g., gallstones, tumors, pancreatitis
- *Post-Necrotic Cirrhosis* – caused by viral hepatitis, exposure to drugs or toxins
- *Metabolic Cirrhosis*—caused by glycogen storage disease, Wilson's disease, α1-antitrypsin deficiency

---

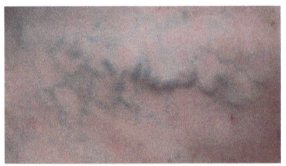

Distended umbilical veins from portal hypertension

- *Hepatorenal syndrome*—renal failure that can accompany advanced liver disease.
- Edema.
- Jaundice.

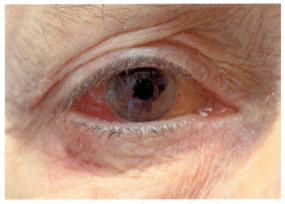

Yellowing of conjunctiva of the eyes with jaundice

- Impaired fat absorption due to reduced synthesis of bile salts by the liver. May lead to a deficiency in fat-soluble vitamins as well.
- *Hepatic encephalopathy*—neurological dysfunction that can accompany advanced liver disease. May be caused in part by the accumulation of ammonia and other toxins in circulation.
- Distention of abdominal and esophageal veins (*esophageal varices*) due to increased portal and venous pressures. *Caput medusae* is a term used to describe the distended abdominal veins that are seen in patients with alcoholic cirrhosis
- Reduced metabolism of circulating sex hormones can result in gynecomastia, menstrual irregularities, and abnormal sexual function
- Coagulopathy due to impaired synthesis of clotting factors and loss of platelets due to splenomegaly
- Liver failure

PORTAL HYPERTENSION

- Elevated portal blood pressure caused by increased resistance to blood flow through the liver as a result of scar tissue replacement.
- The increased portal pressure causes the backing up of blood into the spleen (splenomegaly) as well as collateral blood vessels of the abdomen and esophagus causing varices.
- Symptoms include bleeding of varices, ascites, and splenomegaly with possible destruction of platelets and other blood cells.

9.14.4.2   Treatment of cirrhosis

- Nutritional and vitamin supplementation. A reduced protein diet is useful to decrease ammonia production
- Diuretics to relieve fluid accumulation
- Intubation or shunting to relieve bleeding from accessory blood vessels
- Management of symptoms of liver failure
- Liver transplant

9.14.5   Liver cancer

Tumors originating in the liver are rare but tend to be malignant when they arise. Such primary tumors are usually asymptomatic until they reach a large size. More commonly, tumors arise outside of the liver and spread to it as a result of metastasis. Due to its rich blood supply, the liver provides an excellent site for growth of metastatic tumors. Lung, breast, colon, and pancreatic tumors are the most common source of metastatic tumors to the liver. The clinical manifestations of liver cancer or metastasis will depend primarily upon the rate of tumor growth. As more functional liver tissue becomes involved, the clinical manifestations tend to become more severe. Growing tumors may impair liver blood flow and bile outflow, leading to hepatomegaly and jaundice. *Cachexia* or lean tissue wasting tends to be severe with liver cancer or metastasis. Long-term prognosis is poor.

9.14.6   Disorders of the gallbladder

The gallbladder is a saclike structure that stores bile produced by the liver. The walls of the gallbladder contain smooth muscle and, under the stimulus of the duodenal hormone *cholecystokinin*, can contract to eject bile down the bile duct and into the duodenum. In the duodenum, bile salts emulsify fats to aid in their absorption. Bile is comprised primarily of water, bile salts, cholesterol and bilirubin.

9.14.6.1   Gallstone formation (Cholelithiasis) (see Figure 9.7)

- Cholelithiasis is the most common disorder of the gastrointestinal system
- The gallstones that form in the gallbladder are hardened precipitates of bile that contain predominately cholesterol
- The size of gallstones can range from the size of a grain of sand to several inches in diameter
- Factors such as aging, excess cholesterol, obesity, sudden dietary changes, or abnormal fat metabolism may contribute to gallstone formation
- Gallstones may be detected by a number of techniques including X-ray, ultrasonography, and cholecystoscopy

9.14.6.1.1   Manifestations of gallstone formation

- Symptoms of gallstone formation will generally not occur until the stones have reached sufficient size to block the bile ducts
- Acute and severe abdominal pain
- Nausea, vomiting, fever, chills
- Jaundice from obstruction of bile outflow

9.14.6.1.2   Treatment of gallstones

- Surgical removal of gallbladder (*cholecystectomy*)
- Endoscopic removal of gallstone
- *Lithotripsy*—the use of sound waves to break up the gallstones in the gallbladder
- Low-fat diet for prevention of additional stone formation

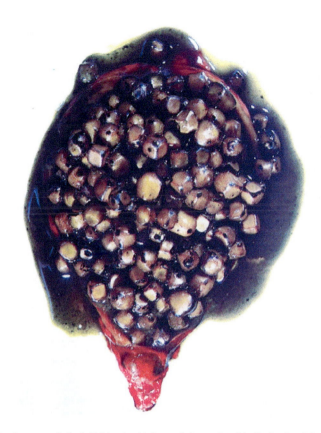

Figure 9.7   Image of cholelithiasis. (Adapted from *Porth's Pathophysiology: Concepts of Altered Health States* by Grossman, Lippincott Williams and Wilkins, 2013.)

9.14.6.2   Cholecystitis

Cholecystitis is an acute or chronic inflammation of the gallbladder. It is most commonly caused by the presence of gallstones in the gallbladder, but may also result from infection or reduced blood flow to the gallbladder. Signs and symptoms are similar to those observed with cholelithiasis. Treatment involves removal of gallstones and antibiotics for treatment of infection if present.

9.14.7   Disorders of the pancreas

9.14.7.1   Pancreatitis

Inflammation of the pancreas that may be acute or chronic. Because the pancreas contains both exocrine and endocrine cells, inflammation of the pancreas can affect both digestive function and the regulation of blood glucose. Possible causes of acute and chronic pancreatitis are listed in the Table 9.10.

Table 9.10   Pancreatitis

Acute
- Many instances do not have a clear cause; often arises in the exocrine acini and involves inflammation due to abnormal release of pancreatic enzymes or reflux of duodenal contents into pancreatic tissues
- May also be caused by blockage of pancreatic outflow through the common bile duct by gallstones
- May be caused in rare instances by certain drugs such as thiazide diuretics, NSAIDS or sulfonamide antibiotics
- May be caused by infectious agents

Chronic
- Alcohol abuse is the most common cause of chronic pancreatitis
- May also be caused by pancreatic tumors or cysts
- May lead to irreversible changes in pancreas structure and function

9.14.7.1.1   Manifestations of pancreatitis
- Epigastric pain
- Fever, nausea, vomiting
- Reduced bowel activity
- Anorexia, malaise
- Intestinal malabsorption, poor digestion of nutrients
- Diabetes mellitus if endocrine function of the pancreas is compromised

9.14.7.1.2   Treatment of pancreatitis
- Prevention of intestinal malabsorption
- Exogenous oral replacement of pancreatic enzymes
- Antibiotics for infection if present
- Pain medication
- Drugs to decrease gastric acid secretion
- Surgical drainage

9.14.7.2   Pancreatic cancer

Approximately 1.5% of individuals will be diagnosed with pancreas cancer during their lifetime. In the United States, pancreatic cancer accounts for about 3% of all cancers in the United States and for about 7% of cancer deaths. The incidence of pancreatic cancer is increasing worldwide. The vast majority of pancreatic cancers arise as adenocarcinomas in the ductal epithelium. Age is a key factor in the development of pancreatic cancer given that it rarely strikes individuals less than 50 years of age. Cigarette smoking, diabetes and chronic pancreatitis also appear to increase the risk of developing pancreatic cancer. Mortality rates are very high and long-term survival is poor.

9.14.7.3   Clinical manifestations of pancreatic cancer

Pancreatic cancers may be asymptomatic until they reach sufficient size to obstruct ductal outflow. Epigastric pain and back pain may occur. Pain may occur with food ingestion. A growing tumor may also obstruct bile outflow and lead to jaundice.

Medical terminology

Ampulla (ăm′pūl-ă): Sac-like dilatation of a duct

Amylase (ăm′ĭ-lās): Enzyme that hydrolyzes or splits starch into smaller molecules

Anus (ā′nŭs): Outlet for body waste from the rectum to the body surface

Bolus (bō′lŭs): A concentrated mass

Cecum (sē′kŭm): Blind pouch forming the first portion of the large intestine

Cephalic (sĕ-făl′ĭk): Referring to the cranium

Cholecystokinin (kō″lĕ-sĭs″tō-kīn′ĭn): Hormone produced in the small intestine in response to the presence of lipids

Chylomicron (kī″lō-mī′krŏn): Lipoprotein molecule formed in the small intestine for the transport of triglycerides in the blood

Chyme (kīm): Food materials mixed with gastric juice forming a thick semi-fluid substance

Colon (kō′lŏn): Large intestine

Enteric (ĕn-tĕr′ĭk): Referring to the small intestine

Esophagus (ē-sŏf′ă-gŭs): Muscular tube that transports ingested materials from the pharynx to the stomach

Feces (fē′sēz): Body waste eliminated from the colon through the anus

Haustrum (haw′strŭm): Sac-like structure in the large intestine

Ileocecal (ĭl′ē-ō-sē′kăl): Referring to the ileum and the cecum

Lacteal (lăk′tē-ăl): Lymphatic capillary found in the villi of the small intestine

Lipase (lī′pās): Enzyme that hydrolyzes or splits triglycerides into mono-glycerides and free fatty acids

Mastication (măs-tĭ-kā′shŭn): Chewing

Mesentery (mĕs′ĕn-tĕr″ē): Serous membrane that attaches organs to the abdominal wall

Micelle (mī′sĕl): Sphere of bile salt molecules needed to transport fatty acids and monoglycerides to the absorptive cells in the small intestine

Mucosa (mū-kō′să): Mucous membrane that lines hollow organs

Peristalsis (pĕr-ĭ-stăl′sĭs): Wave-like muscular contraction that propels chyme along the gastrointestinal tract

Peritoneum (pĕr″ĭ-tō-nē′ŭm): Serous membrane lining the abdominal cavity

Pharynx (făr′ĭnks): Common passageway for food and air

Plexus (plĕks′ŭs): Network of nerves

Pyloric (pī-lor′ĭk): Referring to the junction between the stomach and the duodenum

Secretin (sē-krē′tĭn): Hormone produced in the small intestine in response to the presence of acid

Segmentation (sĕg″mĕn-tā′shŭn): Stationary muscular contraction that mixes chyme with digestive enzymes and exposes chyme to the absorptive surface

Bibliography

Brown, J. H., and Taylor, P., Muscarinic receptor agonists and antagonists, in *Goodman and Gilman's The Pharmacological Basis of Therapeutics*, 11th ed., Brunton, L. L., Lazo, J. S., and Parker, K. L., Eds., McGraw-Hill, New York, 2006, chap. 7.

Fox, S. I., *Human Physiology*, 9th ed., McGraw-Hill, Boston, MA, 2006.

Ganong, W. F., *Review of Medical Physiology*, 19th ed., Appleton & Lange, Stamford, CT, 1999.

Guyton, A. C., and Hall, J. E., *Textbook of Medical Physiology*, 11th ed., W. B. Saunders, Philadelphia, PA, 2006.

Hoogerwerf, W. A., and Pasricha, P. J., Pharmacotherapy of gastric acidity, peptic ulcers, and gastroesophageal reflux disease, in *Goodman and Gilman's The Pharmacological Basis of Therapeutics*, 11th ed., Brunton, L. L., Lazo, J. S., and Parker, K. L., Eds., McGraw-Hill, New York, 2006, chap. 36.

Johnson, L. R., Salivary secretion, in *Gastrointestinal Physiology*, 7th ed., Johnson, L. R., Ed., Mosby, St. Louis, MO, 2007, chap. 7.

Johnson, L. R., Gastric secretion, in *Gastrointestinal Physiology*, 7th ed., Johnson, L. R., Ed., Mosby, St. Louis, MO, 2007, chap. 8.

Johnson, L. R., Pancreatic secretion, in *Gastrointestinal Physiology*, 7th ed., Johnson, L. R., Ed., Mosby, St. Louis, MO, 2007, chap. 9.

Johnson, L. R., Digestion and absorption, in *Gastrointestinal Physiology*, 7th ed., Johnson, L. R., Ed., Mosby, St. Louis, MO, 2007, chap. 11.

Lichtenberger, L. M., Gastrointestinal physiology, in *Physiology Secrets*, Raff, H., Ed., Hanley and Belfus, Inc., Philadelphia, PA, 1999, chap. 5.

Pappano, A. J., and Katzung, B. G., Cholinergic-blocking drugs, in *Basic and Clinical Pharmacology*, 8th ed., Katzung, B. G., Ed., Lange Medical Books/McGraw-Hill, New York, 2001, chap. 8.

Pasricha, P. J., Treatment of disorders of bowel motility and water flux; antiemetics; agents used in biliary and pancreatic disease, in *Goodman and Gilman's The Pharmacological Basis of Therapeutics*, 11th ed., Brunton, L. L., Lazo, J. S., and Parker, K. L., Eds., McGraw-Hill, New York, 2006, chap. 37.

Peery, A. F., Dellon, E. S., Lund, J. et al., 2012. Burden of gastrointestinal disease in the United States: 2012 update. *Gastroenterology*. 143(4):1179–1187.

Sherwood, L., *Human Physiology from Cells to Systems*, 5th ed., Brooks/Cole, Pacific Grove, CA, 2004.

Silverthorn, D. U., *Human Physiology, An Integrated Approach*, 4th ed., Prentice Hall, Upper Saddle River, NJ, 2007.

Taber's Cyclopedic Medical Dictionary, 20th ed., F. A. Davis Co., Philadelphia, PA, 2005.

Weisbrodt, N. W., Regulation: Nerves and smooth muscle, in *Gastrointestinal Physiology,* 7th ed., Johnson, L. R., Ed., Mosby, St. Louis, MO, 2007, chap. 2.

Weisbrodt, N. W., Swallowing, in *Gastrointestinal Physiology,* 7th ed., Johnson, L. R., Ed., Mosby, St. Louis, MO, 2007, chap. 3.

Weisbrodt, N. W., Gastric emptying, in *Gastrointestinal Physiology,* 7th ed., Johnson, L. R., Ed., Mosby, St. Louis, MO, 2007, chap. 4.

Weisbrodt, N. W., Bile production, secretion, and storage, in *Gastrointestinal Physiology,* 7th ed., Johnson, L. R., Ed., Mosby, St. Louis, MO, 2007, chap. 10.

Widmaier, E. P., Raff, H., and Strang, K. T., *Vander's Human Physiology, The Mechanisms of Body Function,* McGraw-Hill, Boston, MA, 2006.

chapter ten

The renal system

Study objectives

- List the vascular components of the nephron and describe their function
- List the tubular components of the nephron and describe their function
- Distinguish between a cortical nephron and a juxtamedullary nephron
- Define the three basic renal processes
- Describe the components of the filtration barrier
- Explain how the filtration coefficient and the figurenet filtration pressure determine glomerular filtration
- Describe the mechanisms by which sodium, chloride and water are reabsorbed
- Describe how each segment of the tubule handles sodium, chloride and water
- Distinguish between the vertical osmotic gradient and the horizontal osmotic gradient
- Describe the functions of the vasa recta
- Describe the process by which potassium ions are secreted and the mechanism that regulates this process
- Define plasma clearance
- Explain how the plasma clearance of inulin is used to determine glomerular filtration rate
- Explain how the plasma clearance of para-aminohippuric acid is used to determine the effective renal plasma flow
- Explain how the myogenic mechanism and tubuloglomerular feedback are responsible for the autoregulation of renal blood flow
- Explain how sympathetic nerves, angiotensin II and prostaglandins affect the resistance of the afferent arteriole
- Describe the factors that regulate the release of renin
- Explain how the control of sodium excretion regulates plasma volume
- Describe the mechanisms by which sodium excretion is controlled
- Explain how the control of water excretion regulates plasma osmolarity
- Describe the mechanisms by which water balance is maintained

- List the various functions performed by the kidneys
- Describe the different methods one can use to assess renal function. What are the pros and cons of each of these?
- Discuss the various mechanisms the kidney uses to help regulate renal blood flow. How can these factors worsen the physiologic changes that accompany renal disease?
- List some possible causes of acute and chronic glomerulonephritis. How does glomerulonephritis differ from pyelonephritis?
- What are renal calculi? What are some factors that can contribute to their formation? What effects might they have on the kidney?
- List prerenal, intrarenal and postrenal causes of renal failure. List the major physiologic effects of renal failure on the various systems of the body. Why does each occur?
- Describe the principle of hemodialysis. What is the role of hemodialysis in renal failure? How does peritoneal dialysis differ from classic hemodialysis? What are the advantages and disadvantages of each type of dialysis?
- List possible causes of urine reflux and neurogenic bladder. What are the possible consequences of each on the kidney?
- Define obstructive uropathy. How can it lead to hydroureter or hydronephrosis?

The kidneys are organs specialized to filter the blood, and as such, contribute importantly to the removal of metabolic waste products as well as to the maintenance of fluid and electrolyte balance. Specific functions of the kidneys include the following:

- Regulation of extracellular fluid volume
- Regulation of inorganic electrolyte concentration in the extracellular fluid
- Regulation of the osmolarity of the extracellular fluid
- Removal of metabolic waste products
- Excretion of foreign compounds
- Maintenance of acid-base balance
- Hormone and enzyme production

The *regulation of extracellular fluid volume*, more specifically plasma volume, is important in the long-term regulation of blood pressure. An increase in plasma volume leads to an increase in blood pressure and a decrease in plasma volume leads to a decrease in blood pressure. Plasma volume is regulated primarily by altering the excretion of sodium in the urine. Other *inorganic electrolytes* regulated by the kidneys include chloride, potassium, calcium, magnesium, sulfate, and phosphate.

The kidneys also *regulate the osmolarity of the extracellular fluid*, specifically plasma osmolarity. The maintenance of plasma osmolarity close to 290 mOsm prevents any unwanted movement of fluid in or out of the body's cells. An increase in plasma osmolarity causes water to leave the cells, leading to cellular dehydration. A decrease in plasma osmolarity causes water to enter the cells, leading to cellular swelling and possibly lysis. Plasma osmolarity is regulated primarily by altering the excretion of water in the urine.

As the major excretory organs in the body, the kidneys are responsible for the *removal of many metabolic waste products*. These include urea and uric acid, which are nitrogenous waste products of amino acid and nucleic acid metabolism, respectively; creatinine, a breakdown product of muscle metabolism; and urobilinogen, a metabolite of hemoglobin that gives urine its yellow color. *Foreign compounds* excreted by the kidneys include drugs (e.g., penicillin, nonsteroidal anti-inflammatory drugs), food additives (e.g., saccharin, benzoate), pesticides, and other exogenous nonnutritive materials that have entered the body. If allowed to accumulate, these substances become quite toxic.

Along with the respiratory system, the renal system *maintains acid-base balance* by altering the excretion of hydrogen ions and bicarbonate ions in the urine. When the extracellular fluid becomes acidic and pH decreases, then the kidneys excrete H^+ ions and conserve HCO_3^- ions. Conversely, when the extracellular fluid becomes alkaline and pH increases, then the kidneys conserve H^+ ions and excrete HCO_3^- ions. Normally, the pH of the arterial blood is 7.4.

Although the kidneys are not considered endocrine glands, per se, they are involved in *hormone production*. Erythropoietin is a peptide hormone that stimulates red blood cell production in the bone marrow. Its primary source is the kidneys. Erythropoietin is secreted in response to renal hypoxia. Chronic renal disease may impair the secretion of erythropoietin, leading to the development of anemia.

The kidneys also *produce enzymes*. The enzyme, renin, is part of the renin-angiotensin-aldosterone system. As will be discussed, these substances play an important role in the regulation of plasma volume and, therefore, blood pressure. Other renal enzymes are needed for the conversion of vitamin D into its active form, 1,25-dihydroxyvitamin D_3, which is involved with calcium balance.

10.1 Functional anatomy of the kidneys

The kidneys lie outside of the peritoneal cavity in the posterior abdominal wall, one on each side of the vertebral column, slightly above the waistline. In the adult human, each kidney is approximately 11 cm long,

6 cm wide, and 3 cm thick. These organs are divided into two regions, the inner *renal medulla* and the outer *renal cortex*.

The functional unit of the kidney is the *nephron* (see Figures 10.1 and 10.2). There are well over 1 million nephrons in each kidney. The nephron has two components:

- Vascular component
- Tubular component

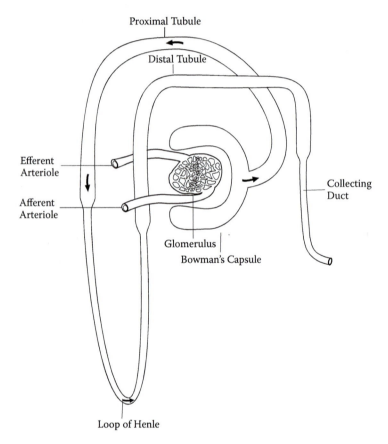

Figure 10.1 The nephron. The functional unit of the kidney is the nephron. It has two components. The vascular component includes the afferent arteriole, which carries blood toward the glomerulus, where filtration of the plasma takes place. The efferent arteriole carries the unfiltered blood away from the glomerulus. The tubular component of the nephron includes Bowman's capsule, which receives the filtrate, the proximal tubule, the Loop of Henle, the distal tubule, and the collecting duct. The tubule processes the filtrate; excreting waste products and reabsorbing nutrient molecules, electrolytes and water.

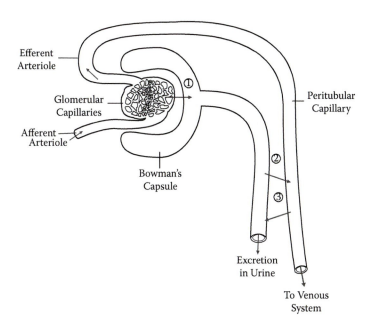

Figure 10.2 Basic renal processes. These processes include filtration, reabsorption and secretion. (1) Filtration is the movement of fluid and solutes from the glomerular capillaries into Bowman's capsule. (2) Reabsorption, which takes place throughout the nephron, is the movement of filtered substances out of the tubule and into the surrounding peritubular capillaries. (3) Secretion is the movement of selected unfiltered substances from the peritubular capillaries into the renal tubule for excretion. Any substance that is filtered or secreted, but not reabsorbed, is excreted in the urine.

10.1.1 Vascular component

Filtration of the plasma takes place at the *glomerulus* (i.e., *glomerular capillaries*), located in the cortical region of the kidney. Water and solutes exit the vascular compartment through these capillaries to be processed by the tubular component of the nephron. Blood is delivered to the glomerulus by the *afferent arterioles*. The glomerular capillaries then join to form a second arteriole referred to as the *efferent arteriole*. All cellular elements of the blood (red blood cells, white blood cells and platelets) as well as the unfiltered plasma continue through this vessel. The efferent arterioles then lead to a second set of capillaries, the *peritubular capillaries*. These capillaries provide nourishment to the renal tissue and return the substances reabsorbed from the tubule to the vascular compartment. Peritubular capillaries are closely associated with all portions of the renal tubules and wrap around them. These capillaries then join to form venules and progressively larger veins that remove the blood from the kidneys.

10.1.2 Tubular component

Approximately 180 L of filtrate is processed by the kidneys each day. Depending upon the volume of fluid intake, about 99% of this filtrate must be reabsorbed from the renal tubule back into the vascular compartment. The movement of substances out of the tubule is facilitated by its structure, which consists of *a single layer of epithelial cells*. As will be discussed, each region of the tubule plays a different role in the reabsorption process.

Upon leaving the glomerular capillaries, the filtrate enters the first portion of the tubule, *Bowman's capsule*. The glomerulus is pushed into Bowman's capsule, much like a fist pushed into a balloon or a catcher's mitt. From Bowman's capsule, the filtrate passes through the *proximal tubule*, which is also located in the cortex of the kidney. The next segment of the tubule is the *Loop of Henle*. This portion of the tubule is found in the medulla of the kidney. The descending limb dips into the medulla and the ascending limb returns toward the cortex. From the Loop of Henle, the filtrate passes through the *distal tubule* in the cortex of the kidney. Finally, up to eight distal tubules empty into a *collecting duct*. The collecting ducts run downward through the medulla. Any filtrate remaining within the tubule at the end of the collecting duct drains through the renal pelvis to the ureters and is excreted as urine.

There are two types of nephrons, which are distinguished by their anatomical characteristics:

- Cortical nephron
- Juxtamedullary nephron

The glomerulus of each *cortical nephron* is in the outer region of the cortex. Furthermore, the Loops of Henle in these nephrons are short and do not penetrate deeply into the medulla. In humans, 70%–80% of the nephrons are of the cortical type.

In contrast, the glomerulus of each *juxtamedullary nephron* is in the inner region of the cortex, close to the medulla. The Loops of Henle in these nephrons are significantly longer, penetrating to the innermost region of the medulla. Within the medulla, the peritubular capillaries of the nephrons are modified to form the *vasa recta*, or straight vessels. Like the Loops of Henle, the vasa recta descend deep into the medulla, form a hairpin loop, and then ascend back toward the cortex. In fact, these vessels run parallel, and in close association, with the Loops of Henle and the collecting ducts. The remaining 20%–30% of the nephrons in the human kidney are of the juxtamedullary type.

10.2 Basic renal processes

There are three basic renal processes performed by the nephron (see Figure 10.2):

- Filtration
- Reabsorption
- Secretion

Filtration is the movement of fluid and solutes from the glomerular capillaries into Bowman's capsule. Filtration is a *nonselective* process, such that everything in the plasma except for the plasma proteins is filtered. Approximately 20% of the plasma is filtered as it passes through the glomerulus. On average, this results in a *glomerular filtration rate (GFR)* of 125 mL/min or 180 L of filtrate per day.

Reabsorption is the movement of filtered substances from the renal tubule into the peritubular capillaries for return to the vascular compartment. This process takes place throughout the tubule. Approximately 178.5 L of filtrate are reabsorbed, resulting in an average urine output of 1.5 L per day.

Secretion is the movement of selected unfiltered substances from the peritubular capillaries into the renal tubule for excretion. Any substance that is filtered or secreted, but not reabsorbed, is *excreted* in the urine.

The maintenance of plasma volume and plasma osmolarity occurs through the regulation of the *renal excretion* of sodium, chloride, and water. Each of these substances is freely filtered from the glomerulus and reabsorbed from the tubule. None of these substances are secreted. Because salt and water intake in the diet may vary widely, the renal excretion of these substances is also highly variable. In other words, the kidneys must be able to produce a wide range of urine concentrations and urine volumes. The most dilute urine produced by humans is 65–70 mOsm/L, and the most concentrated the urine can be is 1,200 mOsm/L (recall that the plasma osmolarity is 290 mOsm/L). The volume of urine produced per day depends largely upon fluid intake. As fluid intake increases, then the urine output increases to excrete the excess water. Conversely, as fluid intake decreases or as an individual becomes dehydrated, then the urine output decreases to conserve water.

On average, 500 mOsm of waste products must be excreted in the urine per day. The minimum volume of water in which these solutes can be dissolved is determined by the ability of the kidney to produce a maximally concentrated urine of 1,200 mOsm/L:

$$\frac{500 \text{ mOsm/day}}{1,200 \text{ mOsm/L}} = 420 \text{ mL water/day}$$

This volume, referred to as *obligatory water loss*, is 420 mL water/day. In other words, 420 mL of water will be lost in the urine each day to excrete metabolic waste products regardless of water intake.

10.3 Glomerular filtration

The first step in the formation of urine is glomerular filtration. The barrier to filtration is designed to facilitate the movement of fluid from the glomerular capillaries into Bowman's capsule without any loss of cellular elements or plasma proteins. There are two advantages to maximizing GFR:

- Waste products are rapidly removed from the body
- All body fluids are filtered and processed by the kidneys several times per day, resulting in the precise regulation of volume and composition of these fluids

10.3.1 Filtration barrier

The *filtration barrier* is composed of three structures:

- Glomerular capillary wall
- Basement membrane
- Inner wall of Bowman's capsule

Like the walls of other capillaries, the *glomerular capillary wall* consists of a single layer of endothelial cells. However, the glomerular endothelial cells are specialized in that they are *fenestrated*; they possess large pores that makes them 100 times more permeable than the typical capillary. These pores are too small, however, to permit the passage of blood cells.

The *basement membrane* is an acellular meshwork consisting of collagen and glycoproteins. The *collagen* provides structural support. The negatively charged *glycoproteins* prevent the filtration of plasma proteins into Bowman's capsule.

The *inner wall of Bowman's capsule* consists of specialized epithelial cells referred to as *podocytes*. This layer of epithelial cells is not continuous. Instead, the podocytes have foot-like processes that project outward. The processes of one podocyte interdigitate with the processes of an adjacent podocyte forming narrow *filtration slits*. These slits provide an ample route for the filtration of fluid.

In summary, the filtrate moves through the pores of the capillary endothelium, through the basement membrane and, finally, through the filtration slits between the podocytes. This route of filtration is completely acellular.

10.3.2   Determinants of filtration

The glomerular filtration rate is influenced by two factors:

- Filtration coefficient
- Net filtration pressure

The *filtration coefficient* is determined by the *surface area* and the *permeability* of the filtration barrier. An increase in the filtration coefficient leads to an increase in GFR and a decrease in the filtration coefficient leads to a decrease in GFR. However, this factor does not play a role in the daily regulation of GFR because its value is relatively constant under normal physiological conditions. On the other hand, chronic, uncontrolled hypertension and diabetes mellitus lead to the gradual thickening of the basement membrane and, therefore, a decrease in the filtration coefficient, a decrease in GFR and impaired renal function.

The *net filtration pressure* is determined by the following forces (see Figure 10.3):

- Glomerular capillary blood pressure
- Plasma colloid osmotic pressure
- Bowman's capsule pressure

Glomerular capillary pressure (P_{GC}) is a hydrostatic pressure that pushes blood out of the capillary. The blood pressure in these capillaries is markedly different from that of typical capillaries. In capillaries located elsewhere in the body, the blood pressure at the arteriolar end is about 30 mmHg and the blood pressure at the venular end is about 10 mmHg (see Chapter 6, section B). These pressures lead to the net filtration of fluid at the inflow end of the capillary and the net reabsorption of fluid at the outflow end of the capillary.

In contrast, blood pressure in the glomerular capillaries is significantly higher and essentially nondecremental. At the inflow end of the capillary near the afferent arteriole, P_{GC} is about 60 mmHg, and at the outflow end of the capillary near the efferent arteriole, P_{GC} is about 58 mmHg. Interestingly, the diameter of the afferent arteriole is larger than that of efferent arteriole. Therefore, the vascular resistance in the afferent arteriole is comparatively low and blood flows readily into the glomerular capillaries, resulting in a higher pressure. Furthermore, the smaller diameter of the efferent arteriole results in an increase in vascular resistance, which limits the flow of blood through this vessel. Consequently, the blood dams up in the glomerular capillaries. The result is a sustained, elevated hydrostatic pressure, which promotes the net filtration of fluid along the entire length of the glomerular capillaries.

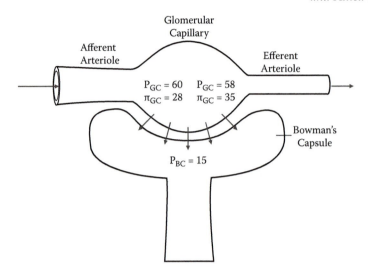

Figure 10.3 Forces determining net filtration pressure. Three forces contribute to the net filtration pressure in the glomerulus. Glomerular capillary blood pressure (P_{GC}) is higher than that of a typical capillary (60 mmHg vs. 30 mmHg). Furthermore, P_{GC} remains high throughout the length of the capillary. This is due to the comparatively small diameter of the efferent arteriole, which causes the blood to dam up within the glomerular capillaries. Glomerular capillary pressure promotes filtration along the entire length of the glomerular capillaries. Plasma colloid osmotic pressure (π_{GC}), generated by the plasma proteins, opposes filtration. This force increases from 28 mmHg at the inflow end of the glomerular capillary to 35 mmHg at the outflow end of the capillary. This is due to the concentration of the plasma proteins as the filtration of the plasma fluid progresses. Bowman's capsule pressure (P_{BC}) is generated by the presence of filtered fluid within Bowman's capsule. This pressure opposes filtration with a force of 15 mmHg.

Plasma colloid osmotic pressure (π_{GC}) is generated by the plasma proteins. These proteins exert an osmotic force on the fluid, which opposes filtration and draws the fluid into the capillary. The π_{GC} is approximately 28 mmHg at the inflow end of the glomerular capillaries. Because 20% of the fluid within the capillaries is filtered into Bowman's capsule, the plasma proteins become increasingly concentrated. Therefore, at the outflow end of the glomerular capillaries, π_{GC} is approximately 35 mmHg.

Bowman's capsule pressure (P_{BC}) is a hydrostatic pressure generated by the presence of filtered fluid within Bowman's capsule. This pressure pushes the fluid out of the capsule and forward toward the remainder of the renal tubule for processing. Bowman's capsule pressure also tends to oppose filtration. On average, P_{BC} is approximately 15 mmHg.

The net filtration pressure may be summarized as follows:

$$\text{Net filtration pressure} = P_{GC} - \pi_{GC} - P_{BC}$$

Therefore, at the inflow end of the glomerular capillaries:

$$\text{Net filtration pressure} = 60 \text{ mmHg} - 28 \text{ mmHg} - 15 \text{ mmHg}$$

$$= 17 \text{ mmHg}$$

At the outflow end of the glomerular capillaries:

$$\text{Net filtration pressure} = 58 \text{ mmHg} - 35 \text{ mmHg} - 15 \text{ mmHg}$$

$$= 8 \text{ mmHg}$$

Under physiological conditions, there is little variation in the values for π_{GC} and P_{BC}. In other words, when plasma protein synthesis is normal and in the absence of any urinary obstruction that would cause the urine to back up and increase P_{BC}, the primary factor that affects glomerular filtration is P_{GC}. An increase in P_{GC} leads to an increase in GFR, and a decrease in P_{GC} leads to a decrease in GFR.

Glomerular capillary pressure is determined primarily by *renal blood flow* (RBF). As RBF increases, then P_{GC} and, therefore, GFR increase. On the other hand, as RBF decreases, then P_{GC} and GFR decrease. Renal blood flow is determined by mean arterial pressure (MAP) and the resistance of the afferent arteriole ($R_{\text{aff art}}$):

$$RBF = \frac{MAP}{R_{\text{aff art}}}$$

10.4 Tubular reabsorption

The process of *tubular reabsorption* is essential for the conservation of plasma constituents that are important to the body: most importantly, electrolytes and nutrient molecules. This process is highly selective in that waste products and substances with no physiological value are not reabsorbed but, instead, are excreted in the urine. Furthermore, the reabsorption of many substances, such as Na^+ ions, H^+ ions, Ca^{++} ions, and water, is physiologically controlled. Consequently, the volume, osmolarity, composition, and pH of the extracellular fluid are precisely regulated.

Throughout its length, the tubule of the nephron is composed of a single layer of epithelial cells. Furthermore, the tubule is close to the peritubular capillaries.

Therefore, reabsorption involves the movement of a substance along the following pathway:

Filtrate within tubular lumen
↓
Across the luminal membrane of the epithelial cell
↓
Through the cytoplasm of the epithelial cell
↓
Across the basolateral membrane of the epithelial cell
↓
Through the interstitial fluid
↓
Across the capillary endothelium
↓
Peritubular capillary blood

This pathway is referred to as *transepithelial transport.*

There are two types of tubular reabsorption:

- Passive
- Active

Tubular reabsorption is considered *passive* when each of the steps in transepithelial transport takes place without the expenditure of energy. In other words, the movement of a given substance is from an area of high concentration to an area of low concentration by way of passive diffusion. Water is passively reabsorbed from the tubules back into the peritubular capillaries.

Active reabsorption occurs when the movement of a given substance across either the luminal surface or the basolateral surface of the tubular epithelial cell requires energy. Substances that are actively reabsorbed from the tubule include glucose, amino acids, Na^+ ions, PO_4^{3-} ions and Ca^{++} ions.

Three generalizations can be made regarding the tubular reabsorption of sodium, chloride, and water:

- Reabsorption of *Na^+ ions* is an *active* process; 80% of the total energy expended by the kidneys is used for sodium transport out of the tubular epithelial cell
- Reabsorption of *Cl^- ions* is a *passive* process; Cl^- ions are reabsorbed based on the electrical gradient created by the reabsorption of Na^+ ions
- Reabsorption of *water* is a *passive* process; water is reabsorbed based on the osmotic gradient created by the reabsorption of Na^+ ions

In other words, when sodium is reabsorbed, chloride and water follow it.

10.4.1 Sodium reabsorption

Sodium is reabsorbed by different mechanisms as the filtrate progresses through the tubule. Sodium ions leave the filtrate and enter the tubular epithelial cell by way of the following processes (see Figure 10.4):

- Na^+-glucose, Na^+-amino acid, Na^+-phosphate and Na^+-lactate symporter mechanisms; Na^+-H^+ antiporter mechanism: first half of the proximal tubule
- Coupled with Cl^- ion reabsorption by way of both transcellular (through the epithelial cell) and paracellular (in between the epithelial cells) pathways: second half of the proximal tubule
- Na^+-K^+-$2Cl^-$ symporter mechanism: ascending limb of the Loop of Henle
- Na^+-Cl^- symporter mechanism: distal tubule
- Na^+ channels: distal tubule, collecting duct

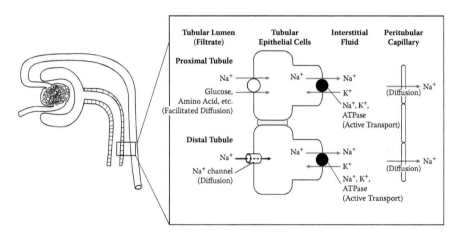

Figure 10.4 Tubular reabsorption of sodium. Sodium ions are actively transported out of the tubular epithelial cell through the basolateral membrane by the Na^+-K^+-ATPase pump. These ions then passively diffuse from the interstitial fluid into the blood of the peritubular capillaries. The active removal of Na^+ ions from the tubular epithelial cells establishes a concentration gradient for the passive diffusion of Na^+ ions into the cells from the tubular lumen. Potassium ions that are actively transported into the epithelial cells of the proximal tubule as the result of this process simply diffuse back into the interstitial fluid through channels located in the basolateral membrane. In the distal tubule and the collecting duct, the K^+ ions diffuse through channels in the luminal membrane into the tubular fluid and are excreted in the urine. The diffusion of sodium may be coupled to the reabsorption of organic molecules, such as glucose or amino acids, in the proximal tubule and the Loop of Henle. It may also occur through Na^+ channels in the distal tubule and the collecting duct.

More simply, in the early regions of the tubule (proximal tubule and Loop of Henle), Na^+ ions leave the lumen and enter the tubular epithelial cells by way of *facilitated transport mechanisms* that are passive. The diffusion of Na^+ ions is coupled with organic molecules or with other ions that electrically balance the flux of these positively charged ions. In the latter regions of the tubule (distal tubule and collecting duct), Na^+ ions diffuse into the epithelial cells through Na^+ channels.

An essential requirement for the diffusion of Na^+ ions is the creation of a concentration gradient for sodium between the filtrate and the intracellular fluid of the epithelial cells. This is accomplished by the *active transport of Na^+ ions* through the basolateral membrane of the epithelial cells (see Figure 10.4). Sodium is moved across this basolateral membrane and into the interstitial fluid surrounding the tubule by the *Na^+-K^+-ATPase pump* and the concentration of Na^+ ions within the epithelial cells is reduced, facilitating the diffusion of Na^+ ions into the cells across the luminal membrane. The movement of K^+ ions into the epithelial cells occurs because of the results of this pump and either diffuse back into the interstitial fluid (proximal tubule and Loop of Henle) or into the tubular lumen for excretion in the urine (distal tubule and collecting duct).

The amount of sodium reabsorbed from the proximal tubule and from the Loop of Henle is held constant:

- Proximal tubule: 65% of the filtered sodium is reabsorbed
- Ascending limb of the Loop of Henle: 25% of the filtered sodium is reabsorbed

This reabsorption occurs regardless of the sodium content of the body. To adjust the *sodium load*, the reabsorption of the remaining 10% of the filtered Na^+ ions from the distal tubule and the collecting duct is physiologically controlled by two hormones:

- Aldosterone
- Atrial natriuretic peptide

Aldosterone, released from the adrenal cortex, *promotes the reabsorption of sodium* from the distal tubule and the collecting duct. The mechanisms of action of aldosterone include:

- Formation of Na^+ channels in the luminal membrane of the tubular epithelial cells (facilitates the passive diffusion of Na^+ ions into the cell)
- Formation of Na^+-K^+-ATPase carrier molecules in the basolateral membrane of the tubular epithelial cells (promotes the extrusion of Na^+ ions from the cells and their movement into the plasma by way of the peritubular capillaries; enhances the concentration gradient for passive diffusion through the Na^+ channels in the luminal membrane)

Atrial natriuretic peptide (*ANP*), released from myocardial cells in the atria of the heart, *inhibits the reabsorption of sodium* from the collecting duct. The mechanisms of action of ANP include:

- Inhibition of aldosterone secretion
- Inhibition of Na^+ channels in the luminal membrane of the tubular epithelial cells

Recall that the reabsorption of Na^+ ions is accompanied by the reabsorption of Cl^- ions, which diffuse down their electrical gradient, and by the reabsorption of water, which diffuses down its osmotic gradient. The net result is an expansion of plasma volume and, consequently, an increase in blood pressure. Therefore, the regulation of sodium reabsorption is important in the long-term regulation of blood pressure.

10.4.2   Chloride reabsorption

Chloride ions are reabsorbed passively based on the electrical gradient established by the active reabsorption of sodium. Chloride ions move from the tubular lumen back into the plasma by two pathways:

- Transcellular: through the tubular epithelial cells
- Paracellular: in between the tubular epithelial cells

Most of the Cl^- ions diffuse between the tubular epithelial cells.

10.4.3   Water reabsorption

Water is reabsorbed passively by way of osmosis from many regions of the tubule. As with sodium and chloride, 65% of the filtered water is reabsorbed from the proximal tubule. An additional 15% of the filtered water is reabsorbed from the descending limb of the Loop of Henle. This reabsorption occurs regardless of the water content of the body. The water enters the tubular epithelial cells through *water channels*, also referred to as *aquaporins*. These channels are always open in the early regions of the tubule.

To adjust the water load, the reabsorption of the remaining 20% of the filtered water from the distal tubule and the collecting duct is physiologically controlled by *antidiuretic hormone* (ADH), also referred to as *vasopressin*. Antidiuretic hormone, synthesized in the hypothalamus and released from the neurohypophysis of the pituitary gland, *promotes the reabsorption of water* from the distal tubule and the collecting duct. The mechanism of action of ADH involves an increase in the permeability of the water channels in the luminal membrane of the tubular epithelial cells.

Water diffuses into these cells and is ultimately reabsorbed back into the plasma by way of the peritubular capillaries.

Recall that the reabsorption of water is important in the regulation of plasma osmolarity. As the levels of ADH increase and more water is reabsorbed from the kidneys, the plasma is diluted and plasma osmolarity decreases. Conversely, as the levels of ADH decrease and more water is lost in the urine, the plasma becomes more concentrated and plasma osmolarity increases.

10.4.4   *Production of urine of varying concentrations*

To effectively regulate plasma volume and osmolarity, the kidneys must be able to alter the volume and the concentration of the urine that is eliminated. Accordingly, the concentration of urine may be varied over a very wide range, depending upon the body's level of hydration. The most dilute urine produced by the kidneys is 65–70 mOsm/L (when the body is overhydrated), and the most concentrated urine is 1,200 mOsm/L (when the body is dehydrated). (Recall that the plasma osmolarity is 290–300 mOsm/L.)

An essential factor in the ability to excrete urine of varying concentrations is the presence of a *vertical osmotic gradient* in the medullary region of the kidney (see Figure 10.5). The osmolarity of the interstitial fluid in the cortical region of the kidney is about 300 mOsm/L. However, the osmolarity of the interstitial fluid in the medulla increases progressively, from 300 mOsm/L in the outer region of the medulla near the cortex, to 1,200 mOsm/L in the innermost region of the medulla. The increase in osmolarity is due to the accumulation of Na^+ ions and Cl^- ions in the interstitial fluid. This vertical osmotic gradient is created by the Loops of Henle of the juxtamedullary nephrons. Recall that the Loops of Henle in these nephrons penetrate deeply into the medulla. The gradient is then utilized by the collecting ducts, along with ADH, to alter the concentration of urine. The following is a summary of the reabsorption of sodium, chloride, and water by each region of the nephron.

Plasma is freely filtered from the *glomerulus*, such that everything in the plasma, except for the plasma proteins, is filtered. Therefore, the initial osmolarity of the filtrate is not different from that of the plasma and is about 300 mOsm/L (see Figure 10.5). Approximately 125 mL/min of the plasma is filtered. As the filtrate flows through the *proximal tubule*, 65% of the filtered Na^+ ions are actively reabsorbed, and 65% of the filtered Cl^- ions and water are passively reabsorbed. Because the water follows the sodium by way of osmosis, there is no change in the osmolarity of the filtrate; only a change in volume. At the end of the proximal tubule, approximately 44 mL of filtrate with an osmolarity of 300 mOsm/L remain in the tubule.

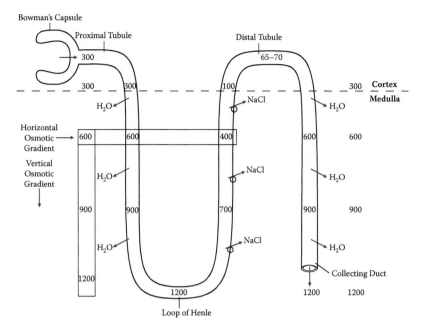

Figure 10.5 Production of urine of varying concentrations. The kidneys are capable of producing urine as dilute as 65–70 mOsm/L and as concentrated as 1,200 mOsm/L. The concentration of the urine is determined by the body's level of hydration. Sodium ions are actively transported from the ascending limb of the Loop of Henle into the interstitial fluid. This active process is used to accumulate Na$^+$ ions and Cl$^-$ ions in the medulla, resulting in a vertical osmotic gradient, in which the interstitial fluid becomes increasingly concentrated, to be established. This gradient is necessary for the reabsorption of water from the collecting duct. Furthermore, a horizontal osmotic gradient of 200 mOsm/L is developed between the filtrate of the ascending limb of the Loop of Henle and the interstitial fluid. As a result, the osmo-larity of the filtrate at the end of the Loop of Henle is 100 mOsm/L. Consequently, the kidney may now excrete a urine that is significantly more dilute than plasma. In this way, when the body is overhydrated, excess water is eliminated. The pres-ence of aldosterone promotes additional reabsorption of Na$^+$ ions from the distal tubule and the collecting duct, which further dilutes the filtrate to 65–70 mOsm/L. The presence of ADH promotes the reabsorption of water from the distal tubule and the collecting duct. Water diffuses out of the collecting duct down its concentration gradient into the interstitial fluid. High levels of ADH may concentrate the filtrate to 1,200 mOsm/L. In this way, when the body is dehydrated, water is conserved.

The *descending limb of the Loop of Henle* is permeable to water only. As this region of the tubule passes deeper into the medulla, water leaves the filtrate down its osmotic gradient until it equilibrates with the increasingly concentrated interstitial fluid (see Figure 10.5) and the filtrate also becomes increasingly concentrated. At the tip of the Loop of Henle, the filtrate has an osmolarity of 1,200 mOsm/L.

The *ascending limb of the Loop of Henle* is permeable to NaCl only. As the filtrate flows upward through this region of the tubule back toward the cortex, Na$^+$ ions are continuously and actively pumped out of the filtrate and into the interstitial fluid. Chloride ions passively follow the sodium and the filtrate becomes increasingly dilute. At the end of the ascending limb of the Loop of Henle, approximately 25 mL of filtrate with an osmolarity of 100 mOsm/L remain in the tubule.

Because the transport of sodium is an active process, it is used to accumulate NaCl in the interstitial fluid of the medulla. In fact, this activity is involved in the initial establishment of the vertical osmotic gradient. Furthermore, sodium is actively transported out of the tubular epithelial cells up its concentration gradient until the filtrate is 200 mOsm/L less concentrated than the surrounding interstitial fluid. This difference between the filtrate and the interstitial fluid is referred to as the *horizontal osmotic gradient*. Because the filtrate at the end of the Loop of Henle has an osmolarity of 100 mOsm/L, the kidneys can produce a urine that is significantly more dilute than the plasma.

As the filtrate progresses through the *distal tubule* and the *collecting duct*, the remaining NaCl (10% of that which was filtered) and water (20% of that which was filtered) are handled. As discussed, the presence of aldosterone enhances the reabsorption of sodium from these regions, resulting in a filtrate that may become as dilute as 65–70 mOsm/L. The presence of ADH enhances the reabsorption of water from these regions. In particular, as the filtrate flows through the collecting duct, it enters a region of increasing osmolarity. The increased permeability of water due to ADH allows the water to diffuse out of the collecting duct and into the interstitial fluid down its concentration gradient. When the levels of ADH are high, the water may continue to leave the tubule until the filtrate equilibrates with the surrounding interstitial fluid. In this case, the filtrate may become as concentrated as 1,200 mOsm/L and a small volume of urine is produced. When the levels of ADH are low, water remains in the collecting duct and a large volume of urine is produced.

PHARMACY APPLICATION: PHYSIOLOGICAL ACTION OF DIURETICS

Diuretics are drugs that cause an increase in urine output. It is important to note that, except for the osmotic diuretics, these drugs typically enhance the excretion of both solutes and water. Therefore, the net effect of most diuretics is to decrease plasma volume but can cause a change in plasma osmolarity. Five classes of diuretics and their major sites of action are as follows:

(Continued)

PHARMACY APPLICATION: PHYSIOLOGICAL
ACTION OF DIURETICS (Continued)

- Osmotic diuretics: proximal tubule and descending limb of the Loop of Henle
- Loop diuretics: ascending limb of the Loop of Henle
- Thiazide diuretics: distal tubule
- Potassium-sparing diuretics: cortical collecting duct
- Carbonic anhydrase inhibitors: proximal tubule

Osmotic diuretics, such as mannitol, act on the proximal tubule and, more specifically, the descending limb of the Loop of Henle portions that are permeable to water. These drugs are freely filtered at the glomerulus, but not reabsorbed. Therefore, the drug remains in the tubular filtrate, increasing the osmolarity of this fluid. This increase in osmolarity keeps the water within the tubule, causing water diuresis. Because they primarily affect water and not sodium, the net effect is a reduction in total body water content more than cation content. Osmotic diuretics are poorly absorbed and must be administered intravenously. These drugs may be used to treat patients in acute renal failure and with dialysis disequilibrium syndrome. The latter disorder is caused by the excessively rapid removal of solutes from the extracellular fluid by hemodialysis.

Loop diuretics, such as furosemide, act on the ascending limb of the Loop of Henle, a portion of the tubule that is permeable to Na^+ and Cl^+ ions. The mechanism of action of these diuretics involves the inhibition of the Na^+-K^+-$2Cl^-$ symporter in the luminal membrane. By inhibiting this transport mechanism, loop diuretics reduce the reabsorption of both NaCl and K^+ ions. Recall that it is the reabsorption of NaCl from the ascending limb of the Loop of Henle that generates and maintains the vertical osmotic gradient in the medulla. Without the reabsorption of NaCl, this gradient is diminished and the osmolarity of the interstitial fluid in the medulla is decreased. When the osmolarity of the medulla is decreased, then the reabsorption of water from the descending limb of the Loop of Henle and the collecting duct is significantly reduced. The net result of the loop diuretics includes reduced NaCl and water reabsorption and, therefore, enhanced NaCl and water loss in the urine. The most potent diuretics available (up to 25% of the filtered Na^+ ions may be excreted), the loop diuretics may cause hypovolemia. These drugs are often used to treat acute pulmonary edema, chronic congestive heart failure and the edema and ascites of liver cirrhosis.

(Continued)

PHARMACY APPLICATION: PHYSIOLOGICAL
ACTION OF DIURETICS (Continued)

Thiazide diuretics, such as chlorothiazide, act on the distal tubule, a portion of the tubule that is permeable to sodium. The mechanism of action of these diuretics involves the inhibition of NaCl reabsorption by blocking the Na^+-Cl^- symporter in the luminal membrane. The thiazide diuretics are only moderately effective due to the location of their site of action. Approximately 90% of the filtered Na^+ ions have already been reabsorbed when the filtrate reaches the distal tubule. These drugs may be used for the treatment of edema associated with heart, liver and renal disease. Thiazide diuretics are also widely used for the treatment of hypertension.

Potassium-sparing diuretics act on the late portion of the distal tubule and on the cortical collecting duct. Because of the location of their action, the potassium-sparing diuretics also have a limited effect on diuresis compared with the loop diuretics (3% of the filtered Na^+ ions may be excreted). However, the clinical advantage of these drugs is that the reabsorption of K^+ ions is enhanced, reducing the risk of hypokalemia.

There are two types of potassium-sparing diuretics with different mechanisms of action. Agents of the first type, which include spironolactone, are also known as aldosterone antagonists. These drugs bind directly to the aldosterone receptor and prevent this hormone from exerting its effects. Agents of the second type, which include amiloride, are inhibitors of the tubular epithelial Na^+ channels. Acting on the Na^+ channels in the luminal membrane, these drugs prevent the movement of Na^+ ions from the filtrate into the epithelial cell. Because this transport of Na^+ ions into the cell is coupled to the transport of K^+ ions out of the cell, less potassium is lost to the filtrate and, therefore, the urine.

Potassium-sparing diuretics are often coadministered with the thiazide or loop diuretics in the treatment of edema and hypertension. In this way, the edema fluid is lost to the urine while K^+ ion balance is better maintained. The aldosterone antagonists are particularly useful in the treatment of primary hyperaldosteronism.

Carbonic anhydrase inhibitors, such as acetazolamide, act in the proximal tubule. These drugs prevent the formation of H^+ ions, which are transported out of the tubular epithelial cell in exchange for Na^+ ions. These agents have limited clinical usefulness because they result in the development of metabolic acidosis.

The *vasa recta* are modified peritubular capillaries. As with the peritubular capillaries, the vasa recta arise from the efferent arterioles. However, these vessels are associated only with the juxtamedullary nephrons and are found only in the medullary region of the kidney. The vasa recta pass straight through to the inner region of the medulla, form a hairpin loop and return straight toward the cortex. This structure allows these vessels to lie parallel to the Loops of Henle and the collecting ducts.

The vasa recta perform several important functions. These vessels:

- Provide oxygen and nourishment to the tubules of the medullary region of the kidneys
- Return the NaCl and water reabsorbed from the Loops of Henle and the collecting ducts back to the general circulation
- Deliver substances to the tubules for secretion
- Maintain the vertical osmotic gradient within the interstitial fluid of the medulla

Blood entering the vasa recta has an osmolarity of about 300 mOsm/L. As the vessels travel through the increasingly concentrated medulla, the osmolarity of the blood within them equilibrates with that of the surrounding interstitial fluid. In other words, the blood also becomes increasingly concentrated. Water leaves the vasa recta down its concentration gradient and NaCl enters the vasa recta down its concentration gradient. Therefore, at the innermost region of the medulla, the osmolarity of the blood is 1,200 mOsm/L. If the process were to be interrupted at this point, all the NaCl that had initially created the vertical gradient would eventually be washed away, or removed from the medulla, by the blood flowing through it. However, like the Loops of Henle, the vasa recta form a hairpin loop and travel back toward the cortex through an increasingly dilute interstitial fluid. Once again, the osmolarity of the blood within them equilibrates with that of the surrounding interstitial fluid. In other words, the blood now becomes increasingly dilute. Water enters the vasa recta down its concentration gradient and NaCl leaves the vasa recta down its concentration gradient. Consequently, when this blood has reached the cortex, its osmolarity has returned to 300 mOsm/L. Therefore, the blood leaving the vasa recta has an osmolarity similar to that of the blood that entered the vasa recta. What does change is the volume of blood that leaves the vasa recta. Once again, the excess NaCl and water reabsorbed from the tubules within the medulla have been picked up by these vessels and returned to the general circulation. It is important to note that this process has been performed without disrupting the vertical medullary gradient.

Tubular secretion is the transfer of substances from the peritubular capillaries into the renal tubule for excretion in the urine. This process is particularly important for the regulation of potassium and hydrogen ions in the body.

It is also responsible for the removal of many organic compounds from the
body. These may include metabolic wastes as well as foreign compounds,
including drugs, such as penicillin. Most substances are secreted by secondary active transport.

10.4.5   Potassium ion secretion

Potassium ions are secreted in the distal tubule and the collecting duct. These
ions diffuse down their concentration gradient from the peritubular capillaries into the interstitial fluid. They are then actively transported up their
concentration gradient into the tubular epithelial cells by way of the Na^+-K^+
pump in the basolateral membrane. Finally, potassium ions exit the epithelial cells by passive diffusion through K^+ channels in the luminal membrane
and enter the tubular fluid to be excreted in the urine.

Potassium secretion is enhanced by aldosterone. As the concentration of
K^+ ions in the extracellular fluid increases, the secretion of aldosterone from
the adrenal cortex also increases. The mechanism of action of aldosterone
involves an increase in the activity of the Na^+-K^+ pump in the basolateral
membrane. Furthermore, aldosterone enhances the formation of K^+ channels in the luminal membrane.

10.4.6   Hydrogen ion secretion

Hydrogen ions are secreted in the proximal tubule, the distal tubule and the
collecting duct. The secretion of hydrogen ions is an important mechanism
in acid-base balance. The normal pH of the arterial blood is 7.4. When the
plasma becomes acidic, H^+ ion secretion increases. Conversely, when the
plasma becomes alkalotic, the secretion of H^+ ions is reduced.

10.5   Plasma clearance

Plasma clearance is defined as the volume of plasma from which a substance is
completely cleared by the kidneys per unit time (milliliter per minute). The calculation of the plasma clearance of certain substances can be used to determine:

- GFR: volume of plasma filtered per minute
- ERPF: effective renal plasma flow

To measure the plasma clearance of a substance, the following variables
must be determined:

- Rate of urine formation (V; mL/min)
- Concentration of the substance in the urine (U; mg/mL)
- Concentration of the substance in the arterial plasma (P; mg/mL)

The plasma clearance of a substance is calculated as follows:

$$\text{Plasma clearance} = \frac{V(\text{mL/min}) \times U(\text{mg/mL})}{P(\text{mg/mL})}$$

To use the *plasma clearance of a substance to determine GFR,* several criteria regarding the substance must be met. The substance must:

- Be freely filtered at the glomerulus
- Not be reabsorbed
- Not be secreted
- Not be synthesized or broken down by the tubules
- Not alter the GFR

A substance that fulfills these criteria is *inulin,* a polysaccharide found in plants. Inulin is administered intravenously to a patient at a rate that results in a constant plasma concentration over the course of at least 1 hour. The urine is collected and its volume and its concentration of inulin are measured.

Consider the following example in which, at the end of 1 hour, 60 mL of urine are produced, the concentration of inulin in the urine is 20 mg/mL and the concentration of inulin in the plasma is 0.16 mg/mL.

$$\text{Plasma clearance of inulin} = \frac{1\,\text{mL/min} \times 20\,\text{mg/mL}}{0.16\,\text{mg/mL}}$$

$$= 125\,\text{mL/min}$$

Because inulin is neither reabsorbed nor secreted, all the inulin in the urine was filtered at the glomerulus. Therefore, the plasma clearance of inulin is equal to the GFR.

Although the measurement of GFR with inulin is quite accurate, it is inconvenient because it requires the continuous infusion of this exogenous substance for several hours. More often, in clinical situations, the plasma clearance of *creatinine* is used to estimate GFR. Creatinine, an end-product of muscle metabolism, is released into the blood at a fairly constant rate. Consequently, only a single blood sample and a 24-hour urine collection are needed. The measurement of the plasma clearance of creatinine provides only an *estimate* of GFR. In fact, this measurement slightly overestimates GFR. A small amount of creatinine is secreted into the urine (about 10% on average). In other words, the concentration of creatinine in the urine is the result of the amount that is filtered (as determined by GFR) *plus* the small amount secreted.

To use the *plasma clearance of a substance to determine the effective rate of plasma flow (ERPF)* through the kidneys, several criteria regarding the substance must be met. The substance must:

- Be freely filtered at the glomerulus
- Not be reabsorbed
- Be secreted into the tubules

A substance that fulfills these criteria is *para-aminohippuric acid* (PAH). All of the PAH that is not filtered at the glomerulus is secreted by the proximal tubule. The net effect is that all the plasma that flows through the nephrons is completely cleared of PAH. It is important to note that about 10%–15% of the total renal plasma flow supplies regions of the kidneys that are not involved with filtration or secretion. Consequently, this plasma cannot be cleared of PAH. Therefore, the plasma clearance of PAH provides a measurement of the *effective* renal plasma flow, that is, the volume of plasma that flows through the nephrons. The ERPF is normally about 625 mL/min. (This value is based on a renal blood flow of about 1.1 L/min and a hematocrit of about 42.)

The *filtration fraction* is the percent of the plasma flowing through the nephrons that is filtered into the tubules. It is calculated using the plasma clearance of inulin (GFR) and the plasma clearance of PAH (ERPF).

$$\text{Filtration fraction} = \frac{\text{GFR}}{\text{ERPF}}$$

$$= \frac{125\ \text{mL/min}}{625\ \text{mL/min}}$$

$$= 20\%$$

On average, 20% of the plasma that flows through the glomerulus is filtered into the tubules.

10.6   Renal blood flow

The kidneys receive a disproportionate fraction of the cardiac output. Although the combined weight of the kidneys accounts for less than 1% of the total body weight, these organs receive 20%–25% of the cardiac output. This magnitude of blood flow, which is in profound excess to their metabolic needs, enables them to carry out their multiple homeostatic functions more efficiently. Assuming a resting cardiac output of 5 L/min, the RBF is approximately 1.1 L/min.

Renal blood flow has a direct effect on GFR, which in turn, has a direct effect on urine output. As RBF increases, the GFR increases and urine output increases. Conversely, as RBF decreases, the GFR decreases and urine output decreases.

Furthermore, any change in urine output affects plasma volume and blood pressure. Therefore, the regulation of RBF and GFR are important considerations.

According to Ohm's Law, $(Q = \Delta P/R)$, RBF is determined by mean arterial pressure (MAP) and the resistance of the afferent arteriole $(R_{aff\ art})$:

$$RBF = \frac{\text{Mean Arterial Pressure}}{R_{\text{afferent arteriole}}}$$

10.6.1 *Autoregulation*

The equation for RBF predicts that an increase in MAP will increase blood flow through the kidneys and a decrease in MAP will decrease blood flow through the kidneys. Physiologically, this response is not always desired. For example, during exercise, MAP increases to increase blood flow to the working skeletal muscles. However, a corresponding increase in RBF would lead to an increase in GFR and an undesired loss of water and solutes in the urine. On the other hand, a profound decrease in MAP could decrease RBF and GFR. In this case, the elimination of wastes would be impaired. Therefore, there are physiological conditions in which maintaining a relatively constant RBF and GFR, even when MAP changes, is advantageous.

Interestingly, RBF remains rather constant when MAP changes in the range of 90–180 mmHg. This ability to maintain a constant blood flow despite changes in MAP is referred to as *autoregulation*. The mechanism of autoregulation involves corresponding changes in the resistance of the afferent arteriole. For example, when there is an increase in MAP, then the resistance of the afferent arteriole increases proportionately so that RBF remains unchanged. It is important to note that the major site of autoregulatory changes is the *afferent arteriole*. As this arteriole constricts, the glomerular capillary pressure and, therefore, the GFR are reduced back toward their normal values.

Autoregulation of RBF is an *intrarenal response*. In other words, the mechanisms responsible for autoregulation function entirely within the kidney and rely on no external inputs. There are two mechanisms that elicit this response:

- Myogenic mechanism
- Tubuloglomerular feedback

10.6.2 *Myogenic mechanism*

As discussed in Chapter 6, *The Circulatory System*, the *myogenic mechanism* involves the contraction of vascular smooth muscle in response to stretch. For example, an increase in MAP would tend to increase RBF. This leads to an increase in pressure within the afferent arteriole and the distension, or stretch, of the vessel wall. Consequently, the vascular smooth muscle of the afferent arteriole contracts, increases the resistance of the vessel and decreases RBF back toward normal.

10.6.3   Tubuloglomerular feedback

Tubuloglomerular feedback involves the activity of the *juxtaglomerular apparatus* (see Figure 10.1). This structure is located where the distal tubule comes into contact with the afferent and efferent arterioles, adjacent to the glomerulus. The juxtaglomerular apparatus is composed of the following:

- Macula densa
- Granular cells

The *macula densa* consists of specialized cells of the distal tubule. These tubular cells are adapted to monitor GFR. In other words, they are sensitive to changes in the rate of filtrate flow through the distal tubule. *Granular cells* are specialized smooth muscle cells of the arterioles, specifically, the afferent arteriole. These cells are adapted to monitor RBF. In other words, they are sensitive to changes in blood flow and blood pressure in the afferent arteriole. As such, they are also referred to as *intrarenal baroreceptors*. It is the granular cells of the juxtaglomerular apparatus that secrete renin. Further discussion of granular cell function is found in a subsequent Section 10.6.6. Angiotensin II. Tubuloglomerular feedback involves the function of the *macula densa*. This mechanism may be summarized with the following example where there is an increase in MAP:

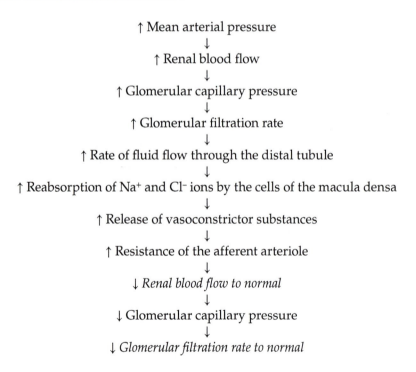

↑ Mean arterial pressure
↓
↑ Renal blood flow
↓
↑ Glomerular capillary pressure
↓
↑ Glomerular filtration rate
↓
↑ Rate of fluid flow through the distal tubule
↓
↑ Reabsorption of Na⁺ and Cl⁻ ions by the cells of the macula densa
↓
↑ Release of vasoconstrictor substances
↓
↑ Resistance of the afferent arteriole
↓
↓ *Renal blood flow to normal*
↓
↓ Glomerular capillary pressure
↓
↓ *Glomerular filtration rate to normal*

An increase in MAP leads to an increase in RBF, an increase in P_{GC} and an increase in GFR and the rate of fluid flow through the distal tubule increases. This leads to an increase in the reabsorption of Na^+ and Cl^- ions by the cells of the macula densa in the distal tubule. Consequently, these cells release vasoconstrictor substances, primarily, *adenosine*. The subsequent increase in the resistance of the nearby afferent arteriole decreases RBF back to normal and P_{GC} and, therefore, GFR decrease back to normal. In this way, the distal tubule regulates its own filtrate flow.

10.6.4   Resistance of the afferent arteriole

Many physiological conditions warrant a change in RBF and GFR, even when MAP is within the autoregulatory range. For example, volume overload is resolved with an increase in RBF, an increase in GFR and an increase in urine output. In this way, excess water and solutes are eliminated. Conversely, volume depletion, such as occurs with hemorrhage or dehydration, is resolved with a decrease in RBF, a decrease in GFR, and a decrease in urine output. In this way, water and solutes are conserved.

The resistance of the afferent arteriole is influenced by several factors including:

- Sympathetic nerves
- Angiotensin II
- Prostaglandins

10.6.5   Sympathetic nerves

The afferent and efferent arterioles are densely innervated by the sympathetic nervous system. Either norepinephrine, released directly from the nerves, or circulating epinephrine, released from the adrenal medulla, stimulate α_1 adrenergic receptors to cause vasoconstriction. The predominant site of regulation is the afferent arteriole. Under normal resting conditions, there is little sympathetic tone to these vessels so that RBF is comparatively high. As discussed previously, this facilitates glomerular filtration. However, the degree of sympathetic stimulation to the kidneys is altered under various physiological and pathophysiological conditions. For example, consider the case where an individual is volume depleted due to hemorrhage or dehydration:

↓ Plasma volume

↓

↓ Mean arterial pressure

↓

Baroreceptor reflex

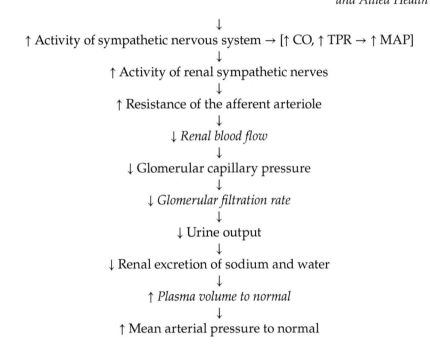

↓
↑ Activity of sympathetic nervous system → [↑ CO, ↑ TPR → ↑ MAP]
↓
↑ Activity of renal sympathetic nerves
↓
↑ Resistance of the afferent arteriole
↓
↓ Renal blood flow
↓
↓ Glomerular capillary pressure
↓
↓ Glomerular filtration rate
↓
↓ Urine output
↓
↓ Renal excretion of sodium and water
↓
↑ Plasma volume to normal
↓
↑ Mean arterial pressure to normal

A loss of plasma volume leads to a decrease in MAP. Baroreceptors located in the aortic and carotid sinuses detect this fall in MAP and elicit reflex responses that include an increase in the overall activity of the sympathetic nervous system. Sympathetic stimulation of the heart and blood vessels leads to an increase in cardiac output (CO) and an increase in total peripheral resistance (TPR). These adjustments, which increase MAP, are responsible for the *short-term regulation of blood pressure*. Although increases in CO and TPR are effective in the temporary maintenance of MAP and blood flow to the vital organs, these activities cannot persist indefinitely. Ultimately, plasma volume must be returned to normal.

An overall increase in sympathetic nervous activity includes an increase in sympathetic input to the kidneys. Consequently, resistance of the afferent arteriole increases, which leads to a decrease in RBF. As discussed, this results in a decrease in P_{GC}, a decrease in GFR and a decrease in urine output. As such, the renal excretion of sodium and water is decreased. In other words, sodium and water are conserved by the body, which increases plasma volume and MAP back toward normal. These changes are responsible for the *long-term regulation of blood pressure*.

Sympathetic stimulation also increases the resistance of the efferent arteriole. This leads to a decrease in the blood pressure in the peritubular capillaries. This fall in pressure facilitates the movement of sodium and water from the tubules into these capillaries.

10.6.6   *Angiotensin II*

Angiotensin II also increases the resistance of the renal arterioles. Consequently, it decreases RBF and GFR.

Angiotensin II is synthesized by the following pathway:

$$\text{Angiotensinogen}$$
$$\downarrow$$
$$\text{Angiotensin I}$$
$$\downarrow$$
$$\text{Angiotensin II}$$

Angiotensinogen, which is synthesized by the liver, is an inactive plasma protein. *Renin*, a hormone secreted by the granular cells of the juxtaglomerular apparatus, promotes the conversion of circulating angiotensinogen into *angiotensin I*. As angiotensin I travels in the blood through the lungs, it is exposed to *angiotensin converting enzyme* (ACE), which is located in the endothelial cells lining the blood vessels of the pulmonary circulation. This enzyme converts angiotensin I into *angiotensin II*.

Angiotensin II has multiple effects throughout the body, all of which directly or indirectly increase MAP. For example, angiotensin II causes the secretion of aldosterone, which enhances sodium reabsorption, expands plasma volume and increases MAP. Angiotensin II is also a potent vasoactive substance that causes widespread vasoconstriction and, therefore, an increase in TPR, which increases MAP. Furthermore, angiotensin II causes powerful vasoconstriction in the renal arterioles that leads to a decrease in RBF and GFR. Consequently, urine output is reduced and water and solutes are conserved by the body. This leads to an increase in plasma volume and, therefore, MAP. Taken together, these effects demonstrate that the production of angiotensin II is beneficial when there has been a fall in blood pressure or blood volume.

The formation of angiotensin II requires the release of renin from the granular cells. Therefore, the factors that affect renin release must be considered:

- Renal sympathetic nerves
- Intrarenal baroreceptors
- Macula densa
- Atrial natriuretic peptide
- Angiotensin II

The sympathetic nervous system increases blood pressure through multiple mechanisms including an increase in cardiac activity and vasoconstriction. Furthermore, stimulation of β_1 *adrenergic receptors* on the granular cells of the afferent arterioles, through the activity of *renal sympathetic nerves* or by circulating epinephrine, has a *direct stimulatory effect on renin secretion*.

The enhanced formation of angiotensin II also increases blood pressure. Specifically, angiotensin II constricts the afferent arteriole, decreases RBF, decreases GFR, decreases urine output, and increases plasma volume and blood pressure. Conversely, a decrease in sympathetic activity results in a decrease in the secretion of renin.

The granular cells that secrete renin also serve as *intrarenal baroreceptors*. These cells monitor blood volume and blood pressure in the afferent arterioles. There is an inverse relationship between arteriolar pressure and renin secretion. In other words, an increase in blood volume causes an increase in arteriolar blood pressure, increased stimulation of the intrarenal baroreceptors and *decreased secretion of renin*. With less angiotensin II-induced vasoconstriction of the afferent arteriole, RBF, GFR and urine output will all increase so that blood volume returns to normal.

The *macula densa*, which is involved in tubuloglomerular feedback, is also a factor in the regulation of renin secretion. In fact, this mechanism involving the macula densa is thought to be important in the maintenance of arterial blood pressure under conditions of decreased blood volume. For example, a decrease in blood volume leads to a decrease in RBF, a decrease in GFR and a decrease in filtrate flow through the distal tubule. The resulting decrease in the delivery of NaCl to the macula densa *stimulates the secretion of renin*. Increased formation of angiotensin II serves to increase MAP and maintain blood flow to the tissues.

Atrial natriuretic peptide is released from myocardial cells in the atria of the heart in response to an increase in atrial filling, or an increase in plasma volume. This hormone *inhibits the release of renin*. With less angiotensin II-induced vasoconstriction of the afferent arteriole, RBF, GFR and urine output all increase. The increased loss of water and solutes decreases blood volume back toward normal.

Angiotensin II directly *inhibits the secretion of renin* from the granular cells. This negative feedback mechanism enables angiotensin II to limit its own formation.

10.6.7   Prostaglandins

The third important factor that influences the resistance of the afferent arterioles is the *prostaglandins*, specifically, PGE_2 and PGI_2. Produced by the kidney, these prostaglandins function as local *vasodilators* that decrease the resistance of the arterioles and increase RBF without changing GFR. Interestingly, the synthesis of PGE_2 and PGI_2 is stimulated by increased activity of the renal sympathetic nerves and by angiotensin II. The vasodilator prostaglandins then oppose the vasoconstrictor effects of norepinephrine and angiotensin II. The net result is a smaller increase in the resistance of the afferent arterioles. This "dampening" effect is important in that it prevents an excessive reduction in RBF, which could lead to ischemia and potential damage of the renal tissues.

10.7   Control of sodium excretion

Sodium is the major extracellular cation. Because of its osmotic effects, changes in sodium content in the body have an important influence on extracellular fluid volume, including plasma volume. For example, excess sodium leads to the retention of water and an increase in plasma volume. An increase in plasma volume then causes an increase in blood pressure. Conversely, sodium deficit leads to water loss and a decrease in plasma volume. A decrease in plasma volume then causes a decrease in blood pressure. Therefore, homeostatic mechanisms involved in the regulation of plasma volume and blood pressure involve the regulation of sodium content, or *sodium balance*, in the body.

Sodium balance is achieved when salt intake is equal to salt output. The intake of salt in the average American diet (10–15 g/day) far exceeds what is required physiologically. Only about 0.5 g/day of salt is lost in the sweat and the feces. The remaining ingested salt must be excreted in the urine.

The *amount of sodium excreted* by the renal system is determined by:

- Amount of sodium filtered at the glomerulus
- Amount of sodium reabsorbed from the tubules

Sodium is freely filtered at the glomerulus. Therefore, any factor that affects GFR will also affect sodium filtration. As discussed previously, GFR is directly related to RBF. In turn, RBF is determined by blood pressure and the resistance of the afferent arteriole (RBF = $MAP/R_{aff\ art}$). For example, an increase in blood pressure or a decrease in the resistance of the afferent arteriole will increase RBF, increase GFR and, consequently, increase the filtration of sodium.

The *amount of sodium reabsorbed* from the tubules is physiologically regulated primarily by aldosterone and, to a lesser extent, by ANP. Aldosterone promotes reabsorption and ANP inhibits it.

The alterations in sodium filtration and sodium reabsorption in response to a decrease in plasma volume are illustrated in Figure 10.6.

A decrease in plasma volume leads to a decrease in MAP, which is detected by the baroreceptors in the carotid sinuses and the arch of the aorta. By way of the vasomotor center, the baroreceptor reflex results in an overall increase in sympathetic nervous activity. This includes stimulation of the heart and of vascular smooth muscle, which causes an increase in cardiac output and in total peripheral resistance. These changes are responsible for the short-term regulation of blood pressure, which temporarily increases MAP back toward normal.

Changes in sodium filtration and sodium reabsorption, which lead to a change in sodium excretion, are responsible for the long-term regulation of blood pressure. These changes are brought about by an increase in the activity of the renal sympathetic nerves. Sympathetic stimulation of α_1 adrenergic

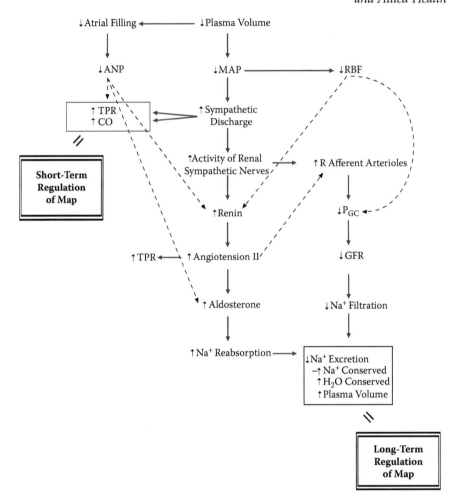

Figure 10.6   The renal handling of sodium.

receptors on renal vascular smooth muscle leads to an increase in the resistance of the afferent arteriole. This causes a decrease in RBF, a decrease in glomerular filtration pressure, a decrease in GFR, and a *decrease in sodium filtration*. If less sodium is filtered, then less sodium is lost in the urine.

Sympathetic stimulation of β_1 adrenergic receptors on the granular cells of the juxtaglomerular apparatus promotes the secretion of renin and, consequently, the formation of angiotensin II. Angiotensin II then causes the following:

- Widespread vasoconstriction
- Increased resistance of the afferent arteriole
- Increased secretion of aldosterone

The widespread vasoconstriction supplements the increase in TPR induced by the sympathetic nervous system. Angiotensin II also causes vasoconstriction of the afferent arteriole, which enhances the decrease in RBF and sodium filtration. Finally, angiotensin II promotes the secretion of aldosterone from the adrenal cortex. Aldosterone then acts on the distal tubule and the collecting duct to increase *sodium reabsorption*.

Sodium reabsorption is also influenced by ANP. The original decrease in plasma volume leads to a decrease in atrial filling and a decrease in the release of ANP from the myocardium. Atrial natriuretic peptide, which acts on vascular smooth muscle, granular cells of the kidney and on the adrenal cortex, normally causes the following:

- Vasodilation
- Decreased renin release
- Decreased aldosterone secretion

Therefore, inhibition of ANP release leads to vasoconstriction and an increase in MAP. Furthermore, less ANP promotes the release of renin and the secretion of aldosterone, which further enhance sodium reabsorption.

Taken together, the homeostatic responses elicited by the initial decrease in plasma volume serve to decrease sodium filtration, increase sodium reabsorption and, consequently, decrease sodium excretion in the urine. This conservation of sodium leads to the conservation of water and an expansion of plasma volume back toward normal.

10.8 Control of water excretion

The regulation of the osmolarity of the extracellular fluid, including that of the plasma, is necessary to avoid osmotically induced changes in intracellular fluid volume. If the extracellular fluid were to become hypertonic (too concentrated), water would be pulled out of the cells. If the extracellular fluid were to become hypotonic (too dilute), water would enter the cells.

The osmolarity of the extracellular fluid is maintained at 290 mOsm/L by way of the physiological regulation of water excretion. As with sodium, *water balance* in the body is achieved when water intake is equal to water output. Sources of water input include:

- Fluid intake
- Water in food
- Metabolically produced water

Sources of water output include:

- Loss from the lungs and non-sweating skin
- Sweating
- Feces
- Urine

The two factors that are controlled physiologically to maintain water balance include fluid intake and urine output. *Fluid intake* is largely influenced by the subjective feeling of *thirst*, which compels an individual to ingest water or other fluids. Urine output is largely influenced by the action of ADH, which promotes the reabsorption of water from the distal tubule and the collecting duct. Thirst and ADH secretion are regulated by the hypothalamus. In fact, three functional regions of the hypothalamus are involved:

- Osmoreceptors
- Thirst center
- ADH-secreting cells

The *osmoreceptors* of the hypothalamus monitor the osmolarity of the extracellular fluid. These receptors are stimulated primarily by an increase in *plasma osmolarity*. The osmoreceptors then provide excitatory inputs to the thirst center and the ADH-secreting cells in the hypothalamus. The threshold for ADH secretion is approximately 285 mOsm/L and the threshold for the stimulation of thirst is approximately 295 mOsm/L. The stimulation of the thirst center leads to an increase of fluid intake. The stimulation of the ADH-secreting cells leads to the release of ADH from the neurohypophysis and, ultimately, an increase in the reabsorption of water from the kidneys and a decrease in urine output. These effects increase the water content of the body and dilute the plasma back toward normal. Plasma osmolarity is the major stimulus for thirst and ADH secretion.

Two other stimuli for thirst and ADH secretion include:

- Decreased extracellular volume
- Angiotensin II

A more moderate stimulus for thirst and ADH secretion is a *decrease in extracellular fluid, or plasma volume*. This stimulus involves the low-pressure receptors in the atria of the heart as well as the baroreceptors in the large arteries. A decrease in plasma volume leads to a decrease in atrial filling, which is detected by the low-pressure receptors, and a decrease in MAP, which is detected by the baroreceptors. Each of these receptors then provides excitatory inputs to the thirst center and to the ADH-secreting cells.

Angiotensin II also stimulates the thirst center, to increase the urge to ingest fluids, and ADH secretion, to promote the reabsorption of water from the kidneys. Other factors that influence ADH-secreting cells (but not the thirst center) include pain, fear, and trauma, which increase ADH secretion, and alcohol, which decreases ADH secretion.

PHARMACY APPLICATION: DRUG-RELATED NEPHROPATHIES

Drug-related nephropathies involve functional or structural changes in the kidneys following the administration of certain drugs. The nephrons are subject to a high rate of exposure to substances in the blood due to the high rate of renal blood flow and the substantial glomerular filtration rate. Furthermore, the kidneys may be involved in the metabolic transformation of some drugs and are, therefore, exposed to their potentially toxic end-products.

Elderly patients are particularly susceptible to kidney damage due to their age-related decrease in renal function. Furthermore, the potential for nephrotoxicity is increased when two or more drugs, capable of causing renal damage, are administered at the same time.

Drugs and toxic end-products of drug metabolism may damage the kidneys by way of the following mechanisms:

- Decrease in renal blood flow
- Direct damage to the tubulointerstitial structures
- Hypersensitivity reactions

Nonsteroidal anti-inflammatory drugs (NSAIDs) may damage renal structures, specifically, the interstitial cells of the medulla. Prostaglandins E_2 and I_2 are vasodilators that help to regulate renal blood flow under normal physiological conditions. Because NSAIDs inhibit the synthesis of prostaglandins, renal damage likely results from an inappropriate decrease in renal blood flow.

Chronic analgesic nephritis (inflammation of the nephrons) is associated with analgesic abuse. Ingredients such as aspirin and acetaminophen have been implicated in this disorder.

Acute drug-related hypersensitivity reactions (allergic responses) may cause tubulointerstitial nephritis, which will damage the tubules and the interstitium. These reactions are most commonly observed with the administration of methicillin and other synthetic antibiotics as well as furosemide and the thiazide diuretics. The onset of symptoms occurs in about 15 days. Symptoms include fever, eosinophilia, hematuria (blood in the urine), and

(Continued)

PHARMACY APPLICATION:
DRUG-RELATED NEPHROPATHIES (Continued)

proteinuria (proteins in the urine). Signs and symptoms of acute renal failure develop in about 50% of the cases. Discontinued use of the drug usually
results in complete recovery. However, some patients, especially the elderly,
may experience permanent renal damage.

10.9 Disorders of the kidney and urinary tract

The kidneys are essential excretory organs that remove the waste products of
metabolism from the body. In addition to their role in excretion, the kidneys
also function in regulation of blood pressure, blood volume and erythropoiesis.
The nephron is the functional unit of the kidney. Each nephron is comprised
of a glomerulus, which acts as a selective filter, and the renal tubules, which
selectively absorb and secrete solutes between the filtrate and blood. In order
for the nephrons to function normally, three things must occur. First, there
must be adequate blood flow through the glomerular capillaries. Second, the
glomerular capillaries, which selectively filter blood, must be intact. Normal
glomeruli allow fluids and small solutes to be filtered into the renal tubules
but not proteins or blood cells. Third, the tubules of the kidney must be able to
selectively reabsorb essential substances from the filtrate while excreting other
substances into the filtrate to be eliminated in the final urine.

10.9.1 Evaluation of renal function

Measurement of the rate at which substances are "cleared" from the plasma
can be a means of evaluating how effectively the kidneys are functioning. In
order to be useful as a measure of renal clearance, the substance measured can
only be filtered by the kidneys and not reabsorbed or secreted by the kidney
tubules. The most widely used method of estimating renal clearance involves
measuring the rate at which *creatinine* is eliminated into the urine over a set
period of time. Creatinine is a by-product of skeletal muscle metabolism and
is present in the plasma at relatively constant levels. The main drawback to
the use of "creatinine clearance" to measure renal function is that any condition that increases skeletal muscle breakdown (e.g., sepsis, muscle injury,
muscle disease) will elevate levels of serum creatinine and invalidate the measure. A second substance that can be used to estimate renal clearance is *inulin*.
Inulin is a polysaccharide that is administered intravenously to the patient and
its elimination in the urine is measured over time. Inulin offers the advantage
that it is not metabolized or formed anywhere in the body and is eliminated
only through renal filtration. The disadvantage to inulin is that it is not an
endogenous substance and must be administered intravenously.

10.9.2   Disorders of the glomerulus

10.9.2.1   Acute glomerulonephritis

- Inflammation of the glomerulus
- Occurs most commonly 7–10 days following an infection with group A streptococcus. Trapping of antibody-antigen complexes in glomerular capillaries causes inflammation of the glomerulus and alters its selective permeability allowing plasma proteins and blood cells to enter the kidney filtrate.
- The active inflammatory process involves infiltration with white blood cells that may enhance the inflammatory process.
- May also be related to systemic conditions such as *lupus erythematosus* and *Berger's disease* where there are excess levels of circulating antibodies or antigen-antibody complexes.
- Glomerular damage may result and certain patients may develop rapidly progressing glomerulonephritis or chronic glomerulonephritis.

10.9.2.2   Rapidly progressing glomerulonephritis

- Occurs most commonly in individuals in their 50s and 60s
- May be idiopathic in origin or the result of acute glomerulonephritis or *Goodpasture syndrome* (see box)
- Presents with rapidly developing inflammation of the glomeruli and dramatic decreases in *glomerular filtration rate*
- Characterized by the formation of proliferative "crescent" that fill Bowman's capsule. Often associated with hematuria
- Rapid degeneration of glomerular function is seen. Prognosis is poor unless diagnosed early and treated effectively. May lead to renal failure

---

GOODPASTURE SYNDROME

- A rare form of rapidly progressing glomerulonephritis caused by antibodies that are produced against cells of the glomerulus
- Leads to extensive inflammation and damage of the glomeruli to the point where renal failure may occur

---

10.9.2.3   IgA nephropathy (Berger's disease)

- A common cause of glomerulonephritis in developed countries, particularly in Asia
- Cause is uncertain but involves the production of an abnormal glycosylated IgA that binds to glomerular tissues and triggers a complement-mediated immune attack

- Rapid glomerular injury is associated with hematuria, and possibly proteinuria
- Treatment may involve immunosuppressive therapy

10.9.2.3.1   *Membranous glomerulonephritis*
- The most common cause of primary glomerulonephrosis in older adults
- Characterized by a thickening of the glomerular basement membrane
- May be associated with the deposition of immune complexes
- Presents with *nephrotic syndrome* (see below)
- Course is highly variable, spontaneous remissions may occur although a significant percentage of cases (30%–40%) may go on to have impaired renal function. Treatment often involves the administration of corticosteroids

10.9.2.3.2   *Chronic glomerulonephritis*
- Chronic inflammation of the glomeruli
- Etiology may be diverse, many patients with chronic glomerulonephritis may have no history of acute renal disease
- May be associated with chronic hypertension, diabetes mellitus
- May remain asymptomatic for a number of years before symptoms of proteinuria, hematuria occur
- Progressive loss of renal function occurs over a number of years, leading to renal insufficiency and renal failure

10.9.2.3.2.1   *Manifestations of glomerulonephritis*
- Proteinuria (appearance of protein in the urine, primarily albumin)
- Hematuria (appearance of blood in the urine)
- With chronic forms of glomerulonephritis, decreased urine volume, and fluid retention may occur as renal insufficiency and renal failure develops
- Hypertension is a possible consequence due to reduced renal blood flow and activation of the renin-angiotensin system

10.9.2.3.2.2   *Treatment of glomerulonephritis*
- Antibiotic therapy if caused by bacterial infection
- Immunosuppressive drugs if autoimmune destruction of glomeruli is occurring
- Management of resulting edema, mineral imbalance and possible hypertension

10.9.3   *Nephrotic syndrome*
- A set of symptoms that occurs when there is damage or inflammation to the glomerulus that leads to significant increases in permeability
- Patients with nephrotic syndrome present with:
  - Massive proteinuria

- Hypoalbuminemia
- Generalized edema due to the loss of colloid osmotic pressure (albumin)
- Hyperlipidemia, lipiduria

10.9.4   Pyelonephritis

- Pyelonephritis is renal disease associated with inflammation of the renal tubules and renal pelvis.
- It occurs when organisms from a lower urinary tract infection enter the kidney.
- Pyelonephritis is more likely to occur in individuals who have a urinary tract obstruction (see below) or urine reflux because these conditions are associated with stasis of urine that may allow bacteria to ascend the urinary tract and enter the kidney.
- Symptoms of pyelonephritis include fever, pain, chills, dysuria, and nausea.
- Appropriate antibiotic therapy will resolve most cases of uncomplicated pyelonephritis.
- Chronic pyelonephritis may occur in patients with chronic urinary tract infections, urinary tract obstruction or urine reflux and may lead to damage of the renal tubules and a progressive loss of renal function.

10.9.5   Urinary tract infections

- Generally bacterial in origin. The most common organisms responsible for urinary tract infection is *E. coli*. Other bacteria that may cause urinary tract infections include *Staphylococcus saprophyticus, Klebsiella, Proteus mirabilis, and Pseudomonas.*
- May occur in any of the urinary tract structures
- Occurs most frequently in females as well as in the elderly of both sexes
- Risk factors for the development of urinary tract infections include:
  - Urine obstruction or reflux
  - Sexual activity
  - Urinary catheterization, instrumentation
  - Neurogenic bladder

10.9.5.1   Manifestations of urinary tract infection
- Painful urination
- Increased urgency and frequency of urination
- *Cystitis*—inflammation of the bladder
- *Pyelonephritis*—inflammation of the renal tubules, pelves and calyces that may be acute or chronic. *Chronic pyelonephritis* may lead to scaring of kidney structures and possible loss of kidney function
- Fever may also occur along with the presence of white blood cells in the urine
- Frequent urinary tract infections in a patient might indicate the presence of a urinary tract obstruction or urine reflux

10.9.5.2   Treatment of urinary tract infection

- Appropriate antibiotics
- Surgical correction of obstruction or structural abnormality that might be causing urine retention

10.9.6   Renal calculi (kidney stones)

- Form mainly in the renal pelves or calyces, but can form anywhere in the kidneys
- Comprised mainly of calcium salts, uric acid and cystine
- Although the exact etiology is unclear, predisposing factors include:
  - Dehydration
  - Changes in urine pH
  - Decreased urine production
  - Excess salt secretion
  - Gout—uric acid stones
  - Obstruction of urine flow

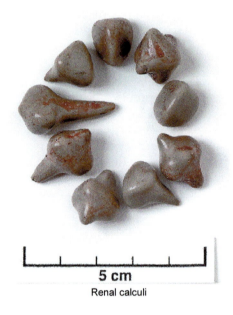

5 cm

Renal calculi

10.9.6.1   Manifestations of renal calculi

- Many renal calculi are asymptomatic until they obstruct kidney structures such as the calyces or pelves
- Severe pain can result from obstruction
- Fever, chills

- Hematuria
- Gastrointestinal symptoms (nausea, vomiting)
- Urine obstruction
- Complications may include damage to renal structures and acute renal failure

10.9.6.2 Diagnosis of renal calculi
- Measurement of stone-forming substances in blood and urine
- X-ray
- Radiography
- Ultrasound

10.9.6.3 Treatment of renal calculi
- Preventative measures include increased fluid intake, acidification of the urine, and reduction of serum uric acid levels
- Surgical removal of stones
- *Lithotripsy*—ultrasonic destruction of stones. Fragmented stones may than pass naturally with the urine

10.9.7 Renal tumors

Tumors of the kidney may be either rare benign *adenomas* or, more commonly, malignant *renal cell carcinomas*. If benign adenomas arise, they tend to be small and usually not clinically significant. The prognosis for renal cell carcinomas depends upon the morphology of the cells involved and the extent of spread outside the kidney. Renal carcinomas may metastasize to the lymphatics, liver, lungs and bone marrow.

Wilm's Tumor (Nephroblastoma) is a rare malignant tumor that arises in infants and children. The tumor presents with unique histology that may resemble embryonic kidney. The tumor generally responds well to chemotherapy but can metastasize rapidly.

10.9.7.1 Manifestations of renal tumors
- Hematuria
- Pain in the flanks
- Weight loss
- Many renal tumors are asymptomatic until the tumor is of advanced size and begins to disrupt renal structures
- Metastatic tumors can occur with advanced disease

10.9.7.2 Treatment of renal tumors
- Chemotherapy, radiation therapy
- Surgical removal of tumors

10.9.8 *Polycystic kidney disease* (see Figure 10.7)

Polycystic kidney disease is a hereditary disorder that can have an *autosomal dominant* (adult form) or *autosomal recessive* (childhood form) pattern of inheritance. Cysts develop in both kidneys and gradually increase in size. Enlarging cysts can destroy normal kidney tissue and lead to a progressive loss of renal function that may culminate in renal failure. The recessive form of the disease may cause renal failure in childhood, whereas the dominant form progresses more slowly and generally does not lead to renal failure until the patient enters their 60s or 70s.

10.9.8.1 *Manifestations of polycystic kidney disease*
- Grossly enlarged kidneys
- Hypertension from activation of the renin-angiotensin system
- Renal insufficiency leading to renal failure
- Pain in the flanks
- Frequent infections

10.9.8.2 *Treatment of polycystic kidney disease*
- Management of renal insufficiency and renal failure with dialysis
- Management of hypertension. Patients may be at particular risk for aneurysms and cerebral hemorrhage
- Renal transplantation
- Antibiotics for frequent infections

10.9.9 *Renal failure*

Renal failure refers to a significant loss of renal function in both kidneys to the point where less than 10%–20% of normal GFR remains. Renal failure may occur as an acute and rapidly progressing process or as a chronic form

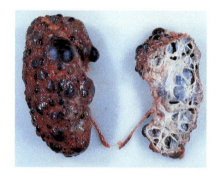

Figure 10.7 A polycystic kidney. (Adapted from *Porth's Pathophysiology: Concepts of Altered Health States* by Grossman, Lippincott Williams and Wilkins, 2013.)

Table 10.1   Causes of acute renal failure

Prerenal Failure
- Caused by impaired or reduced blood flow to the kidney
- Possible causes include shock, hypotension, anaphylaxis, sepsis
- Unless blood flow and oxygen delivery are restored, permanent damage to the kidney will result

Intrarenal Failure
- Results from acute damage to renal structures
- Possible causes include acute glomerulonephritis, pyelonephritis
- May also result from *acute tubular necrosis* (ATN), that is, damage of the kidney structure from exposure to toxins, solvents, drugs, and heavy metals. ATN is the most common cause of acute renal failure

Postrenal Failure
- Results from conditions that block urine outflow
- Possible causes include obstruction of urine outflow by calculi, tumors, prostatic hypertrophy

---

in which there is a progressive loss of renal function over a number of years. Possible causes of renal failure are listed in Table 10.1.

10.9.9.1   Acute renal failure
- Abrupt decrease in renal function
- The possible causes of acute renal failure are shown in the Table 10.1. These causes of acute renal failure may be *prerenal, intrarenal* or *postrenal* in nature. Acute renal failure is often reversible so long as permanent injury to the kidney has not occurred

10.9.9.2   Manifestations of acute renal failure
- *Oliguria* (reduced urine output)
- Possible edema and fluid retention
- Elevated blood urea nitrogen levels (BUN), and serum creatinine
- Alterations in serum electrolytes

10.9.9.3   Treatment of acute renal failure
- Prevention of acute renal failure through support of blood pressure and blood volume
- Correction of fluid and electrolyte imbalances
- *Dialysis* may be employed while the kidneys are in the recovery phase
- Low-protein, high-carbohydrate diet to minimize the formation of nitrogenous wastes

10.9.10   Chronic renal failure

Chronic renal failure is the end result of progressive kidney damage and loss of function. Chronic renal failure is often classified into four progressive

Table 10.2   Stages of chronic renal failure

1. Diminished renal reserve—GFR is decreased to 35%–50% of normal
2. Renal insufficiency—GFR is decreased to 20%–35% of normal
3. Renal failure—GFR is reduced to less than 20% of normal
4. End-stage renal disease—GFR is less than 5% of normal

stages based on the loss of GFR that has occurred (see Table 10.2). Some of the possible causes of chronic renal failure include:

- Chronic glomerulonephritis
- Chronic infections
- Renal obstruction
- Exposure to toxic chemical, toxins, or drugs (see drug box)
- Diabetes
- Hypertension
- *Nephrosclerosis* (atherosclerosis of the renal artery)

AMINOGLYCOSIDE ANTIBIOTICS AND NEPHROTOXICITY

- The aminoglycoside antibiotics are a widely used group of drugs that include agents such as streptomycin, gentamicin and kanamycin.
- The aminoglycosides can be nephrotoxic under certain conditions. Aminoglycoside toxicity is most likely to occur in the elderly, those with renal insufficiency or with chronic use.
- Concurrent use of loop diuretics may also compound the adverse renal effects of the aminoglycosides.

10.9.10.1   Manifestations of chronic renal failure

Because the kidneys play such an essential role in a number of physiologic processes, renal failure is a multisystem disease. The kidneys have a tremendous reserve capacity for function and as a result overt symptoms generally do occur until renal insufficiency is present. The effects of chronic renal failure on the various systems of the body are detailed in Table 10.3.

10.9.10.2   Treatment of renal failure

- Careful management of fluids and electrolytes
- Prudent use of diuretics
- Careful dietary management. Restriction of dietary protein intake is helpful to limit the formation of nitrogenous wastes
- Recombinant erythropoietin to treat anemia
- Renal dialysis (see box and Figure 10.8)
- Renal transplantation

Table 10.3 Effects of chronic renal failure on various systems of the body

System	Effect	Cause
Body Fluids	• Polyuria • Metabolic acidosis • Reduced H^+ excretion • Abnormal levels of Na^+, K^+, Ca^{++}, PO_4^-	• Inability to concentrate urine • Loss of tubular function
Hematologic	• Anemia • Coagulopathies	• Impaired erythropoietin production • Abnormal platelet function
Cardiovascular	• Hypertension • Edema	• Activation of renin-angiotensin system
Gastrointestinal Tract	• Anorexia • Nausea	• Accumulation of metabolic wastes
Neurologic	• Uremic encephalopathy	• Accumulation of ammonia and nitrogenous wastes
Musculoskeletal	• Muscle and bone weakness (renal osteodystrophy)	• Loss of calcium and minerals • Excess PTH activity

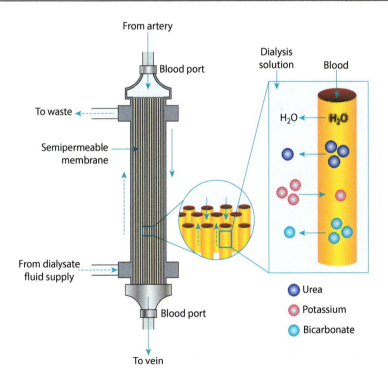

Figure 10.8 Renal dialysis. (Adapted from *Porth's Pathophysiology: Concepts of Altered Health States* by Grossman, Lippincott Williams and Wilkins, 2013.)

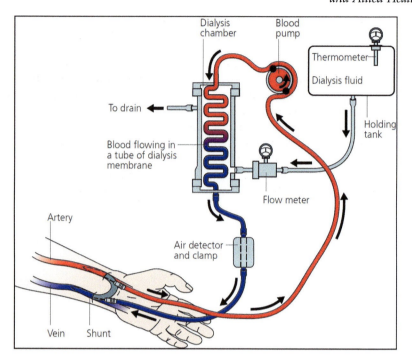

VICIOUS CYCLE OF CHRONIC RENAL FAILURE

There are several physiologic adaptations that occur in the kidneys in response to chronic renal failure. These changes include:

1. Increased renal blood flow and GFR in functional nephrons
2. Hypertrophy of functional nephrons

In the short term, these adaptations may be beneficial; however, in the long term, the increased pressure in the kidneys and increased oxygen demand can further damage the nephrons and worsen renal failure.

HEMODIALYSIS (See the above figure)

- A procedure in which an "artificial kidney" machine takes the place of the patients own failing kidneys.
- Using an indwelling catheter, blood is withdrawn from the patient and passed through a chamber containing a dialysis membrane and

(Continued)

HEMODIALYSIS (See the above figure) (Continued)

clean dialysate solution. Waste products, which are in high concentration in the patients' blood, diffuse across the dialysate membrane and into the dialysate solution. The cleaned blood is then returned to the patient via a second catheter.

- Complications to hemodialysis can include risk of infection, hypotension, and electrolyte imbalance. Patients receiving hemodialysis must undergo the procedure several times per week for 3–6 hours per treatment. Newer high-flux dialysate membranes and improved dialysate solutions have reduced the time of each dialysis session by 1–2 hours.

- An alternative to classic hemodialysis is a technique called *peritoneal dialysis.* A catheter is implanted into the peritoneal cavity and clean dialysate solution is introduced into the peritoneal cavity. The patient's own peritoneum is used as the dialyzing membrane. After a fixed period of time (8–48 hours) the fluid containing the accumulated wastes is removed. Complications may include infections from the catheter, hypotension, edema, and metabolic abnormalities. Peritoneal dialysis offers the advantage that it may be performed in one's own home.

10.10   Disorders of the bladder and urethra

Obstructive uropathy is a general term that refers to conditions that obstruct the outflow of urine (see Figure 10.9). Causes of urinary tract obstruction include stricture of the urethra or ureters, prostatic hypertrophy, and pelvic organ prolapse. When outflow is obstructed from the bladder urine can back up and accumulate in the ureters and lead to their distention. This condition is called *hydroureter*. Prolonged obstruction of urine outflow can cause urine to back up and accumulates in the spaces (pelves and calyces) of the kidney. This is condition is called *hydronephrosis*. The presence of hydronephrosis is more serious than hydroureter because the increased pressure in the renal capsule caused by hydronephrosis can rapidly damage functional structures in the kidney.

10.10.1   Urine reflux

The backward flow of urine from the bladder into the ureters and kidneys (*vesicoureteral reflux*) or from the urethra into the bladder (*urethrovesical reflux*).

- Generally results from congenital abnormalities in the structure or location of the ureters or urethra. May also occur from strictures or scarring.

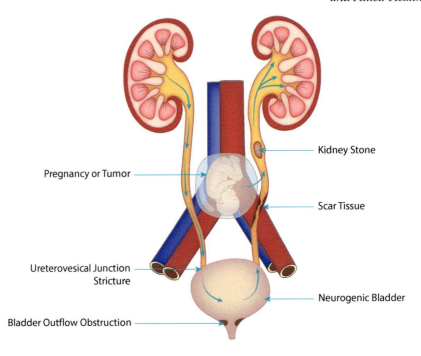

Figure 10.9 Causes of obstructive uropathy. (Adapted from *Porth's Pathophysiology: Concepts of Altered Health States* by Grossman, Lippincott Williams and Wilkins, 2013.)

- Patients often present with urine retention and recurrent urinary tract infections that can lead to *pyelonephritis.*
- Treatment may include antibiotic therapy and possible surgical correction of the structural abnormality.

10.10.2 Neurogenic bladder

- Bladder paralysis that occurs from interruption of nervous input to the muscles of the bladder wall
- Patients are unable to voluntarily or involuntarily empty their bladder
- Causes may include spinal cord trauma, polio, multiple sclerosis and tumors affecting spinal nerves
- Diabetic patients often suffer from peripheral neuropathies that may affect the nerves involved in innervating the bladder muscles and lead to bladder dysfunction
- Manifestations include marked urine retention, frequent urinary tract infections and possible deterioration of renal function (postrenal failure)

10.10.3   Urinary incontinence

The term urinary incontinence refers to the involuntary passage of urine. The risk for urinary incontinence increase with aging and it is a common problem in older adults. Causes of urinary incontinence include:

- Stresses (laughing, coughing, squatting) that increase pressure on the bladder
- *Overactive bladder* (*OAB*) – changes in nervous innervation or bladder muscle function that occur with aging may lead to urinary urgency and incomplete voiding of the bladder
- Bladder overflow—involuntary urine loss that occurs when the bladder is overdistended

10.10.3.1   Treatment of overactive bladder
- Pelvic floor muscle exercises to strengthen the muscle that control urination
- Medications—alpha adrenergic blockers, antimuscarinic agents
- Medical devices, surgery

10.10.4   Bladder cancer

Approximately 74,000 new cases of bladder cancer were diagnosed in the United States in 2015. The average age at diagnosis is 74 years. Men are three to four times more likely to develop bladder cancer than women. The vast majority of bladder cancers arise from the transitional epithelial cells that line the bladder. Tumors may be papillary or flat and have varying degrees of invasiveness. Because the bladder stores urine, the bladder epithelium will be bathed in any carcinogens that are excreted and concentrated into the urine. As such, cigarette smoking is an important risk factor for the development of bladder cancer. Individuals who have been exposed to industrial solvents, toxins and carcinogens likewise have a greater risk for the development of bladder cancer. Most cases of bladder cancer are initially asymptomatic. When symptoms do occur they may include hematuria, urinary urgency, and dysuria. Treatment and prognosis of bladder cancer is dependent upon the type of cancer cells that are present and their invasiveness.

Medical terminology

Acellular (ā-sĕl′ū-lăr): Not containing cells
Aquaporin (ă-kwă-pŏr′ĭn): Water channel
Basolateral (bā-sō-lăt′ĕr-ăl): Referring to the base and side of a cell
Bowman's capsule (bō′măns căp′sūl): Initial portion of the renal tubule that receives the filtrate

Cirrhosis (sĭ-rō'sĭs): Irreversible disease of the liver characterized by the loss of normal hepatic tissue and by scarring

Diuretic (dī"ū-rĕt'ĭk): Substance that increases urine production

Eosinophilia (ē"ō-sĭn-ō-fĭl'ē-ă): Abnormally high number of eosinophils

Fenestrated (fĕn'ĕ-strāt-ĕd): Having openings

Glomerulus (glō-mĕr'ū-lŭs): Capillary network in the kidney where filtration takes place

Hemoturia (hē"mă-tū'rē-ă): Blood in the urine

Hypertonic (hī"pĕr-tŏn'ĭk): Having a higher osmotic pressure

Hypotonic (hī"pō-tŏn'ĭk): Having a lower osmotic pressure

Juxtaglomerular(jŭks"tă-glō-mĕr'ū-lăr): Near the glomerulus

Macula densa (măk'ū-lă dĕn'ză): Specialized cells of the distal tubule forming a portion of the juxtaglomerular apparatus

Natriuretic (nā"trē-ūr-ĕt'ĭk): Substance that increases the excretion of sodium in the urine

Nephritis (nĕf-rī'tĭs): Inflammation of the kidneys

Nephron (nĕf'rŏn): Functional unit of the kidney

Nephropathy (nĕ-frŏp'ă-thē): Disease of the kidney

Nephrotoxin (nĕf"rō-tŏk'sĭn): Substance that damages the kidney

Osmolarity (ŏs"mō-lăr'ĭ-tē): Concentration of osmotic particles in a solution

Osmoreceptor (ŏz"mō-rē-sĕp'tŏr): Receptor sensitive to changes in osmotic pressure

Podocyte (pŏd'ō-sīt): Specialized epithelial cell in Bowman's capsule

Proteinuria (prō"tē-ĭn-ū'rē-ă): Protein in the urine

Tubuloglomerular(tū"bū-lō-glō-mĕr'ū-lăr): Referring to the tubule and the glomerulus of the nephron

Ureter (ū'rĕ-tĕr): Tube that transports urine from the kidney to the bladder

Urethra (ū-rē'thră): Tube that transports urine from the bladder to the outside of the body

Vasa recta (vā'să rĕk'tă): Capillaries that lie parallel to the loops of Henle

Bibliography

Costanzo, L., *Physiology*, 3rd ed., W. B. Saunders Company, Philadelphia, PA, 2006.

Fox, S. I., *Human Physiology*, 9th ed., McGraw-Hill, Boston, MA, 2006.

Guyton, A. C., and Hall, J. E., *Textbook of Medical Physiology*, 11th ed., Elsevier/Saunders, Philadelphia, PA, 2006.

Marieb, E. N., and Hoehn, K., *Anatomy & Physiology*, 3rd ed., Pearson Benjamin Cummings, San Francisco, CA, 2008.

Jackson, E. K., Diuretics, in *Goodman and Gilman's The Pharmacological Basis of Therapeutics*, 11th ed., Brunton, L. L., Lazo, J. S., and Parker, K. L., Eds., McGraw-Hill, New York, 2006, chap. 28.

Koeppen, B. M., and Stanton, B. A., *Renal Physiology*, 4th ed., Mosby, St. Louis, MO, 2007.

Porth, C. M., *Pathophysiology, Concepts of Altered Health States*, 7th ed., Lippincott, Williams & Wilkins, Philadelphia, PA, 2005.

Sherwood, L., *Human Physiology from Cells to Systems*, 5th ed., Brooks/Cole, Pacific Grove, CA, 2004.

Silverthorn, D., *Human Physiology: An Integrated Approach*, 4th ed., Prentice Hall, Upper Saddle River, NJ, 2007.

Stedman's Medical Dictionary for the Health Professions and Nursing, 5th ed., Lippincott Williams & Wilkins, Philadelphia, PA, 2005.

Taber's Cyclopedic Medical Dictionary, 20th ed., F. A. Davis Co., Philadelphia, PA, 2005.

Widmaier, E. P., Raff, H., and Strang, K. T., *Vander's Human Physiology, The Mechanisms of Body Function*, McGraw-Hill, Boston, MA, 2006.

Vander, A. J., *Renal Physiology*, 5th ed., McGraw-Hill, New York, 1995.

chapter eleven

The endocrine system

Study objectives

- Differentiate between the primary functions of the nervous system and the endocrine system
- Describe the biochemical and functional distinctions between steroid hormones, protein/peptide hormones, and amine hormones
- Explain the beneficial effects of the binding of hormones to plasma proteins
- Explain how hormones are eliminated
- Distinguish between a trophic and a nontrophic hormone
- Describe the three types of hormone interactions
- Explain the two primary mechanisms by which hormones carry out their effects
- Describe how the effects of hormones are amplified
- Describe how the pituitary gland is formed during embryonic development
- Describe the anatomical and functional relationships between the hypothalamus and the pituitary gland
- Explain how negative feedback mechanisms limit the release of hormones from the adenohypophysis
- List the functions and describe the mechanisms that regulate the release of hormones from the neurohypophysis
- List the functions and describe the mechanisms that regulate the release of hormones from the adenohypophysis
- Discuss the functions and the factors that regulate the release of the following hormones: thyroid hormones, calcitonin, parathyroid hormone, aldosterone, cortisol, adrenal androgens, insulin and glucagon
- Compare and contrast diabetes insipidus and SIADH in terms of etiology and clinical symptoms
- Discuss the main differences between acromegaly and gigantism
- Distinguish idiopathic short stature from familial short stature
- Distinguish cretinism from myxedema. Why does each occur how do they differ from one another?
- List the main symptoms of hyperthyroidism and hypothyroidism
- Define toxic and nontoxic goiter

- List the main cause and key manifestations of each of the following disorders:

  - Congenital adrenal hyperplasia
  - Addison disease
  - Cushing syndrome
  - Graves' disease

- What is a pheochromocytoma? What effects does it have on the body?
- List the main actions of insulin and glucagon in the body
- List factors that put an individual at risk for developing diabetes mellitus
- Describe the association between the presence of obesity and the development of type 2 diabetes
- Define the three "polys." Why does each occur?
- What are the physiologic manifestations of diabetic ketoacidosis? How might it occur in a patient with type 1 diabetes?
- What is hyperosmolar-hyperglycemic syndrome? How might it occur in a patient with type 2 diabetes?
- Discuss pharmacologic and non-pharmacologic treatment for type 1 and type 2 diabetes mellitus.
- Discuss possible mechanisms of tissue injury in diabetes mellitus
- List the major effects of chronic diabetes mellitus on the body. Why does each occur?
- Define gestational diabetes

There are two major regulatory systems that are the main contributors to homeostasis: the nervous system and the endocrine system. To maintain relatively constant conditions in the internal environment of the body, each of these systems influences the activity of all the other organ systems. Using electrical impulses, the nervous system coordinates rapid, precise responses, such as muscle contractions. However, the effects of the nervous system's impulses are of short duration (milliseconds). Unlike the nervous system, the endocrine system regulates metabolic activity within the cells of the organs and tissues and coordinates activities that require longer duration (hours, days), rather than speed. Examples of such activities include growth, the long-term regulation of plasma volume and blood pressure, and the coordination of menstrual cycles in females.

The endocrine system carries out its effects through the production of *hormones*, chemical messengers that exert a regulatory effect on the cells of the body. Secreted from *endocrine glands*, which are ductless structures, hormones are released directly into the blood. They are then transported by the circulation to the tissues upon which they exert their effects. Because they travel in the blood, the serum concentrations of hormones are very low (10^{-11} to 10^{-9} M); therefore, these molecules must be very potent.

This chapter will consider the hormones secreted from several endocrine glands including the pituitary, thyroid, parathyroid, and adrenal glands, as well as the pancreas. It is important to note, however, that hormones may be secreted from organs and tissues whose primary functions are not endocrine in nature. For example, the hypothalamus synthesizes and releases many hormones that influence the secretion of hormones from the anterior pituitary gland. In addition, the hypothalamus synthesizes the hormones that are subsequently released from the posterior pituitary gland. Other tissues and their hormones include the following:

- Heart: atrial natriuretic hormone (Chapter 7)
- Kidneys: erythropoietin (Chapter 10)
- Stomach: gastrin (Chapter 9)
- Small intestine: secretin, cholecystokinin, gastric inhibitory peptide (Chapter 9)
- Gonads (ovaries and testes): estrogen, progesterone, testosterone (Chapter 12)

Further discussion of these hormones may be found in the chapters as indicated within the parentheses above.

Generally, a single hormone does not affect all the body's cells. The tissues that respond to a hormone are referred to as the *target tissues*. The cells of these tissues possess specific receptors to which the hormone binds. This receptor binding then elicits a series of events that influences cellular activities.

11.1   Biochemical classification of hormones

Hormones are classified into three biochemical categories (see Table 11.1):

- Steroids
- Proteins/peptides
- Amines

Table 11.1   Hormones of the hypothalamus

- *Growth Hormone-Releasing Hormone (GHRH)*—stimulates the release of growth hormone (GH) from the anterior pituitary
- *Gonadotrophin-releasing hormone (GnRH)*—stimulates release of luteinizing hormone (LH) and follicle stimulating hormone (FSH) from the anterior pituitary
- *Thyrotrophin-releasing hormone (TRH)*—stimulates the release of thyroid-stimulating hormone (TSH) and prolactin (PRL) from the anterior pituitary
- *Corticotrophin-releasing hormone (CRH)*—stimulates the release of adrenocorticotrophin (ACTH) from the anterior pituitary
- *Somatostatin*—inhibits the release of growth hormone from the anterior pituitary

Steroid hormones are produced by the adrenal cortex, testes, ovaries, and the placenta. Synthesized from cholesterol, these hormones are lipid soluble. Therefore, they cross cell membranes readily and bind to receptors found intracellularly. However, their lipid solubility renders them insoluble in blood. Therefore, these hormones are transported in the blood bound to proteins. This protein binding protects these hormones from rapid elimination and, thus, steroid hormones tend to have relatively long half-lives.

Steroid hormones are not typically preformed and stored for future use within the endocrine gland. Because they are lipid soluble, they could readily diffuse out of the cells and physiological regulation of their release would not be possible. On a side note, steroid hormones are absorbed easily by the gastrointestinal tract and may be administered orally.

The *protein/peptide hormones* are derived from amino acids and most hormones are of this type. Peptide hormones contain fewer than 100 amino acids (e.g., antidiuretic hormone, oxytocin, insulin, and glucagon). Protein hormones contain more than 100 amino acids (e.g., growth hormone). Glycoprotein hormones are peptide chains containing more than 100 amino acids as well as one or more carbohydrate groups (e.g., follicle-stimulating hormone, luteinizing hormone, thyroid-stimulating hormone).

This class of hormones are preformed and stored for future use in membrane-bound secretory granules with the gland's cells. When needed, they are released by exocytosis. Protein/peptide hormones are water soluble, circulate in the blood predominantly in an unbound form and, therefore, tend to have relatively short half-lives. Because these hormones are unable to cross the cell membranes of their target tissues, they bind to receptors on the membrane surface. Protein/peptide hormones cannot be administered orally because they are easily digested in the gastrointestinal tract. Instead, they are typically administered by injection (e.g., insulin). Small peptides can cross through mucous membranes and, therefore, may be given sublingually or intranasally. For example, Miacalcin®, the synthetic form of the hormone calcitonin, is administered in the form of a nasal spray.

Amine hormones, which are derived from the amino acid tyrosine, include the thyroid hormones and the catecholamines. The thyroid hormones tend to be biologically similar to steroid hormones in that they are mainly insoluble in the blood and are transported predominantly (>99%) bound to proteins. As such, these hormones have longer half-lives (triiodothyronine, $T_3 = 24$ hours; thyroxine, $T_4 = 7$ days). Furthermore, thyroid hormones cross cell membranes to bind with intracellular receptors and may be administered orally (e.g., synthryoid). In contrast to the steroid hormones, however, the thyroid hormones have the unique property of being stored extracellularly in the thyroid gland as part of the thyroglobulin molecule.

The catecholamines are biologically similar to protein/peptide hormones in that these hormones are soluble in the blood and are transported in an unbound form. Therefore, the catecholamines have a relatively short half-life. Because these hormones do not cross cell membranes, they bind to receptors on the membrane surface. Finally, the catecholamines are stored intracellularly in secretory granules for future use.

11.2   Transport of hormones

As discussed in the previous section, steroid and thyroid hormones are transported in the blood bound to plasma proteins. The serum concentrations of free hormone (H), plasma protein (P), and bound hormone (HP) are in equilibrium:

$$[H] \times [P] = [HP]$$

The total hormone concentration in the plasma is the sum of the free hormone and the bound hormone. When the concentration of the free form of a hormone decreases, more of this hormone will be released from the binding proteins. Only the free hormone may diffuse across capillary walls and reach the target cells. Logically, it is the free hormone that is the biologically active form. It binds to the target tissue to cause its actions, and it is involved with the negative feedback control of its secretion.

The binding of hormones to plasma proteins has several beneficial effects including:

- Facilitation of transport
- Prolonged half-life
- Hormone reservoir

The steroid and thyroid hormones are minimally insoluble in the blood. Binding to plasma proteins renders them water soluble and facilitates their transport. Secondly, protein binding prolongs the circulating half-life of these hormones. Because they are lipid soluble, they cross cell membranes easily. As the blood flows through the kidney, these hormones would enter cells or be filtered and lost to the urine if they were not held in the blood by the impermeable plasma proteins. Finally, the protein-bound form of the hormone serves as a "reservoir" of hormone that minimizes the changes in free hormone concentration when hormone secretion from its endocrine gland changes abruptly.

11.3   Functional classification of hormones

Hormones are classified into two functional categories:

- Trophic hormones
- Nontrophic hormones

A *trophic hormone* acts on another endocrine gland to stimulate the secretion of its hormone. For example, thyrotropin, or thyroid-stimulating hormone (TSH), stimulates the secretion of thyroid hormones from the thyroid gland. Adrenocorticotropin, or adrenocorticotropic hormone (ACTH), stimulates the adrenal cortex to secrete the hormone cortisol. Both trophic hormones, TSH and ACTH, are produced by the pituitary gland. In fact, many trophic hormones are secreted by the pituitary. It is for this reason that the pituitary gland is sometimes referred to as the "master gland," as its hormones regulate the activity of other endocrine glands.

A *nontrophic hormone* acts on non-endocrine target tissues. For example, parathormone (parathyroid hormone), released from the parathyroid glands, acts on bone tissue to stimulate the release of calcium into the blood. Aldosterone, released from the cortical region of the adrenal glands, acts on the kidney to stimulate the reabsorption of sodium into the blood.

Once a hormone has carried out its effect, the plasma concentration of the hormone must return to its normal range. The concentration of a hormone in the plasma depends upon its:

- Rate of secretion from the endocrine gland
- Rate of removal from the blood

Removal of a hormone from the blood occurs by either of the following mechanisms:

- Excretion
- Metabolic transformation

These mechanisms are carried out primarily by the liver and the kidneys. For example, hormones may be excreted by way of the bile (liver) or within the urine (kidneys).

In some instances, hormones may be metabolized by the cells of its target tissue. Peptide hormones, in the form of hormone-receptor complexes, may be taken up by the target cell by way of endocytosis. The hormone is then degraded intracellularly and the receptor is subsequently returned to the plasma membrane.

11.4   Hormone interactions

Multiple hormones may affect a single target tissue simultaneously. Therefore, the response of the target tissue depends not only on the effects of each hormone individually, but also on the nature of the interaction of the hormones at the tissue. There are three types of hormone interactions including:

- Synergism
- Permissiveness
- Antagonism

Synergism occurs when two hormones interact at a target tissue such that the combination of their effects is greater than the sum of their separate effects. For example, epinephrine, cortisol, and glucagon are three hormones that each increase the level of blood glucose. The magnitude of their individual effects on glucose levels tend to be low to moderate. However, the simultaneous activity of all three hormones results in an increase in blood glucose that is several times greater than the sum of their individual effects.

In *permissiveness,* one hormone enhances the responsiveness of the target tissue to a second hormone. In other words, the first hormone increases the activity of the second hormone. For example, the normal maturation of the reproductive system requires not only reproductive hormones from the hypothalamus, the pituitary, and the gonads, it also requires the presence of thyroid hormone. Although thyroid hormone by itself has no effect on the reproductive system, if it is absent, the development of this system is delayed. Therefore, thyroid hormone is considered to have a permissive effect on the reproductive hormones, facilitating their actions causing sexual maturation.

The mechanism of permissiveness involves *up-regulation,* or an increase in the number of hormone receptors. In the previous example, thyroid hormone up-regulates the receptors for sex hormones such as estrogen, progesterone, or testosterone.

Antagonism occurs when the actions of one hormone oppose the effects of another. For example, insulin decreases blood glucose and promotes the formation of fat. Glucagon, on the other hand, increases blood glucose and promotes the degradation of fat. Therefore, the effects of insulin and glucagon are antagonistic.

11.5   Mechanisms of hormone action

The binding of a hormone to its receptor initiates intracellular events that direct the hormone's action. Ultimately, all hormones produce their effects by altering intracellular protein activity. However, the mechanism by which this occurs depends on the location of the hormone receptor. Receptors are located on the cell surface, in the cytoplasm of the cell, or in some cases, within a cell's nucleus. There are two general mechanisms by which most hormones carry out their effects. These include:

- Signal transduction and second-messenger systems
- Gene activation

Protein/peptide hormones and the catecholamines are water-soluble substances and, accordingly, are unable to cross the plasma membrane to enter the cell. Therefore, these hormones must bind to their specific receptors on the cell surface. This receptor binding causes a response within the cell by way of *signal transduction* and the production of intracellular *second-messenger molecules*. The original, extracellular hormone is considered to the *first messenger* because it carried the signal to the target tissue.

The most common second messenger activated by the protein/peptide hormones and the catecholamines is *cyclic adenosine monophosphate (cAMP)*. The pathway by which cAMP is formed and alters cellular function is illustrated in Figure 11.1. The process begins when the first messenger binds to its receptor. These receptors are quite large and span the bilayer of phospholipids within the plasma membrane. On the intracellular surface of the membrane, the receptor is associated with a protein called *G protein*, which serves as a transducer molecule. These proteins are referred to as G proteins because they bind with guanosine nucleotides. G protein acts as an intermediary between the receptor and the second messengers that will alter cellular activity. In an unstimulated cell, the inactive G protein binds guanosine diphosphate (GDP). When the hormone binds to its G protein-associated receptor, the G protein releases GDP, and becomes able to bind with *guanosine triphosphate (GTP)*, which is found in the cytoplasm. Upon binding with the GTP, the now activated G protein loses its affinity for the receptor and increases its affinity for the plasma membrane-embedded enzyme, *adenylyl cyclase*. In turn, the adenylyl cyclase becomes activated and splits adenosine triphosphate (ATP) to form cAMP. The cAMP molecule serves as the second messenger that carries out the effects of the hormone inside the cell.

The primary function of cAMP is to activate *protein kinase A*. This kinase then attaches phosphate groups to specific enzymatic proteins in the cytoplasm. The phosphorylation of these enzymes either enhances or inhibits their activity. This results in either the enhancement or the inhibition of specific cellular reactions and processes. Either way, cellular metabolism has been altered.

There are several noteworthy aspects of this mechanism of hormonal action including:

- Onset of hormonal effects
- Multiple pathways

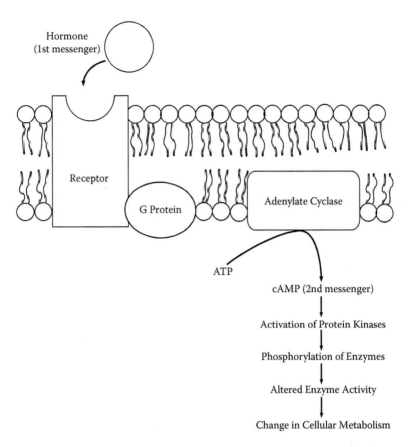

Figure 11.1   The cyclic AMP second-messenger system. The most common second-messenger system activated by the protein/peptide hormones and the catecholamines involves the formation of cAMP. This multistep process is initiated by the binding of the hormone (the first messenger) to its receptor on the cell surface. The subsequent increase in the formation of cAMP (the second messenger) leads to the alteration of enzyme activity within the cell. A change in the activity of these enzymes alters cellular metabolism.

- Cellular specificity
- Amplification of effect
- Prolonged action of hormones

First, the *onset of hormonal effects* to the activation of second-messenger systems is comparatively rapid (within minutes). This mechanism involves changing the activity of *existing* enzymes rather than the production of *new* enzymes, which is a lengthier process. Second, there are *multiple signal transduction and second-messenger pathways*. For example, another signal transduction system involves the opening and closing of ion channels. Furthermore, some tissues use calcium as a second messenger and others use cyclic guanosine monophosphate (cGMP) or inositol triphosphate (IP_3). Third, the *cellular specificity* of a hormone's effect depends on the different kinds of enzyme activity that are ultimately modified in different target tissues. For example, antidiuretic hormone causes the reabsorption of water from the kidneys and the constriction of smooth muscle in blood vessels; two very different effects in two very different tissues caused by one hormone.

Fourth, the effects elicited by second-messenger systems involve a multistep process. This is advantageous because at many of these steps a multiplying or cascading effect takes place, which causes *amplification* of the initial signal. For example, one molecule of the hormone, epinephrine, binding to its receptor on a hepatocyte may result in the production of 10 million molecules of glucose. Finally, *hormonal action is prolonged*. Once an enzyme is activated, the effects are as long-lasting as the enzyme and no longer depend on the presence of the initiating hormone.

PHARMACY APPLICATION: MULTIPLE TARGETS IN THE PHARMACOTHERAPY OF ASTHMA

Asthma is an inflammatory illness characterized by severe bronchoconstriction and wheezing. The pharmacotherapy for this disorder is directed toward a reduction in inflammation and bronchodilation. There are several different pharmacologic approaches and, therefore, different drug classes that may be employed in treating patients with asthma. The two types of asthma medications discussed below are targeted for different points in the signal transduction and second-messenger pathway, which contribute to the regulation of airway smooth muscle tone.

β_2 adrenergic receptor stimulation leads to increased levels of the second messenger, cAMP. An increase in cAMP causes bronchodilation. Albuterol (Proventil®, Ventolin®) is an example of a short-acting β_2 adrenergic receptor agonist. Long-acting medications include salmeterol xinafoate (Serevent®) and formoterol (Foradil®).

Theophylline, a methylxanthine, also increases the levels of the second messenger, cAMP. The mechanism by which it does so is uncertain. One proposed mechanism involves the inhibition of the enzyme, phosphodiesterase. This enzyme breaks down cAMP. Therefore, inhibition of phosphodiesterase leads to an accumulation of cAMP and an increase in signal transduction through this pathway. Another proposed mechanism for the increase in cAMP in response to theophylline involves the antagonism of adenosine receptors. Adenosine receptor stimulation may

(Continued)

**PHARMACY APPLICATION: MULTIPLE TARGETS IN
THE PHARMACOTHERAPY OF ASTHMA (Continued)**

lead to bronchoconstriction in asthmatics. Blockade of these receptors
with theophylline would prevent this effect and lead to bronchodilation.

The importance of theophylline as a therapeutic agent has decreased
over the last several years as other newly developed drugs, such as corticosteroids (fluticasone propionate, Flovent®) and leukotriene receptor
antagonists (montelukast, Singulair®), have come into use. Research continues into the identification of other phosphodiesterase inhibitors that
may be more potent bronchodilators with fewer side effects.

Steroid hormones and thyroid hormones carry out their effects by way of
gene activation. In contrast to the protein/peptide hormones, which alter *existing* enzyme activity, these hormones induce the synthesis of *new* enzymes,
which then influence cellular metabolism.

Hormones in this category are lipophilic and easily enter the cells of
the target tissue by diffusing through the plasma membrane. Typically, the
receptors for steroid hormones are found in the cytoplasm. The hormone
binds to its receptor forming a *hormone-receptor complex*. This complex then
translocates to the cell nucleus. In some cases, unbound receptors are found
in the nucleus and hormone-receptor complexes may be formed there. For
example, receptors for thyroid hormones are found within the nucleus.

In addition to binding with their specific hormones, these receptors are
also capable of binding to DNA at specific attachment sites referred to as the
hormone response elements (HRE). Each of the steroid hormones binds with its
receptor and attaches to a different HRE. A given HRE is located in a DNA
span adjacent to the gene that will be transcribed. Binding of the hormone-
receptor complex to the DNA activates specific genes within the target cell,
resulting in the formation of *mRNA molecules*. The mRNA then diffuses into
the cytoplasm and binds to a ribosome, where protein synthesis takes place.
These new proteins serve as enzymes that regulate cellular reactions and
processes. Once again, intracellular metabolism has been altered.

As with signal transduction and second-messenger systems, the mechanism of gene activation allows for amplification of the hormone's effect. For
example, a single hormone-activated gene induces the formation of many
mRNA molecules and each mRNA molecule may be used to synthesize
many enzyme molecules. Furthermore, the effects of hormones using this
mechanism are prolonged. As long as the newly synthesized enzyme is
active, the effect of the initiating hormone persists.

11.6   The pituitary gland

The *pituitary gland*, or *hypophysis*, is located at the base of the brain just below
the hypothalamus. It is composed of two functionally and anatomically
distinct lobes (see Figure 11.2):

- Neurohypophysis (posterior pituitary)
- Adenohypophysis (anterior pituitary)

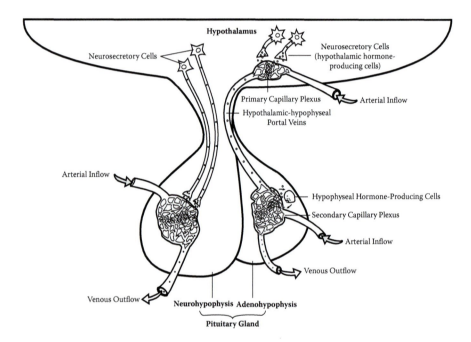

Figure 11.2   Anatomical and functional relationship between the hypothalamus
and the pituitary gland. The neurohypophysis is derived from the hypothalamus.
This anatomical connection allows the hypothalamus to directly influence the function of the neurohypophysis. Action potentials conducted by neurosecretory cells
originating in the hypothalamus cause the release of hormones stored in the neurohypophysis. The adenohypophysis is derived from glandular tissue and, therefore,
has no anatomical connection to the hypothalamus. The release of hormones from
the adenohypophysis is regulated by hypothalamic hormones. These hormones
are carried to the adenohypophysis through the hypothalamic-hypophyseal portal
veins. Hypothalamic hormones enter the tissue of the adenohypophysis and influence the production of adenohypophyseal hormones. Hormones released from both
regions of the pituitary gland, the neurohypophysis and the adenohypophysis, are
removed from the pituitary gland by the venous outflow blood and transported to
target tissues throughout the body.

As its name implies, the *neurohypophysis* is derived embryonically from nervous tissue. It is essentially an outgrowth of the hypothalamus and is composed of bundles of axons, or neural tracts, of neurosecretory cells originating in two hypothalamic nuclei. These neurons are referred to as *neurosecretory cells* because they generate action potentials (*neuro-*) as well as synthesize hormones (*-secretory*). The cell bodies of the neurosecretory cells in the supraoptic nuclei produce primarily antidiuretic hormone (ADH) and the cell bodies of the paraventricular nuclei produce primarily oxytocin. These hormones are then transported down the axons to the neurohypophysis and stored in membrane-bound vesicles in the neuron terminals. Much like neurotransmitters, the hormones are released in response to the arrival of action potentials at the neuron terminal.

The *adenohypophysis* is derived embryonically from glandular tissue, specifically, *Rathke's pouch*. This tissue originates from the oropharynx, or the roof of the mouth. It then migrates toward the embryonic nervous tissue destined to form the neurohypophysis. When these two tissues come into contact, Rathke's pouch loses its connection with the roof of the mouth and the pituitary gland is formed.

Unlike the neurohypophysis, which releases hormones originally synthesized in the hypothalamus, the adenohypophysis synthesizes its own hormones in specialized groups of cells. It is similar to the neurohypophysis, however, in that the release of its hormones into the blood is regulated by the hypothalamus.

11.7   Relationship between the hypothalamus and the pituitary gland

The hypothalamus plays a very important role in the maintenance of homeostasis. It carries out this function in large part, by regulating the activities of the neurohypophysis and the adenohypophysis. For example, the hypothalamus processes signals from other regions of the nervous system including information regarding pain and emotional states, such as depression, anger and excitement. In addition, because it is not protected by the blood-brain barrier, it monitors the composition of the blood and helps to regulate the concentration of nutrients, electrolytes, water and hormones. In other words, it is an important processing center for information concerning the internal environment. This information is then used to control the release of hormones from the pituitary.

Due to their different embryonic origins, the neurohypophysis and the adenohypophysis are regulated by the hypothalamus using two very different mechanisms:

- Nerve signals
- Hormonal signals

As discussed previously, the neurohypophysis has a direct anatomical connection to the hypothalamus. Therefore, the hypothalamus regulates the release of hormones from the neurohypophysis by way of *nerve signals*. Action potentials generated by the neurosecretory cells originating in the hypothalamus are transmitted down the neuronal axons to the nerve terminals in the neurohypophysis and stimulate the release of the hormones into the blood. The tracts formed by these axons are referred to as the *hypothalamic-hypophyseal tracts* (see Figure 11.2). The action potentials are initiated by various forms of sensory input to the hypothalamus. Specific forms of sensory input that regulate the release of ADH and oxytocin are described in subsequent Section 11.9, Neurohypophysis.

The adenohypophysis does not have a direct anatomical connection with the hypothalamus; therefore, regulation of its hormone secretion by way of neuronal signals is not possible. Instead, these two structures are associated by a specialized circulatory system and the secretion of hormones from the adenohypophysis is regulated by *hormonal signals* from the hypothalamus (see Figure 11.2). Systemic arterial blood is directed first to the hypothalamus. The exchange of materials between the blood and the interstitial fluid of the hypothalamus takes place at the *primary capillary plexus*. The blood then flows to the adenohypophysis through the *hypothalamic-hypophyseal portal veins*. Portal veins are blood vessels that connect two capillary beds. The second capillary bed in this system is the *secondary capillary plexus* located in the adenohypophysis.

Located in close proximity to the primary capillary plexus in the hypothalamus are specialized neurosecretory cells. In fact, the axons of these cells terminate on the capillaries. The neurosecretory cells synthesize two types of hormones; *releasing hormones* and *inhibiting hormones* (see Table 11.2). Each of

Table 11.2   Hormones of the pituitary gland

Hormones produced in the anterior pituitary

Growth Hormone (GH)—stimulates growth of long bones, organs, and muscle during development

Adrenocorticotrophin (ACTH)—stimulates the adrenal cortex to produce adrenal hormones such as cortisol

Thyroid-stimulating Hormone (TSH)—regulates secretion of thyroid hormones T_3 and T_4

Luteinizing Hormone (LH)—stimulates steroidogenesis in the gonads, maintains secretory function of the corpus luteum

Follicle-stimulating Hormone (FSH)—stimulates gamete production in the gonads

Prolactin (PRL)—initiates and maintains milk production in the mammary glands postpartum

Hormones released by the posterior pituitary

Oxytocin—stimulates contraction of uterine smooth muscle during labor and delivery as well as milk ejection from the mammary glands

Antidiuretic Hormone (ADH, Vasopressin)—acts upon the kidney to stimulate water reabsorption in the distal tubules and collecting ducts

these hormones helps to regulate the release of a particular hormone from the adenohypophysis. For example, thyrotropin-releasing hormone produced by the neurosecretory cells of the hypothalamus stimulates the secretion of thyrotropin from the thyrotrope cells of the adenohypophysis. The hypothalamic releasing hormone is picked up by the primary capillary plexus, travels through the hypothalamic-hypophyseal portal veins to the anterior pituitary, leaves the blood by way of the secondary capillary plexus and exerts its effect on the appropriate cells of the adenohypophysis. The hypophyseal hormone, in this case, thyrotropin, is then picked up by the secondary capillary plexus, removed from the pituitary by the venous blood and delivered to its target tissue.

A noteworthy feature of this specialized circulation is that the regulatory hypothalamic hormones are delivered directly to the adenohypophysis by the portal system. Therefore, the concentration of these hormones remains very high because they are not diluted in the blood of the entire systemic circulation.

11.8   Negative feedback control

In many cases, hormones released from the adenohypophysis are part of a three-hormone axis that includes:

- The hypothalamic hormone
- The adenohypophyseal hormone
- The endocrine gland hormone

The hypothalamic hormone either stimulates or inhibits the secretion of the adenohypophyseal hormone. The trophic hormone from the adenohypophysis then stimulates the release of a hormone from another endocrine gland. This final endocrine gland hormone not only carries out its effects on its target tissues, it may also exert a *negative feedback* effect on the release of the hypothalamic and/or the adenohypophyseal hormones. In this way, this final hormone regulates its own release (see Figure 11.3). This process is referred to as *long-loop negative feedback*. The adenohypophyseal hormone may also exert a negative feedback effect on the hypothalamic hormone and limit its own release. This process is referred to as *short-loop negative feedback*.

11.9   Neurohypophysis

11.9.1   Antidiuretic hormone

ADH, also referred to as *vasopressin*, has two major effects, both of which are reflected in its names:

- Antidiuresis (decrease in urine formation by the kidney)
- Vasoconstriction of arterioles

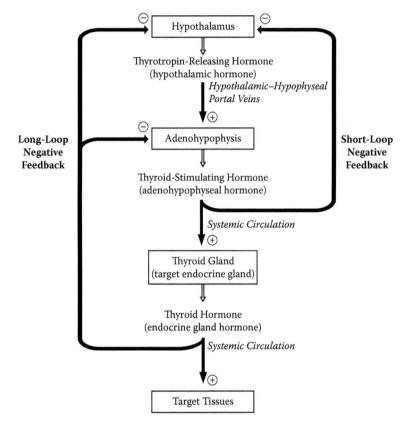

Figure 11.3 Negative-feedback regulation of hormone release. Hormones released from the adenohypophysis are often part of a three-hormone axis that includes the hypothalamic hormone, the adenohypophyseal hormone and the target endocrine gland hormone. Long-loop negative feedback occurs when the final hormone in the axis inhibits the release of the hypothalamic and/or the adenohypophyseal hormones. Short-loop negative feedback occurs when the adenohypophyseal hormone inhibits the release of the hypothalamic hormone. Illustrated in this figure is the thyrotropin-releasing hormone/thyroid-stimulating hormone/thyroid hormone axis.

Antidiuretic hormone promotes the reabsorption of water from the tubules of the kidney, or *antidiuresis*. Specifically, it acts on the collecting ducts and increases the number of water channels, or *aquaporins,* which increases the diffusion coefficient for water. This results in the conservation of water by the body and the production of a low volume of concentrated urine. This process may begin within 5–10 min of the presence of ADH. The reabsorbed water affects both plasma osmolarity and blood volume. The additional water dilutes the plasma and decreases plasma osmolarity. Furthermore, the added water expands blood volume. This effect of ADH on the kidney occurs at relatively low concentrations.

At higher concentrations, ADH causes *constriction of arterioles*. This vaso-constriction serves to increase blood pressure.

Antidiuretic hormone secretion is regulated by several factors:

- Plasma osmolarity
- Blood volume
- Blood pressure
- Alcohol

The primary factor that influences ADH secretion is a change in *plasma osmolarity*. The hypothalamus houses *osmoreceptors* that lie near ADH-producing neurosecretory cells. When plasma osmolarity increases, the osmoreceptors become stimulated, which results in the stimulation of neurosecretory cells, an increase in the frequency of action potentials in these cells, and the release of ADH from their axon terminals in the neurohypophysis. The water con-served, because of ADH effects on the kidney, helps to reduce plasma osmo-larity or dilute the plasma back to normal.

The hypothalamic osmoreceptors have a threshold of 280 mOsM/L. Below this value, the osmoreceptors are not stimulated and little or no ADH is secreted. Maximal ADH levels occur when plasma osmolarity is about 295 mOsM/L. Within this range, the regulatory system is very sen-sitive with measurable increases in ADH secretion occurring in response to 1% changes in plasma osmolarity. The regulation of ADH secretion is an important mechanism by which a normal plasma osmolarity of 290 mOsM/L is maintained. (As discussed in Chapter 5, section A, the maintenance of a normal plasma osmolarity is important in preventing the inappropriate movement of water into or out of the body's cells. This would lead to cellular swelling and possible lysis, or cellular dehydration, respectively.)

Other factors regulating ADH secretion include blood volume and blood pressure. A decrease in *blood volume* of 10%–25% causes an increase in ADH secretion that may be sufficient to cause vasoconstriction as well as antidi-uresis. A decrease in *mean arterial blood pressure* of 5% or more also causes an increase in ADH secretion. The resulting water conservation and vasocon-striction help increase blood volume and blood pressure back to normal. Furthermore, the effect of blood pressure on ADH secretion may be correlated to the increase that occurs during sleep when blood pressure decreases. The result is the production of a low volume of highly concentrated urine, which is less likely to elicit the micturition (urination) reflex and interrupt sleep.

In contrast to these physiological factors, *alcohol* inhibits the secretion of ADH, allowing for the loss of water from the kidney. Therefore, the con-sumption of alcoholic beverages may lead to excessive water loss and dehy-dration instead of volume expansion.

PHARMACY APPLICATION: DIABETES INSIPIDUS

Diabetes insipidus is caused by a decrease in ADH secretion or a decrease in the kidney's response to ADH. This absolute or relative deficiency of ADH leads to excessive urination (polyuria) due to the patient's inability to reabsorb water from the kidneys. The excessive water loss leads to extreme thirst (polydipsia).

The preferred medication for treating diabetes insipidus is desmopressin acetate (synthetic 1-deamino-8-D-arginine vasopressin; DDAVP). Desmopressin may be prepared as a sterile solution for injection or as a nasal solution for intranasal administration. The duration of effect with continued intranasal dosing is 5–24 hours. Desmopressin may also be administered orally. Because this drug is a peptide, it is rapidly inactivated by the enzyme trypsin. Therefore, oral doses of desmopressin are 10–20 times that of the intranasal dose. The typical nasal dosage is 10–40 μg daily and the oral dosage is 0.1–0.2 mg every 12–24 hours.

11.9.2   Oxytocin

The second hormone synthesized in the hypothalamus and secreted from the neurohypophysis is oxytocin. This hormone also exerts its major effects on two different target tissues. Oxytocin stimulates:

- Contraction of uterine smooth muscle
- Contraction of myoepithelial cells in the mammary glands

Oxytocin stimulates *contraction of the smooth muscle in the wall of the uterus*. During labor, this facilitates the delivery of the fetus while during intercourse, it may facilitate the transport of the sperm through the female reproductive tract for fertilization of the ovum. Oxytocin also causes *contraction of the myoepithelial cells* surrounding the alveoli of the mammary glands. This results in *"milk-letdown"* or the expulsion of milk from deep within the gland into the larger ducts from which the milk can be obtained more readily by the nursing infant.

The secretion of oxytocin is regulated by *reflexes elicited by cervical stretch and by nursing*. Normally, as labor begins, the fetus is positioned head down. This orientation exerts pressure on the cervix and causes it to stretch. Sensory neurons in the cervix are thereby activated to transmit signals to the hypothalamus that will stimulate the release of oxytocin from the neurohypophysis. This hormone then enhances uterine contraction, which causes further pressure and stretch of the cervix. Additional oxytocin is released, and so on, until there is adequate pressure build up so that delivery takes place. In the lactating breast, nursing activates sensory neurons in the nipple to transmit signals to the hypothalamus to stimulate oxytocin release from the neurohypophysis and, therefore, milk-letdown. Interestingly, this reflex may also be triggered through a conditioned response where the sight or sound of the hungry infant is sufficient to enhance oxytocin secretion. In contrast, the release of oxytocin from the neurohypophysis may be inhibited by pain, fear or stress.

The function of oxytocin in males is not clearly understood but may be associated with ejaculation.

PHARMACY APPLICATION: INDUCTION AND PREVENTION OF PARTURITION

Agents designed to stimulate uterine contractions are used to induce or augment parturition (labor). Circumstances that warrant the induction of labor include Rh problems (see Chapter 5, section C), maternal diabetes, premature rupture of membranes, and preeclampsia. Synthetic oxytocin (Pitocin®, Syntocinon®) is the clinical drug of choice. This medication is administered intravenously.

Preterm labor may be treated with oxytocin receptor antagonists. The drug Atosiban decreases the frequency of uterine contractions and reduces the likelihood of preterm delivery.

11.10   Adenohypophysis

11.10.1   Gonadotropins

The gonadotropins, follicle-stimulating hormone and luteinizing hormone, exert their effects on the gonads (ovaries in the female and testes in the male). Taken together, the gonadotropins stimulate the gonads to:

- Produce gametes (ova and sperm)
- Secrete sex hormones (estrogen, progesterone, and testosterone)

Follicle-stimulating hormone (FSH), as its name indicates, stimulates the development of the ovarian follicles in females. It is within the follicles that the ova, or eggs, develop. This hormone also induces the secretion of estrogen from the follicle. In males, FSH acts on the Sertoli cells of the testes, which are involved with the production of sperm, or spermatogenesis.

Luteinizing hormone (LH) is also named for its effects in the female. It stimulates the rupture of the follicle to release the ovum and causes the conversion of the ovarian follicle into a *corpus luteum* (Latin, *"yellow body"*). LH also induces the secretion of estrogen and progesterone from the corpus luteum. In males, LH acts on the Leydig cells of the testes to stimulate the secretion of testosterone.

Both FSH and LH are produced by the same cell type in the adenohypophysis, the gonadotrope. The release of FSH and LH is regulated by the hypothalamic releasing hormone, *gonadotropin-releasing hormone (GnRH)*.

11.10.2   Thyroid-stimulating hormone (TSH)

Also known as thyrotropin, this hormone regulates the growth and metabolism of the thyroid gland. Furthermore, it stimulates the synthesis and release of the thyroid hormones, T_3 and T_4. The release of TSH from the thyrotrope cells of the adenohypophysis is induced by *thyrotropin-releasing hormone (TRH)*.

11.10.3   Adrenocorticotropic hormone (ACTH)

Also known as adrenocorticotropin, this hormone stimulates growth and steroid production in the adrenal cortex. Specifically, it stimulates the secretion of cortisol and other glucocorticoids that are involved with carbohydrate metabolism. The release of ACTH from the adenohypophysis is influenced by more than one factor. *Corticotropin-releasing hormone (CRH)* from the hypothalamus stimulates the secretion of ACTH. In addition, ACTH secretion follows a *diurnal pattern*, with a peak in the early morning and a valley late in the evening.

11.10.4   Prolactin

The hormone *prolactin (PRL)*, which is produced by the lactotrope cells of the adenohypophysis, is involved with the initiation and maintenance of lactation in females. Its function in males is uncertain. Lactation involves three processes:

- Mammogenesis
- Lactogenesis
- Galactopoeisis

Mammogenesis is the growth and development of the mammary glands, which produce the milk. This process requires the actions of many hormones, including estrogens and progestins, in addition to PRL. *Lactogenesis* is the initiation of lactation. During pregnancy, lactation is inhibited by the high levels of estrogens and progestins. At delivery, the levels of these two hormones fall, allowing PRL to initiate lactation. *Galactopoeisis* is the maintenance of milk production. This process requires both PRL and oxytocin.

The release of PRL from the adenohypophysis is normally inhibited by *prolactin-inhibiting hormone (PIH, dopamine)* from the hypothalamus. PRL secretion is also controlled by *prolactin-releasing factor (PRF)*. The release of PRF from the hypothalamus is mediated by reflexes elicited by suckling and breast stimulation.

11.10.5   Growth hormone (GH)

Also known as somatotropin, this is one of the few hormones that exerts its effects on organs and tissues throughout the body. Growth hormone is essential for the normal growth and development of the skeleton as well as visceral, or soft, tissues from birth until young adulthood. Growth of the skeleton involves both an increase in bone thickness and an increase in bone length. The mechanism of this growth involves the stimulation of osteoblast (bone-forming cell) activity and the proliferation of the epiphyseal cartilage in the ends of the long bones. The growth of visceral tissues occurs by *hyperplasia* (increasing the number of cells) and *hypertrophy* (increasing the size of cells). Growth hormone causes hyperplasia by stimulating cell division and by inhibiting apoptosis (programmed cell death). Growth hormone causes cellular hypertrophy by promoting protein synthesis and inhibiting protein degradation.

The growth-promoting effects of GH are carried out by *somatomedins*, which are peptides found in the blood. At least four somatomedins have been identified and described. The two most important somatomedins, which are structurally and functionally similar to insulin, are referred to as *insulin-like growth factors I and II (IGF-I and IGF-II)*. Growth hormone stimulates the production of IGF-I in the liver, which is the predominant source of that found in the circulation. Local production of IGF-I also occurs in many target tissues. It is IGF-I that is thought to mediate the growth-promoting effects of GH throughout life. Levels of both GH and IGF-I increase in parallel during puberty and other periods of growth in children. In contrast, IGF-II production does not depend on GH. Instead, IGF-II is thought to be important during fetal growth and development and is secreted in response to PRL. The role of IGF-II in the adult is unknown.

Growth hormone also has many metabolic actions in the body:

- Protein metabolism
- Increase in tissue amino acid uptake
- Increase DNA transcription
- Increase RNA translation
- Increase in protein synthesis
- Decrease in catabolism of proteins and amino acids
- Lipid metabolism
- Stimulation of lipolysis

- Inhibition of lipogenesis
- Increase in blood fatty acids
- Increase in the utilization of fats over carbohydrates for energy production
- Carbohydrate metabolism
- Decrease in glucose uptake and utilization by muscle
- Increase in the hepatic output of glucose (glycogenolysis)
- Increase in blood glucose

The net effects of these actions include enhanced growth due to protein synthesis, enhanced availability of fatty acids for use by skeletal muscle as an energy source and glucose sparing for the brain, which can use only this nutrient molecule as a source of energy.

The release of GH from the adenohypophysis is regulated by two hypothalamic hormones, *growth hormone-releasing hormone* (*GHRH*) and *growth hormone-inhibiting hormone* (*GHIH, somatostatin*). Any factor or condition that enhances the secretion of GH could do so by stimulating GHRH release or by inhibiting GHIH release. The secretion of GH follows a diurnal rhythm with GH levels low and constant throughout the day and with a marked burst of GH secretion approximately 1 hour following the onset of sleep (deep or stages III and IV sleep). Other factors that stimulate GH secretion include exercise, stress, trauma, hypoglycemia and starvation, especially with severe protein deficiency. Factors that inhibit GH secretion include hyperglycemia and aging. In most individuals, the production of GH decreases after 30 years of age and falls to about 25% of the adolescent level in very old age. This decrease in GH production is likely a critical factor in the loss of lean muscle mass at a rate of 5% per decade and the gain of body fat at the same rate after 40 years of age.

11.11   Thyroid gland

The thyroid gland is a butterfly-shaped structure lying over the anterior surface of the trachea just below the larynx. This gland produces two classes of hormones synthesized by two distinct cell types:

- Thyroid hormones (T_3 and T_4), synthesized by follicular cells
- Calcitonin, synthesized by parafollicular cells

11.11.1   Thyroid hormones

Internally, the thyroid consists of *follicles* that are spherical structures whose walls are formed by a single layer of epithelial cells called *follicular cells*. The center of each follicle contains a homogenous gel referred to as *colloid*. Thyroid hormones are stored here as a component of the larger molecule, *thyroglobulin*. The amount of the thyroid hormones stored within the colloid is enough to supply the body for 2–3 months.

Thyroid hormones, derived from the amino acid tyrosine, are unique because they contain *iodine*. At this time, its incorporation into thyroid hormones is the only known use for iodine in the body. There are two thyroid hormones, named for the number of iodides added to the tyrosine residues of the thyroglobulin, *triiodothyronine* (T_3) and *tetraiodothyronine* (T_4, *thyroxine*). Although significantly more T_4 is synthesized by the thyroid gland, T_3 is the active hormone. At the target tissue, T_4 is converted to the more potent T_3 by the removal of an iodine.

The thyroid hormones are lipophilic and are relatively insoluble in the plasma. Therefore, they are transported throughout the circulation bound to plasma proteins such as *thyroxine-binding globulin* (75%) and albumins (25%). Approximately 99.96% of circulating thyroxine is protein bound. Bound hormone is not available to cause any physiological effects; however, it is in equilibrium with the remaining 0.04%, which is unbound. It is this free form of the hormone that binds to receptors on the target tissues and cause its effects.

Thyroid hormone's primary action is to alter cellular metabolism. In fact, complete lack of thyroid hormone secretion causes the basal metabolic rate to fall 40%–50% below normal. Significant excess of thyroid hormone secretion may increase basal metabolic rate to 60%–100% above normal. Some of the many metabolic effects of thyroid hormone in the body include the following:

- Growth and maturation
- Perinatal lung maturation
- Normal skeletal growth
- Neurological
- Normal fetal and neonatal brain growth and development
- Regulation of neuronal proliferation and differentiation, myelinogenesis, neuronal outgrowth and synapse formation
- Normal central nervous system function in adults
- Sympathetic nervous system function
- Increase in the number of β-adrenergic receptors
- Increase in heart rate
- Tremor
- Sweating
- Cardiovascular system
- Vasodilation
- Increase in heart rate
- Increase in myocardial contractility
- Increase in cardiac output
- Metabolism
- Increase in the number and activity of mitochondria
- Increase in the rate of ATP formation
- Increase in basal metabolic rate
- Stimulation of all metabolic pathways, both anabolic and catabolic

- Increase in carbohydrate uptake and utilization
- Increase in glycolysis and gluconeogenesis
- Increase in lipolysis and fatty acid mobilization
- Increase in oxygen consumption
- Increase in the rate and depth of breathing
- Increase in heat production

As mentioned previously, thyroid hormones are secreted at a relatively steady rate. The secretion of hormones from the thyroid gland is regulated by negative feedback in the hypothalamic-pituitary-thyroid axis. The hypothalamus secretes thyrotropin-releasing hormone (TRH), which stimulates the release of TSH from the adenohypophysis of the pituitary. Thyroid-stimulating hormone then stimulates the release of T_3 and T_4 from the thyroid. In this hormone axis, negative-feedback inhibition is exerted primarily at the level of the pituitary. As the intracellular concentration of T_3 in the thyrotrope cells of the pituitary increases, then there is a decrease in the responsiveness of these TSH-producing cells to TRH. The mechanism of this decreased responsiveness involves the downregulation, or a decrease in the number, of TRH receptors. This results in a decrease in the secretion of TSH, and, consequently, a decrease in the secretion of T_3 and T_4. The excess of intracellular T_3, which elicits the negative feedback control of secretion comes from two sources; 80% from the removal of iodine from serum T_4 within the thyrotrope cells and 20% from serum T_3. Other factors that alter the release of TRH and, therefore, thyroid hormones, include exposure to cold (increased secretion) as well as anxiety (decreased secretion).

PHARMACY APPLICATION: HYPOTHYROIDISM

A deficiency in thyroid hormone production leads to hypothyroidism. In regions of the world where there is sufficient iodine in the diet, the most common cause of this disorder is Hashimoto's thyroiditis. This is an autoimmune disease characterized by the production of antibodies directed against the thyroid gland. Clinical manifestations of hypothyroidism are related to myxedema (fluid accumulation, which is most obvious in the face) and the hypometabolic state. Specifically, symptoms include the gradual onset of weakness and fatigue, weight gain, and nervous system dysfunction (e.g., mental dullness, lethargy, impaired memory).

Hypothyroidism is treated pharmacologically with synthetic preparations of thyroid hormones. Levothyroxine sodium (L-T4, Synthroid®, Levoxyl®) is typically administered in a tablet form. Because it is an amine hormone, absorption of this medication from the small intestine is variable and incomplete, such that 50%–80% of the dosage is absorbed.

11.11.2   Calcitonin

This hormone, which is also secreted from the thyroid gland, is synthesized by the *parafollicular cells* (C cells) located between the follicles. The primary effect of *calcitonin* is to decrease the blood levels of calcium and phosphate. The mechanism of action involves the direct inhibition of osteoclast activity, which decreases bone resorption, or the breakdown of bone. This results in less demineralization of the bone and, therefore, a decrease in the release of calcium and phosphate from the bone into the blood. Calcitonin has no direct effect on bone formation by osteoblasts.

The release of calcitonin from the thyroid is regulated by plasma calcium levels through negative feedback. An increase in the level of calcium in the blood stimulates the secretion of calcitonin and a decrease in the level of calcium in the blood inhibits secretion.

**PHARMACY APPLICATION: THERAPEUTIC
EFFECTS OF CALCITONIN**

The normal physiological effects of calcitonin are relatively weak. However, when used pharmacologically, the effects of this hormone are very important. Paget's disease is characterized by a significant increase in osteoclast activity and, therefore, a high rate of bone turnover and hypercalcemia. Because there is minimal species variation, human calcitonin or calcitonin from other species may be used to treat this disorder. Therefore, pharmacological intervention includes the administration of salmon calcitonin (Miacalcin®), which will depress the bone resorption and ease the symptoms of Paget's. Salmon calcitonin, which is 20 times more potent than human calcitonin, has also been approved for therapeutic use in patients with postmenopausal osteoporosis.

11.12   Parathyroid glands

There are four small parathyroid glands embedded on the posterior surface of the thyroid gland as it wraps around the trachea. *Parathyroid hormone* (PTH, parathormone) is the principle regulator of calcium metabolism. The overall effects of PTH include:

- Increase in blood levels of calcium
- Decrease in blood levels of phosphate

Parathyroid hormone carries out these effects through multiple mechanisms of action:

- Decrease in calcium excretion in the urine
- Increase in phosphate excretion in the urine
- Increase in bone resorption
- Activation of vitamin D_3

Calcium is freely filtered along with the other components of the plasma through the nephrons of the kidney. Most of this calcium is reabsorbed back into the blood from the proximal tubule of the nephron. However, because the kidneys produce about 180 L of filtrate per day, the amount of calcium that is filtered is substantial. Therefore, the physiological regulation of even a small percentage of calcium reabsorption may have a significant effect on the amount of calcium in the blood. Parathyroid hormone acts primarily on the distal tubules and the collecting ducts to increase the reabsorption of calcium from these segments of the tubule and decrease the amount excreted in the urine. This activity conserves calcium and increases its concentration in the blood.

Phosphate, which is also freely filtered with the plasma through the nephrons of the kidney, is reabsorbed into the blood from the proximal tubule. Parathyroid hormone acts on this segment to decrease phosphate reabsorption and increase the amount excreted in the urine.

Parathyroid hormone stimulates bone resorption by increasing the number and the activity of osteoclasts. This demineralization process in the bone releases both calcium and phosphate into the blood. Although the action of PTH on the bone appears to increase blood phosphate, its action on the kidney, which increases phosphate excretion in the urine, more than compensates for this increase and the net effect is a decrease in serum phosphate.

The final mechanism of action of PTH involves the activation of vitamin D_3 through the stimulation of 1α-hydroxylase in the kidney. In the gastrointestinal tract, vitamin D_3 is essential for the absorption of calcium. Enhanced absorption of calcium from dietary sources serves to further increase the concentration of calcium in the blood. Many foods, in particular dairy products, which are rich in calcium, are fortified with vitamin D.

The release of PTH from the parathyroid glands is regulated by plasma calcium levels through negative feedback. A decrease in the level of calcium in the blood stimulates the secretion of PTH within minutes. If the calcium deficiency persists, the parathyroid glands will hypertrophy as much as 5-fold or more. An increase in the level of calcium in the blood inhibits secretion. Persistent calcium excess may cause the parathyroid glands to reduce in size.

11.13   Adrenal glands

There are two adrenal glands, one located on the superior surface of each kidney. These glands are composed of two distinct anatomical and, therefore, functional regions:

- Adrenal medulla
- Adrenal cortex

11.13.1   Adrenal medulla

The adrenal medulla, derived from neural crest tissue, forms the inner portion of the adrenal gland. It is the site of production of the *catecholamines*, epinephrine and norepinephrine. The catecholamines serve as a circulating counterpart to the sympathetic neurotransmitter, norepinephrine, which is released directly from sympathetic neurons to the tissues. As such, the adrenal medulla and its hormonal products play an important role in the activity of the sympathetic nervous system. This is fully discussed in Chapter 14.

11.13.2   Adrenal cortex

The adrenal cortex, forming the outer portion of the adrenal gland, accounts for 80%–90% of the weight of the gland. It is the site of synthesis of many types of steroid hormones including:

- Mineralocorticoids
- Glucocorticoids
- Adrenal androgens

11.13.3   Mineralocorticoids

The primary mineralocorticoid is *aldosterone*. The actions of this hormone include:

- Stimulation of renal retention of sodium
- Promotion of renal excretion of potassium

Total lack of aldosterone secretion results in death within several days due to the rapid loss of sodium and chloride from the body (as much as 10%–20% of the total sodium in the body per day). This sodium deficiency results in a decrease in blood volume and, therefore, cardiac output. Death ensues from cardiogenic shock. The loss of sodium is accompanied by the marked accumulation of potassium in the body fluids.

Aldosterone acts on the distal tubule of the nephron to increase sodium reabsorption (Figure 10.4). The mechanism of action involves an increase in the number of sodium-permeable channels on the luminal surface of the distal tubule and an increase in the activity of the Na^+-K^+-ATPase pump on the basilar surface of the tubule. Sodium diffuses down its concentration gradient out of the lumen and into the tubular cells. The pump then actively removes the sodium from the cells of the distal tubule and into the extracellular fluid so that it may diffuse into the surrounding capillaries and return to the circulation. Due to its osmotic effects, the retention of sodium is accompanied by the retention of water. In other words, wherever sodium goes, water follows. As a result, aldosterone is very important in the regulation of blood volume and blood pressure. The retention of sodium and water expands the blood volume and, consequently, increases mean arterial pressure. The maximum effect is reached only after several hours.

The retention of sodium is coupled to the excretion of potassium. For every three Na^+ ions reabsorbed, two K^+ ions and one H^+ ion is excreted.

The release of aldosterone from the adrenal cortex is regulated primarily by two important factors:

- Serum potassium levels
- Renin-angiotensin system

The mechanism by which *potassium* regulates aldosterone secretion is unclear; however, this ion appears to have a direct effect on the adrenal cortex. A small increase in the level of potassium in the blood results in a several-fold increase in the release of aldosterone. The action of aldosterone on the kidney then decreases the level of potassium back to normal.

Angiotensin II is a potent stimulus for the secretion of aldosterone. The formation of angiotensin II occurs by the following process:

Angiotensinogen

↓ Renin

Angiotensin I

↓ ACE

Angiotensin II

This multistep process is initiated by the enzyme, renin. Angiotensinogen is a precursor peptide molecule released into the circulation from the liver. In the presence of renin, an enzyme produced by specialized cells in the kidney, angiotensinogen is split to form angiotensin I. This prohormone is then acted upon by angiotensin-converting enzyme (ACE) as the blood passes through the lungs to form angiotensin II. Angiotensin II acts directly on the adrenal cortex to promote aldosterone secretion.

Because this process will not occur without renin, it is important to understand the factors involved in its release from the kidney. These factors include:

- Decrease in blood volume
- Decrease in blood pressure
- Sympathetic stimulation

A decrease in either blood volume or blood pressure may result in a decrease in the blood flow to the kidney. The kidney monitors renal blood flow by way of stretch receptors in the blood vessel walls. A decrease in renal blood flow stimulates the release of renin. The subsequent secretion of aldosterone causes the retention of sodium and water and, therefore, an increase in blood volume and blood pressure back to normal. An increase in renal blood flow tends to cause the opposite effect.

Sympathetic nerve activity causes an increase in blood pressure through many mechanisms including an increase in cardiac activity and vasoconstriction. Activation of the sympathetic system also causes the stimulation of β_1-adrenergic receptors on the renin-producing cells, which promotes renin release.

11.13.4   Glucocorticoids

The primary glucocorticoid is *cortisol*. Receptors for the glucocorticoids are found in all tissues. The overall effects of these hormones include:

- Increase in blood glucose
- Increase in blood free fatty acids

Cortisol increases blood glucose by several mechanisms of action including:

- Decrease in glucose utilization by many peripheral tissues (especially muscle and adipose tissue)
- Increase in availability of gluconeogenic substrates
  - Increase in protein catabolism (especially muscle)
  - Decrease in amino acid transport into extrahepatic cells
  - Increase in amino acid transport into hepatic cells
  - Increase in lipolysis
- Increase in hepatic gluconeogenesis (as much as 6- to 10-fold)

Cortisol-induced lipolysis not only provides substrates for gluconeogenesis (formation of glucose from noncarbohydrate sources), but it also increases the amount of free fatty acids in the blood. Thus, the fatty acids are used by muscle as a source of energy and glucose is spared for use by the brain to form energy.

The release of cortisol from the adrenal cortex is regulated by several factors including:

- Circadian rhythm
- Stress
- Negative-feedback inhibition by cortisol

Corticotropin-releasing hormone (CRH) secreted from the hypothalamus stimulates the release of ACTH from the adenohypophysis. This pituitary hormone then stimulates the release of cortisol from the adrenal cortex. The hormones of this hypothalamic-pituitary-adrenocortical axis exhibit marked diurnal variation. This variation is due to the diurnal secretion of CRH. The resulting secretion of cortisol increases at night and peaks in the early morning, approximately 1 hour after rising (6 a.m.–8 a.m.). The levels of cortisol then gradually fall during the day to a low point late in the evening, between 8 p.m. and 12 a.m. This rhythm is influenced by many factors including light-dark patterns, sleep-wake patterns and eating. After an individual changes time zones, it takes about 2 weeks for this rhythm to adjust to the new time schedule, which may account for some aspects of jet lag.

Cortisol is an important component of the body's response to stress, both physical and psychological. Some of the types of stress that stimulate cortisol secretion include trauma, infection, intense heat or cold, surgery, debilitating disease and physical restraint. Nervous signals regarding stress are transmitted to the hypothalamus and the release of CRH is stimulated. The resulting increase in cortisol increases the levels of glucose, free fatty acids and amino acids in the blood, providing the metabolic fuels that enable the individual to cope with the stress.

A potent inhibitor of this system is cortisol itself. This hormone exerts a negative-feedback effect on both the hypothalamus and the adenohypophysis and inhibits the secretion of CRH and ACTH, respectively.

PHARMACY APPLICATION: THERAPEUTIC EFFECTS OF CORTICOSTEROIDS

When administered in pharmacological concentrations (greater than physiological), cortisol and its synthetic analogs (hydrocortisone, prednisone) have potent anti-inflammatory and immunosuppressive effects. In fact, these steroids inhibit almost every step of the inflammatory response including decreased release of vasoactive and chemoattractive factors, decreased secretion of lipolytic and proteolytic enzymes,

(Continued)

**PHARMACY APPLICATION: THERAPEUTIC
EFFECTS OF CORTICOSTEROIDS (Continued)**

decreased extravasation of leukocytes to areas of injury, and ultimately, decreased fibrosis. Typically, the inflammatory response is quite beneficial in that it limits the spread of infection. However, there are many clinical conditions, such as rheumatoid arthritis and asthma, where the response itself becomes a destructive process. Therefore, although the glucocorticoids have no effect on the underlying cause of disease, the suppression of inflammation by these agents is very important clinically.

Corticosteroids also exert inhibitory effects on the overall immune process. These drugs impair the function of the leukocytes responsible for antibody production and destruction of foreign cells. Corticosteroids are used therapeutically in the prevention of organ transplant rejection.

The therapeutic use of corticosteroids should be undertaken with caution. Because they suppress the inflammatory response and the activity of the immune system, the patient is more susceptible to infection. Other adverse effects include the development of gastric ulcers, hypertension, atherosclerosis, and weight gain.

11.13.5   Adrenal androgens

The predominant androgens, or male sex hormones, produced by the adrenal cortex are *dehydroepiandrosterone (DHEA)* and *androstenedione*. These steroid hormones are moderately active androgens; however, in the peripheral tissues they can be converted to more powerful androgens, such as testosterone, or even to estrogens. The quantities of these hormones that are released from the adrenal cortex are very small. Therefore, the contribution of this source of these hormones to androgenic effects in the male are negligible compared with that of the testicular androgens. However, it is likely that a portion of the early development of male sex organs results from the secretion of these hormones during childhood.

The adrenal gland is the major source of androgens in females. These hormones stimulate pubic and axillary (underarm) hair development in pubertal females. In pathological conditions where adrenal androgens are overproduced, masculinization of females may occur.

11.14   Pancreas

The pancreas is both an exocrine gland and an endocrine gland. The exocrine tissue produces a bicarbonate solution and digestive enzymes. These substances are transported to the small intestine where they play a role in the chemical digestion of food. These functions are fully discussed in Chapter 9.

Scattered throughout the pancreas, surrounded by exocrine cells, are small clusters of endocrine cells referred to as the *islets of Langerhans*. These islets make up only 2%–3% of the mass of the pancreas. However, their blood supply has been modified so that they receive 5–10 times more blood than the exocrine pancreas. Furthermore, this blood, carrying the pancreatic hormones, is then transported through the hepatic portal vein and delivered directly to the liver where the hormones, in a relatively high concentration, carry out many of their metabolic effects. The most important hormones produced by the pancreas that regulate glucose metabolism are insulin and glucagon.

11.14.1 Insulin

Insulin is a peptide hormone produced by the beta cells of the islets of Langerhans, which constitute approximately 60% of all the cells of the islets. Insulin is an important anabolic hormone secreted at times when the concentration of nutrient molecules in the blood is high, such as periods following a meal. Its overall effects include allowing the body to use carbohydrates as an energy source and to store nutrient molecules. Specifically, insulin exerts its important actions on the following tissues:

- Liver:
  - Increase in glucose uptake
  - Increase in glycogenesis (formation of glycogen, the storage form of glucose)
  - Increase in lipogenesis (formation of triglycerides, the storage form of lipids)
- Adipose tissue:
  - Increase in glucose uptake
  - Increase in free fatty acid uptake
  - Increase in lipogenesis
- Muscle:
  - Increase in glucose uptake
  - Increase in glycogenesis
  - Increase in amino acid uptake
  - Increase in protein synthesis

Insulin is the only hormone that lowers blood glucose (epinephrine, growth hormone, cortisol, and glucagon all increase blood glucose). It does so by stimulating the uptake of glucose from the blood into the liver, adipose tissue and muscle. This glucose is first used as an energy source and then it is stored in the form of glycogen in the liver and in muscle. Excess glucose is stored as fat in adipose tissue.

Insulin also plays a role in fat metabolism. In humans, most fatty acid synthesis takes place in the liver. The mechanism of action of insulin involves directing excess nutrient molecules toward metabolic pathways leading to fat synthesis. These fatty acids are then transported to storage sites, predominantly adipose tissue. Finally, insulin stimulates the uptake of amino acids into cells where they are incorporated into proteins.

The secretion of insulin from the pancreas is regulated primarily by the circulating concentration of glucose. When serum glucose increases, the secretion of insulin is stimulated; and when serum glucose decreases, the secretion of insulin is inhibited. Insulin secretion typically begins to increase within 10 min following the ingestion of food and reaches a peak in 30–45 min. This increased insulin stimulates the uptake of glucose into the body's cells and lowers serum glucose levels back to normal. Other factors affecting insulin secretion include circulating amino acids and free fatty acids; several gastrointestinal hormones, including gastrin, secretin, cholecystokinin, and gastric inhibitory peptide (which is likely the most important of these hormones); and the parasympathetic nervous system. Each of these factors stimulates the secretion of insulin. Sympathetic nervous stimulation inhibits insulin secretion.

11.14.2   Glucagon

Also a peptide hormone, *glucagon* is produced by the alpha cells of the islets of Langerhans, which constitute approximately 25% of the cells of the islets. The overall effects of glucagon include:

- Increase in hepatic glucose production
  - Glycogenolysis
  - Gluconeogenesis
- Stimulation of lipolysis in the liver and in adipose tissue

The effects of glucagon on glucose metabolism are generally opposite to those of insulin. Acting primarily on the liver, glucagon stimulates glycogenolysis (breakdown of glycogen, the storage form of glucose) and gluconeogenesis, which increase blood glucose levels within minutes. This hormone also stimulates lipolysis, which increases the circulating concentration of free fatty acids. These molecules may then be used as an alternative energy source by muscle or they may serve as gluconeogenic substrates in the liver. Finally, glucagon stimulates the hepatic uptake of amino acids that also serve as substrates for gluconeogenesis.

Factors that stimulate glucagon secretion include a decrease in blood glucose, an increase in blood amino acids, sympathetic nervous stimulation, stress and exercise. Factors that inhibit glucagon secretion include insulin and an increase in blood glucose.

Table 11.2 summarizes the major functions of the hormones discussed in this chapter.

11.15   Endocrine disorders

Glands of the endocrine system secrete various hormones that play a key role in maintaining normal homeostasis as well as allowing the body to deal with periods of physiologic stress. Abnormalities of endocrine glands generally fall into one of the several categories:

Hypersecretion
- Excess activity of a specific hormone or hormones
- May be due to overproduction of a hormone due to abnormal glandular function, glandular hypertrophy/hyperplasia or the presence of tumors that secrete hormone

Hyposecretion
- Reduced activity of a specific hormone or hormones
- May be due to atrophy of glandular tissue or damage from autoimmune attack, infection or neoplasia; may also occur as a result of reduced hormonal stimulation of a gland

Altered Responsiveness of a Tissue to a Specific Hormone
- Tissue no longer responds to a specific hormone
- May involve down-regulation of receptors or altered receptor/secondary messenger function
- Circulating levels of hormone may be normal or even elevated (e.g., type 2 diabetes)

11.15.1   Abnormalities of the hypothalamus/pituitary glands

The *hypothalamus* is often referred to as the "master gland" of the body due to its regulatory role over other glands. The hypothalamus lies at the base of the brain and receives neural input from a number of higher brain regions. These neural connections allow the hypothalamus to integrate many of the interactions between the autonomic nervous system and endocrine system. The hypothalamus is connected to the *pituitary* gland through a stalk called the *infundibulum*. Hypothalamic releasing hormones are carried by a blood vessel portal system found within the infundibulum to the anterior pituitary, where they, in turn, stimulate the release of specific hormones from the anterior pituitary. Two hormones of the posterior pituitary (oxytocin and vasopressin) are actually synthesized in neuron clusters within the hypothalamus and transported down axons to the posterior pituitary where they are released. A summary of the hypothalamic and pituitary hormones is given in Tables 11.1 and 11.2.

Injury to the hypothalamus can lead to a decreased production of hypothalamic hormones. In light of the many hormones released in response to hypothalamic releasing hormones, manifestations of abnormal hypothalamic function will be numerous. Release of pituitary hormones (e.g., LH, FSH, GH, ACTH) will be impaired as will release of thyroid hormones as a result of TRH deficiency.

11.15.1.1 Hypopituitarism

- Decreased activity of the pituitary gland along with hyposecretion of one or more pituitary hormones. If all pituitary hormones are lacking it is termed *panhypopituitarism*
- Most commonly results from damage to the pituitary (trauma, infection, ischemia) or tumors
- Manifestations are highly variable and will depend upon the hormone or hormones that are lacking. For the effects of specific hormone deficiency see the following sections.

11.15.2   Disorders of the anterior pituitary gland

11.15.2.1 Alterations of growth hormone secretion

Growth hormone is a polypeptide that is synthesized and secreted by the anterior pituitary gland. Growth hormone stimulates the release of *insulin-like growth factor (IGF-1)* from the liver. It is IGF-1 that is responsible for stimulating the growth of cartilage, long bones, muscle and organs during childhood development.

11.15.2.1.1 Measurement of growth hormone   Serum GH and IGF-1 levels can be measured directly. GH release occurs over a 24-hour period with peak release occurring in the early morning hours. The induction of hypoglycemia with insulin or the administration of GHRH or levodopa can be used to stimulate the release of GH for diagnostic purposes. Serum levels of IGF-1 will generally parallel those of GH release.

11.15.2.1.2 Growth hormone hyposecretion

- In children and adolescents, GH secretion occurs in a pulsatile fashion at night and during sleep. Daytime levels of GH are very low and not indicative of overall GH release. In order to evaluate GH secretion in a particular patient it is important to take samples throughout a 24-hour period.
- Deficiency of GH secretion may occur from a congenital defect in the pituitary gland or may be acquired as a result of injury or tumor

growth. Growth hormone deficiency is also seen in congenital conditions such as Turner syndrome and Down syndrome. Many cases of GH deficiency are *idiopathic,* meaning their cause cannot be clearly identified.

11.15.2.1.3   Manifestations of growth hormone deficiency
- The major manifestation of growth hormone deficiency in children is short stature
- Delayed development of muscle and bone may also occur

GROWTH HORMONE, THE FOUNTAIN OF YOUTH?

Growth hormone secretion decreases as we age. There is a significant body of evidence that this drop in growth hormone secretion contributes to the loss of muscle and skin tone that we experience as we age. A number of studies in reputable journals have reported that supplemental growth hormone administration can slow and even reverse some of the undesirable effects of aging on the body. In certain countries, "spas" have even arisen that include growth hormone replacement therapy as part of their youth-restoring regimens.

However, long-term growth hormone replacement therapy is very expensive and may be associated with the development of glucose intolerance, diabetes and even certain types of cancers. Does the risk outweigh the potential benefits?

11.15.2.1.4   Treatment of growth hormone deficiency
- Many patients with idiopathic growth hormone deficiency and resulting short stature will benefit from GH replacement therapy in terms of final height and development.
- The use of GH supplementation in children with *familial short stature* (children who are normal, but who will be short because their parents were short) is controversial. Although these children might experience some modest increase in final height, GH replacement therapy is very expensive and may be associated with an increased risk of diabetes and leukemia.

11.15.2.1.5   Growth hormone hypersecretion
Gigantism and Acromegaly
- Gigantism results from the excess production of growth hormone before the epiphyseal growth plates of the long bones fuse (around puberty)

- Acromegaly is due to a growth hormone excess that occurs after the epiphyseal growth plates of the long bones fuse
- Both conditions are most commonly caused by an adenoma of the anterior pituitary gland

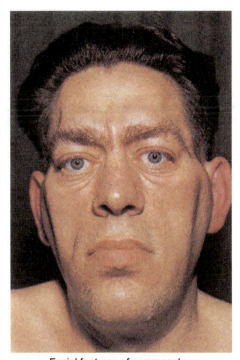

Facial features of acromegaly

Manifestations of Growth Hormone Hypersecretion
- Extremely tall stature with gigantism due to excessive growth of the long bones
- Overgrowth of connective tissues with acromegaly. Although bones can no longer grow in length, they can grow in thickness. Patients present with thickening and deformation of the hands, face, skull, feet
- Patients also tend to have very oily skin
- Central nervous system disturbances (headache, vision changes) abnormalities may occur
- Cardiovascular disease in the form of hypertension and coronary artery disease represents a significant source of mortality in these patients

Treatment of Growth Hormone Hypersecretion

- Surgical removal of tumor. Note that secretion of other pituitary hormones may be altered as a result of tumor removal
- Radiation therapy of the tumor may be performed if surgery is not feasible

11.15.3   Disorders of the posterior pituitary

11.15.3.1   Syndrome of inappropriate ADH (SIADH)

- A condition characterized by excess production of ADH from the posterior pituitary
- May be caused by pituitary tumors or injury. Cancers cells found in the lungs, prostate or pancreas may also produce ADH. Can also occur transiently due to physiologic stress or the administration of certain drugs such as carbamazepine

11.15.3.1.1   Manifestations of SIADH

- Excessive water retention
- Serum hypoosmolality
- Urine hyperosmolality
- Weight gain due to water accumulation
- Decreased serum sodium levels due to *dilutional hyponatremia*

11.15.3.1.2   Treatment of SIADH

- Fluid restriction
- Diuretics
- Removal of tumor if present

11.15.3.2   Diabetes insipidus

- A condition caused by decreased production of ADH and not related to the condition of diabetes mellitus, which involves insulin deficiency
- The word diabetes is derived from ancient Greek and means "siphon" to reflect the copious amounts of urine that are lost with this condition. Insipidus is derived from Latin and implies the urine is "tasteless," diluted and devoid of solutes
- May result from defects in the hypothalamus/pituitary or from a tumor or trauma (*neurogenic form*)
- A *nephrogenic* form of diabetes insipidus also occurs in which ADH production is normal but the kidneys do not respond to the effects of ADH. Nephrogenic diabetes insipidus may occur with renal inflammation or injury

---

QUESTION?

How would you distinguish the nephrogenic form of diabetes insipidus from the neurogenic form of diabetes insipidus?

11.15.3.2.1   Manifestations of diabetes insipidus

- Production of excessive amounts of very dilute urine (urine hypoosmolality)
- Increased serum osmolality
- Possible hypotension and reflex tachycardia
- Possible dehydration and excessive thirst (*polydyspsia*)

11.15.3.2.2   Treatment of diabetes insipidus
The synthetic vasopressin analog *desmopressin acetate* (oral or nasal administration) can be administered for the neurogenic form of diabetes insipidus. ADH replacement is generally lifelong.

11.15.4   Alteration of thyroid function

There are two main hormones produced by the thyroid gland *thyroxin* (T_4) and *triiodothyronine* (T_3). Both of these hormones are derived from the amino acid *tyrosine* and contain *iodine* that is extracted from the blood. The release of thyroid hormones from the anterior pituitary is regulated by TRH secreted from the hypothalamus. The main actions of T_3 and T_4 are to increased basal metabolic rate and help maintain normal metabolic function. Normal levels of thyroid hormone are also important for normal development of the nervous system in the fetus and newborn.

11.15.4.1   Tests of thyroid function
A diagnosis of primary hypothyroidism is made when levels of TSH are elevated while levels of T_3 and T_4 are decreased. In secondary hypothyroidism where the cause is pituitary insufficiency, levels of TSH would also be decreased. A diagnosis of primary hyperthyroidism is made when levels of T_3 and T_4 are elevated while TSH is decreased. TSH would also be increased in cases of secondary hyperthyroidism. A radioiodine (^{123}I)-uptake test may be used to determine how effectively the thyroid gland is taking up and concentrating iodine from the blood. The presence of anti-thyroid antibodies may also be tested for in patients with Hashimoto or Graves' disease.

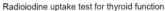
Radioiodine uptake test for thyroid function

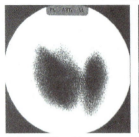 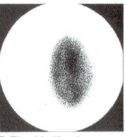 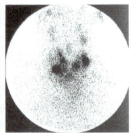

A. Normal thyroid   B. Thyroid with only one   C. Thyroid with reduced
                         functional lobe   function in both lobes

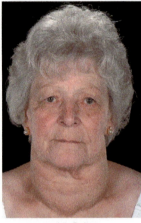

(a) Goiter

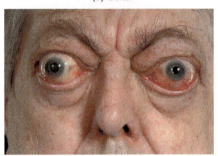

(b) Exophthalmos

11.15.4.2 Hypothyroidism

- May be a primary condition resulting from a defect within the thyroid itself or can be secondary to a lack of stimulation by TSH.
- Dietary deficiency of *iodine* may lead to hypertrophy of the thyroid gland that presents as a *goiter* (see Box). Hypothyroidism will also occur in patients who have undergone a *thyroidectomy* or who are taking antithyroid drugs such as methimazole or propylthiouracil.

- The most common cause of hypothyroidism in adults is an autoimmune condition called *Hashimoto's thyroiditis* (autoimmune thyroiditis) in which antibodies are produced against the tissue of the thyroid. Although the exact etiology of this autoimmune disorder is unknown, it can lead to progressive destruction of the thyroid gland and loss of thyroid function. Hashimoto's thyroiditis occurs predominately in women. It may present with a toxic goiter due to inflammation of the thyroid gland caused by autoimmune attack.

TOXIC AND NONTOXIC GOITER

Nontoxic Goiter—hypertrophy of the thyroid gland that is not accompanied by excess secretion of thyroid hormones. May occur as a result of dietary iodine deficiency. Symptoms are those of hypothyroidism.

Toxic Goiter—hypertrophy of the thyroid that is accompanied by excess thyroid production. May be associated with Graves' disease. Symptoms are those of hyperthyroidism. Thyrotoxicosis is a term that is used to describe the "toxic" effects of excess thyroid hormones on the body.

11.15.4.2.1 Manifestations of hypothyroidism
- Cold intolerance
- Weight gain
- Fatigue
- Bradycardia
- Cool, dry skin
- Anorexia
- Constipation
- *Myxedema*—edema of the face (swelling around the eyes), hands and ankles. Drooping eyelids.
- Possible long-term complications of untreated hypothyroidism may include cardiac hypertrophy, heart failure, and *myxedematous coma* that presents with hypothermia, seizures and respiratory depression. Myxedematous coma is most likely to occur during winter months in elderly patients with poorly managed or undiagnosed hypothyroidism.

11.15.4.2.2 Congenital hypothyroidism—cretinism
- Hypothyroidism that occurs during fetal development
- May occur as a result of a congenital defect in thyroid development
- Severe developmental delays and mental retardation can occur if left untreated

11.15.4.2.3   Treatment of hypothyroidism   Thyroid hormone replacement therapy. A variety of synthetic and natural T_3/T_4 preparations are available for use orally. *Levothyroxine*, a synthetic form of T_4, is currently the preferred drug of choice for thyroid hormone replacement therapy.

11.15.4.3   Hyperthyroidism

Hyperthyroidism results from the increased synthesis and release of the thyroid hormones T_3 and T_4. Hyperthyroidism may be a primary condition that results from an overactive thyroid gland or it may occur secondary to excessive stimulation of the thyroid by TSH from the pituitary. Secondary hyperthyroidism is a rare condition that may be caused by a pituitary adenoma. Hyperthyroidism is also referred to as *thyrotoxicosis* due to the range of serious physiologic alterations that occur as a result of increased circulating thyroid hormone levels. One of the most common causes of hyperthyroidism is *Graves' disease* (see below). In rare cases carcinomas arising outside of the thyroid may produce thyroid hormone or TSH.

11.15.4.3.1   Graves' disease   Graves' disease is an autoimmune condition in which patients with produce antibodies that bind TSH receptors on the thyroid and mimic the actions of TSH. This effect leads to the excess production of thyroid hormones. As a result of the high levels of circulating thyroid hormone, the release of TSH and TRH is suppressed.

11.15.4.3.2   Manifestations of hyperthyroidism
- Increased basal metabolic rate
- Increased heat production, patient always feels "hot"
- Tachycardia
- Increased catecholamine sensitivity. Patients are at risk for cardiac arrhythmias
- Warm skin, thin hair
- Increased appetite
- Weight loss
- Enhanced bowel activity
- Behavioral changes including possible nervousness and hyperactivity
- *Exophthalmos*—bulging around the eyes cause by fluid accumulation
- *Pretibial myxedema*—accumulation of fluids around the tibia and knee region
- *Toxic goiter*

11.15.4.3.3   Thyroid storm   Thyroid storm is an extreme, life-threatening episode of hyperthyroidism. It is most likely to occur in newly diagnosed or poorly managed patients with hyperthyroidism that are subjected to a period of physiologic or emotional stress. Manifestations include hypertension, tachycardia, high fever and pronounced central nervous system effects such as agitation, anxiety, and delirium. Patients may experience dangerous arrhythmias and high-output cardiac failure.

11.15.4.3.4 Treatment of hyperthyroidism
- β-blocking drugs to blunt the effects of excess adrenergic stimulation.
- Anti-thyroid drugs (*propylthiouracil, methimazole*) that block production of thyroid hormone.
- *Radioiodine*—given orally and taken up by hormone producing cells of the thyroid as if it were normal iodine. The cytotoxic actions of the β and γ radiation destroy the hormone producing cells of the thyroid. After treatment, the patient usually becomes hypothyroid and must be managed with thyroid hormone replacement therapy. Radioactive iodine should not be used in patients of childbearing age due to the possible effects on offspring. High-energy ^{131}I is used to selectively destroy thyroid tissue, whereas lower-energy ^{123}I is used to diagnose thyroid function.
- Surgical ablation of a portion of the thyroid may also be used. Following surgery, patients may likewise become hypothyroid and require thyroid hormone replacement therapy.

11.15.5 Disorders of the adrenal glands

The adrenal glands are small triangular shaped structures that lie on top of the kidneys. Anatomically, the adrenal glands may be divided into two parts, the *adrenal medulla* and the *adrenal cortex*. The adrenal medulla contains cells that secrete the *catecholamine's* epinephrine and norepinephrine. Cells of the adrenal cortex secrete the *glucocorticoids* (mainly *cortisol*), the *mineralcorticoids* (*aldosterone*) and small amounts of *testosterone*. The physiologic functions of the adrenal hormones are shown in Table 11.3.

11.15.5.1 Hyposecretion of adrenal hormones
11.15.5.1.1 Congenital adrenal hypoplasia (CAH)
- An autosomal recessive disorder in which the enzyme(s) necessary for cortisol synthesis are deficient or absent. The most common enzyme lacking in patients with CAH is *21-hydroxylase*. In a smaller percentage of cases (~10%), the 11-β hydroxylase may be absent or deficient.
- Lack of cortisol negative feedback on the pituitary gland leads to excess ACTH production, which, in turn, causes adrenal

Table 11.3 Physiologic effects of adrenal hormones

Hormones from the adrenal medulla

Catecholamines (epinephrine and norepinephrine):
- Involved in the "fight-or-flight" response
- Interact with α and β receptors in the body
- Increase heart and respiratory rate
- Increase energy availability; stimulate glycogenolysis in the liver as well as plasma levels of free fatty acids
- Reduce gastrointestinal activity

Hormones from the adrenal cortex

Glucocorticoids (cortisol):
- Stimulate the synthesis and storage of glycogen
- Increase gluconeogenesis and blood glucose levels
- Exert catabolic effects in muscle and fat tissue
- Anti-inflammatory action; used clinically as anti-inflammatory agents

Mineralcorticoids (aldosterone):
- Acts on the distal tubules and collecting ducts of the kidney to increase reabsorption of sodium
- Increase plasma volume
- Increase renal excretion of potassium and protons

---

hyperplasia and increases the synthesis and release of androgens from the adrenal cortex.
- Aldosterone production may also be altered depending upon the severity of the enzyme defect.

11.15.5.1.2 Manifestations of CAH
- Masculinization of the female external genitals (*pseudohemaphroditism*), enlarged penis in males, early puberty
- Short stature and poor growth due to premature fusion of the epiphyseal growth plate in the long bones
- With certain forms of CAH, a lack of aldosterone production may lead to significant "salt wasting" (sodium losses) and dehydration
- Weight loss
- Diagnosis is made by measurement of metabolites

11.15.5.1.3 Treatment of CAH
- Administration of cortisone/hydrocortisone will reduce ACTH levels and block the subsequent production of excess androgens
- Serum electrolyte levels should be closely monitored and corrected, particularly in the salt-wasting form of CAH. Mineralcorticoid replacement in patients who are "salt wasters"

- Reconstructive surgery of the genitals may be necessary in females to alter the male characteristics

11.15.5.1.4   Addison's disease
- A primary condition associated with atrophy of the adrenal glands
- The majority of cases arise from autoimmune destruction of the adrenal glands. Some cases may occur as a result of adrenal gland injury due to by infection or tumors
- Addison's disease is a rare condition that affects 1 in 100,000 individuals, mostly in the range of 30–50 years of age
- The result is decreased production of cortisol, aldosterone and androgens from the adrenal glands
- Decreased levels of glucocorticoids (cortisol) results in a compensatory increase in levels of ACTH

11.15.5.1.5   Manifestations of Addison's disease
- The manifestations of Addison's disease are due to deficiency of all three hormone groups produced by the adrenal gland (glucocorticoids, mineralcorticoids and androgens)
- Weakness and fatigue
- Increased pigmentation of the skin due to an ACTH-induced increased in *melanocyte* (skin pigment cell) activity
- Weight loss, anorexia, hypometabolism, cold intolerance
- Cardiovascular changes—hypotension, orthostatic hypotension, ECG changes
- Changes in EEG and mental function
- Although androgen production from the adrenal glands is reduced, androgen production from other sites in the body (testis) is sufficient to maintain normal sexual function and development

---

ADRENAL CRISIS

An episode of severe hypotension, vascular collapse, acute renal failure and hypothermia caused by a combined lack of cortisol and aldosterone.

It may be precipitated by infection, trauma and dehydration in individuals with Addison's disease and can be life threatening.

11.15.5.1.6   Treatment of Addison's disease
- Lifelong replacement therapy with glucocorticoids (cortisone/hydro-cortisone) and mineralcorticoids (aldosterone).

11.15.5.1.7   Cushing syndrome (Figure 11.4)
- A condition characterized by excess production of glucocorticoids
- May be caused by excess ACTH secretion due to pituitary tumors or less commonly as a result of a cortisol-producing tumor of the adrenal gland itself. In rare instances, ACTH or cortisol-producing malignant tumors may occur in the body outside of the pituitary or adrenal glands themselves
- An *iatrogenic* form of Cushing syndrome may also occur in patients receiving therapeutic levels of glucocorticoids (corticosteroids)

QUESTION?

How would you determine if a patient's Cushing syndrome was caused by the adrenal gland or the pituitary gland?

11.15.5.1.8   Diagnosis of Cushing syndrome   A diagnosis of Cushing syndrome is based on excess excretion of cortisol in the urine over a 24-hour period. Plasma levels of ACTH may also be evaluated. Imaging studies would be of value in determining the presence of pituitary or adrenal tumors.

11.15.5.1.9   Manifestations of Cushing's syndrome
- The effects of Cushing syndrome are primarily those of excess cortisol levels
- Characteristic "Moon face," "buffalo hump" patterns of abnormal fat distribution along with abdominal adiposity
- Glucose intolerance and possible diabetes mellitus
- Thin, atrophied skin
- Poor wound healing, impaired immune function, increased susceptibility to infection
- Hypertension
- Muscle weakness and wasting
- Reduced bone density, hypercalciuria with possible development of renal calculi
- Alterations in mental function and personality
- Increased androgen levels in females with possible "virilization"
- Mortality is approximately 50% within 5 years if left untreated

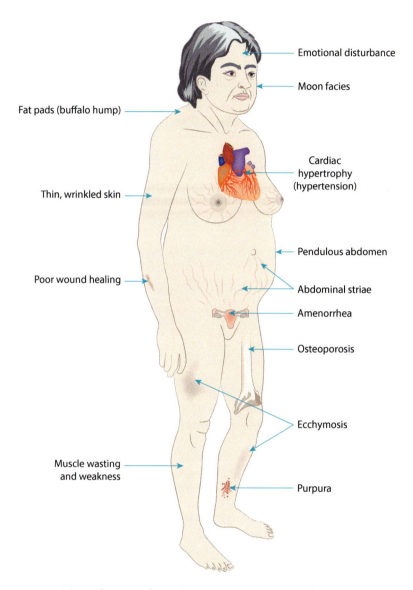

Figure 11.4 Major feature of Cushing's disease. (Adapted from *Porth's Pathophysiology: Concepts of Altered Health States* by Grossman, Lippincott Williams and Wilkins, 2013.)

11.15.5.1.10 Treatment of Cushing's disease
- Surgical removal of tumors
- Radiation therapy
- Drug therapy may be used to inhibit steroid synthesis if tumor is inoperable or ectopic. *Mitotane* is a compound that is structurally similar to

the insecticide DDT. It is used because of its selective toxicity for cells of the adrenal cortex to treat tumors arising in this tissue

11.15.6 Disorders of the adrenal medulla

The adrenal medulla is responsible for secreting catecholamines (epinephrine, norepinephrine) in response to activation of the sympathetic nervous system ("fight or flight")

11.15.6.1 Pheochromocytoma

- A tumor (usually benign) that arises in the *chromaffin* cells of the adrenal medulla that produce the catecholamines
- Symptoms are those of excess catecholamine production and can be life threatening
- Excess catecholamine production may be continual or occur in episodes ("bursts") during periods of stress when the sympathetic ("fight or flight") nervous system is activated

11.15.6.2 Diagnosis of pheochromocytoma

A diagnosis of pheochromocytoma is made base upon elevated circulating blood levels or urine metabolites of catecholamines. Imaging studies are used to confirm the presence of pheochromocytoma.

11.15.6.3 Manifestations of pheochromocytoma

- Hypertension often occurs with episodic increases in blood pressure
- Tachycardia and an increased risk of arrhythmia
- Severe headache
- Nausea and vomiting
- Hypermetabolism, heat intolerance, weight loss
- Excess sweating (*diaphoresis*)
- Palpitations
- Anxiety
- Risk of stroke due to marked hypertension

11.15.6.4 Treatment of pheochromocytoma

- β and α blocking drugs to blunt catecholamine effects
- Surgical removal of tumor

11.16 Diabetes

Diabetes mellitus is the most common endocrine disorder. Approximately 800,000 new cases of diabetes are diagnosed each year. The prevalence of diabetes is 8.2% among all men and women in the United States. The frequency of the disease increases to 18.4% in individuals 65 years of age or

Table 11.4   Risk factors for diabetes mellitus

- Obesity (risk for type 2 diabetes)
- Sedentary lifestyle (risk for type 2 diabetes)
- Familial history of diabetes mellitus
- Increasing age
- Ethnicity—high-risk groups include African Americans, Hispanics, and American Indians
- Dietary Factors

older. Diabetes is a disease of the *endocrine pancreas*. Some risk factors for diabetes mellitus are presented in Table 11.4.

11.16.1   The endocrine pancreas

Throughout the pancreas, endocrine are cells found in scattered clusters called *islets of Langerhans*. These endocrine cells can be classified into three distinct types: *alpha cells* that produce the hormone *glucagon*; *beta cells* that produce *insulin* and *delta cells* that produce *somatostatin* (see Table 11.5). The major regulator of insulin and glucagon release from the pancreas is blood glucose level. An increase in blood glucose (as occurs after a meal) will stimulate the release of insulin and inhibit the release of glucagon. Conversely, decreases in blood glucose (during fasting for example) will stimulate the release of glucagon and inhibit the release of insulin. When released, the main effect of insulin is to lower blood glucose levels by enhancing the utilization and uptake of insulin. Glucagon directly counters the effects of insulin by decreasing glucose utilization and uptake as well as stimulating the formation of new glucose from

Table 11.5   Hormones of the endocrine pancreas

Glucagon
Increases glycogen breakdown in liver
Increases lipolysis in adipose tissue
Increases gluconeogenesis in liver
Increases proteolysis in skeletal muscle. Liberated amino acids may in turn be converted to glucose
Insulin
Increases glucose transport into tissues
Increases glycogen synthesis in liver and muscle
Increases triglyceride synthesis in adipose tissue and liver
Increases amino acid uptake and protein synthesis
Somatostatin
Inhibits the release of glucagon and insulin locally
Inhibits the release of growth hormone from the anterior pituitary

glycogen and amino acids. The major target tissues for insulin and glucagon action are liver, skeletal muscle and fat.

11.16.2   Diabetes mellitus

Diabetes mellitus is a group of disorders characterized by abnormalities of insulin. The term "diabetes" is derived from the Greek word "siphon," which represents the copious amounts of urine (polyuria) produced by patients with diabetes mellitus (and *diabetes insipidus,* see the endocrine chapter). The term mellitus is derived from the Latin word for "honeyed" or sweet and represents the high levels of glucose present in the urine of patients with diabetes mellitus. There are two main types of diabetes mellitus, *type 1 diabetes mellitus* and *type 2 diabetes mellitus.*

11.16.2.1   Types of diabetes
11.16.2.1.1   Type 1 diabetes
- Most commonly occurs in children and young adults less than 20 years of age.
- Associated with a progressive autoimmune destruction of the pancreatic beta cells. Patients with type 1 diabetes often have immune cell (lymphocytes, macrophages) infiltration of their pancreatic beta cells. Autoantibodies against insulin and the pancreatic beta cells may also be present.
- Although the exact etiology of type 1 diabetes is not fully understood, there is an increased incidence in individuals with certain HLA subtypes (HLA-DQ and HLA-DR). Environmental factors such as certain types of viral infections and exposure to cow's milk proteins may also stimulate the production of autoantibodies in susceptible individuals.
- Little or no insulin secretion occurs, therefore, patients are dependent upon the administration of exogenous insulin for their survival.

11.16.2.1.2   Manifestations
- Hyperglycemia
- Weight loss
- The three "polys"—*polyuria, polydipsia, polyphagia* (see Box)
- Weakness and fatigue due to poor energy utilization and skeletal muscle catabolism

- An acute complication of type 1 diabetes may be *diabetic ketoacidosis (DKA)*. DKA is the accumulation of acidic ketone bodies in the blood due to an increase in fatty acid metabolism. Due to a lack of insulin tissues cannot effectively utilize glucose for energy. As a result, cells turn to increased fat mobilization, fatty acid release and ketogenesis for energy. This in turn results in the generation of excess amounts of acidic ketone bodies that now cause acidosis. The effects of DKA are shown in Table 11.6

THE THREE "POLYS"

Polyuria—excess blood glucose filtered by the kidneys cannot be reabsorbed and is eliminated at the expense of water.

Polydipsia—excessive thirst caused by the osmotic diuresis of glucose and subsequent tissue dehydration. The thirst response is mediated by the hypothalamus in response to increased serum osmolarity.

Polyphagia—poor utilization of carbohydrates (due to the lack of insulin) results in depletion of stores fats, proteins and carbohydrates.

11.16.2.1.3 Treatment of type 1 diabetes
- Insulin replacement therapy
- Dietary management

Table 11.6 Symptoms of diabetic ketoacidosis

Diabetic Ketoacidosis
- Decreased blood pH levels
- Ketonuria—appearance of excess ketones in the urine
- Lethargy
- Anorexia, nausea, vomiting
- Markedly increased respiratory rate as an attempt to correct decreased blood pH
- Acetone breath—acetone is a volatile ketone body that is eliminated via the lungs. It may be noticeable in the exhaled air during diabetic ketoacidosis
- Central nervous system depression, coma and possible death

Treatment includes administration of insulin and replacement of fluids and electrolytes.

INSULIN THERAPY

Insulin preparations were originally derived from bovine or porcine sources but now are supplied as a pure human form made by recombinant DNA technology or modification of porcine insulin. Insulin must be administered by injection because an oral form would be degraded in the gastrointestinal tract. Insulin is generally available in three preparations:

1. Short-acting forms—peak action in 2–4 hours, duration 6–8 hours.
2. Intermediate-acting forms—peak action in 6–12 hours, duration 12–24 hours.
3. Long-acting form—peak action 8–24 hours, duration 24–36 hours.

11.16.2.1.4 Somogyi effect A complication that is more likely to occur in patients with type 1 diabetes mellitus. The Somogyi effect is an episode of rebound hyperglycemia that can occur after a period of hypoglycemia. Such hypoglycemia may occur after a patient with diabetes injects insulin. When hypoglycemia occurs, hormones such as cortisol, growth hormones and glucagon stimulate gluconeogenesis and glycogenolysis, which now raises blood glucose. Diabetic patients will also often ingest glucose in order to counter their hypoglycemia, which further raises their blood glucose. The dose and timing of insulin injection may need to be adjusted in diabetic patients who experience Somogyi effect.

11.16.2.1.5 Dawn phenomenon The dawn phenomenon refers to a rise in blood glucose that occurs in the early morning hours. It likely occurs as a result of circadian variations in growth hormone and may occur in patients with type 1 or type 2 diabetes. The dawn phenomenon may occur in conjunction with the Somogyi effect if there is overnight hypoglycemia and lead to significant hyperglycemia in the morning hours. The dose and timing of insulin injection may need to be adjusted in diabetic patients to prevent this occurrence.

11.16.2.2   Type 1 diabetes (Figure 11.5)
- Greater prevalence than type 1 diabetes
- The primary manifestation is "insulin resistance," which is a lack of responsiveness by tissues and the pancreas itself to insulin. The exact etiology of the insulin resistance is unknown but may be linked to abnormalities of insulin receptors, intracelluar signaling pathways or glucose transporters
- Obesity appears to be an important contributing factor to development of type 2 diabetes. Tissues (liver, fat and muscle) in obese individuals have an altered responsiveness to the effects of insulin
- May be associated with *metabolic syndrome* (see box)

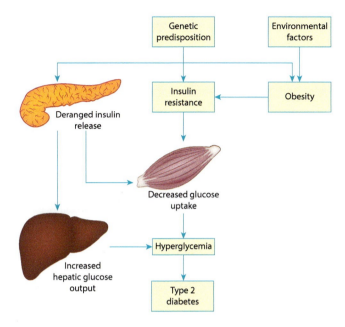

Figure 11.5   Etiology of Type II diabetes. (Adapted from *Porth's Pathophysiology: Concepts of Altered Health States* by Grossman, Lippincott Williams and Wilkins, 2013.)

- Most commonly occurs in obese men between 40 and 60 years of age
- A strong genetic component is also present
- Insulin secretion may be normal or even elevated at the time of diagnosis
- The continued overproduction of insulin by the beta-cells can eventually lead to beta-cell "burnout" and destruction
- An acute complication of type 2 diabetes may be *hyperglycemic hyperosmolar syndrome* (see Table 11.7)

METABOLIC SYNDROME

A group of conditions that includes:

- Abdominal adiposity
- Elevated triglyceride levels
- Low HDL levels
- Hypertension
- Hyperglycemia

In order to be diagnosed with metabolic syndrome, a patient must exhibit three of the above conditions.

A patient's risk for heart disease, stroke and diabetes increases in direct proportion to the number of the above conditions they exhibit.

Table 11.7   Hyperglycemic-Hyperosmolar-Nonketotic Syndrome (HHNKS)

A syndrome of type 2 diabetes mellitus that can result from acute insulin deficiency. Caused by a lack of insulin or insulin effect. Ketosis does not occur because the amount of insulin required to prevent the breakdown of fats is less than that needed to lower blood glucose.

Manifestations include:

- Severe dehydration
- Extreme thirst
- Serum osmolarity over 300 mOsm.
- Osmotic diuresis of glucose
- Depressed neurologic function
- Possible shock, coma, and death
- Generally a more dangerous condition than diabetic ketoacidosis

Treatment includes insulin therapy, fluid replacement and correction of electrolyte imbalances if present.

11.16.2.2.1   Manifestations of type 2 diabetes

- Manifestations of type 2 diabetes may include many of those seen in type 1 diabetes including polyuria, polydipsia, polyphagia, fatigue, and weakness. Other manifestations of type 2 diabetes tend to be more generalized and can include:
- Hyperinsulinemia
- Visual changes
- *Paresthesia* (abnormal sensations such as tingling or burning, often occurs in the extremities)
- Recurrent infections
- Ketoacidosis is rare with type 2 diabetes

11.16.2.2.2   Treatment of type 2 diabetes

- Weight loss can improve insulin sensitivity in obese individuals with type 2 diabetes.
- Exercise may also enhance glucose utilization and improve glucose control in patients with type 2 diabetes, thus reducing the risk of diabetic complications.
- Dietary management.
- Oral hypoglycemic drugs (see Table 11.8).
- Insulin replacement may be necessary during later stages of the disease when beta cells are destroyed to maintain normal metabolic function (see *Insulin Therapy Box*).

11.16.3   Long-term complications of diabetes

There are a number of long-term complications of diabetes that contribute significantly to the mortality and morbidity that is seen with this disease.

Table 11.8   Oral Hypoglycemic Agents

---

1. *Sulfonylureas* (e.g., Glyburide):
   • Simulate insulin secretion from the beta cells
   • Only effective if some beta cells are still functional

2. *Biguanides* (e.g., Metformin):
   • Reduces glucose production by the liver
   • May increase insulin-mediated glucose uptake by peripheral tissues

3. *Thiazolidinedione Derivatives* (e.g., Pioglitazone):
   • Increase insulin sensitivity in peripheral tissues
   • Increase glucose uptake and oxidation in muscle and adipose tissues independent of insulin

4. *Incretin Hormone Mimetic* (e.g., Exenatide, Liraglutide)
   • Inhibit the actions of glucagon
   • Stimulate postprandial insulin release
   • Slow gastric emptying, increase satiety

5. *Alpha Glucosidase Inhibitors* (e.g., Acarbose)
   • Inhibit the digestion of complex carbohydrates in the gut

6. *Glucose Transport Inhibitors* (e.g., Canagliflozin)
   • Inhibits the reuptake of filtered glucose in the renal tubules

---

The etiology of the complications is likely multifactorial and involves tissue injury related to chronically elevated blood glucose levels. Some possible mechanisms of tissue injury in chronic diabetes mellitus are listed in Table 11.9. The occurrence of these long-term complications can be greatly reduced by proper management of blood glucose levels. Chronic diabetes can lead to injury in a number of different target organs and tissues including nerves, kidney, blood vessels and eyes. Diabetic patients may also have impaired wound healing and be at increased risk for infections. Comprehensive evaluation and effective management of the diabetic patient is essential for to prevent the long-term complications that can accompany diabetes mellitus. A key component of comprehensive diabetic care includes prompt diagnosis and routine monitoring (see Table 11.10).

11.16.3.1   Diabetic neuropathy
• Diabetes is the most common cause of neuropathy in the United States
• It is associated with abnormalities of nerve conduction and function
• Diabetic neuropathy often effects peripheral nerves, but it can also involve sensory, motor and autonomic nerves

Table 11.9   Mechanisms of tissue injury in diabetes

---

1. Glycosylation of Proteins—attachment of glucose to proteins in the eye, blood vessel walls, and kidney membranes will change their structure and may lead to altered function and eventual damage of these tissues. Circulating glycosylated proteins may also be trapped in the glomeruli of the kidney leading to inflammation and injury.
2. Formation of Alcohol Sugars (e.g., sorbitol) that, unlike glucose, do not easily diffuse out of tissues. Because these alcohol sugars are osmotically active they can lead to swelling and damage of tissues. The accumulation of other sugars such as galactose might also contribute to this phenomenon.
3. Poor Blood Flow and Oxygen Delivery to Tissues—glycosylation of hemoglobin alters its affinity for oxygen, whereas progressive vascular disease can reduce overall blood flow to tissues leading to ischemic tissue injury.

Table 11.10   Diagnosis and Monitoring of Diabetes Mellitus

Diagnosis of Diabetes

- Presence of the three "polys" as well as significant weight loss.
- Elevated fasting blood glucose levels (>140 mg/dL).
- Presence of glucose in the urine.

Monitoring of Diabetes

- Frequent measurement of blood glucose levels.
- Measurement of *glycosylated hemoglobin* (Hb A_{1c}, hemoglobin that has glucose bound to it) that forms at a rate that increases with increasing blood glucose. It is a useful measure of blood glucose control in diabetic patients.
- Measurement of urine ketone levels in patients with insulin-dependent diabetes mellitus is also useful to assess disease management.
- Screening for the presence of protein in the urine, which might indicate renal disease.
- Routine eye exams.

- May also affect nerves responsible for gastrointestinal motility and bladder emptying and lead to *diabetic gastroparesis* and *diabetic bladder*
- Sensory neuropathies may manifest as *paresthesias,* with symptoms of numbness, tingling, and pain
- Diabetic neuropathy is often progressive and irreversible

11.16.3.2   *Diabetic nephropathy*

- Diabetes is the leading cause of end-stage renal disease in the United States
- Glomerular injury is the key feature of diabetic nephropathy. The glomerular injury is characterized by thickening of the glomerular basement membrane and *glomerulosclerosis*

- Although the exact etiology is unclear, trapping of glycosylated proteins in the glomeruli appears to be a key contributing factor.
- The appearance of protein (albumin) in the urine is an early indicator of altered glomerular permeability.
- Renal function may continue to deteriorate as glomerular filtration decreases. Signs and symptoms of renal insufficiency will appear as renal function continues to decline.

11.16.3.3   Vascular disease
- Chronic diabetes mellitus is associated with significant increases in the incidence of coronary artery disease, cerebrovascular disease and peripheral vascular disease.
- Vascular disease may result from a number of factors including elevated serum lipid levels, vascular injury, and enhanced atherogenesis (formation of atherosclerotic lesions).
- Coronary artery disease, and stroke are significant sources mortality and morbidity in diabetic patients. Peripheral vascular disease can lead to gangrene and amputations (particularly of the toes and feet) in diabetics. Diabetes mellitus is the leading cause of nontraumatic amputations in the United States.

11.16.3.4   Diabetic retinopathy
- Diabetes is the leading cause of acquired blindness in the United States.
- The most serious consequence of long-term diabetes on the eye is retinal damage. The retina is a highly metabolic tissue that is especially vulnerable to the effects of chronic hypoxia and diabetes. Hemorrhage of eye capillaries and chronic inflammation is common and can lead to increases in intraocular pressure that scar the retina and impair vision. This phenomenon is usually progressive and can lead to blindness.
- Diabetes is also associated with an increased incidence of glaucoma and cataract formation.

11.16.3.5   Impaired healing and increased infections risk
- As a result of peripheral vascular disease, injuries in diabetic patients do not heal properly. Poor blood flow limits the delivery of leukocytes and oxygen to the injured area while impairing removal of debris and infectious organisms.
- The high glucose levels serve as a nutrient to support the growth of microorganisms.
- Peripheral neuropathies may impair diabetic patients awareness that they are injured or that an injury might be getting infected.
- Diabetic patients might also be more susceptible to physical injuries due to impaired vision and sensory perception.

11.16.3.6   Increased risk of infection

Diabetic patients are at an increased risk for infections as a result of several factors, including:

- Poor wound healing
- Peripheral vascular disease
- Elevated blood and tissue glucose, which can serve as a nutrient for bacterial growth
- Neuropathies that can impair detection of injuries or injuries that have become infected
- Impaired activity of immune cells

11.16.4   Diabetes in pregnancy

11.16.4.1   Gestational diabetes

- Glucose intolerance occurs in about 1%–6% of all pregnancies
- May present with variable severity
- Most commonly seen during the third trimester of pregnancy
- Resolves itself in most patients after birth, but a certain percentage (50%–60%) will go on to develop diabetes mellitus in the years following the pregnancy
- Gestational diabetes may be associated with an increased risk of fetal abnormalities
- It is currently recommended that all pregnant women be screened for the presence of gestational diabetes

Medical terminology

Amplification (ăm″plĭ-fĭ-kā′shŭn): Enlargement, magnification

Anabolism (ă-năb′ō-lĭzm): Building of body tissue; metabolic reactions in which substances are synthesized

Androgenic (ăn″drō-jĕn-ĭk): Causing masculinization

Antagonism (ăn-tăg′ŏn-ĭzm): Contrary or opposing action

Antidiuretic (ăn″tĭ-dĭ-ū-rĕt′ĭk): Decreasing urine formation

Cardiogenic (kăr″dē-ō-jĕn′ĭk): Originating in the heart

Catabolism (kă-tăb′ō-lĭzm): Breaking down of body tissue; metabolic reactions in which substances are degraded

Cervix (sĕr′vĭks): Neck of the uterus

Diurnal (dī-ŭrn′ăl): Repeating once every 24 hours

Down-regulate (down-rĕg′ūlāt″): To decrease the number of receptors on a cell membrane

Extravasation (ĕks-trăv″ă-sā′shŭn): Escape of fluid from the vascular compartment into the tissue spaces

Follicle (fŏl'ĭ-kl): In the ovary, structure that releases the mature ovum

Gamete (găm'ēt): Mature female or male reproductive cell (e.g., ovum, sperm)

Gluconeogenesis (gloo″kō-nē″ō-jĕn'ĕ-sĭs): Formation of glucose from precursors other than carbohydrates (gastrointestinal., amino acids, lactic acid)

Glycogenesis (glī″kō-jĕn'ĕ-sĭs): Formation of glycogen from glucose molecules

Glycogenolysis (glī″kō-jĕn-ŏl'ĭ-sĭs): Breakdown of glycogen into its component glucose molecules

Gonad (gō'năd): Reproductive organ (e.g., ovary in the female; teste in the male)

Half-life (hăf'līf): Time required to eliminate half of a chemical substance

Hypercalcemia (hī″pĕr-kăl-sē'mē-ă): Presence of excess calcium in the blood

Hyperglycemia (hī″pĕr-glī-sē'mē-ă): Presence of excess glucose in the blood

Hypertrophy (hī-pĕr'trŏ-fē): Excessive development or growth of an organ or tissue

Hypoglycemia (hī″pō-glī-sē'mē-ă): Abnormally low level of glucose in the blood

Intranasal (ĭn″tră-nā'zl): Within the nasal cavity

Lipogenesis (līp″ō-jĕn'ĕ-sĭs): Formation of fat

Lipolysis (līp″-ŏl'ĭ-sĭs): Breakdown of fat to release fatty acids

Neurosecretory cell (nū″rō-sē'krĕ-tor-ē sĕl): In the hypothalamus, neuron that secretes a hormone from its axon terminal in response to an action potential

Osteoblast (ŏs'tē-ō-blăst): Cell that causes bone formation

Osteoclast (ŏs'tē-ō-klăst): Cell that causes bone resorption or bone breakdown

Ovum (ō'vŭm): Female reproductive cell; egg

Parturition (păr-tū-rĭsh'ŭn): Process of giving birth to offspring

Plexus (plĕks'ŭs): Network of nerves or blood vessels

Polydipsia (pŏl″ē-dĭp'sē-ă): Excessive thirst

Polyuria (pŏl″ē-ū'rē-ă): Excessive urination

Portal vein (pŏr'tăl vān): A vein that provides circulatory communication between two capillary beds

Postmenopausal (pōst″mĕn-ō-paw'zăl): Occurring after permanent cessation of menstruation

Potent (pō'tĕnt): Highly effective medicinally

Proteolytic (prō″tē-ō-lĭt'ĭk): Causing the breakdown of proteins

Reservoir (rĕz'ĕr-vwor): A place for storage

Resorption (rē-sorp'shŭn): In the bone, demineralization, or the removal of bone tissue

Sperm (spĕrm): Male reproductive cell

Sublingual (sŭb-lĭng'gwăl): Beneath the tongue

Synergism (sĭn'ĕr-jĭzm): Coordinated action between two or more agents so that the combined action is greater than the sum of each acting separately

Translocate (trăns-lō′kāt): To move from one region to another
Tremor (trĕm′or): Quivering or involuntary movement of the muscles
Up-regulate (ŭp-rĕg′yŭ-lāt): To increase the number of receptors on a cell membrane
Vasoactive (vās″ō-ăk′tĭv): Causing constriction of blood vessels

Bibliography

Boushey, H. A., Drugs used in asthma, in *Basic & Clinical Pharmacology*, 8th ed., Katzung, B. G., Ed., McGraw-Hill, New York, 2001, chap. 20.

Farwell, A. P., and Braverman, L. E., Thyroid and antithyroid drugs, in *Goodman and Gilman's, The Pharmacological Basis of Therapeutics*, 11th ed., Brunton, L. L., Lazo, J. S., and Parker, K. L., Eds., McGraw-Hill, New York, 2006, chap. 56.

Fitzgerald, P. A., Hypothalamic & pituitary hormones, in *Basic & Clinical Pharmacology*, 8th ed., Katzung, B. G., Ed., McGraw-Hill, New York, 2001, chap. 37.

Friedman, P. A., Agents affecting mineral ion homeostasis and bone turnover, in *Goodman and Gilman's, The Pharmacological Basis of Therapeutics*, 11th ed., Brunton, L. L., Lazo, J. S., and Parker, K. L., Eds., McGraw-Hill, New York, 2006, chap. 61.

Fox, S. I., *Human Physiology*, 9th ed., McGraw-Hill, Boston, MA, 2006.

Golan, D. E., Tashjian, A. H., Armstrong, E. J., Galanter, J. M., Armstrong, A. W., Arnout, R. A., and Rose, H., Integrative inflammation pharmacology: Asthma, in *Principles of Pharmacology, The Pathophysiologic Basis of Drug Therapy*, Lippincott Williams & Wilkins, Philadelphia, PA, 2005, chap. 45.

Guyton, A. C., and Hall, J. E., *Textbook of Medical Physiology*, 11th ed., Elsevier/Saunders, Philadelphia, PA, 2006.

Iversen, S., Iversen, L., and Saper, C. B., The autonomic nervous system and the hypothalamus, in *Principles of Neural Science*, 4th ed., Kandel, E. R., Schwartz, J. H., and Jessell, T. M., Eds., McGraw-Hill, New York, 2000, chap. 49.

Jackson, E. K., Vasopressin and other agents affecting the renal conservation of water, in *Goodman and Gilman's, The Pharmacological Basis of Therapeutics*, 11th ed., Brunton, L. L., Lazo, J. S., and Parker, K. L., Eds., McGraw-Hill, New York, 2006, chap. 29.

Kettyle, W. M., and Arky, R. A., *Endocrine Pathophysiology*, Lippincott-Raven Publishers, Philadelphia, PA, 1998.

Matfin, G., Kuenzi, J. A., and Guven, S., Disorders of endocrine control of growth and metabolism, in *Pathophysiology, Concepts of Altered Health States*, 7th ed., Porth, C. M., Ed., Lippincott Williams & Wilkins, Philadelphia, PA, 2005, chap. 42.

Page, C. P., 1999. Recent advances in our understanding of the use of theophylline in the treatment of asthma. *J Clin Pharmacol.* 39:237–240.

Parker, K. L., and Schimmer, B. P., Pituitary hormones and their hypothalamic releasing factors, in *Goodman and Gilman's, The Pharmacological Basis of Therapeutics*, 11th ed., Brunton, L. L., Lazo, J. S., and Parker, K. L., Eds., McGraw-Hill, New York, 2006, chap. 55.

Porterfield, S. P., *Endocrine Physiology*, 2nd ed., Mosby, Inc., St. Louis, MO, 2001.

Porth, C. M., *Pathophysiology, Concepts of Altered Health States*, 7th ed., Lippincott Williams & Wilkins, Philadelphia, PA, 2005.

Schimmer, B. P., and Parker, K. L., Adrenocorticotropic hormone; Adrenocortical steroids and their synthetic analogs; Inhibitors of the synthesis and actions of adrenocortical hormones, in *Goodman and Gilman's, The Pharmacological Basis of Therapeutics*, 11th ed., Brunton, L. L., Lazo, J. S., and Parker, K. L., Eds., McGraw-Hill, New York, 2006, chap. 59.

Sherwood, L., *Human Physiology from Cells to Systems*, 5th ed., Brooks/Cole, Pacific Grove, CA, 2004.

Silverthorn, D., *Human Physiology: An Integrated Approach*, 4th ed., Prentice Hall, Upper Saddle River, NJ, 2007.

Stedman's Medical Dictionary for the Health Professions and Nursing, 5th ed., Lippincott Williams & Wilkins, Baltimore, MD, 2005.

Taber's Cyclopedic Medical Dictionary, 20th ed., F. A. Davis Co., Philadelphia, PA, 2005.

Undem, B. J., Pharmacotherapy of asthma, in *Goodman and Gilman's, The Pharmacological Basis of Therapeutics*, 11th ed., Brunton, L. L., Lazo, J. S., and Parker, K. L., Eds., McGraw-Hill, New York, 2006, chap. 27.

Widmaier, E. P., Raff, H., and Strang, K. T., *Vander's Human Physiology, The Mechanisms of Body Function*, McGraw-Hill, Boston, MA, 2006.

chapter twelve

The reproductive system

Study objectives

- Explain the process and the purpose of gametogenesis
- Describe the location and the function of each of the organs and structures in the male reproductive system including the testes, seminiferous tubules, testicular interstitial tissue, scrotum, epididymides, vas deferens, ejaculatory ducts, penis, prostate gland, seminal vesicles, and bulbourethral glands
- Distinguish between Sertoli cells and Leydig cells
- List the functions of testosterone in the male
- Describe the location and the function of each of the organs and structures in the female reproductive system including the ovaries, fallopian tubes, uterus, endometrium, myometrium, and the vagina
- Distinguish between granulosa cells and thecal cells
- Explain the events of the follicular phase of the ovarian cycle including changes in hormone (FSH, LH, estrogen, and progesterone) secretion, follicular development and the endometrium
- Explain the events of the luteal phase of the ovarian cycle including changes in hormone (FSH, LH, estrogen, and progesterone) secretion, corpus luteum development, and the endometrium
- Describe how FSH, LH, estrogen, and progesterone regulate the ovarian cycle
- List the other functions of the female sex hormones
- Describe the major disorders associated with the male reproductive system
- Describe the major disorders associated with the female reproductive system
- List the most common sexually transmitted diseases
- Identify the organism associated with each of the most common sexually transmitted diseases
- Describe the main symptoms and possible long-term consequences for each of the most common sexually transmitted diseases

Unlike the other organ systems discussed in this textbook, the reproductive system does not contribute to the maintenance of homeostasis; it is responsible for the formation of *offspring*. Reproduction is the process of passing genetic material from one generation to the next. As such, reproduction involves *gametogenesis*, or the production of sex cells (*gametes*). The male gamete, or *sperm*, contains 23 chromosomes and the female gamete, or *ovum*, also contains 23 chromosomes. The fertilization of the ovum by the sperm results in the formation of a *zygote* with the full human complement of 46 chromosomes. This chapter will discuss the following:

- Gametogenesis (spermatogenesis and oogenesis)
- Male reproductive system
- Testosterone
- Female reproductive system
- Ovarian cycle

12.1   Gametogenesis

12.1.1   Spermatogenesis

Male germ cells are referred to as *spermatogonia*. At puberty, the germ cells, which are found in the *Sertoli cells* of the testes, divide. Some of the cells reproduce by way of *mitosis* while some may also undergo *meiosis* and become *primary spermatocytes*. Meiotic division by one primary spermatocyte eventually leads to the formation of four *spermatozoa*, or *sperm*. This development process takes about 64 days.

12.1.2   Oogenesis

Germ cells, found in the ovaries in the female, are referred to as *oögonia*. These cells undergo complicated replication. The first stage of meiosis, which involves the replication of the cell's DNA to form *primary oocytes*, occurs during fetal development. At birth, each ovary holds about 1 million primary oocytes, each of which is contained within its own hollow ball referred to as an *ovarian follicle*.

Meiotic division resumes at puberty, at which point the number of oocytes and follicles has been reduced to about 400,000. This next meiotic process produces two to three *polar bodies* and one egg, or *ovum*. The polar bodies will eventually disintegrate and the ovum will mature and ultimately be released from the ovary by the process of *ovulation* (discussed in a subsequent section in this chapter). Approximately 400 of the oocytes will ovulate during a female's reproductive years; the rest will die by way of *apoptosis*. Oogenesis ceases entirely when the female reaches *menopause*, or the period that marks the permanent cessation of menstrual activity. Menopause typically occurs between 35 and 58 years of age (95% by the age of 55).

12.2 Male reproductive system

The male reproductive system includes the following organs and structures:

- Testes
- Epididymides
- Vas deferens
- Ejaculatory ducts
- Penis
- Prostate gland
- Seminal vesicles
- Bulbourethral glands

12.2.1 Testes

The testes are paired, ovoid structures located in the *scrotum*. A component of the external *genitalia*, the scrotum is a sac-like structure into which the testes migrate during fetal development. The testes function in *spermatogenesis*, the formation of sperm, and in the production of testosterone. The location of the testes outside of the abdominal cavity is necessary to produce viable sperm, which require a temperature 2°F–3°F lower than the core body temperature.

The testes have two compartments:

- Seminiferous tubules
- Interstitial tissue

The *seminiferous tubules* account for approximately 90% of the weight of the testes in the adult. Each tubule contains two types of cells:

- *Spermatogonia* in various stages of spermatogenesis: The spermatogonia in different regions of the tubule are at different stages of development. In this way, sperm production is staggered and can remain relatively constant at a rate of 200 million sperm per day (about the number of sperm released in a single ejaculation).
- *Sertoli cells*: Spermatogenesis in the Sertoli cells is stimulated by the hormones follicle-stimulating hormone (FSH) and testosterone.

The *interstitial tissue* is found between the seminiferous tubules. *Leydig cells*, which secrete testosterone, are located here. Testosterone secretion by the Leydig cells is stimulated by luteinizing hormone (LH).

12.2.2 Epididymides

Spermatozoa are drained from each testis by the *epididymis* (pleural: epididymides). At this point, the sperm are nonmotile and will undergo maturational changes as they pass through the epididymis. For example, they become more resistant to changes in pH and temperature. The epididymis also serves as a storage site for sperm between ejaculations.

12.2.3 Vas deferens

Spermatozoa are drained from the epididymis by the *vas deferens* (also referred to as the *ductus deferens*). This structure transports the sperm out of the scrotum and into the pelvic cavity.

12.2.4 Ejaculatory ducts

Spermatozoa are drained from the vas deferens by the *ejaculatory ducts*. These ducts enter the *prostate* and quickly merge with the *urethra*.

12.2.5 Penis

The urethra, which is a common passageway for urine and sperm, is found in the *penis*. *Emission* refers to the movement of semen into the urethra and *ejaculation* refers to the forcible expulsion of the semen out of the penis. Emission and ejaculation occur as the result of peristaltic contractions of the tubular system, contractions of the seminal vesicles and prostate, and contractions of muscles at the base of the penis. These actions are the result of sympathetic nerve stimulation. *Erection*, which involves increased blood flow into the penis, is mediated by parasympathetic nerve activity and the release of nitric oxide.

    Semen consists of the sperm as well as fluid (99%) secreted from the three male accessory sex organs: prostate gland, seminal vesicles, and bulbourethral glands.

12.2.6 Prostate

The doughnut-shaped prostate gland surrounds the neck of the bladder and the urethra. Its ducts open into the prostatic portion of the urethra. The slightly alkaline fluid produced by the prostate during ejaculation neutralizes the pH of the vagina so that the sperm are fully motile and become capable of fertilizing an ovum.

12.2.7 Seminal vesicles

These large sac-like glands are located below the urinary bladder. The duct from each gland merges with the vas deferens to form the ejaculatory duct. The fluid produced by the seminal vesicles, which accounts for about 60% of the volume of the semen, is rich in fructose and nourishes the sperm.

12.2.8 Bulbourethral glands

The small bulbourethral glands are located below the prostate. The ducts of these glands drain into the urethra just after it leaves the prostate. The fluid produced by the bulbourethral glands contains mucus, which acts as a lubricant, and buffers, which assist in neutralizing the acidic environment of the vagina.

PHARMACY APPLICATION: ERECTILE DYSFUNCTION

Erectile dysfunction (ED) is defined by the National Institutes of Health (NIH) Consensus Development Panel on Impotence as "the inability to achieve and maintain an erection sufficient to permit satisfactory sexual intercourse." Although ED is more common in older males, it is not a natural part of the aging process. In fact, 20%–46% of men 40–69 years of age have self-reported moderate or complete erectile dysfunction. Until the late 1990s, there were no truly effective oral medications for ED. More recently, a class of drugs referred to as phosphodiesterase-5 (PDE-5) inhibitors have been developed for the treatment of ED. These medications include sildenafil (Viagra®), vardenafil (Levitra®), tadalafil (Cialis®), and avanafil (Stendra®). Differences between these drugs involve the onset and duration of their therapeutic effects.

Recall from the previous discussion, erection results from increased blood flow into the penis and is mediated by parasympathetic nerve activity and the release of nitric oxide. Nitric oxide causes vasodilation by increasing the formation of cGMP within vascular smooth muscle cells. Vasodilation causes an increase in blood flow, engorgement, swelling, and stiffening of the penis or, in other words, an erection. The mechanism of action of the PDE-5 inhibitors involves blocking the breakdown of cGMP. This effect enhances the accumulation of cGMP and, therefore, improves erectile function.

Testosterone is produced primarily by the Leydig cells of the testes. A small amount (5%) is secreted by the adrenal cortex. In many target cells, testosterone must be converted to *dihydrotestosterone* (*DHT*) to be effective; this derivative is more potent than testosterone.

Testosterone secretion may begin as early as 8 weeks after conception. Secretion reaches a peak at 12–14 weeks and then declines to very low levels by about 21 weeks. Testosterone secretion during fetal development plays a very important role in sex differentiation and the masculinizing of the embryonic structures. Secretion of testosterone begins again at puberty and is necessary for spermatogenesis, the development of secondary sex characteristics, and several anabolic effects. Secretion declines gradually and to varying degrees in males over 50 years of age. The mechanism of this decline is not known. A summary of the actions of testosterone is found in Table 12.1.

Table 12.1 Actions of testosterone in the male

Sex Differentiation

- Development of the fetal *Wolffian ducts* into the epididymides, vas deferens, seminal vesicles, and ejaculatory ducts
- Development of the fetal urogenital sinus into the prostate gland
- Development of the external genitalia (fetal genital tubercle into the penis; fetal labioscrotal swellings into the scrotum)

Initiation and Maintenance of Spermatogenesis in the Sertoli Cells
Secondary Sex Characteristics

- Growth and maintenance of accessory sex organs
- Growth of penis
- Growth of facial and axillary hair
- Body growth
- Inhibition of action of estrogen on breast growth
- Stimulation of sex drive and enhancement of aggressive behavior

Anabolic Effects

- Protein synthesis and muscle growth
- Growth of bones and other organs and tissues (including the larynx)
- Cessation of bone growth
- Secretion of erythropoietin from the kidneys

Miscellaneous

- Inhibition of gonadotropin releasing hormone (GnRH) from the hypothalamus
- Inhibition of LH from the adenohypophysis
- Maintenance of relatively constant testosterone secretion from the testes

---

12.3   Female reproductive system

The female reproductive system includes the following organs and structures:

- Ovaries
- Fallopian tubes
- Uterus
- Vagina

12.3.1   Ovaries

The ovaries are paired, almond-sized organs located in the lower left and lower right quadrants of the abdominal cavity. As with the testes in the male, these female gonads have two primary functions:

- Production of gametes (ova)
- Secretion of sex hormones (estrogen, progesterone)

12.3.2 Fallopian tubes

Ova released from ovarian follicles are transported to the uterus by way of the *fallopian tubes*. Also referred to as *oviducts*, these tubes are 20–25 cm in length and about the diameter of a typical pencil. Ciliated epithelial cells lining the fallopian tubes assist with the movement of the ova toward the uterus.

12.3.3 Uterus

A muscular, hollow, pear-shaped organ located in the center of the pelvic cavity, the uterus is responsible for maintaining the fetus during gestation and for expelling it at the end of the pregnancy. Prior to the occurrence of a pregnancy, the uterus is relatively small and is about 3-in. long, 2-in. wide, and 1-in. thick. The uterus has three layers:

- Perimetrium
- Myometrium
- Endometrium

The *perimetrium* is the outermost layer. This serous layer of connective tissue is continuous with the visceral peritoneum that covers the abdominopelvic organs.

The *myometrium* is the thick, middle layer of smooth muscle in the uterus. Contraction of the smooth muscle wall is responsible for *parturition*, or delivery of the fetus.

The *endometrium* is the innermost layer of the uterus. It is highly vascularized and nutrient-rich. Endometrial cells accumulate lipids and glycogen, which provide nourishment to a developing embryo prior to the formation of the placenta. This layer includes a stratified squamous epithelium that lines the uterus and alternately proliferates and sloughs off. This layer also includes a basal layer of connective tissue where the blood vessels and *endometrial glands* are located. The secretions from the endometrial glands are necessary for the implantation of the embryo in the uterine wall. Furthermore, these glands provide a source of nutrients and growth factors during the first trimester of human pregnancy. After this period, the placenta, which is not fully established until 10–12 weeks of pregnancy, takes over the support of the fetus.

12.3.4 Vagina

A muscular, expandable tube that connects the uterus to the external surface of the body. The vagina is lined with stratified squamous epithelium that is resistant to bacterial colonization. This structure serves as a passageway for the insertion of the penis, the reception of semen, the discharge of menstrual flow, and the delivery of the fetus.

The *ovarian cycle* alternates between two phases:

- Follicular phase
- Luteal phase

The average cycle lasts about 28 days. However, the length of the ovarian cycle varies among women and among cycles in any particular woman.

12.3.5 Follicular phase

Includes the development of the primary follicle into a mature follicle, also known as a *Graafian follicle*, as well as ovulation, or the release of the ovum from the follicle. The steps involved in the follicular phase are:

- *Primary oocytes* (46 chromosomes) are contained within *primary follicles* (40 μm): This follicle consists of a single layer of follicular cells, specifically, *granulosa cells.*
- Development of the *secondary follicle*:
  - Follicular cells proliferate: Granulosa cells proliferate forming several layers of cells that surround the primary oocyte.
  - Formation of the *zona pellucida*: Granulosa cells secrete a thick gel-like layer of proteins and polysaccharides that lies between the inner layer of these cells and the primary oocyte. Cytoplasmic processes of the inner layer of granulosa cells penetrate the zona pellucida and form gap junctions with the oocyte. Nutrients and chemical messengers (e.g., factors that maintain meiotic arrest such as *oocyte maturation-inhibiting substance*) are delivered to the primary oocyte through these passageways.
  - Formation of *thecal cells*: Concurrent with granulosa cell proliferation is the differentiation of surrounding ovarian connective tissue into thecal cells. The follicular cells of the secondary follicle, which now includes granulosa cells and thecal cells, secrete estrogen.
  - Formation of the *antrum*: A fluid-filled space referred to as the antrum begins to form within the granulosa layer. This fluid is derived from the granulosa cells and begins to accumulate some of the estrogen secreted by these cells. As the antrum increases in size, so does the follicle, which reaches a diameter of 12–16 mm in the mature follicle.
- Formation of the mature follicle: One primary follicle will typically grow more rapidly than other follicles and develop into the mature follicle within about 14 days after the onset of follicular development. This follicle is dominated by the antrum. The enclosed oocyte completes the first stage of meiotic division so that it is now a *secondary oocyte* (23 chromosomes). (The second meiotic division is completed after ovulation only if fertilization has occurred.)

- Ovulation: The mature follicle bulges on the surface of the ovary. The follicular cells release enzymes (e.g., collagenase) that digest the thin layer of connective tissue in the wall of the ovary that significantly weakens it. Following the LH surge and the rupture of the follicle, the ovum is swept into the fallopian tube by the antral fluid. Any other follicles that had been developing simultaneously in the ovary will undergo *atresia*, or degeneration. If the released ovum is not fertilized within a few days of its release, it will also degenerate.

12.3.6 Luteal phase

The follicular cells left behind in the ruptured follicle are transformed into a *corpus luteum* (*corpus*, body; *luteum*, yellow), so named for the abundant storage of cholesterol within the granulosa cells that will be used to form sex hormones. Copious quantities of progesterone and smaller amounts of estrogen are secreted from the corpus luteum. If fertilization and implantation occur, then the corpus luteum grows larger and continues to secrete the hormones necessary to maintain the pregnancy until the placenta is fully developed. If fertilization and implantation do not occur, then the corpus luteum will degenerate within 14 days of its formation.

12.3.7 Hormonal regulation of the ovarian cycle

The ovarian cycle is regulated by the complex interaction of hypothalamic, pituitary, and ovarian hormones:

- GnRH: gonadotropin releasing hormone; produced by the hypothalamus
- FSH and LH: follicle-stimulating hormone and luteinizing hormone (gonadotropins); produced by the adenohypophysis
- Estrogen and progesterone: produced by the ovaries

The secretion of these hormones, and their effects during the cycle, are summarized in Figure 12.1, Table 12.2, and in the following discussion. Day 1 of the ovarian cycle is the first day of *menstruation*, or the bleeding caused by the sloughing of the lining of the uterus. This day was chosen because menstrual discharge provides an easily observed sign.

During the *follicular phase*, hormonal secretion and actions include the following:

- *Gonadotropin* secretion increases during the end of the previous luteal phase and the beginning of the new follicular phase. *FSH*, in particular, stimulates the development of several follicles within the ovary.
- As the primary follicle grows, *FSH* and *LH* stimulate the secretion of estrogen from the granulosa cells and the thecal cells, respectively.

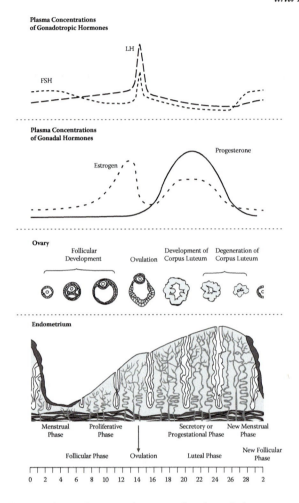

Figure 12.1   The correlation between hormone levels and changes in the ovary and the endometrium during the ovarian cycle.

Table 12.2   Actions of sex hormones in the female

GnRH, Gonadotropin-Releasing Hormone
- Stimulates the secretion of FSH and LH from the adenohypophysis

FSH, Follicle-Stimulating Hormone
- Stimulates the development of ovarian follicles
- Stimulates the secretion of estrogen from the granulosa cells of the primary follicle

LH, Luteinizing Hormone
- Stimulates thecal cells to secrete androgen that is converted to estrogen in thegranulosa cells

(Continued)

Table 12.2 (*Continued*) Actions of sex hormones in the female

---

- LH surge
  - Inhibits estrogen synthesis by follicular cells
  - Reinitiates meiosis in the oocyte by inhibiting the release of oocyte maturation-inhibiting substance
  - Elicits the production of prostaglandins that induce ovulation
  - Causes differentiation of follicular cells into luteal cells
  - Stimulates steroid hormone secretion from the corpus luteum

Estrogen, during the Follicular Phase of the Ovarian Cycle
- Inhibits the secretion of GnRH, FSH, and LH
- Enhances its own secretion from the granulosa cells
- Causes the endometrium to thicken
- Induces the production of progesterone receptors in the myometrium
- Triggers the surge in LH secretion at mid-cycle

Estrogen, during Pregnancy
- Stimulates the growth of the myometrium and increases uterine strength which is necessary for parturition
- Helps to prepare the mammary glands for lactation following parturition by promoting the development of the ducts through which milk will be ejected
- Inhibits the effects of prolactin during the last half of pregnancy and, thereby, prevents milk secretion prior to parturition

Estrogen, Days before Parturition
- Promotes the formation of gap junctions between uterine smooth muscle cells so that the myometrium may contract in a coordinated fashion during parturition
- Markedly increases the number of receptors for oxytocin in uterine smooth muscle cells

Estrogen, Miscellaneous
- Stimulates the growth and maintenance of the entire reproductive tract
- Enhances the transport of sperm to the fallopian tubes by stimulating upward contractions of the uterus

Estrogen, Miscellaneous
- Promotes fat deposition
- Increases bone density
- Closes epiphyseal plates

Progesterone
- Inhibits the secretion of GnRH, FSH, and LH during the luteal phase of the ovarian cycle
- Elicits the secretory phase in the endometrium and provides a suitable, nurturing environment for an implanted embryo
- Promotes the formation of a mucus plug in the cervix
- Stimulates breast development during pregnancy
- Inhibits the effects of prolactin during pregnancy
- Prevents miscarriage by inhibiting uterine contractions during pregnancy

---

- *Estrogen* secreted from the follicle during the follicular phase:
  - Inhibits GnRH secretion from the hypothalamus and FSH and LH secretion from the adenohypophysis, which inhibits the development of new follicles and ovulation during the follicular phase of that particular cycle.
  - Enhances estrogen secretion from the granulosa cells, which allows hormone secretion to continue even as levels of FSH decrease.
  - Causes the endometrium to thicken, or the *uterine proliferative phase.*
  - Induces the production of progesterone receptors in the endometrium.
  - Estrogen secretion peaks near the end of the follicular phase. The high levels of estrogen at this point elicit a surge in LH production at mid-cycle. Ovulation occurs about 16–24 hours after the LH surge.

During the *luteal phase*, hormonal secretion and actions include the following:

- *LH* promotes:
  - The production of locally acting prostaglandins, which cause the rupture of the follicle.
  - Transformation of granulosa cells and thecal cells into the luteal cells of the corpus luteum, a process referred to as *luteinization.*
- The corpus luteum secretes abundant *progesterone* as well as some *estrogen.* Although low levels of estrogen tend to stimulate the secretion of GnRH from the hypothalamus and FSH and LH from the adenohypophysis, these effects are overwhelmed by the actions of progesterone that inhibit the secretion of these hormones. As a result, new follicular maturation and ovulation during the luteal phase of that particular cycle are prevented.
- *Progesterone* from the corpus luteum acts on the endometrium to produce vascular and secretory changes that will provide a suitable and nurturing environment for an implanted embryo. This is referred to as the *secretory*, or *progestational phase.* Specifically, progesterone:
  - Stimulates blood vessel growth in the connective tissue layer.
  - Elicits endometrial gland growth and coiling.
  - Stimulates endometrial cells to accumulate lipids and glycogen within their cytoplasm.
  - Causes cervical mucus to thicken, forming a plug that blocks the opening of the uterus and prevents the admission of bacteria and sperm.
- Degeneration of the corpus luteum causes *progesterone* and *estrogen* secretion to decrease. As a result:
  - Inhibition of GnRH, FSH and LH secretion is removed, which leads to a new follicular phase.
  - Maintenance of a secretory endometrium ceases. Blood vessels in the surface layer of the endometrium constrict. The resulting

decrease in the delivery of oxygen and nutrients causes the cells of this layer to die. About two days after the corpus luteum ceases to function, the surface layer of the endometrium sloughs off and menstruation begins. Menstrual discharge consists of about 80 mL of blood, serous fluid and cellular debris. It typically lasts 3–7 days, well into the follicular phase of the next ovarian cycle.

PHARMACY APPLICATION: ORAL CONTRACEPTIVES

Oral contraceptives are among the most widely used class of drugs in the United States and throughout the world. They are convenient, accessible and reliable. The most commonly used agents contain a combination of both estrogen-like and progestin-like steroids. The preparations come in 28-day packs. The first 21 pills contain the active steroids and the last 7 days contain inert ingredients.

The mechanism of action of the steroids involves the inhibition of GnRH, FSH, and LH secretion. Thus, follicular development and ovulation do not occur. The endometrium thickens and develops secretory capacity, as it would normally do under the influence of endogenously produced estrogen and progesterone. Then during the last 7 days when the steroids are withdrawn, the endometrium sloughs and menstruation occurs as it would normally upon degeneration of the corpus luteum.

12.4   Disorders of the male reproductive system

12.4.1   Disorders of the penis

12.4.1.1   Peyronie's disease
A disease associated with progressive fibrosis of the tunica albuginea as a result of a localized inflammatory vasculitis. It is a slow-developing condition characterized by the development of tough fibrous tissue on the dorsal side of the penis. The cause is uncertain. Peyronie's disease may be associated with painful erection and possibly impotence. There is no cure, but the disease may spontaneously resolve and often responds to various pharmacologic therapies.

12.4.1.2   Priapism
A condition associated with prolonged (>4 hours), involuntary and painful erection. The cause is idiopathic in the majority of patients but may also be related to neurologic injury, sickle cell disease or the use of certain drugs such as those for erectile dysfunction. Priapism is considered a urologic emergency because prolonged erection may be associated with ischemia and

damage to erectile tissues. Treatment includes cold saline enemas, irrigation of the corpus cavernosum, alpha-adrenergic blocking drugs and possible surgical intervention.

12.4.1.3   Impotence

Impotence or erectile dysfunction is associated with the inability of obtaining an erection necessary for successful sexual activity. Occasional erectile dysfunction, while stressful, is normal and may be related to daily life issues such as stress or lack of sleep. The majority of men experience some degree of erectile dysfunction as they age. However, the regular occurrence of erectile dysfunction may indicate the presence of an underlying physiologic or psychologic disorder and the patients should seek evaluation and treatment. Physiologic causes of erectile dysfunction may include hypertension, vascular disease, diabetes, obesity, neurologic disorders, sleep disorders, tobacco use, and surgery/treatment for prostate disorders. Psychologic causes of erectile dysfunction may include depression, anxiety and stress. A thorough physical examination with blood work and urinalysis can often identify the most common physiologic causes of erectile dysfunction. There a number of pharmacologic and non-pharmacologic interventions that have demonstrated efficacy in the treatment of erectile dysfunction.

12.4.2   Disorders of the testis and scrotum

12.4.2.1   Spermatocele
- Painless cyst that develops at the end of the epididymis
- Cysts are filled with sperm
- They generally do not require treatment unless they cause pain
- The cause is uncertain but the generally do not impact fertility

12.4.2.2   Varicocele
- Dilation of veins within the spermatic cord; often the result of a congenital malformation
- The majority occur on the left side and may be tender or painful to touch; palpation has been compared with touching "a bag of worms"
- Varicoceles can interfere with blood flow to testis and impair fertility; distended veins may be surgically ligated

12.4.2.3   Testicular cancer
The incidence of testicular cancer is rare when compared with other types of cancers. It is most common in men between 15 and 35 years of age.

12.4.2.3.1 Symptoms
- The presence of a lump in either testicle
- A feeling of heaviness in the scrotum
- Pain in the scrotum, back or abdomen

12.4.2.3.2 Diagnosis
- Physical examination
- Blood tests to detect tumor markers specifically associated with testicular cancer
- Ultrasound
- There are two main forms of testicular cancer:
  - *Seminoma*—most common form, particularly in older men. Slower growing, less invasive form
  - *Nonseminoma*—Develops earlier in life and tends to be a more rapidly growing and invasive cancer

12.4.2.3.3 Treatment
- Surgery to remove testicle and any affected lymph nodes in the region
- Chemotherapy
- Radiotherapy
- The long-term prognosis is generally very good if the tumor is localized to the testis and has not spread

12.4.3 Disorders of the prostate

12.4.3.1 Prostatitis

Prostatitis is inflammation of the prostate. It may be commonly caused by infection with bacteria such as *E.coli*, *Klebsiella*, *Proteus*, and *Enterobacter*. Bacterial prostatitis may be acute or chronic. Common symptoms may include cloudy urine, discharge, urinary urgency, perineal discomfort and possibly lower back pain. Diagnosis may be made through urine culture. Treatment includes the use of appropriate antibiotics that may need to be administered for an extended period of time due to poor penetration of the drug into the prostate. Nonbacterial prostatitis (*prostatodynia*) may also occur with significant frequency, possibly as a result of urinary reflux.

12.4.3.2 Benign prostatic hyperplasia (BPH)

BPH is a condition of prostatic enlargement that occurs in men as they get older. The prevalence of BPH in men 60 years of age and older is 40%–50%, but increases to 90% in men 80 years of age and older.

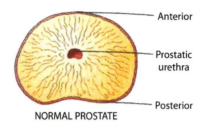

NORMAL PROSTATE

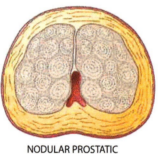

NODULAR PROSTATIC HYPERPLASIA

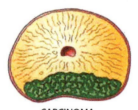

CARCINOMA OF PROSTATE

12.4.3.2.1   Symptoms
- Difficulty urinating
- Incomplete urination
- Weak urine stream
- Nocturia—increased frequency of nighttime urination
- The frequency of BPH is less in Asian men when compared with white or black men

12.4.3.2.2   Long-term complications of untreated BPH
- Urinary retention
- Increased risk of urinary tract infections
- Dilation of the bladder and ureters (*hydroureter*) and possible damage to the kidneys as a result of increased pressure and urine backflow (*hydonephrosis*)
- Formation of *bladder stones*

12.4.3.2.3   Diagnosis
- Digital rectal examination to determine size and texture of the prostate
- *Prostate-specific antigen (PSA) test*—circulating levels of this protein are increased as the prostate grows. Elevated PSA levels may also be indicative of prostate cancer or prostatitis
- Urine outflow studies to measure the strength and volume of urine flow
- Neurological examination—to rule out neurologic causes of impaired urination

12.4.3.2.4   Treatment
- Medications such as alpha-adrenergic blockers can relax muscle in the bladder neck and to ease the passage of urine. 5α-Reductase inhibitors such as finasteride can reverse prostate growth by inhibiting the enzyme that converts testosterone to dihydrotestosterone. These drugs may however take up to 6 months to be fully effective. A number of minimally invasive surgical procedures may also be performed to reduce prostate size and enhance urine outflow.

12.4.3.3   Prostate cancer

Prostate cancer is one of the most common cancers affecting males and will account for approximately 10% of all new cancer cases in the coming year. The incidence of prostate varies greatly by geographic region. The lowest incidence is seen in men from Asia and parts of Africa. Although the highest rates of prostate cancer are observed in men from North America and Europe. Risk factors for the development of prostate cancer include increasing age, family history of prostate cancer, high-fat diet, and obesity. Race also appears to be a significant factor because the incidence of prostate cancer in black men is significantly greater than that of white men. In addition, black men are more likely to develop a more aggressive form of prostate cancer.

12.4.3.3.1   Symptoms
- Prostate cancer may not yield overt symptoms until the condition is well advanced
- Difficulty urinating, reduced urine stream
- Incomplete voiding
- Pelvic pain
- Bloody semen
- Impotence

12.4.3.3.2   Diagnosis
- Digital rectal exam—may be used to detect changes in prostate size, shape and texture

- PSA test—PSA levels are significantly elevated with prostate cancer; however, PSA levels may also increase as a result of BPH and prostatitis
- Ultrasound
- Prostate biopsy—if cancer cells are detected, the cancer is staged with regard to size, spread and aggressiveness (see Table 12.1)

12.4.3.3.3   Treatment
- Once prostate cancer is confirmed by biopsy, genetic testing may be done to determine how aggressive the cancer cells are in terms of their growth and potential for spread.
- Imaging tests (MRI, ultrasound, PET scan, bone scan) and lymph node biopsies will also be performed to determine if the cancer has spread from the prostate to surrounding or distal tissues.
- Treatment is guided by the aggressiveness of the cancer that is found. For men diagnosed with low-risk prostate cancer, treatment may not be needed at first. If a treatment plan is decided upon, it may include surgical removal, radiation therapy, chemotherapy, hormonal therapy to reduce the effects of testosterone, or immunologic therapy.
- The long-term prognosis will depend upon the stage at which the tumor was discovered and the aggressiveness of the cancer cells. The 5-year survival for men with low-risk prostate cancer and no treatment approaches 100%.

12.5   Disorders of the female reproductive system

12.5.1   Disorders of the vagina, cervix, and uterus

12.5.1.1   Vaginitis
Inflammation of the vagina. Most commonly caused by infection with bacteria, yeast (*Candida*), and parasites such as *Trichomonas vaginalis*. Some of these organisms may be transmitted by sexual activity. The decreases in estrogen levels that occur with menopause may also lead to changes in the vaginal flora and pH that make the tissues there more susceptible to inflammation, irritation and infection. Symptoms typically include vaginal discharge, burning, itching, and pain during urination or intercourse. The treatment will depend upon the cause of the vaginitis.

12.5.1.2   Cervical lesions and cervical cancer
Cervical cancer is the second most common cancer in women. The mortality from cervical cancer has decreased significantly in recent years as a result of early detection and improved treatments. Infection with the Human Papillomavirus (HPV) has been associated with the development of cervical cancer In particular, two HPV subtypes, 16 and 18, are associated most

frequently with the development of cervical cancer. The HPV subtypes 6 and 11 appear to be a lower risk for causing cervical cancer but are associated with the development of genital warts. Other risk factors for cervical cancer include early sexual activity, multiple sex partners, and impaired immune function.

12.5.1.2.1 Diagnosis

- Pap test—cells from the cervix are removed and examined under a microscope for abnormalities. Cervical cancers arise from precancerous lesions in the cervix. Under microscopic examination, these precancerous cells present with *dysplastic* changes that include variation in shape and size as well as abnormal cellular components (e.g., nucleus). The more significant the dysplasia that is observed, the greater the risk for the development of cancer.
- HPV DNA testing may be done to determine if a woman is infected with HPV and if the variants that are present pose a significant risk for cervical cancer.
- Biopsy of the cervix may be performed to obtain tissue for examination if cancer is suspected.
- The most common form of cervical cancer is *squamous cell carcinoma*. A second, less common form of cervical cancer is *adenocarcinoma*, which arises from the glandular cells lining the cervix.
- Staging of cervical cancer is based on the size, spread and type of cancer detected. Stage I cervical cancers are those that are confined to the cervix. Increasing stage numbers (II, II, IV) indicate a greater size and spread of the cancer.
- Early diagnosis is crucial. The 5-year survival for patients with Stage IA cervical cancer is 93%.

12.5.1.2.2 Treatment

- A *hysterectomy* (surgical removal of the cervix and uterus) can cure early-stage cervical cancer. Chemotherapy and radiotherapy are also treatment options for all stages of cervical cancer.

12.5.1.3 Endometriosis

Endometriosis is a condition in which normal endothelial tissue that normally lines the uterus grows outside of the uterus. The condition most commonly affects the fallopian tubes, ovaries and lining of the pelvis. The cause of endometriosis is uncertain. The incidence of endometriosis is approximately 5%–10% percent of women who are of reproductive age. Risk factors include never giving birth, early onset of menses, late onset of menopause, and family history of endometriosis.

12.5.1.3.1 Symptoms
- Painful menstruation
- Excessive bleeding
- Pain with urination and defecation
- Cyst formation in the fallopian tubes if they are affected
- Infertility

12.5.1.3.2 Diagnosis A number of conditions may be associated with pelvic pain; these should be ruled out as well. The presence of endometriosis may be detected through a combination of methods including pelvic examination, ultrasound and laparoscopy.

12.5.1.3.3 Treatment
- Pain management that usually includes use of nonsteroidal anti-inflammatory agents (NSAIDs).
- Hormonal therapy may reduce the tissue enlargement and pain that is associated with endometriosis but will not reverse or cure the condition. Hormonal therapy may include oral contraceptives, gonadotrophin-releasing hormone analogs and androgenic agents such as danazol.
- Surgery may be used to remove the abnormal tissue in cases of severe pain or if the patient is trying to become pregnant.

12.5.1.4 Endometrial (Uterine) cancer
Endometrial cancer is the most common female reproductive cancer in the United States and the fourth most common cancer in women. Endometrial cancer occurs most frequently in postmenopausal women. The average age at diagnosis is 60 years. In addition to age, other risk factors include hormonal abnormalities, menstruation at an early age or menopause at a later age, never being pregnant, and obesity. There are three types of endometrial cancer: *endometroid adenocarcinoma*, which is the most common form; *uterine carcinosarcoma*; and *uterine sarcoma*, which is the less common form that begins in the muscle of the uterine walls.

12.5.1.4.1 Symptoms
- Unusual vaginal bleeding or discharge
- Pelvic pain
- Unexplained weight loss

12.5.1.4.2 Diagnosis
- Blood tests are available for certain endometrial cancer protein markers such as CA 125
- Imaging studies
- Biopsy

12.5.1.4.3 Treatment The treatment of endometrial cancer will depend upon the type of cancer present and the amount it has spread. Treatment options may include surgery, chemotherapy, radiotherapy, and hormonal therapy. Early detection is key and long-term outcomes for patients diagnosed with early stage endometrial cancer are quite good.

12.5.1.5 Uterine fibroids

Uterine fibroids are benign growths that form in the uterus of women of childbearing age. Many women may have them and not be aware of their presence due to a lack of symptoms. They do not progress to uterine cancer nor do they increase a woman's risk for developing uterine cancer. If symptoms do occur, they are generally heavy menstrual bleeding, prolonged menstruations, impaired bladder emptying, and pelvic pain. They may be diagnosed though pelvis exam, ultrasound, and imaging tests. Most do not require treatment, but if they do, the options include hormonal therapy and surgery. A newer noninvasive option is MRI-guided focused ultrasound surgery, which uses high energy sound waves to destroy regions of fibrous tissue.

12.5.1.6 Uterine prolapse

Uterine prolapse is a condition that occurs when the muscle and ligaments that support the uterus stretch and weaken. As a result, the uterus can enter the vagina and even protrude externally. The condition is most likely to occur in women who had multiple vaginal deliveries. Mild prolapse may not require treatment and may be improved with specific exercises. More severe cases will likely require surgical correction.

12.5.2 Disorders of the ovaries

12.5.2.1 Polycystic ovary syndrome

Polycystic ovary syndrome is a hormonal condition that affects approximately 5%–10% of women of childbearing years. Although the actual cause of the condition is uncertain, patients affected by the condition present with numerous small fluid-filled follicles.

12.5.2.1.1 Symptoms
- Irregular menstrual periods.
- Excess production of male hormones (androgens). Excess androgens may produce symptoms such as hirsutism, acne and thinning hair.
- Impaired ovary function. The fluid-filled follicles that surround the ovaries may impair ovum release (*anovulation*) and lead to infertility.
- The condition may also be associated with the presence of marked obesity. Many women with polycystic ovary syndrome may exhibit hyperinsulinemia and signs of *metabolic syndrome*.

12.5.2.1.2   Complications
- Infertility
- Type II diabetes
- Metabolic syndrome and increased risk for cardiovascular disease
- Increased risk for endometrial cancer as a result of hormonal imbalance

12.5.2.1.3   Diagnosis
- Measurement of circulating hormone levels
- Pelvic ultrasound

12.5.2.1.4   Treatment
- Lifestyle changes—weight loss, exercise, management of blood pressure, blood glucose and dyslipidemia
- Birth control pills to help regulate menstrual cycle
- Progestin therapy to help regulate the menstrual cycle and reduce the risk of endometrial cancer
- Spironolactone to antagonize the effects of androgens
- Treatments to increase ovulation and fertility if the patient wishes to become pregnant

12.5.2.2   Ovarian cancer
Even though ovarian cancer accounts for only 3% of all cancers in women, it is responsible for more deaths each year than any other cancer of the female reproductive system. Most cases of ovarian cancer occur in women 50 years of age and over.

12.5.2.2.1   Risk factors
- Age over 50 years
- *BRCA1* or *BRCA2* gene mutations that are also associated with an increased risk of developing breast cancer
- Early menses and late menopause
- Estrogen replacement therapy
- Family history of ovarian cancer

12.5.2.2.2   Symptoms
- May be asymptomatic initially or may present with nonspecific symptoms that can make early diagnosis difficult
- In later stages, one may see pelvic pain, changes in bowel function and weight loss

12.5.2.2.3 *Diagnosis*
- Blood test for the detection of CA-125 tumor antigen. However, this marker has a low specificity for ovarian cancer
- Ultrasound
- Biopsy

12.5.2.2.4 *Treatment*
- Treatment will depend upon the stage at which the cancer was detected but generally includes surgery and chemotherapy. The overall 5-year survival for all patients diagnosed with ovarian cancer is 46.5%.

12.5.3 *Menstrual disorders*

The "normal" menstrual cycle varies from woman to woman. The duration and timing of a woman's menstrual cycle may vary within a broad range from one month to the next. Factors such as contraceptive use and heavy physical exertion can significantly alter the menstrual cycle. Normal variations in the menstrual cycle also occurs as a woman ages.

12.5.3.1 *Amenorrhea*
Amenorrhea is said to occur when a woman misses three successive menstrual cycles. This can occur naturally if a woman is pregnant, breastfeeding or entering menopause. It may also be caused by the use of oral contraceptives or other medications such as antidepressants, antipsychotics, antihypertensives and chemotherapy agents. Heavy exercise or physical exertion and marked reductions in body fat can also cause amenorrhea. All of the above would be classified as *secondary* causes of amenorrhea. *Primary* causes of amenorrhea would include abnormalities of the hypothalamus or pituitary gland or genetic abnormalities such as Turner syndrome. Diagnosis is generally made through measurement of circulating hormones and imaging studies to rule out other causes. Treatment will depend upon the cause of the amenorrhea and may involve hormonal therapy.

12.5.3.2 *Dysmenorrhea*
Dysmenorrhea is defined as pain or discomfort associated with menstruation. Some degree of dysmenorrhea is generally associated with normal menstruation. Worsening dysmenorrhea may also be a sign of uterine fibroids, endometriosis, or infection. Patients with severe dysmenorrhea may undergo imaging studies to identify underlying disorders. Treatment for simple dysmenorrhea normally involves the use of pain medications such as NSAIDs or acetaminophen. Surgical procedure may be necessary to correct any underlying conditions that are diagnosed.

12.5.3.3 Menopause

Menopause is the cessation of menstruation that occurs as women age. The average age of menopause for women in the United States is 51. Prior to the actual occurrence of menopause (*perimenopause*), a woman's menstrual cycle generally becomes irregular and she begins to experience some of the symptoms of menopause outlined below. Although the process of menopause is a natural occurrence, it may be accompanied by numerous symptoms that can be upsetting and uncomfortable. Fortunately, a number of these symptoms can be readily treated.

12.5.3.4 Symptoms
- Irregular periods
- Night sweats
- Hot flashes, headache, dizziness
- Vaginal dryness
- Mood changes
- Sleep disturbances
- Weight gain
- Thinning hair, dry skin
- A long-term complication of menopause can be *osteoporosis* due to decreasing estrogen levels

12.5.3.5 Treatment
- Topical estrogen is used to treat vaginal dryness and atrophy.
- Hormonal therapy may be used for the treatment of menopause symptoms and osteoporosis; however, there is evidence that long-term hormonal (estrogen) therapy may increase the risk for cancer certain cancers such as breast cancer. Selective estrogen receptor modulators (SERMs) may be used in place of estrogen because they do not affect breast tissue.

12.5.4 Disorders of the breast

A number of conditions may affect breast tissue. Some conditions such as mastitis are benign, whereas other types of lesions may be precancerous. Breast cancer is currently the most common cancer to affect females after skin cancer.

12.5.4.1 Mastitis

Mastitis is inflammation of breast tissue. It may occur in women who are lactating, but it may also result from bacterial infections that may or may not be related to breastfeeding. Symptoms generally include breast swelling and tenderness, pain with breastfeeding and possible fever. If milk ducts become blocked, an abscess or cyst may develop in the breast. Treatment includes antibiotics, pain relievers and warm compresses.

12.5.4.2 Fibrocystic changes

Fibrocystic changes refer to changes in breast texture or morphology. Fibrocystic changes are common in breast tissue and do not increase a woman's risk of developing breast cancer. In some women, these changes may be associated with breast pain and tenderness.

12.5.4.3 Proliferative changes

Several types of benign breast changes may increase a patients risk for developing breast cancer. These include "proliferative lesions without atypia," and "proliferative lesions with atypia." Both of these conditions involve tissues of the milk ducts and lobules that are growing more rapidly than they should. The presence of proliferative lesions without atypia can double a woman's risk for breast cancer. The presence of proliferative lesions with atypia can increase woman's risk for breast cancer 4- to 5-fold because "atypia" is associated with the presence of abnormal cells that may be precancerous. Women diagnosed with either condition should have more frequent breast screenings and may be prescribed hormonal therapy with drugs such as tamoxifen, a SERM that has been shown to reduce the risk of developing certain types of breast cancer.

12.5.5 Breast cancer

Approximately 300,000 new cases of breast cancer will be diagnosed this coming year in the United States. As a result of enhanced early detection and improved treatments, the death rate from breast cancer has been dropping in women over 50 years of age.

12.5.5.1 Risk factors for breast cancer

- Increasing age
- Family history of breast cancer
- Atypical hyperplasia of the breast
- Hormone replacement therapy
- Smoking
- Genetic factors:
  - It is estimated that 5%–10% of breast cancers are due to an inherited genetic mutation. The presence of mutations in two breast cancer genes *BRCA1* or *BRCA2* can increase a woman's risk for breast cancer significantly. Fifty to sixty-five percent of women with the *BRCA1* mutation will develop breast cancer by 70 years of age. Although approximately 45% of women with the *BRCA2* mutation will develop breast cancer by this same age. The presence of these gene mutations can also significantly increase woman's risk for developing ovarian cancer. The *BRCA1* and *BRCA2* genes normally produce tumor-suppressor proteins; however, the protective effect of these genes appears to be lost if they are mutated.

12.5.5.2   Diagnosis
- Breast examination
- Mammogram
- Ultrasound
- Breast MRI
- Breast biopsy
- Tumors are classified based on their histologic characteristics. Staging of tumors is based on size, involvement of the lymph nodes and distal spread

12.5.5.3   Treatment
- Treatment of breast cancer is dependent upon cancer characteristic, size, stage and sensitivity to certain hormones
- Surgical option may include removal of the cancerous tumor (*lumpectomy*) or removal of the breast (*mastectomy*). Local lymph nodes may also be removed and analyzed for the presence of cancer cells
- Radiation therapy
- Chemotherapy
- Hormonal therapy—may include medications that block the effects of estrogen (i.e., SERMs) or those that inhibit the formation of estrogen (i.e., *aromatase inhibitors*)
- Targeted therapies:
  - Antibody drugs that bind to and block the human epidermal growth factor-2 receptor (HER2). Certain breast cancers may overexpress this receptor and thus exhibit accelerated growth due to activation for epidermal growth factor

12.5.5.4   Prognosis
The long-term prognosis is dependent upon the characteristics of the cancer cells, and stage at which the cancer was detected. The 5-year survival rate for localized breast cancer that has not spread is 99%. For cancers that have spread regionally but not to distal tissues, the 5-year survival rate is 85%. Survival rates are significantly lower in patients whose breast cancer has spread to distal tissues.

12.6   Sexually transmitted diseases
Sexually transmitted diseases (STDs) are those that are transmitted from person to person through sexual contact. Organisms responsible for these sexually transmitted diseases may be spread from person to person through blood, semen, vaginal and other body fluids. Some STDs may not cause obvious symptoms or the symptoms may take months to years to manifest. Bacteria are the organisms most commonly responsible for causing STDs. Other STDs may be caused by viruses or parasites.

12.6.1 Diagnosis

The actual symptoms associated with various STDs will vary depending upon the organism that is responsible. General symptoms of STD include:

- Sores, lesions, or bumps associated with the penis or vagina
- Abnormal discharge from the penis or vagina
- Painful urination or intercourse
- Abdominal pain
- Vaginal bleeding

12.6.2 Risk factors

- Unprotected sex
- Multiple sex partners
- Certain STDs such as gonorrhea, syphilis, chlamydia and HIV may be passed from the mother to the infant during pregnancy and delivery

12.6.2.1 Bacterial STDs

- Chlamydia:
  - Caused by the bacteria *chlamydia trachomatis*
  - Most common STD in the United States
  - May be asymptomatic. If symptoms are present that may be similar to those observed with gonorrhea
- Gonorrhea:
  - Caused by the bacteria *N. gonorrhea*
  - Second most commonly reported STD in the United States
  - Symptoms manifest 3–5 days after exposure and include purulent milky discharge from the genitals
- Syphilis:
  - Caused by the bacterial spirochete *Treponema pallidum*
- The course of the disease is divided into three stages: *primary, secondary and tertiary*
  - *Primary syphilis*—characterized by the presence of a small *chancre* or sore on the penis. May not be easily observed in the vagina or rectum
  - *Secondary syphilis*—rash on trunk, palms or soles of the feet that may spread to entire body. Symptoms usually resolve spontaneously after several weeks and the organism enters a latent phase that may last for a number of weeks to a year. During this latent phase, patients generally do not experience overt symptoms
  - *Tertiary syphilis*—untreated organism enters eyes, brain, nervous system, joints and blood vessels leading to death

12.6.2.2 Viral STDs

12.6.2.2.1 Genital herpes

- Caused by the *herpes simplex virus*
- Initial symptoms may be sores, eruptions, pain and swelling in the genital area. Many cases may initially be asymptomatic. The herpes virus may become latent and cause no obvious symptoms for a period of time. Even though symptoms are not evident during the latent phase, individuals can still transmit the virus to others
- The virus may also be transmitted from the mother to the newborn during the delivery process. Herpes infection in a newborn can have serious consequences including central nervous system damage and blindness
- In immunocompromised individuals, the herpes virus cause meningitis and eye damage

12.6.2.2.2 Human papillomavirus (HPV)

There are a number of different HPV variants that infect various tissues of the body. Most type of HPV are associated with benign warts on the hands, feet, face and neck. A number of HPV variants can infect the genitalia and cause a range of conditions from genital warts to cervical dysplasia. Low-risk HPV variants such as types 6 and 11 are responsible for most cases of benign genital warts (*condylomata acuminate*). Although genital warts are benign, they are also highly contagious through intimate contact. High-risk variants of HPV such as 16 and 18 are associated with an increased risk for cervical, anal, and oropharyngeal cancers. A DNA test is available to determine if an individual is infected with a high-risk variant of HPV. A pap test is also useful for detecting abnormal changes in cervical tissue that may be a precursor to cervical cancer. A highly effective vaccine is available against high-risk HPV strains and is recommended for all young boys and girls 11–12 years of age.

12.6.2.3 Other STDs

12.6.2.3.1 Trichomoniasis

Trichomoniasis is caused by the aerobic parasitic protozoa *Trichomoniasis vaginalis*. According to the CDC, 3.7 million individuals in the United States have trichomoniasis. The majority of women infected (85%) and most infected men have no symptoms. If symptoms are present, they usually include foul-smelling discharge, painful urination, erythema and itching. Diagnosis is made through microscopic examination of fluids or by testing for protozoa antigen or DNA. Treatment involves the use of the agents metronidazole and tinidazole. Untreated infection in pregnant women has been associated with an increased risk of preterm delivery and low birth weights.

12.6.2.4 Long-term consequences of STDs

- Infertility
- *Pelvic inflammatory disease*—infection of a woman's reproductive organs. Can lead to pain, infertility, ectopic pregnancy and the formation of scar tissue
- Infection of the newborn
- Increased risk for certain cancers
- Systemic effects
- Neurologic and central nervous system damage from syphilis

12.6.2.4.1 Diagnosis of STDs

- Physical examination
- Symptoms
- Culture
- Tests to detect antigens or nucleic acids form the organism

12.6.2.4.2 *Treatment of STDs* Antibiotics, antivirals, and antiprotozoal agents are available to treat and cure most STDs. Some STDs such as herpes and HIV cannot yet be cured but can be suppressed through the use of appropriate antiviral therapy. Growing drug resistance is becoming a major concern with some STDs such as gonorrhea and syphilis.

Medical terminology

Antrum (ăn′trŭm): In the reproductive system, the fluid-filled cavity of a developing ovarian follicle

Atresia (ă-trē′zē-ă): In the reproductive system, the normal death of an ovarian follicle

Corpus luteum (kor′pŭs lū′tŭm): Yellow structure that forms within a ruptured ovarian follicle and secretes progesterone and estrogen

Ejaculation (ē-jăk″ū-lā′shŭn): Ejection of semen from the male urethra

Emission (ē-mĭsh′ŭn): Movement of semen into the urethra

Endometrium (ĕn-dō-mē′trē-ŭm): Lining of the uterus where implantation of the embryo takes place

Erection (ē-rĕk′shŭn): State of swelling and stiffness of the penis due to its engorgement with blood

Estrogen (ĕs′trō-jĕn): Female sex hormone

Fertilization (fĕr-tĭl-ĭ-zā′shŭn): Fusion of the sperm with an ovum

Gamete (găm′ēt): Mature male (sperm) or female (ovum) reproductive cell

Gametogenesis (găm″ĕt-ō-jĕn′ē-sĭs): Formation of gametes

Genitalia (jĕn-ĭ-tāl′ē-ă): Reproductive organs

Graafian follicle (grăf′ē-ăn): Mature ovarian follicle

Granulosa cell (grăn″ū-lōsă): Estrogen producing cell within the ovarian follicle

Implantation (ĭm″plăn-tā′shŭn): Embedding of the embryo within the endometrium

Leydig cell (lī′dĭg): Testosterone-producing cell of the testes

Luteinization (lū″tē-ĭn-ī-zā′shŭn): Formation of the corpus luteum within a ruptured follicle

Meiosis (mī-ō′sĭs): Process where oögonia or spermatogonia undergo cell division to produce the gametes, ova and sperm

Menopause (měn′ō-pawz): Permanent cessation of menstruation

Menstruation (měn-stroo-ā′shŭn): Sloughing of the endometrium

Mitosis (mī-tō′sĭs): Process where cells divide to reproduce themselves

Myometrium (mī″ō-mē′trē-ūm): Smooth muscle layer of the uterine wall

Oogenesis (ō″ō-jěn′ě-sĭs): Formation of a mature ovum

Oögonium (ō″ō-gō′nē-ŭm): Stem cell from which an oocyte originates

Ovulation (ŏv″ū-lā′shŭn): Rupture of the follicle and discharge of the ovum

Parturition (păr-tū-rĭsh′ŭn): Process of giving birth to offspring

Placenta (plă-sěn′tă): Uterine structure that provides nourishment and oxygen to a developing fetus

Progesterone (prō-jěs′těr-ōn): Female sex hormone

Puberty (pū′běr-tē): Stage in life where an individual becomes capable of reproduction

Scrotum (skrō′tŭm): Pouch that contains the testes external to the pelvic cavity

Semen (sē′měn): Fluid discharge from the male containing sperm

Sertoli cell (sěr-tō′lē): Sperm-producing cell of the testes

Spermatogenesis (spěr″măt-ō-jěn′ě-sĭs): Formation of mature sperm

Spermatogonium (spěr″măt-ō-gō′nē-ŭm): Stem cell from which sperm originate

Spermatozoa (spěr″măt-ō-zō′ă): Sperm

Testosterone (těs-tŏs′těr-ōn): Male sex hormone

Thecal cell (thē′kăl): Androgen-producing cell in the ovarian follicle

Zona pellucida (zō′nă pěl-lū′sĭă): Thick layer surrounding the oocyte

Zygote (zī′gōt): Fertilized ovum

Bibliography

Ansong, K. S., Lewis, C., Jenkins, P., Bell, J., 2000. Epidemiology of erectile dysfunction: A community-based study in rural New York state. *Ann Epidemiol.* 10:293–296.

Fox, S. I., *Human Physiology*, 9th ed., McGraw-Hill, New York, 2006.

Gray, C. A., Taylor, K. M., Ramsey, W. S., Hill, J. R., Bazer, F. W., Bartol, F. F., and Spencer, T. E., 2001. Endometrial glands are required for preimplantation conceptus, elongation and survival. *Biol Reprod.* 64(6):1608–1613.

Hempstock, J., Cindrova-Davies, T., Jauniaux, E., and Burton, G., 2004. Endometrial glands as a source of nutrients, growth factors and cytokines during the first trimester of human pregnancy: A morphological and immunohistochemical study. *Reprod Biol Endocrinol.* 2:58.

Erectile Dysfunction. 2017, April 25. Retrieved from http://www.nlm.nih.gov/medlineplus/erectiledysfunction.html.

Kantor, J., Bilker, W. B., Glasser, D. B., and Margolis, D.J., 2002. Prevalence of erectile dysfunction and active depression: An analytic cross-sectional study of general medical patients. *Am J Epidemiol.* 156:1035–1042.

Loose, D. S., and Stancel, G. M., Estrogens and progestins, in *Goodman and Gilman's The Pharmacological Basis of Therapeutics*, 11th ed., Brunton, L. L., Lazo, J. S., and Parker, K. L., Eds., McGraw-Hill, New York, 2006, chap. 57.

Matfin, G., Disorders of the male genitourinary system, in *Pathophysiology, Concepts of Altered Health and Disease*, 7th ed., Porth, C. M., Ed., Lippincott, Williams & Wilkins, Philadelphia, PA, 2005.

Michel, T., Treatment of myocardial ischemia, in *Goodman and Gilman's The Pharmacological Basis of Therapeutics*, 11th ed., Brunton, L. L., Lazo, J. S., and Parker, K. L., Eds., McGraw-Hill, New York, 2006, chap. 31.

NIH Consensus Development Panel on Impotence, NIH Consensus Conference: Impotence. *JAMA.* 270:83–90, 1993.

Sherwood, L., *Human Physiology from Cells to Systems*, 5th ed., Brooks/Cole, Pacific Grove, CA, 2001.

Silverthorn, D. U., *Human Physiology, An Integrated Approach*, 4th ed., Prentice Hall, Upper Saddle River, NJ, 2007.

Taber's Cyclopedic Medical Dictionary, 20th ed., F. A. Davis Co., Philadelphia, PA, 2005.

Widmaier, E. P., Raff, H., and Strang, K. T., *Vander's Human Physiology, The Mechanisms of Body Function*, McGraw-Hill, Boston, MA, 2006.

chapter thirteen

The nervous system

Study objectives

- Describe the organization of the nervous system including the central nervous system (CNS) and the peripheral nervous system (PNS)
- Distinguish between the three types of neurons: afferent neurons, efferent neurons and interneurons
- Describe the functions of the neuroglial cells
- List the three major levels of CNS function and describe their activities
- Distinguish between the three types of tracts in the CNS: projection tracts, association tracts, and commissural tracts
- Describe the activity of each of the functional areas of the cerebral cortex
- Explain how language is processed in the cerebral cortex
- Describe the lateral specialization that occurs in the cerebral cortex
- Describe the function of the basal ganglia, the thalamus, the hypothalamus and the brainstem
- Describe the function of the limbic system
- Distinguish between the three regions of the cerebellum and their functions
- Compare and contrast the exchange of materials between the blood and peripheral tissues with that of the blood and the brain
- Explain the functions of the blood-brain barrier
- Explain the functions of cerebrospinal fluid
- Define *cauda equina* and explain how it is formed
- Distinguish between a nerve and a tract
- Explain the function of the gray matter of the spinal cord
- Describe the location and function of each of the four types of neurons found in the gray matter of the spinal cord
- Explain the function of the white matter of the spinal cord
- Describe the composition of the ascending tracts, including both the origin and termination of each of the neurons
- Distinguish between corticospinal tracts and multineuronal tracts
- Discuss the mechanisms by which spinal anesthesia and epidural anesthesia exert their effects
- Define the various categories of reflexes
- List the components of the reflex arc

- Explain the mechanism of the withdrawal reflex
- Explain the mechanism of the crossed-extensor reflex
- Describe the major features of brain injury
- Compare and contrast the various types of bleeds associated with brain injury
- List symptoms associated with increased intracranial pressure
- List symptoms associated with various types of brain ischemia
- Compare and contrast hemorrhagic stroke and occlusive stroke with regard to etiology, symptoms and treatments
- Discuss how encephalitis differs from meningitis. List some organisms that might cause each
- Describe the various types of tumors that can occur in the CNS
- Compare and contrast the various types of seizure that can occur with regard to their symptoms and manifestations. Discuss why *status epilepticus* is so dangerous
- List the various types of headaches that can occur along with the major features of each
- Compare and contrast the various neurodegenerative disorders with emphasis on their etiology, manifestations and clinical course
- List the major symptoms associated with spinal cord injury

The nervous system is one of the two regulatory systems in the human body that influences the activity of all the other organ systems. It consists of literally billions of neurons that are interconnected in a highly organized circuitry. It is the number of neurons and the way they are interconnected within a circuit that distinguishes one region of the brain from another and the brain of one individual from that of another person. In addition, *plasticity,* the ability to alter circuit connections and function, in response to sensory input and experiences, adds further complexity and distinctiveness to our neurological responses and behavior.

The nervous system is divided into two anatomically distinct regions:

- Central nervous system
- Peripheral nervous system

The *central nervous system* (CNS) consists of the brain and the spinal cord. The *peripheral nervous system* (PNS) consists of the 12 pairs of cranial nerves that arise from the brainstem and the 31 pairs of spinal nerves that arise from the spinal cord. These peripheral nerves carry information between the CNS and the tissues of the body.

The PNS consists of two divisions:

- Afferent division
- Efferent division

The *afferent division* carries sensory information toward the CNS, and the *efferent division* carries motor information away from the CNS toward the effector structures (muscle tissue and glands). The efferent division is further divided into two components: the somatic nervous system, which consists of the motor neurons that innervate skeletal muscles, and the autonomic nervous system, which innervates cardiac muscle, smooth muscle and glands.

13.1 Neurons

There are three functional classes of neurons in the human nervous system:

- Afferent neurons
- Efferent neurons
- Interneurons

Afferent neurons lie predominantly in the PNS (see Figure 13.1). Each has a sensory receptor that is activated by a particular type of stimulus, a cell body located adjacent to the spinal cord, and an axon. Two regions of an axon exist: the *peripheral axon* extends from the receptor to the cell body and the *central axon* continues from the cell body into the spinal cord. Afferent neurons transmit sensory information from receptors in the periphery of the body to the CNS.

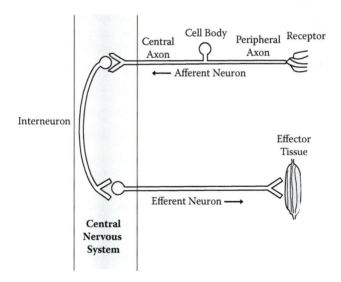

Figure 13.1 Types of neurons. Afferent neurons, which transmit impulses toward the CNS, and efferent neurons, which transmit impulses away from the CNS, lie predominantly in the peripheral nervous system. Interneurons, which process sensory input and coordinate motor responses, lie entirely within the central nervous system.

Efferent neurons also lie predominantly in the PNS. In this case, the cell bodies are found in the CNS in either the spinal cord or the brainstem, and the axons extend out into the periphery of the body where they innervate the effector tissues. By way of convergence, the centrally located cell bodies may receive inputs from several different regions of the brain and the spinal cord that will influence their activity. Efferent neurons transmit information from the CNS to muscles and glands.

Interneurons, the third class of neurons, lie entirely within the CNS. The human brain and spinal cord contains well over 100 billion neurons, and interneurons account for approximately 99% of all the neurons within the body. Interneurons lie between afferent and efferent neurons and are responsible for integrating sensory input and coordinating a motor response. In the simplest condition, interneurons process responses at the level of the spinal cord in the form of *reflexes*, which are automatic, stereotyped responses to given stimuli. For example, stimulation of pain receptors generates action potentials in their associated afferent neurons. These impulses are transmitted to the spinal cord where the afferent neurons stimulate interneurons. These interneurons then stimulate efferent neurons that cause skeletal muscle contraction in the affected area to move the body part away from the painful stimulus. This *withdrawal reflex* involves comparatively few interneurons and does not require any input from higher nervous centers in the brain. On the other hand, a response to some other stimulus may involve more sophisticated neurological phenomena such as memory, motivation, judgment and intellect. This type of response is not automatic, is clearly far more complex and may require the activity of millions of interneurons in many regions of the brain prior to the stimulation of motor neurons to carry out the desired effect.

13.2   Level of CNS function

There are three major levels of CNS function:

- Spinal cord
- Brainstem
- Cerebrum and the cerebral cortex

The *spinal cord* is the most anatomically inferior portion of the CNS, and its functions are at the lowest level of sophistication (see Table 13.1). As mentioned previously, the spinal cord receives sensory input from the periphery of the body and contains the cell bodies of motor neurons responsible for both voluntary and involuntary movements. Once again, the involuntary and neurologically simple reflexes are processed entirely at the level of the spinal cord. Voluntary, deliberate movements are initiated and controlled by thought processes in the cerebrum. The second important

Table 13.1 Major levels of CNS function

Spinal Cord	Processes reflexes, transmits nerve impulses to and from brain
Brainstem	Receives sensory input and initiates motor output, controls life-sustaining processes (e.g., respiration, circulation, digestion)
Cerebrum and Cerebral Cortex	Processes, integrates, and analyzes information; involved with the highest levels of cognition, voluntary initiation of movement, sensory perception, and language

function of the spinal cord is to *transmit nerve impulses* to and from the brain. *Ascending pathways* carry sensory input to higher levels of the CNS, and *descending pathways* carry impulses from the brain to motor neurons in the spinal cord.

The *brainstem*, which consists of the medulla, pons and midbrain, is, in evolutionary terms, the oldest and smallest region of the brain. Continuous with the spinal cord, the brainstem receives sensory input and initiates motor output by way of cranial nerves III through XII, which are functionally analogous to the 31 pairs of spinal nerves. Whereas the spinal cord processes sensory and motor activities in the trunk of the body and the limbs, the brainstem processes these activities primarily in the head, neck and face. The brainstem also controls many basic life-sustaining processes, including respiration, circulation, and digestion. Even with the loss of higher cognitive function, this lower level of the brain can sustain bodily functions essential for survival.

The *cerebrum and the cerebral cortex*, which account for 80% of the total brain weight in humans, constitute the highest functional level of the CNS. As our species became more cognitively sophisticated, the cerebral cortex became larger and more highly folded. These convolutions or folds serve to increase the surface area of the cerebral cortex, thus allowing for a greater number of neurons. For example, the total surface area of the cerebral cortex for the rat, cat and human are 6, 83, and 2,500 cm^2, respectively. It is not unexpected that the cerebrum is the most highly developed in the human. Responsible for the highest levels of processing, integration and analysis of information, the cerebral cortex plays an important role in the most elaborate neurological functions including intellect, thought, personality, voluntary initiation of movement, final sensory perception, and language.

13.3 The brain

The brain is the integrative portion of the nervous system that serves to receive, process, and store sensory information and then plan and orchestrate the appropriate motor response. It is divided into several anatomically

Table 13.2   Adult brain structures

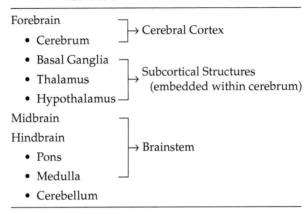

and functionally distinct regions (see Table 13.2). The forebrain consists of the cerebrum, the basal ganglia, the thalamus and the hypothalamus. The midbrain along with the pons and the medulla of the hindbrain compose the functional region referred to as the brainstem. The cerebellum is also considered a component of the hindbrain but is functionally distinct from the brainstem. A summary of the functions of the major components of the brain can be found in Table 13.3.

The *cerebrum* is composed of two hemispheres, the left and the right, which are anatomically connected to ensure intercommunication. Two types of tissue compose each hemisphere (see Figure 13.2):

- Gray matter
- White matter

The *gray matter*, which contains the unmyelinated cell bodies of neurons, is on the outer surface of the cerebrum and forms the *cerebral cortex*. The *white matter*, which is composed of the myelinated axons of neurons, is found underlying the cortex in the core of the cerebrum. These axons are bundled together according to function and organized into units referred to as *tracts*. There are three types of tracts in the cerebrum:

- Projection tracts
- Association tracts
- Commissural tracts

Projection tracts may be *descending* and carry motor nerve impulses from the cerebral cortex to lower regions of the brain or spinal cord or they may be *ascending* and carry sensory impulses from lower regions of the brain or spinal cord to the cortex. *Association tracts* transmit nerve impulses from one

Table 13.3 Summary of the functions of the major components of the brain

Forebrain

Cerebral Cortex
- Sensory perception
- Voluntary movement of skeletal muscle
- Language
- Intellect, personality, judgment, behavior, memory

Basal Ganglia
- Inhibition of skeletal muscle tone
- Coordination of slow, sustained movements

Thalamus
- Relay station for sensory input
- Role in awareness

Hypothalamus
- Regulation of the autonomic nervous system
- Regulation of endocrine system function
- Thermoregulation
- Regulation of plasma volume, plasma osmolarity, thirst, hunger, urine output
- Influence on behavior and emotions

Brainstem

Medulla
- Cardiovascular, respiratory, digestive control centers

Pons
- Relay station for cerebrum and cerebellum
- Assists medulla in control of breathing

Midbrain
- Contributes to control of eye movements
- Relay station for auditory and visual reflexes

Reticular Formation
- Cortical awareness, ability to direct attention, sleep
- Coordination of orofacial motor activities
- Coordination of eating and breathing
- Response to pain

Cerebellum

- Maintenance of balance
- Control of eye movements
- Regulation of skeletal muscle tone
- Coordination of skilled voluntary movements
- Contributes to planning, programming, and initiation of voluntary skeletal muscle activity
- Procedural memory and motor learning

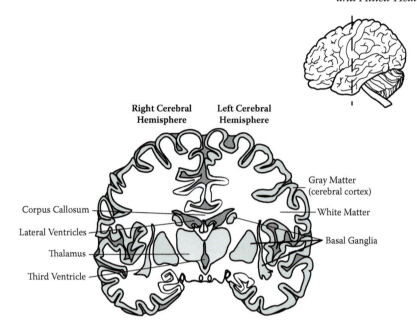

Figure 13.2 Frontal section of the brain. The cerebrum is composed of two types of tissue: the internal white matter and the external gray matter that forms the cerebral cortex. Embedded within the cerebral hemispheres are other masses of gray matter, the basal ganglia and the thalamus. The ventricles are filled with cerebrospinal fluid (CSF).

functional region of the cerebral cortex to another within the same hemisphere. *Commissural tracts* transmit impulses from one hemisphere to the other. The primary example of this type of tract is the corpus callosum, the thick band of tissue connecting the left and the right hemispheres and consisting of more than 100 million neurons. The communication provided by each of these types of tracts facilitates the integration, processing and storage of information among the various regions of the brain.

The cerebral cortex is not a smooth surface but, instead, is highly folded and has a furrowed appearance (see Figure 13.3). A convolution formed by these folds is referred to as a *gyrus (pl. gyri)*. Each gyrus is separated from another by a *sulcus (pl. sulci)*, which is a shallow groove, or a *fissure*, which is a deeper groove. The functional importance of gyri, sulci, and fissures is they significantly increase the surface area of the cerebral cortex, providing space for a greater number of neurons.

Both hemispheres of the cerebrum consist of four lobes including the:

- Frontal lobes
- Parietal lobes
- Occipital lobes
- Temporal lobes

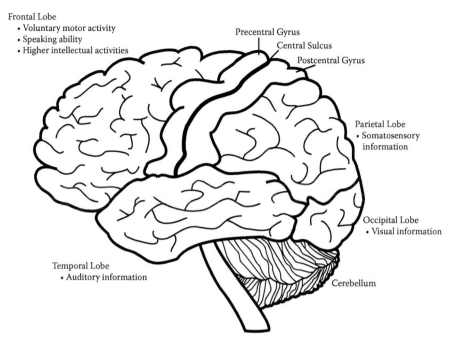

Frontal Lobe
- Voluntary motor activity
- Speaking ability
- Higher intellectual activities

Precentral Gyrus

Central Sulcus

Postcentral Gyrus

Parietal Lobe
- Somatosensory information

Occipital Lobe
- Visual information

Temporal Lobe
- Auditory information

Cerebellum

Figure 13.3   Lateral view of the four lobes of the cerebral cortex.

Named for the bones of the cranium, under which they lie, the lobes are conspicuously defined by prominent sulci of the cortex, which have a relatively constant position in human brains. Each lobe is specialized for different activities (see Figure 13.3, Table 13.4). The *frontal lobes*, located in the anterior portions of the hemispheres, are responsible for voluntary motor activity, speaking ability

Table 13.4   Functions of the lobes of the cerebral cortex

Frontal Lobe
- Voluntary movement of skeletal muscle
- Speaking ability
- Higher intellectual abilities, personality, judgment, behavior

Parietal Lobe
- Processing and integration of somatosensory information
- Understanding spoken and written language
- Formulating coherent patterns of speech (or writing) to express thoughts and emotions

Occipital Lobe
- Processing and integration of visual information

Temporal Lobe
- Processing and integration of auditory information

and higher intellectual activities. The *parietal lobes*, located posterior to the frontal lobes, process and integrate sensory information. The *occipital lobes* in the posterior-most aspects of the cerebrum process visual information, and the *temporal lobes*, located laterally, process auditory information.

The cerebral cortex is organized into several functionally discrete areas (see Figure 13.4). However, it is important to note that no single area functions in isolation. The activity in each area depends on neurons in other areas for incoming and outgoing messages.

The *somatosensory cortex* is located within the postcentral gyrus, which is the anterior-most region of the parietal lobes (see Figure 13.3). This region contains the terminations of ascending pathways that transmit nerve impulses concerning temperature, touch, pressure, pain and proprioception. The latter is the awareness of posture, movement, changes in equilibrium and the position of one's body parts, particularly in reference to surrounding objects. As such, the somatosensory cortex is the site for initial cerebral processing of these types of inputs.

Each section of this region of cortex receives sensory input from a specific area of the body in a highly organized and sequential manner. It is organized in a "foot-to-tongue" pattern along the medial-to-lateral axis (top-to-bottom of the gyrus). Interestingly, the size of the region of the cortex devoted to different areas of the body is quite disproportionate. For example, the trunk of the body and the legs are not densely innervated with sensory neurons. As a result, the axonal terminations of the pathways originating

Cortical Area	Function
Sensory Input ↓	Relayed from afferent neuronal receptors.
Primary Sensory Areas ↓	Initial cortical processing of sensory input.
Unimodal Association Areas ↓	Further processing of information from a single sensory modality.
Multimodal Sensory Association Areas ↓	Highest level of processing, integration, and interpretation of diverse sensory input for planning purposeful action.
Multimodal Motor Association Areas ↓	Neuronal programming of movements according to cortical and subcortical input.
Primary Motor Cortex	Transmission of impulses to somatic efferent motor neurons in spinal cord to initiate voluntary contraction of skeletal muscle.

Figure 13.4 Potential route of transmission of electrical impulses through association pathways of the cerebral cortex.

in these body parts are limited in number and take up only a small portion of the somatosensory cortex. Conversely, the face, the tongue and the hands are very densely innervated with sensory neurons. Therefore, the terminations of pathways originating in these body parts are numerous and are represented in a much larger portion of the somatosensory cortex. The proportion of cortex devoted to a given body part is determined by the degree of sensory perception associated with that body part as well as the importance of the sensory input from that part of the body. The somatosensory cortex not only localizes the source of sensory input, it also perceives the intensity of the stimulus.

These ascending sensory pathways cross from one side of the CNS to the other so that sensory input from the left side of the body is transmitted to the somatosensory cortex of the right cerebral hemisphere and vice versa. Therefore, damage to a region of cortex in a given hemisphere results in sensory deficits such as numbness and tingling in the opposite side of the body.

In addition to the somatosensory cortex, there are special senses areas in the cerebral cortex involved with the primary or initial processing of a specific type of stimulus. The *primary visual cortex* (sight) is located within the occipital lobes, the *primary auditory cortex* (hearing) and the *primary olfactory cortex* (smell) are found within the temporal lobes and the *primary gustatory* or *taste cortex* is located at the base of the somatosensory cortex in the parietal lobes.

Each of these primary areas is surrounded by a "higher order" sensory area or a *unimodal association area* that further integrates information from a single sensory modality and provides more complex aspects of the input. For example, the primary visual cortex is the first site of processing of visual information. Association tracts originating in this area then project to the surrounding unimodal association area for higher level processing of this visual input. In fact, the visual unimodal association cortex occupies the remaining portion of the occipital lobes.

The *posterior parietal cortex* is located posterior to the somatosensory cortex and serves as its unimodal association area. In addition to the further processing of somatosensory input, information from the somatosensory cortex is integrated with visual inputs in this region as association tracts from both of these functional areas terminate here. This activity is important for planning complex movements and for hand (proprioception)–eye (visual) coordination.

The unimodal association areas in turn project to *multimodal sensory association* areas that integrate information about more than one sensory modality. Activity in the multimodal sensory association areas helps to create a complete understanding of one's surroundings. It is in these areas that the highest level of cognitive brain function takes place. Not only do these areas process, integrate and interpret several different forms sensory information, they then link this data to the planning of movement and goal-directed action.

The *prefrontal multimodal association area* is located within the anterior-most region of the frontal lobe. It is involved with some of the most distinctly human intellectual traits including memory and planning of motor activity, long-term planning and judgment, foresight, a sense of purpose, a sense of responsibility, a sense of social propriety, personality traits and behavior. Consistent with this notion, lesions to this association area result in profound cognitive deficits, impaired motor activity, and changes in personality and social behavior. These patients do not respond to environmental stimuli as non-affected, normal individuals do. They have a lack of consistency of purpose, a lack of foresight, and a lack of ambition. In other words, they tend to achieve less in life; an outcome that suggests their ability to plan and organize everyday activities is impaired. Interestingly, however, their general intelligence, perception and long-term memory remain somewhat intact.

The *posterior multimodal association area* is located at the junction of the parietal, temporal and occipital lobes. It pools and integrates somatic, auditory and visual stimuli for complex perceptual processing. As such, this area is involved primarily with visuospatial localization, language and attention. Lesions here interfere with awareness of one's body position and of the space in which it moves as well as the ability to integrate and make sense of the elements of a visual scene. In other words, these patients have normal visual acuity but cannot focus on an object of interest.

The *limbic multimodal association area* is partially located in each of the temporal, parietal and frontal lobes. It is concerned with emotional expression and memory storage. Although these functions appear to be unrelated, it is important to remember that the emotional impact of an event is a major determinant of whether the event is remembered. Damage here may cause profound changes in emotional expression with little change in perception or intelligence. Tumors in this region have been associated with emotional disturbances, including fear, irritability, and depression. Once again, it is important to remember that although each of these multimodal association areas has their own characteristic functions, they are highly interconnected and work together toward an end result.

The multimodal sensory association areas then project to the *multimodal motor association areas* located in the frontal lobes, including the *premotor cortex* and the *supplementary motor cortex*. Neurons here are active during preparation for a movement. These regions receive input from the basal ganglia, the cerebellum, the somatosensory cortex and the posterior multimodal association cortex (all of which provide information about the ongoing movement) as well as the prefrontal multimodal association area. As such, these areas are important in the programming of complex sequences of movements and in orienting the body and limbs toward a specific target. For example, the motor planning for opening a door includes turning the body toward the door and extending the arm and hand toward the doorknob. Lesions in these multimodal motor association areas interfere with the coordination and the performance of complex integrated movements.

Following the development of the motor program, neurons originating in the multimodal motor association areas transmit impulses by way of association tracts to the neurons of the primary motor cortex. The *primary motor cortex* is located within the precentral gyrus, which is the posteriormost region of the frontal lobe adjacent to the multimodal motor association areas (see Figure 6.3). It is this area that initiates voluntary contractions of specific skeletal muscles. Neurons whose cell bodies reside here transmit impulses by way of descending projection tracts to the spinal cord where they synapse with alpha motor neurons (which innervate skeletal muscles).

As with the somatosensory cortex, neurons here are highly organized, with each section of the cortex innervating specific body parts in a sequential manner. Once again, the map is laid out in a "foot-to-tongue" pattern. Also like the somatosensory cortex, the size of the region of the primary motor cortex devoted to different parts of the body is quite disproportionate. Large portions of the primary motor cortex innervate the muscles of the hands, which perform complex movements, as well as the muscles responsible for speech and eating. On the other hand, little cortex is devoted to motor pathways terminating in the trunk of the body or the lower extremities, which are not capable of complex movements. Therefore, the distortions in cortical representation parallel the importance of a particular part of the body in terms of complexity of motor skills. Although electrical activity in a specific region of the primary motor cortex will result in the contraction of its associated muscle, recent studies have shown that many muscles, particularly those distal muscles of the upper extremities, are regulated from more than one cortical location. Therefore, in addition to the area of the cortex devoted to the arm, other arm-specific neurons are located diffusely in other areas of the motor cortex.

A third similarity between the primary motor cortex and the somatosensory cortex is that the projection tracts cross from one side of the CNS to the other. Therefore, activity of motor neurons in the left cerebral hemisphere causes muscle contraction on the right side of the body and vice versa. As the commands for muscle contraction originate in the primary motor cortex, lesions in this region of cortex, within a given hemisphere, will result in paralysis in the opposite side of the body.

The exchange of information among individuals is largely limited to species with advanced nervous systems and is found predominantly in birds and mammals. In humans, communication takes place primarily through *language* or the use of spoken or written words to convey a message. The processing of language requires a large network of interacting brain areas, both cortical and subcortical. However, the two predominant cortical areas are Wernicke's area and Broca's area. In approximately 96% of people, these cortical areas for language skills are found only in the left hemisphere.

Even languages such as American Sign Language, which rely on visuomo-tor abilities instead of auditory speech abilities, depend primarily on the left hemisphere.

Sensory input to the language areas comes from either the auditory cor-tex (hearing) or the visual cortex (reading). This input goes first to *Wernicke's area*, which is located within the left cerebral cortex near the junction between the parietal, temporal and occipital lobes. This area is involved with lan-guage comprehension and is important for understanding both spoken and written messages. It is also responsible for formulating coherent patterns of speech. In other words, this area enables an individual to attach mean-ing to words and to choose the appropriate words to convey their thoughts. Impulses are then transmitted to *Broca's area*, which is found in the left fron-tal lobe in close association with the motor areas of the cortex that control the muscles necessary for articulation. Broca's area is, therefore, responsible for the mechanical aspects of speaking.

A patient with a lesion in Wernicke's area is unable to understand any spoken or visual information. Furthermore, the patient's own speech, while fluent, is unintelligible because of frequent errors in the choice of words. This condition is known as *receptive aphasia*. On the other hand, a patient with a lesion in Broca's area is able to understand spoken and written lan-guage but is unable to express their response in a normal manner. Speech in this patient is nonfluent and requires great effort because they cannot establish the proper motor command to articulate the desired words. This condition is known as *expressive aphasia*.

The *basal ganglia* consist of several nuclei or masses of gray matter embed-ded within the white matter of each cerebral hemisphere (see Figure 13.2). As with the cerebral cortex, this gray matter consists of functional aggrega-tions of neuronal cell bodies. An important function of the basal ganglia involves their contribution to the control of voluntary movement. The axons of neurons originating in the primary motor cortex travel through descend-ing projection tracts to the spinal cord where they stimulate motor neurons to cause skeletal muscle contraction. At the same time, by way of divergence, these neurons transmit impulses to the basal ganglia. It is these impulses that form the primary source of input to these structures. In turn, the basal ganglia send impulses to the brainstem, which also transmits impulses to motor neurons in the spinal cord as well as the thalamus, which then trans-mits impulses back to the motor areas of the cerebral cortex.

The activity of the basal ganglia tends to be inhibitory. The thalamus positively reinforces motor activity in the cerebral cortex. Impulses from the basal ganglia modulate this effect. Through their inputs to the brainstem and, ultimately the motor neurons in the spinal cord, the basal ganglia inhibit muscle tone (recall that the degree of skeletal muscle contraction and tone is determined by the summation of excitatory and inhibitory inputs to the motor neurons). They also contribute to the coordination of slow, sustained contractions, especially those related to posture and body support. Motor disturbances associated with the basal ganglia include tremor and other involuntary movements; changes in posture and muscle tone, such as muscle rigidity; and slowness of movement without paralysis. Thus, disorders of the basal ganglia may result in either diminished movement (hypokinesias, such as Parkinson's disease) or excessive movement (hyperkinesias, such as Huntington's disease).

The *thalamus* is located between the cerebrum and the brainstem. Lying along the midline of the brain, it consists of two oval-shaped masses of gray matter, one in each cerebral hemisphere (see Figure 13.2). The thalamus is often described as a *relay station* as ascending tracts transmitting upward from the spinal cord, as well as sensory tracts from the eyes and the ears, extending ultimately to the cerebral cortex pass through it. In fact, all sensory fiber tracts, except olfactory tracts, that transmit impulses to the cerebral cortex first synapse with neurons in the thalamus. Therefore, the thalamus may be considered the functional "gateway" to the cerebral cortex.

The thalamus acts as a *filter* for information to the cortex by either preventing or enhancing the passage of specific information depending upon its significance to the individual. In fact, more than 99% of all sensory information transmitted toward the brain is discarded, as it is considered irrelevant and unimportant. This selection activity is accomplished largely at the level of the thalamus. As such, it plays an important role in general arousal and focused attention. For example, an individual may easily sleep through the noise of city traffic as this sensory input has been previously determined to be unimportant. However, this same individual may also be immediately aroused by the ever so quiet arrival of their teenager home late in the evening. This sensory is quite important to a parent and passes readily through the filter of the thalamus.

As mentioned previously in the discussion of the basal ganglia, the thalamus also plays a role in the regulation of skeletal muscle contraction by positively reinforcing voluntary motor activity initiated by the cerebral cortex.

As its name suggests, the *hypothalamus* lies beneath the thalamus and above the pituitary gland. Although it is quite small, accounting for only about 4 g of the total 1,400 g of the adult human brain (<1% of the total brain mass), it plays a vital role in the maintenance of homeostasis in the body. It is composed of numerous cell groups and fiber pathways, each with a specific function.

The hypothalamus plays a particularly important role in regulating the autonomic nervous system, which innervates cardiac muscle, smooth muscle and glands. Many of these effects involve ascending or descending pathways of the cerebral cortex passing through the hypothalamus. (Regulation of autonomic nervous system activity is discussed in detail in Chapter 14.) Endocrine activity is also regulated by the hypothalamus by way of its control over pituitary gland secretion. (Hypothalamic regulation of endocrine secretion is discussed in detail in Chapter 11.)

Recent studies have demonstrated that the hypothalamus serves to integrate autonomic nervous system responses and endocrine function with behavior, especially behavior associated with basic homeostatic requirements. The hypothalamus provides this integrative function by regulating the following:

- Blood pressure and electrolyte composition by regulating mechanisms involved with urine output, thirst, salt appetite, maintenance of plasma osmolarity and vascular smooth muscle tone
- Body temperature by regulating metabolic thermogenesis (e.g., shivering), cutaneous vasoconstriction or vasodilation, and behaviors that cause an individual to seek a warmer or cooler environment
- Energy metabolism by regulating food intake, digestion and metabolic rate
- Reproduction by way of hormonal control of sexual activity, pregnancy and lactation
- Responses to stress by altering blood flow to skeletal muscles and other tissues as well as enhancing the secretion of hormones from the adrenal cortex (glucocorticoids) whose metabolic activities enable the body to physically cope with stress

The hypothalamus regulates these physiological parameters by a three-step process involving negative feedback mechanisms (Chapter 2). First, the hypothalamus has access to and monitors sensory information from the entire body. Second, it compares this information to the various biological set points that have been established for optimal cellular function. Finally, if a deviation from set point for a given parameter is detected, the hypothalamus elicits a variety of autonomic, endocrine and behavioral responses to return the parameter to its set point and reestablish homeostasis. For example, blood glucose levels are monitored by the hypothalamus. When blood glucose is low (<50 mg glucose/100 mL blood), it mediates the sensation of hunger to drive the individual to ingest food.

The functional region known as the *brainstem* consists of the midbrain and the pons and medulla of the hindbrain. It is continuous with the spinal cord and serves as an important connection between the brain and the spinal cord because all sensory and motor pathways pass through it. The brainstem consists of numerous neuronal clusters or *centers*, each of which controls vital, life-supporting processes.

The *medulla*, which is immediately superior to and continuous with the spinal cord, contains control centers for subconscious, involuntary functions such as cardiovascular activity, respiration, swallowing, and vomiting. The primary function of the *pons* is to serve as a relay for the transfer of information between the cerebrum and the cerebellum. Along with the medulla, it also contributes to the control of breathing. Continuing rostrally from the medulla and pons, the *midbrain* controls eye movement and relays signals for auditory and visual reflexes. It also provides linkages between components of the motor system including the cerebellum, the basal ganglia, and the cerebrum.

In addition, the brainstem contains a diffuse network of neurons known as the *reticular formation*. This network is best known for its role in cortical alertness, ability to direct attention and sleep. It is also involved with the coordination of orofacial motor activities, particularly with activities involved with eating and the generation of emotional facial expressions. Other functions include the coordination of eating and breathing, blood pressure regulation and the response to pain. In addition to forming a diffuse network with far-reaching functions in the brainstem, some reticular formation neurons may cluster together, forming nuclei or control centers. These centers contribute to the regulation of the gastrointestinal system (including swallowing and vomiting), the respiratory system (including the initiation and modulation of respiratory rhythm, coughing, hiccupping and sneezing), and the cardiovascular system.

The *cerebellum* (Latin, little brain) is part of the hindbrain and is attached to the dorsal surface of the upper region of the brainstem. Although it constitutes only 10% of the total volume of the brain, it contains more than half of all its neurons. Its surface consists of a thin cortex of gray matter with extensive folding, a core of white matter and three pairs of nuclei embedded within it. The cerebellum is immature at birth but continues to develop throughout childhood and adolescence.

The specialized function of the cerebellum is to coordinate movement by evaluating differences between intended movement and actual movement. It carries out this activity while a movement is in progress as well as during repetitions of the same movement. Three important aspects of the cerebellum's organization enable it to carry out this function. First, it receives extensive sensory input from somatic receptors in the periphery of the body (proprioceptors) and from receptors in the inner ear providing information regarding equilibrium and balance. Second, output from the cerebellum is transmitted to the premotor and motor systems of the cerebral cortex and the brainstem, systems that control spinal interneurons and motor neurons. Finally, circuits within the cerebellum exhibit significant plasticity, which is necessary for motor adaptation and learning. Examples of motor learning include riding a bicycle, playing a musical instrument, and throwing a football.

The cerebellum consists of three functionally distinct parts:

- Vestibulocerebellum
- Spinocerebellum
- Cerebrocerebellum

The *vestibulocerebellum* receives sensory input regarding motion of the head and its position relative to gravity as well as visual input. Outputs control axial muscles (primarily head and neck muscles) and limb extensors assuring balance while standing still and during movement. Outputs also control eye movements and coordinate movement of the head and eyes. Lesions here affect an individual's balance. The ability to use the incoming sensory information to control eye movements when the head is rotating and movements of the limbs and body during standing and walking is also impaired.

The *spinocerebellum* influences muscle tone and coordinates skilled voluntary movements. It receives sensory input from interneurons in the spinal cord transmitting somatic information, in particular, from muscle and joint proprioceptors providing data regarding body movements and positions that are actually taking place. It also receives input from the cortical motor areas providing information regarding the intended or desired movement. The spinocerebellum then compares these inputs. If the actual status of a body part differs from the intended status, the spinocerebellum transmits impulses back to the motor areas of the brain to make the appropriate adjustments in the activation of the associated skeletal muscles.

The *cerebrocerebellum* is involved with the planning, programming and initiation of voluntary activity. It also participates in procedural memories or motor learning. This region of the cerebellum receives input from and provides output to the cortical motor areas directly. Lesions of the cerebrocerebellum cause delays in initiating movements and irregularities in the timing of multistep movements.

Disorders of the human cerebellum result in three types of abnormalities. The first is *hypotonia* or reduced muscle tone. Another includes abnormalities in the execution of voluntary movements or *ataxia* (defective muscular coordination). The third type of muscular malfunction is *intention tremors*. These tremors differ from the resting tremors of Parkinson's disease in that they occur *during* a movement and are most pronounced at the end of the movement when the patient attempts to terminate it.

PHARMACY APPLICATION: CENTRALLY ACTING DRUGS

Combinations of centrally acting drugs are frequently used to achieve a desired therapeutic effect, particularly when the agents used have different mechanisms of action. For example, a patient with Parkinson's disease may be treated with one drug that blocks the effects of the neurotransmitter, acetylcholine, and second drug that enhances the activity of another neurotransmitter, dopamine. However, potentially detrimental effects may occur when the agents used have additive effects.

(Continued)

PHARMACY APPLICATION: CENTRALLY
ACTING DRUGS (Continued)

The effect of a CNS stimulant or depressant is additive with the effects of all other categories of stimulant and depressant drugs. For example, the combination of benzodiazepines (diazepam, Valium®) or barbiturates (pentobarbital, Nembutal®) with ethanol is not only additive, it may be fatal. Each of these drugs, especially the barbiturates, has a depressant effect on the respiratory center in the brainstem, such that high doses may cause the cessation of breathing. The effect of a CNS drug is also additive with the physiological state of the patient. For example, anesthetics and antianxiety drugs are less effective in a hyperexcitable patient compared with a normal patient.

Glial cells outnumber neurons in the nervous system and account for 90% of the cells within the CNS. However, because they do not branch as much as neurons, these cells occupy only 50% of the volume of the brain. Glial cells do not transmit electrical impulses. Instead, these cells serve as the connective tissue of the CNS providing structural and metabolic support for the neurons. As such, glial cells maintain an appropriate microenvironment essential for optimal neuronal function.

There are several types of glial cells in the CNS:

- Astrocytes
- Oligodendrocytes
- Microglia
- Ependymal cells

The most abundant type of glial cell is the *astrocyte*. Found throughout the CNS, astrocytes are highly branched cells with processes that extend to the surfaces of neuronal dendrites and cell bodies. Expansions of these processes, referred to as *end-feet*, also form a complete lining around the outer surface of the brain and spinal cord where these structures come into contact with the pia mater, the innermost meningeal membrane that encloses the CNS. In addition, end-feet are found surrounding the small blood vessels of the CNS. These glial cells have many important functions within the brain. Astrocytes:

- Provide a pathway for neuronal migration during fetal development
- Enhance synapse formation and synaptic transmission
- Provide structural support by holding neurons together in their proper framework
- Induce formation of the blood-brain barrier in CNS capillaries

- Secrete growth factors necessary for neuronal function
- Form an astrocytic scar in response to brain injury
- Maintain electrolyte concentration (in particular, K⁺ ions) and the pH of the interstitial fluid in the CNS
- Participate in neurotransmitter metabolism and removal

Oligodendrocytes are functionally analogous to the Schwann cells of the peripheral nervous system. These glial cells are responsible for the formation of the myelin sheath that surrounds the neuronal axons in the CNS. However, in contrast to the Schwann cell, oligodendrocytes send out several processes that enable them to provide myelin to many axons at the same time.

Microglia are the immune effector cells of the CNS and are the predominant glial cells involved with CNS inflammation. Functionally analogous to macrophages in the periphery of the body, these glial cells serve as phagocytic scavengers in the brain. Like the macrophage, microglia are derived from monocytes. These cells migrate into the CNS during embryonic development.

In a healthy individual, microglia account for only 1% of the cells in the CNS. In this case, they are considered to be quiet or resting and remain stationary until activated by infection or injury. When activated, the microglia become highly mobile and migrate toward the site of damage. At that time, they proliferate and phagocytose cellular debris.

Ependymal cells line the internal cavities of the CNS, including the ventricles of the brain and the central canal of the spinal cord. As such, these cells form a selectively permeable epithelial layer that separates the fluid compartments of the CNS (cerebrospinal fluid vs. interstitial fluid). In the ventricles, the ependymal cells contribute to the formation of cerebrospinal fluid (CSF). Furthermore, these cells contain cilia whose beating contribute to the flow of CSF throughout the ventricles. Ependymal cells also serve as neural stem cells with the potential of forming other glial cells.

13.4 Blood-brain barrier

The movement of substances between the blood and the extracellular fluid surrounding the cells in most tissues of the body occurs very readily. This exchange takes place at the level of the capillaries, the smallest blood vessels in the cardiovascular system whose walls are formed by a single layer of endothelial cells. Lipid-soluble substances move across this layer of endothelial cells at any point because they can move directly *through* the plasma membrane by passing between the phospholipid molecules of the bilayer. The movement of water-soluble substances is limited to the multiple pores found *between* the cells; however, it also takes place rapidly and efficiently.

This nonselective exchange of materials, which includes all substances except plasma proteins, does not occur in all vascular beds, however. Many substances found in the blood are potentially harmful to the CNS. Therefore, the brain and the spinal cord are protected from these substances by the *blood-brain barrier.* In the capillaries of the brain and spinal cord, there are no pores between the endothelial cells. Instead, there are *tight junctions*, which fuse the cells together. As mentioned previously, astrocytes also play a role in the formation of the blood-brain barrier. As a result, exchange between the blood and the extracellular fluid of the brain is altered. Lipid-soluble substances, such as oxygen, carbon dioxide, steroid hormones, most anesthetics and alcohol, continue to move directly through the plasma membrane and, therefore, remain very permeable. Because the blood-brain barrier anatomically prevents the movement of materials between the cells, it is impermeable to water-soluble substances, such as glucose, amino acids and ions. These substances are exchanged between the blood and the extracellular fluid of the brain by way of highly selective membrane-bound protein carriers.

There are several benefits to the presence of this barrier. It protects the neurons of the CNS from fluctuations in plasma components. For example, a change in the K^+ ion concentration could alter neuronal function due to its effect on membrane potential. Second, the barrier minimizes the possibility that harmful blood-borne substances reach the CNS. Finally, it prevents any blood-borne substances that could function as neurotransmitters from reaching the brain and causing inappropriate neuronal stimulation.

The blood-brain barrier exists in all areas of the brain and spinal cord except the hypothalamus and some regions of the brainstem. The absence of the barrier in these regions coincides with the functions of the areas. For example, the hypothalamus contributes to homeostasis by monitoring the concentration of various blood-borne substances such as glucose and hormones. Glucose and amino acid-derived hormones are hydrophilic and would be unable to come into contact with hypothalamic neurons if the barrier were present. Another instance includes the vomit center of the medulla whose neurons detect the presence of potentially toxic substances in the blood. This center prevents the further absorption of these substances from the gastrointestinal tract by inducing vomiting. Once again, neurons in this region need to be exposed to any hydrophilic toxins in order to carry out this function.

PHARMACY APPLICATION: ANTIHISTAMINES AND THE BLOOD-BRAIN BARRIER

Antihistamine drugs have long been used to treat symptoms of allergy such as sneezing, itching, watery discharge from the eyes and nose and possibly wheezing. The older or first-generation histamine H_1 receptor antagonists such as Benadryl® and Tavist® effectively relieve

(Continued)

> **PHARMACY APPLICATION: ANTIHISTAMINES**
> **AND THE BLOOD-BRAIN BARRIER (Continued)**
>
> these peripheral symptoms. However, these medications, of the drug
> class ethanolamines, are very lipophilic and readily cross the blood-
> brain barrier to interact with histamine H_1 receptors in the CNS as well.
> As a result, they also cause central effects such as diminished alert-
> ness, slowed reaction times and sedation. The newer or nonsedating
> antihistamines such as Claritin® and Allegra® have been chemically
> designed to be less lipophilic and not cross the blood-brain barrier at
> therapeutic doses. Therefore, these medications, which are of the drug
> class piperidines, eliminate the peripheral symptoms of allergy with-
> out depressing CNS activity.

13.5   Cerebrospinal fluid

Embedded within the brain are four *ventricles* or chambers that form a continuous fluid-filled system. In the roof of each of these ventricles is a network
of capillaries referred to as the *choroid plexus*. It is from the choroid plexuses of
the two lateral ventricles (one in each cerebral hemisphere) that *cerebrospinal
fluid* is primarily derived. Due to the presence of the blood-brain barrier, the
selective transport processes of the choroid plexus determine the composition of the CSF. Therefore, the composition of the CSF is markedly different
from the composition of the plasma. However, the CSF is in equilibrium with
the interstitial fluid of the brain and contributes to the maintenance of a consistent chemical environment for the neurons, which serves to optimize their
function.

The CSF flows through the ventricles in a downward pattern through
the central canal of the spinal cord and then upward, back toward the brain
through the subarachnoid space surrounding the brain and spinal cord. As
the CSF flows over the superior surface of the brain, it leaves the subarachnoid space and is absorbed into the venous system. Although CSF is actively
secreted at a rate of 500 mL/day, the volume of this fluid in the system is
approximately 140 mL. Therefore, the entire volume of CSF is turned over
three to four times per day.

The one-way flow of the CSF and its constant turnover facilitate its
important function of *removing potentially harmful brain metabolites*. The CSF
also protects the brain from impact by serving as a *shock-absorbing system*
that lies between the brain and its bony capsule. Finally, because the brain
and the CSF have about the same specific gravity, the brain floats in this
fluid. This *reduces the effective weight of the brain* from 1,400 g to less than 50 g
and prevents compression of neurons on the inferior surface of the brain.

13.6   The spinal cord

The lowest level of the CNS, both anatomically and functionally, is the *spinal cord*. Continuous with the brainstem, the spinal cord exits the skull through the opening in the occipital bone called the *foramen magnum* and then passes through the *vertebral foramen* of each individual vertebra that form the vertebral column, to the level of the first or second lumbar vertebrae.

The spinal cord is divided into four anatomical regions: cervical, thoracic, lumbar, and sacral. These regions are named according to the vertebrae adjacent to them during embryonic development. Each region is further subdivided into 31 functional segments: 8 cervical (C) segments, 12 thoracic (T) segments, 5 lumbar (L) segments, 5 sacral (S) segments, and 1 coccygeal (Co) segment. A pair of spinal nerves extends from each segment, with 1 nerve from the left side of the spinal cord and 1 nerve from the right side. Spinal nerves exit the CNS through the *intervertebral foramina*, or openings, between adjacent vertebrae. There are 31 pairs of spinal nerves:

- 8 cervical
- 12 thoracic
- 5 lumbar
- 5 sacral
- 1 coccygeal

In terms of sensory input, each specific region of the body surface innervated by a given spinal nerve is referred to as a *dermatome.* These spinal nerves may also branch off and innervate a deeper internal organ as well. Dermatomes are highly organized and begin at the level of the head and proceed downward to the feet, and vary significantly in size and shape.

Spinal nerves arising from the *cervical level* of the spinal cord are involved with sensory perception and motor function and innervate dermatomes located at the back of the head, the neck and the arms. Nerves arising from the *thoracic level* innervate dermatomes found on the anterior surface of the trunk (chest and abdomen) as well as the upper back. Spinal nerves from the *lumbar region* innervate dermatomes of the lower back and the anterior surface of the legs and feet. Finally, spinal nerves from the *sacral region* of the cord innervate dermatomes located at the external genitalia, the buttocks, the posterior surface of the legs and the bottom of the feet.

Lesions of the spinal cord interrupt sensation and motor function. The affected regions of the body are those innervated by spinal nerves below the level of the lesion. For example, damage to the spinal cord at the functional level of T_{12}, or the twelfth thoracic spinal nerve, would result in paralysis and numbness of the lower back and legs. Interestingly, the phrenic nerves, which innervate the diaphragm, the major muscle of inspiration, arise from spinal cord segments C_3 through C_5. Therefore, only lesions high in the cervical region will affect breathing.

The human spinal cord and the vertebral column initially grow at the same rate during embryonic development. In this way, the spinal segments and the vertebral bones for which they are named are aligned. Therefore, the spinal nerves emerge from the vertebral column through the intervertebral foramina at the same level as the spinal cord segment from which they arise. However, after the third month of gestation, each vertebral bone becomes larger compared with the associated spinal segment. Therefore, the vertebral column grows approximately 25 cm longer than the spinal cord. (This explains why the spinal cord extends only as far as the upper lumbar vertebrae.) Thus, the spinal cord segment from which each pair of spinal nerves arise is no longer aligned with its associated vertebral bone. Because the vertebral column is now longer than the spinal cord, the intervertebral foramina have shifted downward relative to their corresponding spinal cord segment. Therefore, the spinal nerve roots arising from each segment must extend downward through the vertebral canal to reach their points of exit. This is the case for the spinal nerves arising from the lumbar and sacral regions of the cord. Only spinal nerve roots are found in the vertebral canal below the level of the first or second lumbar vertebrae. Because of its appearance, this bundle of nerve roots is collectively referred to as the *cauda equina*, or "horse's tail." A sample of cerebrospinal fluid may be obtained from this region by way of a *lumbar puncture* or "spinal tap." A needle may be safely inserted into the vertebral canal without the possibility of penetrating the spinal cord. The spinal nerve roots are easily pushed aside by the needle, significantly reducing the possibility of puncturing one of these nerves.

The spinal nerves associate with the spinal cord by way of two branches, or roots:

- Dorsal root
- Ventral root

The *dorsal root* contains afferent, or sensory, neurons. Impulses in these neurons travel from peripheral tissues toward the spinal cord. The dorsal root joins the spinal cord laterally, toward the posterior surface of the cord (Figure 13.5). The *ventral root* contains efferent, or motor, neurons. Impulses in these neurons travel away from the spinal cord toward the peripheral tissues. The ventral root exits the spinal cord laterally, toward the anterior surface of the cord.

It is important to note that a *nerve* is defined as a bundle of neuronal axons; some are afferent and some are efferent. A nerve does not consist of entire neurons, only their axons. Furthermore, nerves are found only in the peripheral nervous system. Bundles of neurons with similar functions located within the CNS are referred to as *tracts*. Therefore, technically speaking, there are no nerves within the brain or within the spinal cord.

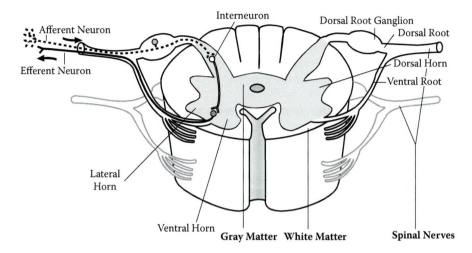

Figure 13.5 Cross-sectional view of the spinal cord. In contrast to the brain, the gray matter of the spinal cord is located internally, surrounded by the white matter. The gray matter consists of nerve cell bodies and unmyelinated interneuron fibers. This component of the spinal cord is divided into three regions, the dorsal horn, the lateral horn and the ventral horn. The white matter consists of bundles of myelinated axons of neurons, or tracts. Each segment of the spinal cord gives rise to a pair of spinal nerves. These nerves contain both afferent and efferent neurons. Afferent neurons enter the spinal cord through the dorsal root and efferent neurons exit the spinal cord through the ventral root.

13.6.1   Functions of the spinal cord

The spinal cord is responsible for two vital CNS functions:

- *Conducts nerve impulses* to and from the brain
- Processes sensory input from the skin, joints and muscles of the trunk and limbs and *initiates reflex responses* to this input

13.6.1.1   Composition of the spinal cord
The spinal cord consists of the following:

- Gray matter
- White matter

The *gray matter* is composed of nerve cell bodies and unmyelinated interneurons. The location of the gray matter in the spinal cord is opposite to that of the brain. In the brain, the gray matter of the cerebrum and the cerebellum is found externally forming a cortex, or covering, over the internally located white matter. In the spinal cord, the gray matter is found internally and is surrounded by the white matter.

A cross-sectional view of the spinal cord reveals that the gray matter has an H-shape (also referred to a butterfly shape) (see Figure 13.4) and is divided into three regions called horns.

- Dorsal horn (posterior, toward the back)
- Ventral horn (anterior, toward the front)
- Lateral horn (toward the side)

There are 1 billion neurons in the human spinal cord. Accordingly, each spinal segment contains millions of neurons within the gray matter. Functionally, there are four types of neurons:

- Second-order sensory neurons
- Somatic motor neurons
- Visceral motor neurons
- Interneurons

The cell bodies of *second-order sensory neurons* are found in the dorsal horn. These neurons receive input from afferent neurons (*first-order sensory neurons*) entering the CNS from the periphery of the body through the dorsal root of the spinal nerve. The function of the second-order sensory neuron is to transmit nerve impulses to higher levels in the CNS. The axons of these neurons leave the gray matter and travel upward in the appropriate ascending tracts of the white matter.

The cell bodies of *somatic motor neurons* are found in the ventral horn. The axons of these neurons exit the CNS through the ventral root of the spinal nerve and innervate skeletal muscles. There are two types of motor neurons located in the ventral horn:

- *Alpha motor neurons*: innervate skeletal muscle fibers to cause contraction
- *Gamma motor neurons*: innervate intrafusal fibers of the muscle spindle to cause contraction, which allows the muscle spindle to remain sensitive to changes in muscle length

The spatial organization of the cell bodies of the motor neurons follows a *proximal-distal rule*. Motor neurons that innervate the most proximal muscles (axial muscles of the neck and trunk) lie most medially in the gray matter. Motor neurons that innervate the most distal muscles (wrists, ankles, digits) lie most laterally in the gray matter.

The cell bodies of *visceral motor neurons* are found in the lateral horn. The axons of these neurons form the efferent nerve fibers of the autonomic nervous system (ANS). The ANS innervates cardiac muscle, smooth muscle and glands (see Chapter 14). The axons of these neurons exit the spinal cord by way of the ventral root.

Numerous *interneurons* are found in all areas of the gray matter of the spinal cord. These neurons are small, unmyelinated, and highly excitable. Interneurons receive input from higher levels of the CNS as well as from sensory neurons entering the CNS through the spinal nerves. Many inter- neurons in the spinal cord synapse with motor neurons in the ventral horn. These interconnections are responsible for the integrative functions of the spinal cord including reflexes.

Afferent neurons that transmit sensory information toward the spinal cord are referred to as *first-order sensory neurons*. The cell bodies of these neurons are found in the *dorsal root ganglia*. These ganglia form a swelling in each of the dorsal roots just outside of the spinal cord. The portion of the axon between the distal receptor and the cell body is referred to as the *peripheral axon* and the portion of the axon between the cell body and the axon terminal within the CNS is referred to as the *central axon*.

Upon entering the spinal cord, the first-order sensory neurons may enter the gray matter. The neurons may then synapse with one or more of the fol- lowing neurons:

- Second-order sensory neuron: transmits impulses to higher levels of the CNS
- Alpha motor neuron: transmits impulses to skeletal muscles
- Interneurons: transmits impulses to motor neurons

Synapses between the first-order sensory neurons and the alpha motor neurons, either directly or by way of interneurons, result in spinal cord reflexes. Reflexes are discussed in more detail in a subsequent Section 13.6.2, Spinal reflexes.

Alternatively, the first-order sensory neurons may initially enter the white matter of the spinal cord. In this case, the axons of these neurons may ascend the cord to the medulla or travel up or down the cord to a different spinal segment. Upon reaching its destination, the axon then enters the gray matter of the spinal cord and synapses with one or more of the neurons discussed above.

The *white matter* of the spinal cord consists of the myelinated axons of neurons. These axons may travel up the spinal cord to a higher spinal seg- ment or to the brain, whereas other axons may travel down the spinal cord to a lower spinal segment. The axons of neurons that carry similar types of impulses are bundled together to form tracts. *Ascending tracts* carry sensory information from the spinal cord toward the brain. *Descending tracts* carry motor impulses from the brain toward the interneurons of the spinal cord or the motor neurons in the lateral or ventral horns of the spinal cord gray matter. In general, these tracts are named based on their origin and termi- nation. For example, the ventral spinocerebellar tract is an ascending tract carrying information regarding unconscious muscle sense (proprioception) from the spinal cord to the cerebellum. On the other hand, the ventral corticospinal tract is a descending tract carrying information regarding voluntary muscle control from the cerebral cortex to the spinal cord.

13.6.1.2   Ascending tracts

Ascending tracts contain three successive neurons:

- First-order neurons
- Second-order neurons
- Third-order neurons

The *first-order neuron* is the afferent neuron that transmits impulses from a peripheral receptor toward the CNS. Its cell body is found in the dorsal root ganglion. A first-order neuron synapses with the *second-order neuron* whose cell body is located in the dorsal horn of the spinal cord or in the medulla of the brainstem. The second-order neuron then synapses with the *third-order neuron* whose cell body is found in the thalamus. Limited processing of sensory information takes place in the thalamus. Finally, the third-order neuron terminates in the somatosensory cortex where more complex, cortical processing begins.

All ascending tracts cross to the opposite side of the CNS. For example, sensory input entering the left side of the spinal cord ultimately terminates on the right side of the cerebral cortex. These tracts may cross at the level of entry into the spinal cord, a few segments above the level of entry, or within the medulla of the brainstem. The locations of specific ascending tracts are illustrated in Figure 13.6.

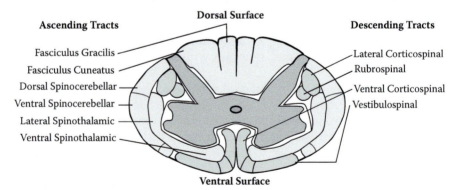

Figure 13.6   Ascending and descending tracts in the white matter of the spinal cord. Tracts are formed of bundles of neuronal axons that transmit similar types of information.

PHARMACY APPLICATION: SPINAL ANESTHESIA

The injection of a local form of anesthetic into the cerebrospinal fluid surrounding the spinal cord causes spinal anesthesia. This injection is made below the level of the second lumbar vertebra and is used to minimize direct nerve trauma. Spinal anesthesia is effective in the control of pain during lower body surgical procedures, such as knee surgery. Currently, the drugs most commonly used in the United States include lidocaine, bupivacaine, and tetracaine. The choice of anesthetic is determined by the duration of anesthesia required. Lidocaine is used for short procedures; bupivacaine is chosen for procedures of intermediate length, and tetracaine is used for procedures of long duration.

The mechanism of action of these anesthetics involves the blockade of Na^+ channels in the membrane of the second-order sensory neuron. The binding site for these anesthetics is on a subunit of the Na^+ channel located near the internal surface of the cell membrane. Therefore, the agent must enter the neuron in order to effectively block the Na^+ channel. Without the influx of sodium, neurons cannot depolarize and generate an action potential (see Chapter 4). Therefore, the second-order sensory neuron cannot be stimulated by impulses elicited by pain receptors associated with the first-order sensory neuron. In other words, the pain signal is effectively interrupted at the level of the spinal cord and does not travel any higher in the CNS. In this way, the brain does not perceive pain.

Interestingly, the second-order sensory neurons are the neurons of the spinal cord gray matter that are most susceptible to the effects of spinal anesthesia. These neurons have a small diameter and are unmyelinated. The small diameter allows the drug to locate its binding site on the Na^+ channel more readily due to a higher concentration of the drug within the neuron. Furthermore, unmyelinated neurons have a greater number of Na^+ channels located over a larger surface area. Alpha motor neurons in the ventral horn are susceptible to these anesthetics only at high doses. This is because alpha motor neurons have a large diameter and are myelinated. The larger diameter results in a lower concentration of the drug within the neuron. Myelination limits the number and availability of Na^+ channels upon which the anesthetic can exert its effect.

13.6.1.3 Descending tracts

Voluntary movement of skeletal muscles is controlled by two types of descending tracts. Neurons in both tracts terminate on and influence the activity of the alpha motor neurons in the ventral horn. The two types of tracts include:

- Corticospinal (pyramidal) tracts
- Multineuronal (extrapyramidal) tracts

The *corticospinal (pyramidal) tracts* originate in the cerebral cortex. Due to their triangular shape, the neurons of the primary motor cortex are referred to as *pyramidal cells*. Most of the axons of these neurons descend directly to the alpha motor neurons in the spinal cord. In other words, these are primarily monosynaptic pathways. This type of synaptic connection is particularly important for the movement of individual fingers. A primary function of these tracts is to regulate fine, discrete, voluntary movements of the hands and fingers. Recall the extensive area of the cerebral cortex devoted to the hands and fingers, which indicates the density of innervation of the muscles in these tissues.

Another descending pathway that accompanies the corticospinal tracts is the *corticobulbar pathway*. This pathway begins in the cerebral cortex and travels to the brainstem (bulbar, pertaining to the brainstem). This pathway influences the neurons that innervate muscles of the eyes, face, tongue and throat. As such, the corticobulbar pathway is the primary source of control for voluntary movement of the head and neck.

As with the ascending tracts, descending tracts cross from one side of the CNS to the other. Most of the tracts cross over in the medulla of the brainstem. Therefore, the right side of the brain influences the activity of the alpha motor neurons and, therefore, the skeletal muscles on the left side of the body.

The *multineuronal (extrapyramidal) tracts* originate in many regions of the brain including the motor regions of the cerebral cortex, the cerebellum, and the basal ganglia. Impulses from these various regions are transmitted to nuclei in the brainstem, in particular, the reticular formation and the vestibular nuclei. The axons of neurons in these nuclei descend to the alpha motor neurons in the spinal cord. Therefore, in contrast to the corticospinal tracts, these pathways are polysynaptic. The multineuronal tracts regulate overall body posture, balance and walking. Specifically, these tracts control subconscious movements of large muscle groups in the trunk and in the limbs. Some of the pathways originating in the brainstem cross to the other side of the spinal cord to affect muscles on the opposite side of the body. However, most remain uncrossed (e.g., vestibulospinal tract, Table 13.5).

These two types of descending motor tracts do not function in isolation. They are extensively interconnected and cooperate in the control of movement. For example, to be able to grasp a doorknob to open a door, there needs to be subconscious positioning of the body to face the door (multineuronal tracts) and extension of the arm toward the doorknob (corticospinal tracts).

The locations of specific descending tracts are illustrated in Figure 13.5. A summary of the functions of each of these tracts is found in Table 13.5.

Table 13.5 Ascending and descending tracts in the white matter of the spinal cord

Ascending pathway	Function
Fasciculus Gracilis	Fine touch discrimination (ability to recognize the size, shape, and texture of objects and their movement across the skin), proprioception, vibration from legs and lower trunk; crossed
Fasciculus Cuneatus	Fine touch discrimination, proprioception, vibration from neck, arms, upper trunk; crossed
Dorsal Spinocerebellar	Proprioception (important for muscle tone and posture); uncrossed
Ventral Spinocerebellar	Proprioception; crossed
Lateral Spinothalamic	Pain, temperature; crossed
Ventral Spinothalamic	Light touch, pressure; crossed

Descending pathway	Function
Lateral Corticospinal	Voluntary control of skeletal muscles; crossed
Rubrospinal	Originates in brainstem, subconscious control of skeletal muscle (muscle tone, posture); crossed
Ventral Corticospinal	Voluntary control of skeletal muscles; uncrossed
Vestibulospinal	Originates in brainstem, subconscious control of skeletal muscle (muscle tone, balance, equilibrium); uncrossed

PHARMACY APPLICATION: EPIDURAL ANESTHESIA

Epidural anesthesia is administered by injecting local anesthetic into the epidural space. Located outside of the spinal cord on its dorsal surface, the epidural space contains fat and is highly vascular. Therefore, this form of anesthesia can be administered safely at any level of the spinal cord. Furthermore, a catheter may be placed into the epidural space, allowing for either continuous infusions or repeated bolus administrations of anesthetic.

The primary site of action of epidurally administered agents is on the spinal nerve roots. As with spinal anesthesia, the choice of drug to be used is determined primarily by the duration of anesthesia desired. However, when a catheter has been placed, short-acting drugs can be administered repeatedly. Bupivacaine is typically used when a long duration of surgical block is needed. Lidocaine is used most often for intermediate length procedures. Chloroprocaine is used when only a very short duration of anesthesia is required.

(Continued)

PHARMACY APPLICATION: EPIDURAL ANESTHESIA (Continued)

An important difference between epidural anesthesia and spinal anesthesia is that agents injected into the epidural space may readily enter the blood due to the presence of a rich *venous plexus* in this area. This is an important consideration when epidural anesthesia is used to control pain during labor and delivery. The agents used are capable of crossing the placenta to enter the fetal circulation and exert a depressant effect on the neonate.

13.6.2   Spinal reflexes

This section will examine the mechanism of simple spinal reflexes that control skeletal muscles.

Reflexes may be classified in several ways and may be named according to the effector tissues that carry out the reflex response:

- *Skeletal muscle reflexes*: control skeletal muscles
- *Autonomic reflexes*: control cardiac muscle, smooth muscle and glands

Other reflexes are named pertaining to the region of the CNS that integrates incoming sensory information and elicits the reflex response:

- *Cranial reflexes*: processed within the brain
- *Spinal reflexes*: processed at the level of the spinal cord

Finally, reflexes may be either classified as either innate or learned:

- *Simple* or *basic reflexes*: preprogrammed (built-in), unlearned responses (e.g., blinking, pulling a hand from a hot surface)
- *Acquired* or *conditioned reflexes*: learned responses that require experience or training (e.g., driving a car, catching a ball)

A reflex occurs when a stimulus elicits an automatic, involuntary response—a response that occurs without conscious effort. Reflexes are specific and predicable, and purposeful. For example, the withdrawal reflex causes a body part to be pulled away from a painful stimulus. In this way, tissue injury is avoided.

Spinal reflexes require no input from the brain because they are elicited entirely at the level of the spinal cord. However, while the reflex is underway, nervous impulses are transmitted to the brain for further processing. In fact, input from the brain may modulate a reflex, or alter the response to a stimulus through conscious effort.

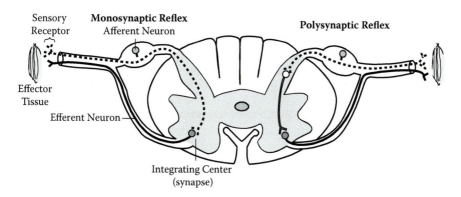

Figure 13.7   Components of a reflex arc. As illustrated by the components of the reflex arc, reflexes may be processed entirely at the level of the spinal cord with no need for input from the brain. A monosynaptic reflex has a single synapse between the afferent and the efferent neurons. A polysynaptic reflex has two or more synapses between the afferent and efferent neurons. In this case, interneurons lie between the sensory and motor neurons. The more interneurons involved, the more complex the response.

A reflex response requires an intact neural pathway that connects the stimulated area and the responding muscle and is referred to as a *reflex arc*. All reflex arcs include the following components (see Figure 13.7):

- Sensory receptor
- Afferent or first-order sensory neuron
- Integrating center in the spinal cord (synapses)
- Efferent or motor neuron
- Effector tissue (skeletal muscle)

A reflex is initiated by the stimulation of a *sensory receptor* located at the peripheral end of an afferent or first-order sensory neuron. This *afferent neuron* transmits impulses to the gray matter of the spinal cord, which serves as an *integrating center* for the sensory input. It is within the gray matter that the afferent neuron will synapse with a neuron. When the afferent neuron synapses directly with an efferent or *motor neuron*, it forms a *monosynaptic reflex*. An example of this type of reflex is the stretch reflex. When the afferent neuron synapses with an interneuron, which then synapses with the motor neuron, it forms a *polysynaptic reflex*. An example of this type of reflex is the withdrawal reflex. Most reflexes are polysynaptic. The motor neuron then exits the spinal cord to innervate an *effector tissue* that carries out the reflex response.

13.6.2.1   Withdrawal reflex
The *withdrawal reflex* is elicited by a painful or tissue-damaging stimulus. The response is to quickly move the body part away from the source of the

stimulus, usually by flexing a limb. Any of the major joints and, therefore, muscle groups, may be involved in a reflex depending upon the point of stimulation. For example, all joints of a limb are involved when a digit, such as a finger, is stimulated (e.g., finger, wrist, elbow, shoulder). Withdrawal reflexes are powerful reflexes and may override other nervous impulses, such as those regarding locomotion, or walking.

An example of the mechanism of the withdrawal reflex is illustrated in Figure 13.8. When a painful stimulus activates a sensory receptor on the right foot, action potentials are transmitted along the afferent neuron to the spinal cord. By way of divergence, this neuron synapses with several other neurons within the gray matter of the spinal cord:

- Excitatory interneuron
- Inhibitory interneuron
- Second-order sensory neuron

The *excitatory interneuron* then synapses with the alpha motor neuron that innervates the *flexor muscles* of the right leg. Consequently, stimulation of the excitatory interneuron leads to stimulation of the alpha motor neuron, which

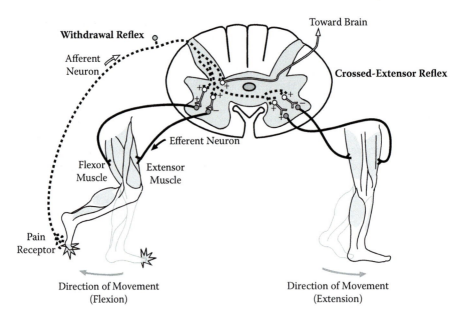

Figure 13.8 The withdrawal reflex coupled with the crossed-extensor reflex. A painful stimulus will elicit the withdrawal reflex. This reflex causes flexor muscles to contract and move the affected body part away from the stimulus. At the same time, the crossed-extensor reflex causes extensor muscles in the opposite limb to contract.

then stimulates the flexor muscles to contract and pick up or withdraw the foot from the painful stimulus.

The *inhibitory interneuron* synapses with the alpha motor neuron that innervates the *extensor muscles* of the right leg. Therefore, stimulation of the inhibitory interneuron leads to the inhibition of the alpha motor neuron and the extensor muscles relax.

The flexor muscles and the extensor muscles are *antagonistic*. In other words, they cause opposite effects. Therefore, when one of these groups of muscles is activated, the other group must be inhibited. This is referred to as *reciprocal inhibition*. In this way, activation of the withdrawal reflex leads to unimpeded flexion.

The *second-order sensory neuron* transmits impulses ultimately to the left side of the brain. This permits the awareness of pain, the identification of its source and, if necessary, postural adjustment. As discussed, impulses in this pathway do not play a role in the reflex per se.

13.6.2.2 Crossed-extensor reflex

Where appropriate, the withdrawal reflex may be accompanied by the *crossed-extensor reflex*. In the example discussed, when the right leg is flexed or lifted, the left leg must be extended or straightened to support the body. In addition to stimulating interneurons on the right side of the spinal cord to influence skeletal muscle activity on the right side of the body, the afferent neuron may also stimulate interneurons on the left side of the spinal cord to influence skeletal muscle activity on the left side of the body. Once again, both excitatory and inhibitory interneurons are involved. However, in this case, these interneurons influence the activity of the opposite muscle groups. Stimulation of the excitatory interneuron on the left side of the spinal cord leads to the stimulation of the alpha motor neuron that innervates the extensor muscles. This causes the left leg to straighten. Stimulation of the inhibitory interneuron on the left side of the spinal cord leads to the inhibition of the alpha motor neuron that innervates the flexor muscles. This results in unimpeded extension of the left leg and the support of the body during the withdrawal of the right leg.

13.7 Disorders of the nervous system

Disorders of neural function include those conditions that affect the brain, spinal cord and associated nerves. Such disorders may include traumatic injury, hypoxic injury, infections, tumors, neurodegenerative diseases and seizure disorders. Injuries to the spinal cord are also discussed.

13.7.1 Disorders of the brain

13.7.1.1 Brain injury

Injury to the brain can result from a number of factors including trauma, increased intracranial pressure, ischemia, stroke, infection, and tumors.

13.7.1.2   Traumatic brain injury

Various injuries to the head such as blunt force trauma, skull fractures, whiplash and penetrating wounds can result in traumatic brain injury. Because the brain floats freely within the skull, blunt force trauma to the head can cause the brain to bang against the skull as it accelerates and decelerates within the brain case. *Contusions* or bruises of brain tissue can occur in regions of the brain that impact the skull. Small contusions may cause limited clinical symptoms, whereas large contusions may produce significant neurologic defects. Traumatic brain injury may also be associated with damaged cerebral blood vessels and bleeding around or into the brain, leading to the formation of intracranial *hematomas*.

CONCUSSION

- A temporary alteration of neurologic function that can occur following a blow to the head. Most patients suffering a concussion remain conscious. Concussions require time to fully heal and are generally not associated with long-term neurologic deficits if they are mild. However, the cumulative effect of multiple concussions can be permanent neurologic deficit.

13.7.1.3   Intracranial hematoma

An intracranial hematoma is a collection of blood that occurs in or around the brain, often as a result of a head injury. Hematomas may cause injury to brain tissue because they can compress the brain and increase intracranial pressure. There are three main types of intracranial hematomas: (Figure 13.9)

1. *Epidural hematoma:*
   - Occurs when blood accumulates between the covering of the brain (the *dura mater*) and the brain tissue.
   - Because the bleeding is often the result of an arterial tear, epidural hematoma may compress brain tissue and lead to neurologic deficits.
   - Patients generally remain conscious during the early stages but progressively become drowsy and unresponsive if the bleeding continues.
2. *Subdural hematoma:*
   - Occurs when blood accumulates between the *dura mater* and brain tissue.
   - Generally involves damage to bridging veins and, as a result, the subdural hematoma develops more slowly than an epidural hematoma.

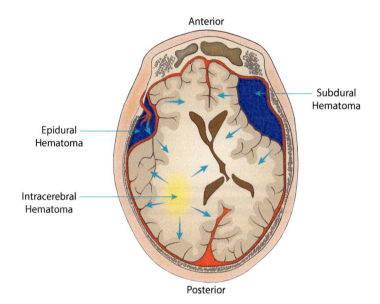

Anterior

Subdural
Hematoma

Epidural
Hematoma

Intracerebral
Hematoma

Posterior

Figure 13.9 Types of intracranial hematomas: (a) Epidural; (b) Subdural; (c) Intracerebral.

- Subdural hematomas are subclassified as:
  - *Acute*—symptoms generally occur within 24 hours. Associated with high mortality rates due to a rapid rise in intracranial pressure.
  - *Subacute*—symptoms may take days to weeks to occur. A period of symptom improvement may be followed by rapid deterioration if the hematoma is not treated.
  - *Chronic*—caused by a slow leakage of blood. Symptoms may take weeks to occur and, as a result, patients may not recall the head injury that was originally responsible for triggering the bleed.
3. *Intracerebral or intraparenchymal hematoma:*
  - Occurs when blood accumulates within the brain tissue.
  - More common in elderly patients whose cerebral vessels are more fragile.
  - May be associated with white matter shear injuries and torn neuronal axons.
  - Clinical symptoms depend upon the size and location of the hematoma as well as its effect on intracranial pressure.

13.7.1.4 Increased intracranial pressure

The skull contains the brain matter (~80%), cerebrospinal fluid (CSF, ~10%) and blood (~10%). Each of these components contributes to the overall intracranial pressure (ICP). The normal intracranial pressure is approximately 5–15 mm Hg. According to the *Monroe–Kellie Hypothesis*, expansion of any of one of the elements within the skull (i.e., brain matter, blood or CSF) must be offset by a concomitant compression of the other elements within the skull. Because an intact skull is rigid and inexpandable, significant accumulations of fluid or blood will cause an increase in the intracranial pressure, which in turn can compress and injure brain tissue. Increases in ICP are associated with conditions such as hemorrhagic stroke, ruptured aneurysm, head trauma, encepha-

---

HYDROCEPHALUS

- A condition associated with the accumulation of excess fluids in the brain.
- The condition may be caused by excess production of CSF or a blockage of the CSF outflow.
- Other causes of hydrocephalus include meningitis, head injury, tumors, and subarachnoid hemorrhage.

---

litis, meningitis, status epilepticus, and hydrocephalus (see box).

13.7.1.5 Symptoms of increased ICP

- Severe headache
- Impaired consciousness
- Lethargy
- Vomiting without nausea
- Papilledema (edema of the optic disk)
- Neurologic defects, including weakness, numbness, vision effects
- *Cheyne–Stokes respiration*—breathing pattern characterized by cycles of apnea followed by deep, labored breathing. Likely occurs when CO_2 accumulates in the brain and begins to drive the breathing patterns.

13.7.1.6 Treatment of increased ICP

Medical management of increased ICP may include sedation, surgical drainage of accumulated fluid, and perfusion of the brain with the osmotic diuretic mannitol. If possible, the underlying cause of the increased ICP must be addressed as well.

13.7.1.7 Brain ischemia and hypoxia

The brain is a one of the most metabolic active organs in the body. Despite accounting for only 2% of the total body mass, the brain utilizes over 20% of the body's total oxygen consumption. Glucose is the major fuel for the brain. However, little glucose is actually stored in the brain and, as a result, the majority of glucose used by the brain must be supplied by circulation. The highly metabolic nature of the brain makes it very susceptible to injury from ischemia and hypoxia. Because the brain does not store significant quantities of oxygen or glucose, the brain becomes deficient in both within minutes of blood flow cessation. Various regions of the brain are more or less susceptible to the effects of ischemia and hypoxia. Regions with highly active neurons are more susceptible to such injury based on their greater demand for oxygen and glucose. Brain neurons further from blood vessels or those in "watershed" areas supplied by distal branches of cerebral blood vessels are particularly vulnerable to ischemic injury when brain perfusion pressures are low.

13.7.1.8 Causes of brain ischemia or hypoxia

- Impairment of cerebral blood flow—e.g., occlusive stroke, atherosclerosis of carotid arteries
- Shock or reduced cardiac output
- Severe anemia, increased CO_2 or CO exposure
- Severe pulmonary or cardiovascular disease

13.7.1.9 Manifestations of cerebral ischemia or hypoxia

- *Cellular effects*:
    - A shift to anaerobic metabolism that can lead to lactic acid accumulation and acidosis
    - Lack of ATP, which in turn may impair function of energy-dependent ion pumps (i.e., Na^+- and Ca^{++}-ATPases) and lead to electrolyte imbalances
    - Neurotransmitter imbalance—the normal balance between excitatory (i.e., glutamate) neurotransmitters and inhibitory neurotransmitters is lost and may result in "excitotoxicity"
    - Calcium accumulation that can activate various calcium-dependent enzymes that can damage cellular components
    - Free radical accumulation
- *Clinical manifestations*:
    - Impaired sensory, motor, and autonomic functions
    - Loss of consciousness

COMA

- Coma is a condition of prolonged unconsciousness
- Coma is associated with brain injury that may result from many factors, including head injury, brain tumors, stroke, drug or alcohol intoxication, and infections
- A coma generally last less than several weeks
- Patients in a coma may exhibit varying degrees of responsiveness that may be prognostic indicators of eventual outcome (see Glasgow Coma Scale) (Table 13.6)
- Patients with a coma lasting weeks to months may transition to a persistent vegetative state with a poor prognosis

---

13.7.2   Stroke

Strokes are also referred to as cerebral vascular accidents (CVAs). According to the Centers for Disease Control and Prevention (CDC) 795,000 individuals in the United States have strokes each year and nearly 130,000 Americans each year will die from them. The most common form of stroke (87%) is

Table 13.6   Glasgow coma scale

Test	Score
Eye(s) Opening	4
• Spontaneous	3
• To speech	2
• To pain	1
• No response	
Verbal Response	5
• Oriented to time, place, person	4
• Confused/disoriented	3
• Inappropriate words	2
• Incomprehensible sounds	1
• No response	
Motor Response	6
• Obeys commands	5
• Moves in response to localized pain	4
• Flexion withdraws from pain	3
• Abnormal flexion	2
• Abnormal extension	1
• No response	
Best Response	15
Comatose	8 or less
Totally Unresponsive	3 or less

Table 13.7 Risk factors for stroke

Nonmodifiable
- Increasing age
- Female sex—because females live longer than males, they are more likely to die from stroke
- Family history
- Black or Hispanic race

Modifiable
- Hypertension—the higher the blood pressure, the greater the risk for stroke
- Dyslipidemia
- Smoking
- Obesity
- Diabetes mellitus
- Increased risk for blood clots—atrial fibrillation, DVT, immobility

"occlusive" or "ischemic" stroke, which is caused by a blockage of blood flow to the brain. Occlusive strokes may result from an embolism that lodges in the cerebral vasculature of from a thrombus that forms *in situ*. Complete occlusion of cerebral blood vessels will lead to injury and death of neuronal tissue. Transient ischemic attacks (TIAs) or "mini-strokes" lasting several minutes may also occur as a result of a developing thrombus or transient occlusion by thrombotic particle. The remainder of strokes are hemorrhagic in nature meaning they are caused by bleeding into the brain. Causes of hemorrhagic stroke include a ruptured cerebral aneurysm or damage to blood vessels. Table 13.7 lists risk factor for stroke.

ATRIAL FIBRILLATION AND STROKE RISK

Atrial fibrillation is an atrial arrhythmia that affects over 2 million individuals each year in the United States. The abnormal atrial contractions that accompany this condition can lead to pooling of blood in the atria, where it can form a clot. If this clot is ejected from the heart, it can travel through the circulation and lodge in the cerebral vasculature to cause an occlusive stroke

---

13.7.2.1 Symptoms of stroke
Occlusive stroke:
- Symptoms develop progressively as the ischemia progresses
- Numbness on one side (hemiparesis)
- Confusion
- Difficulty speaking
- Blurred vision

- Loss of coordination
- Difficulty walking

Hemorrhagic stroke:
- Symptoms develop rapidly
- Excruciating headache
- Loss of consciousness

13.7.2.2 Complications of stroke

Disabilities caused by a stroke may be temporary or permanent and may include:

- Paralysis
- Difficulty talking
- Difficulty swallowing (dysphagia)
- Memory loss, cognitive difficulties
- Pain, paresthesia
- Emotional changes

13.7.2.3 Diagnosis of stroke

- Symptoms
- CT scan
- MRI

13.7.2.4 Treatment of stroke

- With an occlusive stroke, "time is brain." The more rapidly blood flow is restored, the greater the possibility of preserving brain function. Hemorrhagic stroke must be ruled out before clot-dissolving drugs or aspirin are used.
- Fibrinolytic drugs such as tissue plasminogen activator (tPA) may be use (ideally within 3 hours) to dissolve any clots that may be present and restore blood flow
- Aspirin may be given immediately to inhibit platelet aggregation and prevent the formation of additional clots
- For hemorrhagic stroke, drugs may be administered to lower intracranial pressure or blood pressure. Surgery may be required or surgical shunts implanted to remove accumulated blood and reduce intracranial pressure.

13.7.3 CNS infections

Infections of the CNS may be bacterial or viral in origin and target the meninges (*meningitis*), brain tissue (*encephalitis*) or spinal cord (*myelitis*). Bacterial meningitis is a common CNS infection. Organisms such as *Streptococcus pneumoniae, Hemophilus influenzae,* and *Nisseria meningitides* may cause acute forms of meningitis. Chronic forms of meningitis may be associated with syphilis, Lyme disease or advanced tuberculosis and may also affect adjacent brain tissue. Most cases of encephalitis are viral in origin and may be caused by viruses such as herpes simplex virus, West Nile virus, arborvirus, and rabies virus.

(a) Around the brain

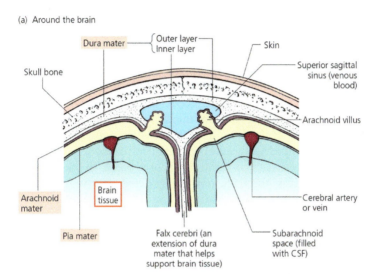

Note: Arachnoid and pia mater are connected by a network of bridging strands (called trabeculae) that help to maintain the patency of the subarachnoid space

(b) Around the spinal cord

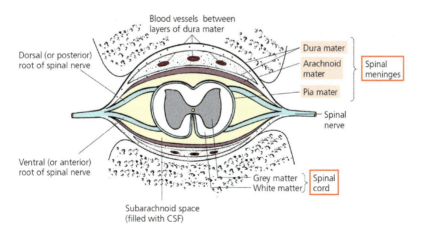

13.7.3.1   Manifestations of CNS infections

- Common symptoms of bacterial meningitis include fever, chills, stiff neck, headache, nausea and vomiting, confusion, light sensitivity, seizures. Long-term effects of untreated bacterial meningitis may be brain damage, seizures, hearing loss, and permanent neurologic deficits. Viral meningitis presents with similar symptoms as bacterial meningitis but usually has a less severe outcome and is often self-limiting.
- Common symptoms of encephalitis include fever, headache, muscle aches, fatigue, and weakness. More serious symptoms may include hallucinations, paralysis, altered vision, seizures, and unconsciousness.

13.7.3.2   Diagnosis of CNS infections

Blood samples may be drawn to culture for a suspected bacterial pathogen. A definitive diagnosis of bacterial meningitis is made by lumbar puncture and subsequent analysis of the CSF. In patients with meningitis, the CSF is often cloudy and contains large numbers of neutrophils along with increased levels of protein and decreased concentrations of glucose. In the case of viral meningitis or encephalitis, the CSF may be collected and analyzed for the presence of a specific virus. With viral meningitis, the CSF generally contains only modest elevations of protein, glucose levels may be normal and infiltration is often with lymphocytes instead of neutrophils.

13.7.3.3   Treatment of CNS infections

Treatment of bacterial CNS infections requires antibiotic therapy. Treatment should not be delayed until a definitive identification of the organism is made, but rather should begin as soon as possible with a broad-spectrum antibiotic with good CNS penetration (i.e., third generation cephalosporin). Treatment of viral encephalitis is mainly supportive and directed at treating any seizures that may occur and preventing increases in intracranial pressure.

MAD COW DISEASE

More accurately known as *bovine spongiform encephalopathy*, it is caused by transmission of a *prion*, which is a normal protein that is structurally modified. The first cases were identified in the 1970s and were linked to feeding of cattle with meat and bone meal from prion-infected sheep.

13.7.4   CNS tumors

Tumors in the brain can only arise from mitotic cells such as oligodendrocytes, Schwann cells, astrocytes and ependymal cells. According to the

American Brain Tumor Association (http://www.abta.org/about-us/news/brain-tumor-statistics/) nearly 70,000 new cases of brain tumor are diagnosed each year. Brain and other CNS tumors are the most common cancers among children 0–19 years of age. The majority of primary brain tumors occur within the meninges, with the second greatest incidence occurring in the various lobes of the cerebral cortex.

13.7.4.1 Type of CNS tumors

13.7.4.1.1 Glial cell tumors Fall into two categories, *astrocytoma* and *oligodendrogliomas:*

- *Astrocytoma:*
    - Tumor arising from the astrocytes. Represents 30% of brain tumors, 80% of malignant tumors
    - Most commonly found in the cerebral hemispheres
    - Progression and prognosis is affected by the degree of anaplasia the tumor cells exhibit. The least differentiated and most aggressive form is the *glioblastoma multiforme.*
- *Oligodendrogliomas:*
    - Tumor arising from the oligodendrocytes
    - Represent 2% of all primary brain tumors. Most common in middle life
    - Prognosis is highly variable and depends upon the location of the tumor and degree of anaplasia.
- *Ependymoma*
    - Tumor derived from the endothelial ependymal cells that line the ventricles and central canal of the spinal cord
    - Most likely to occur early in life
    - Prognosis depends upon the degree of anaplasia and location of the tumor
- *Meningioma*
    - Tumor that develops from cells in the arachnoid membrane
    - Most commonly occur in middle-to-later life
    - Often benign, slow growing, good prognosis

13.7.4.2 Manifestations of CNS tumors

- Localized or generalized increases in intracranial pressure:
    - Vomiting, papilledema
- Seizures
- Headache
- Neurologic deficits—speech, motor, sensory
- Fatigue, depression
- Behavioral changes

13.7.4.3   Diagnosis of CNS tumors
- MRI
- CT scan

13.7.4.4   Treatment of CNS tumors
- Radiation therapy
- Chemotherapy
- Surgical excision

13.7.5   Seizure disorders

A seizure is a sudden and uncontrolled increase in brain activity. A seizure is not a disease in itself and can be caused by a number of factors such as high fever, electrolyte imbalances, CNS infections, brain injury, hepatic encephalopathy, metabolic abnormalities, strokes, and drug toxicity. Depending upon the location of the seizure within the brain, manifestations may be motor, sensory, autonomic or psychic. The majority of seizures occur within the cerebral cortex.

13.7.5.1   Epilepsy
Epilepsy is a disease that is characterized by uncontrolled seizure activity. Although the mechanism of seizure activity in patients with epilepsy is uncertain, there are several possible mechanisms by which they may occur:

1. Imbalance occurs between inhibitory CNS neurotransmitters such as gamma-aminobutyric acid (GABA) and excitatory amino acids such as glutamate such that levels of the inhibitory neurotransmitters are decreased, whereas levels of excitatory neurotransmitters are increased.
2. Abnormal activity of CNS ion channels (C^{++}, K^+, Na^+) leads to altered resting membrane potential or abnormal depolarizations

13.7.5.2   Type of seizures
Seizures are classified based on how the abnormal activity in the brain begins. The two main classifications of seizures are *focal seizures* and *generalized seizures*.

13.7.5.3   Focal seizures
Focal seizures occur in a specific area (foci) of the brain. Focal seizures are further divided into two subcategories based on the presentation of the seizure:

- *Simple partial seizure:*
  - No loss of consciousness, patients are fully aware the seizure is occurring

- Symptoms depend upon the region of the brain affected by the seizure and may include *sensory disturbances* (altered sensations, tastes, smells, vision), *motor disturbances* (abnormal movements on the contralateral side), *autonomic disturbances* (flushing, diaphoresis, tachycardia).
- *Complex partial seizure:*
  - Patients exhibit impaired consciousness
  - Often referred to as *psychomotor seizures* to reflect the motor and psychic manifestations
  - Symptoms may include *automatisms* that are repetitive behaviors such as hand rubbing, swallowing, grimacing or walking in circles. Complex visual, and auditory hallucinations may occur. Patients often report a feeling of *déjà vu.*

13.7.5.4 Generalized seizures

The most common form of seizure is a generalized seizure that involves both lobes of the cerebral cortex. Generalized seizures may start as seizure activity that involves the entire cerebral cortex (*primary generalized*), or they may occur as a result of a focal seizure that has spread throughout the cerebral cortex (*secondary* generalized). Generalized seizures are subdivided into several classifications: *tonic-clonic, myoclonic, clonic, tonic, atonic, and absence.*

Tonic-Clonic seizure
- Previously referred to as *grand mal* seizures
- Involves uncontrolled stiffening of muscles (tonic) followed by alternating contraction and relaxation (clonic)
- Patients are unconscious during the seizure. They may lose their bladder control and bite their tongue
- As a result of the widespread seizure activity, the brain may become depleted in oxygen and nutrients. During the period after the seizure (*postictal stage*), patients often sleep for several hours and may experience a period of confusion after awakening.

Aura or Prodrome
Some patients with seizure disorders may experience a "feeling" or "sensation" that warns them they are about to have a seizure. In some instances a simple partial seizure may precede complex partial or generalized tonic-clonic seizure and possibly serve as a warning or aura to that particular patient

---

Status Epilepticus
- A state of continuous seizure activity that last greater than 5 min
- Termed convulsive status epilepticus if it involves generalized tonic-clonic seizures
- Considered a medical emergency due to brain hypoxia
- May result in permanent brain damage and even death if not treated medically
- Often treated with intravenous benzodiazepines

Myoclonic
- Presents as sudden, brief twitches or jerks of arm and leg muscles. May be generalized in terms of presentation or limited to muscles of face, extremities or trunk

Clonic
- Associated with rhythmic jerking muscle movements. May begin with a loss of consciousness and hypotonia

Tonic
- Sudden stiffening of muscles in the back, arms and legs that may cause patients to fall to the ground

Atonic
- Sudden loss of muscle tone that may cause patient to droop or fall to the ground. Also known as "drop" seizures

Absence
- Previously called *petit mal* seizures
- Occur primarily in children and may resolve in adulthood
- Characterized by repeated periods of blank staring coupled with subtle automatisms such as lip smacking or rapid movement of the eyelids
- Patients appear awake but are unresponsive during the seizure
- Each seizure lasts only a few seconds but they may occur repeatedly throughout the day

13.7.5.5   Diagnosis of seizure disorders

- Neurologic examination
- Electroencephalogram (EEG). Changes in brain wave patterns may be evident even if a seizure is not occurring. Absence seizures present with a unique EEG pattern similar to that observed during slow-wave sleep.
- MRI to detect lesions or abnormalities in the brain.
- Positron emission tomography (PET scan) to visualize active areas of the brain

13.7.5.6   Treatment of seizure disorders

Numerous anti-seizure medications are currently available. A number such as phenytoin and carbamazepine work by blocking cortical Na^+ channels. Others such as ethosuximide block cortical Ca^{++} channels. Agents such as the benzodiazepine, barbiturates and gabapentin enhance the inhibitory effects of GABA. The choice of agent(s) will depend upon the seizure type and severity. Ideally, patients should be treated with monotherapy to reduce potential side effects and interactions; however, this may not always be feasible.

13.7.6   Headache

The vast majority of headaches are benign occurrences associated with pain in any region of the head. The presentation of pain may be unilateral or bilateral. Pain may be a dull and throbbing or sharp and radiating. The duration of a typical headache may also vary greatly. Simple headaches may be the result of stress, excess alcohol consumption, smoking, and fatigue and are easily treated with aspirin and quiet rest. The etiology of more complex headaches remains poorly understood and may be related to abnormal nerve activity, regional alterations in brain blood flow, or the inappropriate release of pain transmitting neuropeptides. Headaches may be classified into two main categories: *primary headaches* and *secondary headaches.*

13.7.6.1   Primary headaches

The most common forms of primary headaches are *cluster headaches, migraine headaches,* and *tension headaches*:

Cluster headache:
- Occur in cyclical patterns or "clusters"
- Occur more commonly in men than women
- Intense pain around one eye or in a region of the head that often wakes individuals in the middle of the night
- Clusters of frequent headaches may be followed by long periods with no headaches
- Given their short duration, cluster headaches are treated with inhaled medications such as triptan drugs (e.g., sumatriptan), and intranasal local anesthetics (e.g., lidocaine)

Migraine headache:
- Intense throbbing or pulsing sensation in one area of the head
- Often accompanied by severe nausea and vomiting, as well as sensitivity to light
- Attacks may last hours to days
- Migraine headaches may be preceded an *aura* that includes sensory symptoms such as flashing lights or tingling in a extremity

- Certain foods or odors may act as "triggers" for migraines and should be avoided
- Women are three times more likely to have migraines than men. Up to 90% of individuals who have migraines have a family history of migraines
- Treatment of mild migraines includes the use of NSAIDs, aspirin and acetaminophen/caffeine combinations (e.g., Excedrin). More severe migraines often require the use of triptan drugs or ergot alkaloids (ergotamine plus caffeine). Prophylactic agents such as beta-blockers, as well as certain antidepressants, and certain anti-seizure medications may be used help prevent migraines that become very severe or frequent.

Tension headache:
- A very common form of mild-to-moderate headache that is often described as a tight band around the head
- Pain is often dull and diffuse
- Most commonly triggered by stress. Tension headaches were thought to be related to muscle tension in the head and neck region; however, research has not supported this idea
- Treatment normally involves over-the counter pain medications such as aspirin, ibuprofen and acetaminophen

13.7.6.2 Secondary headaches

Secondary headaches may result from a serious brain conditions such as brain cancer, brain aneurysm, encephalitis, concussion, or hemorrhagic stroke or more benign processes such as sinus infection, influenza, ear infections or excess alcohol consumption.

13.7.7 Degenerative disorders of the brain and CNS

Neurodegenerative diseases are those that are associated with progressive loss of neurons and nervous function and include conditions such as Parkinson's disease, Alzheimer's disease, multiple sclerosis, amyotrophic lateral sclerosis (ALS), and Huntington's disease.

13.7.7.1 Parkinson's disease

Dr. James Parkinson wrote the first accurate medical description of Parkinson's disease in 1817. In his essay he described a condition that was characterized by involuntary tremors, muscle weakness, abnormal gait and difficulty walking. Today we know that Parkinson's disease is a progressive neurologic condition that results from destruction of dopaminergic neurons in the *substantia nigra* and *basal ganglia* regions of the brain. These areas play an important role in both controlling and initiating voluntary movements. The basal ganglia also plays a role in regulating activity of the autonomic nervous system.

Although the exact etiology of Parkinson's disease is still unknown, evidence suggests that certain genetic variations or environmental exposures may increase and individuals risk for developing Parkinson's disease. It is likely that Parkinson's disease develops as a result of complex interactions between genes and environmental factors. One potential causative gene mutation is found on chromosome 4 in a gene that codes for the protein *α-synuclein*, a major component of the abnormal accumulations called *Lewy bodies* that are found in the affected dopaminergic neurons of patients with Parkinson's disease. Other gene mutations associated with Parkinson's disease include those in *LRRK2, PARK2, PARK7, PINK1,* and *SNCA* genes. Environmental exposure to substances such as manganese (in welders) and pesticides as well as brain injury (boxers) have also been associated with an increased risk for the development of Parkinson's disease

13.7.7.1.1   Clinical manifestations of Parkinson's disease (see Figure 13.10)
- Tremor—at rest in the hands and extremities
- Bradykinesia (slowed movements)—difficulty initiating voluntary movements, shuffling gait, difficulty walking
- Muscle rigidity
- Impaired posture and balance
- Shuffling gait
- Autonomic function may also be affected in patients because the basal ganglia interacts with the autonomic nervous system. Symptoms of autonomic dysfunction include excess sweating, constipation, orthostatic hypotension, constipation and urinary incontinence.
- As the disease progresses, disorders of cognitive function, psychiatric disorders and sleep disorders may occur.
- Patients usually have a significantly shortened life span.

13.7.7.1.2   Diagnosis of Parkinson's disease   A diagnosis is usually made based on physical and neurologic examination as well as a review of the symptoms. Brain imaging studies such as MRI are generally of little value in diagnosing Parkinson's disease.

13.7.7.1.3   Treatment of Parkinson's disease
- There is no cure for Parkinson's disease and treatment is mainly used to reduce symptoms. The mainstays of drug therapy for Parkinson's disease are agents that enhance dopamine levels or signaling within the brain. Because dopamine does not cross the blood-brain barrier, the precursor to dopamine, L-DOPA is administered. The combination drug *levodopa/*

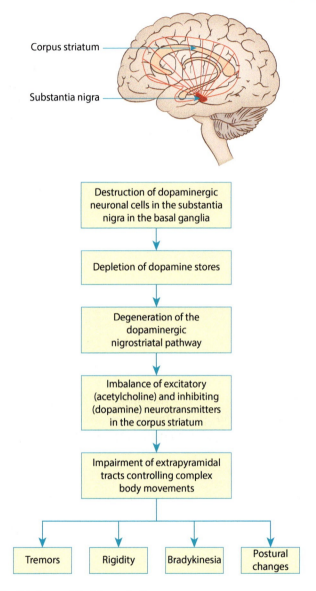

Corpus striatum

Substantia nigra

Destruction of dopaminergic neuronal cells in the substantia nigra in the basal ganglia

↓

Depletion of dopamine stores

↓

Degeneration of the dopaminergic nigrostriatal pathway

↓

Imbalance of excitatory (acetylcholine) and inhibiting (dopamine) neurotransmitters in the corpus striatum

↓

Impairment of extrapyramidal tracts controlling complex body movements

| Tremors | Rigidity | Bradykinesia | Postural changes |

Figure 13.10   Etiology of Parkinson's disease.

carbidopa (Sinemet) contains L-DOPA along with an enzyme inhibitor that prevents the peripheral conversion of L-DOPA to dopamine. Agents such as *ropinirole* and *pramipexole* directly stimulate dopamine receptors in the brain, whereas other agents such as *selegiline* and *rasagiline* inhibit the MAO-B enzyme that degrades dopamine in the brain. Anticholinergic agents such as *benztropine* are also useful for treating tremor and rigidity.

13.7.7.2 Alzheimer's disease

Alzheimer's disease is the leading cause of dementia in elderly patients and is the sixth leading cause of death in the United States. According to estimates, nearly 5.3 million Americans were living with Alzheimer's disease in 2015. Two thirds of theses affected patients were women. The risk of developing Alzheimer's increases proportionally with increasing age. However, a small percentage (<5%) of individual may develop an early-onset form of Alzheimer's disease that manifests in their 40s and 50s.

13.7.7.2.1 Etiology of Alzheimer's disease Alzheimer's disease is associated with a marked atrophy of neurons in the cerebral cortex that is accompanied by enlargement of the brain ventricles. Areas of the cortex affected include those involved in speech, memory, and cognition. Decreased levels of the neurotransmitter acetylcholine occur as a result of reduced neuronal synthesis.

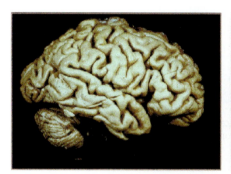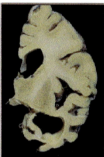

Atrophy of cortex in Alzheimer's disease

Although the exact cause of Alzheimer's disease is still uncertain, great strides have been made in recent years to enhance our understanding of the disease process. Two pathologic "hallmarks" found in the brains of patients with Alzheimer's disease are the presence of *beta amyloid plaques*, and *neurofibrillary tangles*. Beta amyloid plaques form from accumulations of a brain protein called amyloid beta. This protein is derived from a larger protein called *amyloid precursor protein (APP)*. There is evidence that improper cleavage or "proteolysis" of the APP leads to the formation of amyloid beta proteins that subsequently accumulate in CNS neurons and alters their function. Neurofibrillary tangles are twisted accumulations of a protein called *tau* that form in the cytoplasm of affected neurons. Because the cytoplasm is essential for the transport of nutrients and other essential substances in the neuron, the presence of neurofibrillary tangles may interfere with this and damage the neuron.

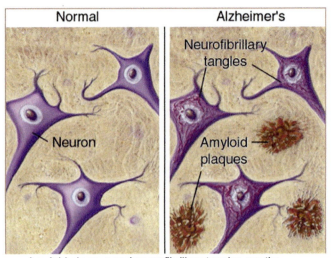

Amyloid plaques and neurofibrillary tangles are the
hallmark of Alzheimer's disease

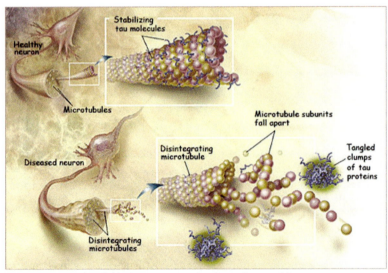

Amyloid plaques may arise from abnormal *tau*
proteins in neuronal microtubules.

Family history is also a risk factor for Alzheimer's disease. Research has shown that individuals who have a close relative affected with Alzheimer's disease have a greater risk of developing the disease themselves. Variations in genes for *APP, presenillin proteins* (*PS*-1 and *PS*-2) and *APOE4* have also been associated with an increased risk for the development of Alzheimer's disease and in some cases the development of early-onset Alzheimer's disease. A strong association has also been made between the occurrence of serious head trauma and an increased risk for the development of Alzheimer's disease in later life.

13.7.7.2.2   *Clinical manifestations of Alzheimer's disease*
- Increasing forgetfulness
- Difficulty organizing thoughts
- Short-term memory loss
- Mild personality changes
- Social withdrawal
- Impaired decision-making
- As the disease progresses, there may be significant cognitive and language impairments, marked disorientation, sleep disorder, and a lack of personal hygiene. Significant psychological changes can occur and may include anxiety, agitation, anger, suspicion and aggressive behavior. An interesting syndrome called "sundowning" can occur in which symptoms of confusion, anxiety and aggression worsen later in the day. The exact cause of sundowning is uncertain.

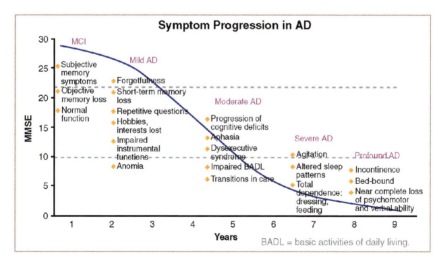

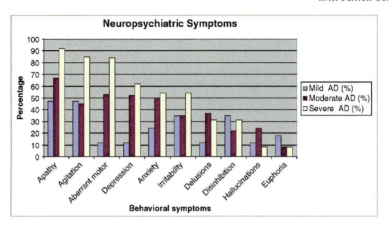

- In later stages individuals generally become bedridden. The average life span for individuals after first being diagnosed with Alzheimer's disease is approximately 8–10 years

13.7.7.2.3 Diagnosis of Alzheimer's disease   A diagnosis of Alzheimer's disease is made primarily from the presentation and progression of symptoms. Other possible causes of dementia, such as poor cerebral blood flow (*vascular dementia*), should also be ruled out. There are currently no blood test or imaging studies that can provide a definitive diagnosis of Alzheimer's disease.

13.7.7.2.4 Treatment of Alzheimer's disease   The current drug therapy for Alzheimer's disease is directed at improving memory loss and cognitive function. *Acetylcholinesterase inhibitors* such as donepezil (Aricept) are commonly prescribed and may provide modest improvement of symptoms early in the disease process. *Memantine* (Namenda), an NMDA receptor antagonist, is also used to slow the progression of symptoms in moderate-to-severe Alzheimer's disease. The blockade of NMDA receptors blunts the effects of the excitatory neurotransmitter glutamate. Some evidence suggests that "excitotoxicity" caused by excessive activity of excitatory neurotransmitters such as glutamate may contribute to the disease process in Alzheimer's disease. Antipsychotic drugs may be helpful for dealing with some of the psychiatric and behavioral manifestations of the disease as it progresses.

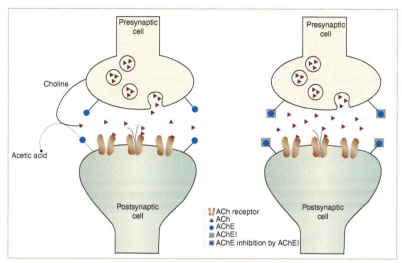

Acetylcholinesterase inhibitors block the enzyme that degrades acetylcholine in the synapse

13.7.7.3 Huntington's disease

Huntington's disease is an inherited disorder that is characterized by a progressive destruction of brain neurons. The disease is inherited as an autosomal recessive disorder. Most patients begin to exhibit symptoms in their 30s to 40s. The condition affects a broad range of CNS neurons and, as a result, the disease can affect voluntary movements, cognitive function, and emotional stability. The genetic defect associated with Huntington's disease is located on chromosome 4 in a gene that encodes for a protein called the *huntingtin* protein. Although the physiologic function of the normal huntingtin protein is uncertain, the abnormal huntingtin protein is larger in size than the normal protein and may not be properly processed or degraded within the CNS neurons. Accumulation of abnormal huntingtin protein fragments may alter neuronal function and lead to cell death.

13.7.7.3.1 Manifestations of Huntington's disease
- Involuntary jerking and writhing movements (*chorea*)
- Muscle rigidity
- Impaired posture and speech
- Difficulty swallowing and talking

- Cognitive impairments that eventually progress to the point of dementia
- Psychological changes that may include depression, impulsive behavior, mania, social withdrawal, and insomnia
- The time from onset of the disease to death is approximately 10–30 years. Pneumonia is a common cause of mortality in patients with advanced disease.

13.7.7.3.2　Diagnosis of Huntington's disease　Diagnosis of Huntington's disease is mainly based upon symptoms and neurologic examination. Brain imaging may reveal changes in areas of the brain that are typically affected by the disease process. Genetic counseling is highly recommended, especially if there is a family history of the disease.

13.7.7.3.3　Treatment of Huntington's disease　There is currently no cure for Huntington's disease. Antipsychotic drugs and agents such as tetrabenazine (Xenazine) may be helpful for treating involuntary movements.

13.7.7.4　Amyotrophic lateral sclerosis

ALS is also known as Lou Gehrig's disease after the hall of fame New York Yankees' baseball player who was afflicted with this condition. ALS is a progressive neurologic condition that primarily affects motor neurons in the anterior (motor) horns of the spinal cord. The term "amyotrophy" refers to the degeneration and shrinkage of motor neurons and subsequent wasting of skeletal muscle that occurs as a result of nervous innervation. The "sclerosis" in the name refers to the hardened or scarred appearance of the neurons at autopsy. ALS affects approximately 5,600 individuals each year in the United States. The average age of onset is 55 and the disease is more prevalent in men than women. Although the exact cause of ALS is uncertain, 5%–10% of cases are inherited. The remaining percentage of non-inherited cases may be possibly related to inappropriate immune response, excess levels of excitatory neurotransmitters such as glutamate, or the accumulation of abnormal proteins in nerve cells. There is currently no cure for ALS, and the average life expectancy after diagnosis is generally 3–5 years. The most common cause of death for patients with ALS is respiratory failure.

13.7.7.4.1　Symptoms of ALS
- Heaviness in legs and feet, difficulty walking
- Hand weakness
- Muscle cramps in arms and shoulders
- Uncontrolled muscle twitches
- Difficulty swallowing and talking
- Progressive weakness of respiratory muscles

13.7.7.4.2   Complications of ALS
- Dysphagia
- Pneumonia
- Loss of speech
- Respiratory failure
- Some patients with ALS may also experience a cognitive decline and dementia

13.7.7.4.3   Diagnosis of ALS   There are no specific tests for ALS. A definitive diagnosis is made based upon a detailed physical and neurologic examination.

13.7.7.4.4   Management of ALS   There is currently no cure for ALS, but specific medications may be used to treat specific symptoms of the disease. Physical therapy, respiratory therapy and nutritional care are essential components of ALS management, as is nutritional, psychological, and social support.

13.7.7.5   Multiple sclerosis
Multiple sclerosis (MS) is a progressive neurologic disease characterized by autoimmune demyelination of CNS neurons. Areas of neuronal demyelination are called "plaques." The presence of insulating myelin sheaths on nerve fibers allows for a rapid "salutatory" conduction of impulses that are able jump between bare areas called the nodes of Ranvier. Loss of the myelin sheath slows and impairs normal electrical conduction in myelinated neurons. Because MS can affect multiple types of CNS neurons, symptoms may include sensory, motor and autonomic dysfunction. Although the exact cause of MS is unknown, there is a very strong autoimmune component with the patient's immune system destroying the myelin sheath covering nerve fibers.

MS currently affects approximately 2.3 million individuals worldwide. Most patients are between 20 and 50 years of age when first diagnosed with MS. Women are two to three times more likely to develop MS than men. The risk of developing MS is also higher in white populations of Northern European descent and in individuals with a first-degree relative who was diagnosed with the disease.

The majority of patients who are first diagnosed with MS present with a relapsing-remitting form of the disease in which they experience episodes of worsening symptoms that develop over days to weeks but usually resolve spontaneously. The course of the disease between exacerbations is stable. Approximately 60%–70% of patients with the relapsing-remitting form of MS will go on to develop a secondary-progressive form of MS that is characterized by a steady progression of symptoms with or without superimposed acute relapses.

13.7.7.5.1   Symptoms and complications of MS

- Numbness or weakness in various muscle groups
- Vision effects such as partial vision loss or double vision
- *Paresthesias* characterized by numbness, tingling or burning sensations
- Tremor
- Speech difficulties
- Generalized fatigue
- Alterations in bladder or bowel function
- Sexual dysfunction
- Mental changes, depression
- Difficulty walking, paralysis of the legs
- Seizures are possible

13.7.7.5.2   Diagnosis of MS

Given the wide variety of potential symptoms, MS may difficult to diagnose. The diagnosis of MS often first begins with clinical and diagnostic tests to rule out other causes of CNS dysfunction. A lumbar puncture may be performed to analyze cerebrospinal fluid for abnormalities in certain antibodies that may be associated with MS. MRI studies of the brain and spinal cord may reveal lesions and plaques on nerve fibers. Evoked potential studies may be conducted in which electrical impulses from CNS neurons are measured following the application of a stimulus. This test can measure the speed at which electrical impulses pass along the patient's nerve pathways.

13.7.7.5.3   Treatment of MS

There is currently no cure for MS. Drug treatment may involve the use of *corticosteroids, beta interferons* and other immune-modifying agents that can reduce the rate of relapses. *Glatiramer acetate* is a drug that mimics the body's myelin proteins and can help block the immune system's attack on myelin. Other drugs may be used as needed to treat muscle spasm (baclofen), bladder issues (cholinergic agents), and depression (antidepressants). Physical and occupational therapy are also of value in patients with MS.

13.7.8   Spinal injury

Injuries to the vertebral column may include fractures, dislocations or subluxations of the vertebrae. Such injuries may occur as a result of sudden impacts, compression of the vertebrae or penetrating injuries or through nontraumatic means such as a growing cancer, inflammation or infection. Damage to the bony structure of the spinal column may result in injury to the spinal cord that is encased within. The effects of spinal cord injury will depend upon the location and extent of the damage that has occurred. Additional damage may occur in the days following an acute spinal cord injury as a result of the bleeding, inflammation and swelling that can occur. Spinal cord injury may result in a partial or complete loss of sensory, motor or autonomic function below the area of the injury. Loss of motor and/or sensory function in the trunk, legs and pelvic organs is referred to as *paraplegia*. Loss of motor and/or sensory function in the arms, legs, trunk and pelvis is referred to as *quadriplegia or tetraplegia*.

13.7.8.1 Manifestations of spinal cord injury
- Loss of motor function
- Loss of sensory or autonomic reflexes
- Paralysis below the level of the injury
- Loss of bowel and bladder function
- Loss of sexual function
- Neuropathic pain due to damaged nerve fibers

13.7.8.2 Treatment of spinal cord injury
- *Spinal shock* is a reversible form or spinal cord trauma that may occur with blunt force trauma (e.g., football injury). However, severe damage to the spinal cord is irreversible.
- Steroids such as intravenous methylprednisolone may be administered early in the course of spinal injury to reduce potential inflammation at the site of the injury.
- Immobilization is essential for anyone suspected of having a spinal injury because it may reduce further injury to the area of damage.

Medical terminology

Afferent neuron (ăf′ĕr-ĕnt nĕr′ŏn): Nerve cell that transmits sensory information from the periphery of the body to the central nervous system

Anesthesia (ăn″ĕs-thē′zē-ă): Localized or generalized loss of sensation following the administration of an anesthetic agent

Antagonist (ăn-tăg′ō-nĭst): A muscle that counteracts the function of the prime mover or agonist muscle (e.g., the triceps brachii muscles are antagonistic to the action of the biceps brachii muscles)

Aphasia (ă-fā′zē-ă): Impairment in the ability to communicate through language

Ataxia (ā-tăk′sē-ă): Defective skeletal muscle coordination

Cauda equina (kaw′dă ē-kwīn′ă): Bundle of spinal nerve roots extending inferiorly through the vertebral canal below the level of the second lumbar vertebra

Dermatome (dĕr′mă-tōm): A region of the body surface supplied by a single spinal nerve

Disproportionate (dĭs-prō-pŏr′shŭn-ăt): Unequal in size

Efferent neuron (ĕf′ĕr-ĕnt): Nerve cell that transmits motor information from the central nervous system to muscle cells and glands

Epidural space (ĕp″ĭ-dūr′ăl spās): Area between the dura mater (outer meningeal covering of the spinal cord) and the vertebrae that is filled with fatty tissue and blood vessels

Fissure (fĭs′ĕr): Deep furrow in the brain

Foramen magnum (for-ā′mĕn măg′nŭm): Large opening in the base of the occipital bone
through which the spinal cord exits the skull

Ganglion (găng′lē-ŏn): Mass of neuronal cell bodies in the peripheral nervous system

Gray matter (grā măt′ĕr): Regions in cerebrum and cerebellum containing neuronal cell bodies and unmyelinated neurons

Gyrus (gī′rŭs): Convolution of the cerebral cortex

Hyperkinesia (hī″pĕr-kĭ-nē′zē-ă): Enhanced motor response or activity

Hypokinesia (hī″pō- kĭ-nē′zē-ă): Reduced motor response or activity

Hypotonia (hī″pō-tō′nē-ă): Reduced muscle tone

Interneuron (ĭn′tĕr-nĕr″ŏn): Nerve cell located entirely within the central nervous system

Multimodal (mŭlt″ē-mōd′ăl): Of more than one type

Nerve (nĕrv): Bundle of neurons that transmits electrical impulses from the central nervous system (brainstem or spinal cord) to the organs and tissues of the body

Nucleus (nū′klē-ŭs): Mass of neuronal cell bodies in the central nervous system

Plasticity (plăs-tĭs′ĭ-tē): Ability to be changed in form

Proprioception (prō′prē-ō-cĕp″shŭn): Awareness of body position and movement

Reciprocal inhibition (rĭ-sĭp′rō-kăl ĭn″hĭ-bĭsh′ŭn): Inhibition of a muscle or muscle group that is antagonistic to the muscle or muscle group being stimulated

Reflex (rē′flĕks): Predictable, stereotyped, involuntary response to a given stimulus

Sulcus (sŭl′kŭs): Small groove or depression of the cerebral cortex

Tract (trăkt): Bundle of neurons that transmits electrical impulses within the central nervous system (brain and spinal cord)

Unimodal (ūn″ē-mōd′ăl): Of one type

Unimpeded (ŭn-ĭm-pēd′ĕd): Unobstructed

White matter (whīt măt′ĕr): Regions in cerebrum and cerebellum consisting of myelinated axons of neurons

Bibliography

Amaral, D. G., The anatomical organization of the nervous system, in *Principles of Neuroscience*, 4th ed., Kandel, E. R., Schwartz, J. H. and Jessell, T. M., Eds., McGraw-Hill, New York, 2000, chap.17.

Bear, M. F., Connors, B. W., and Paradiso, M. A., *Neuroscience, Exploring the Brain*, 3rd ed., Lippincott Williams & Wilkins, Philadelphia, PA, 2007.

Bloom, F. E., Neurotransmission and the central nervous system, in *Goodman and Gilman's, The Pharmacological Basis of Therapeutics*, 11th ed., Brunton, L. L., Lazo, J. S. and Parker, K. L., Eds., McGraw-Hill, New York, 2006, chap. 12.

Garoutte, B. *Neuromuscular Physiology*, 4th ed., Mill Valley Medical Publishers, Millbrae, CA, 1996.

Ghez, C., and Thach, W. T., The cerebellum, in *Principles of Neuroscience*, 4th ed., Kandel, E. R., Schwartz, J. H. and Jessell, T. M., Eds., McGraw-Hill, New York, 2000, chap. 42.

Laterra, L., and Goldstein, G. W., Ventricular organization of cerebral spinal fluid: Blood-brain barrier, brain edema, and hydrocephalus, in *Principles of Neuroscience*, 4th ed., Kandel, E. R., Schwartz, J. H. and Jessell, T. M., Eds., McGraw-Hill, New York, 2000, appendix B.

Lynch, J. C., The cerebral cortex, in *Fundamental Neuroscience for Basic and Clinical Applications*, Haines, D. E., Ed., Churchill Livingstone/Elsevier, Philadelphia, PA, 2006, chap. 32.

Ma, T. P., The basal nuclei, in *Fundamental Neuroscience for Basic and Clinical Applications*, Haines, D. E., Ed., Churchill Livingstone/Elsevier, Philadelphia, PA, 2006, chap. 26.

Mihailoff, G. A., and Haines, D. E., The diencephalon, in *Fundamental Neuroscience for Basic and Clinical Applications*, Haines, D. E., Ed., Churchill Livingstone/ Elsevier, Philadelphia, PA, 2006, chap. 15.

Mihailoff, G. A., and Haines, D. E., Motor system II: Corticofugal systems and the control of movement, in *Fundamental Neuroscience for Basic and Clinical Applications*, Haines, D. E., Ed., Churchill Livingstone/Elsevier, Philadelphia, PA, 2006, chap. 25.

Naftel, J. P., Ard, M. D., Fratkin, J. D., and Hutchins, J. B., The cell biology of neurons and glia, in *Fundamental Neuroscience for Basic and Clinical Applications*, Haines, D. E., Ed., Churchill Livingstone/Elsevier, Philadelphia, PA, 2006, chap. 2.

Nieuwenhuys, R., Ten Donkelaar, H. J., and Nicholson, C., *The Central Nervous System of Vertebrates*, vol. 3, Springer, Berlin, Germany, 1998.

Rechtschaffen, A., and Siegel, J., Sleep and dreaming, in *Principles of Neuroscience*, 4th ed., Kandel, E. R., Schwartz, J. H. and Jessell, T. M., Eds., McGraw-Hill, New York, 2000, chap. 47.

Saper, C. B., Brain Stem, Reflexive behavior, and the cranial nerves, in *Principles of Neuroscience*, 4th ed., Kandel, E. R., Schwartz, J. H. and Jessell, T. M., Eds., McGraw-Hill, New York, 2000, chap. 44.

Saper, C. B., Iversen, S., and Frackowiak, R., Integration of sensory and motor function: The association areas of the cerebral cortex and the cognitive capabilities of the brain, in *Principles of Neuroscience*, 4th ed., Kandel, E. R., Schwartz, J. H. and Jessell, T. M., Eds., McGraw-Hill, New York, 2000, chap. 19.

Sherwood, L., *Human Physiology, From Cells to Systems*, 5th ed., Brooks/Cole, Pacific Grove, CA, 2004.

Sherwood, L., Klandorf, H., and Yancey, P. H., *Animal Physiology, From Genes to Organisms*, Brooks/Cole, Pacific Grove, CA, 2005.

Silverthorn, D. U., *Human Physiology, An Integrated Approach*, 4th ed., Prentice Hall, Upper Saddle River, NJ, 2007.

Skidgel, R. A., and Erdos, E. G., Histamine, Bradykinin and their antagonists, in *Goodman and Gilman's, The Pharmacological Basis of Therapeutics*, 11th ed., Brunton, L. L., Lazo, J. S. and Parker, K. L., Eds., McGraw-Hill, New York, 2006, chap. 24.

Taber's Cyclopedic Medical Dictionary, 20th ed., F. A. Davis Co., Philadelphia, PA, 2005.

Warren, S., Capra, N. F., and Yezierski, R. P., The somatosensory system I: Tactile discrimination and position sense, in *Fundamental Neuroscience for Basic and Clinical Applications*, Haines, D. E., Ed., Churchill Livingstone/Elsevier, Philadelphia, PA, 2006, chap. 17.

Widmaier, E. P., Raff, H., and Strang, K. T., *Vander's Human Physiology, The Mechanisms of Body Function*, McGraw-Hill, Boston, MA, 2006.

chapter fourteen

The autonomic nervous system

Study objectives

- Explain how various regions of the central nervous system regulate autonomic nervous system function
- Explain how autonomic reflexes contribute to homeostasis
- Describe how the neuroeffector junction in the autonomic nervous system differs from that of a neuron-to-neuron synapse
- Compare and contrast the anatomical features of the sympathetic and parasympathetic systems
- For each neurotransmitter in the autonomic nervous system, list the neurons that release them and the type and location of receptors that bind with them
- Describe the mechanism by which neurotransmitters are removed
- Distinguish between cholinergic and adrenergic receptors
- Describe the overall and specific functions of the sympathetic system
- Describe the overall and specific functions of the parasympathetic system
- Explain how the effects of catecholamines differ from those of direct sympathetic stimulation

The *autonomic nervous system (ANS)* is also known as the visceral or involuntary nervous system. It functions without conscious, voluntary control. Because it innervates cardiac muscle, smooth muscle, and various endocrine and exocrine glands, this nervous system influences the activity of most of the organ systems in the body. Therefore, it is evident that the ANS makes a significant contribution to homeostasis. The regulation of blood pressure, gastrointestinal responses to food, contraction of the urinary bladder, focusing of the eyes and thermoregulation are just a few of the many homeostatic functions regulated by the ANS. Several distinguishing features of the ANS and the somatic nervous system, which innervates skeletal muscle, are summarized in Table 14.1.

Table 14.1   Distinguishing features of the somatic and autonomic nervous systems

Somatic nervous system	Autonomic nervous system
Conscious control, voluntary	Unconscious control, involuntary
Skeletal muscle	All innervated structures except skeletal muscle (e.g., cardiac muscle, smooth muscle, glands)
Movement, respiration, posture	Visceral functions (e.g., cardiac activity, blood flow, digestion)
No peripheral ganglia; synapses located entirely within cerebrospinal axis	Peripheral ganglia located outside of cerebrospinal axis
Alpha motor neuron	Preganglionic neuron and postganglionic neuron
Myelinated, large diameter (9–13 μm)	Nonmyelinated, small diameter (~1 μm)
Neurotransmitter: acetylcholine only	Neurotransmitters: acetylcholine and norepinephrine
Cell bodies in ventral horn of spinal cord	Cell bodies in brainstem, lateral horn of spinal cord
Axon divides; each axon terminal innervates a single muscle fiber directly	No discreet innervation of individual effector cells
Motor end-plate or neuromuscular junction = axon terminal in close apposition to a specialized surface of the muscle cell membrane	Axon terminal with multiple varicosities releases neurotransmitter over a wide surface area affecting many tissue cells
No gap junctions between effector cells; no spread of electrical activity from one muscle fiber to another	Gap junctions allow the spread of electrical activity throughout the tissue

14.1   Regulation

The efferent nervous activity of the ANS is regulated by several regions in the central nervous system (CNS):

- Hypothalamus and brainstem
- Cerebral cortex and limbic system
- Spinal cord

The efferent nervous activity of the ANS is largely regulated by autonomic reflexes. In many of these reflexes, sensory information is transmitted to homeostatic control centers, such as those located in the hypothalamus and the brainstem. Much of the sensory input from the thoracic and abdominal viscera is transmitted to the brainstem by afferent fibers of cranial nerve X, the vagus nerve. Other cranial nerves also contribute sensory input to the hypothalamus and the brainstem. This input is integrated and a response is carried out by the transmission of nerve signals that modify the activity of preganglionic autonomic neurons. Many important variables in the body are monitored and regulated in the hypothalamus and the brainstem including heart rate, blood pressure, gastrointestinal peristalsis and glandular secretion, body temperature, hunger, thirst, plasma volume, and plasma osmolarity.

An example of this type of autonomic reflex is the baroreceptor reflex. Baroreceptors act as sensory receptors that monitor blood pressure and are found in some of the major systemic arteries. When a person has a sudden drop in blood pressure (e.g., standing up), the decreased blood pressure is sensed by the baroreceptor as a decrease in tension and the baroreceptor will decrease in the firing of impulses. This causes the vasomotor center to increase sympathetic activity in the heart and blood vessels and decrease vagal tone (parasympathetic influence on the cardiac SA node), causing an increase in heart rate.

These neural control centers in the hypothalamus and the brainstem may also be influenced by higher brain areas. Specifically, the cerebral cortex and the limbic system influence ANS activities associated with emotional responses by way of hypothalamic-brainstem pathways. For example, blushing during an embarrassing moment, a response most likely originating in the frontal association cortex, involves vasodilation of blood vessels to the face. Other emotional responses influenced by these higher brain areas include fainting, breaking out in a cold sweat, and a racing heart rate.

Some autonomic reflexes may be processed at the level of the spinal cord. These include the micturition reflex (urination) and the defecation reflex. Although these reflexes are subject to influence from higher nervous centers, they may occur without input from the brain.

14.2 Pathways

The efferent pathways of the ANS consist of two neurons that transmit impulses from the CNS to the effector tissue. The *preganglionic neuron* originates in the CNS with its cell body in the lateral horn of the gray matter of the spinal cord or in the brainstem. The axon of this neuron travels to an autonomic ganglion located outside of the CNS where it synapses with a *postganglionic neuron*. It is this neuron that innervates the effector tissue. (A *ganglion* is a cluster of nerve cell bodies in the peripheral nervous system. A *nucleus* is a cluster of nerve cell bodies in the central nervous system.)

Synapses between the autonomic postganglionic neuron and the effector tissue, the *neuroeffector junction*, differ greatly from the neuron-to-neuron synapses discussed previously in Chapter 13 (see Table 14.1). The postganglionic fibers in the ANS do not terminate in a single swelling like the synaptic knob, nor do they synapse directly with the cells of a tissue. Instead, where the axons of these fibers enter a given tissue, they contain multiple swellings called *varicosities*. When the neuron is stimulated, these varicosities release neurotransmitter along a significant length of the axon and, therefore, over a large surface area of the effector tissue. The neurotransmitter diffuses through the interstitial fluid to wherever its receptors are in the tissue. This diffuse release of the neurotransmitter affects many tissue cells simultaneously. Furthermore, cardiac muscle and most smooth muscle have *gap junctions* between the cells. These specialized intercellular communications allow for the spread of electrical activity from one cell to the next. Thus, the discharge of a single autonomic nerve fiber to an effector tissue may alter the activity of the entire tissue.

14.3   Divisions

The ANS is composed of two anatomically and functionally distinct divisions, the *sympathetic system* and the *parasympathetic system*. Two important features of these divisions include:

- Tonic activity
- Dual innervation

Both systems are *tonically active*. In other words, they provide some degree of nervous input to a given tissue on a continued basis. Therefore, the frequency of discharge of neurons in both systems can either increase or decrease and tissue activity may be either enhanced or inhibited. This characteristic of the ANS improves its ability to more precisely regulate a tissue's function. Without tonic activity, nervous input to a tissue could only increase.

Many tissues are *innervated by both systems*. Because the sympathetic system and the parasympathetic system typically have opposing effects on a given tissue, increasing the activity of one system while simultaneously decreasing the activity of the other results in very rapid and precise control of a tissue's function. For example, sympathetic nervous stimulation increases heart rate and parasympathetic nervous stimulation decreases heart rate. Under conditions of exercise where it is beneficial to increase heart rate and pump more blood to the skeletal muscles, there is a simultaneous increase in sympathetic activity and decrease in parasympathetic activity to the heart. Both effects serve to increase heart rate. Therefore, the activity of a given tissue is the result of the balance of the input from these two opposing systems. Several distinguishing features of these two divisions of the ANS are summarized in Table 14.2.

Each system is dominant under certain conditions. The sympathetic system predominates during emergency "fight-or-flight" reactions and during exercise. The overall effect of the sympathetic system under these conditions is to prepare the body for strenuous physical activity.

Table 14.2 Distinguishing features of the sympathetic and parasympathetic systems

Sympathetic system	Parasympathetic system
Originates in the thoracic and lumbar regions of the spinal cord (T_1–L_2)	Originates in the brainstem (cranial nerves III, VII, IX, and X) and the sacral region of the spinal cord (S_2–S_4)
Ganglia located in paravertebral sympathetic ganglion chain or in collateral ganglia	Terminal ganglia located near or embedded within target tissue
Short cholinergic preganglionic fibers	Long adrenergic postganglionic fibers
Long cholinergic preganglionic fibers	Short cholinergic postganglionic fibers
Ratio of preganglionic fibers to postganglionic fibers is 1:20	Ratio of preganglionic fibers to postganglionic fibers is 1:3
Divergence coordinates activity of neurons at multiple levels of the spinal cord	Limited divergence
Activity often involves mass discharge of entire system	Activity normally to discrete organs
Predominates during emergency "fight-or-flight" reactions and exercise	Predominates during quiet "rest and digest" conditions

More specifically, sympathetic nervous activity will increase the flow of blood that is well oxygenated and rich in nutrients to the tissues that need it, such as the working skeletal muscles. The parasympathetic system predominates during quiet, resting conditions. The overall effect of the parasympathetic system, under these conditions, is to conserve and store energy, and to regulate basic body functions such as digestion and urination (*"rest and digest"*).

The preganglionic neurons of the sympathetic system arise from the thoracic and lumbar regions of the spinal cord (segments T_1 through L_2) (see Figure 14.1). Most of these preganglionic axons are short and synapse with postganglionic neurons within ganglia found in the *sympathetic ganglion chains*. These ganglion chains, which run parallel immediately along either side of the spinal cord, each consist of 22 ganglia. The preganglionic neuron may exit the spinal cord and synapse with a postganglionic neuron in a ganglion at the same spinal cord level from which it arises. The preganglionic neuron may also travel more rostrally or caudally (upward or downward) in the ganglion chain to synapse with postganglionic neurons in ganglia at other levels. In fact, a single preganglionic neuron may synapse with several postganglionic neurons in many different ganglia. Overall, the ratio of preganglionic fibers to postganglionic fibers is about 1:20. The long postganglionic neurons originating in the ganglion chain then travel outward and terminate on the effector tissues.

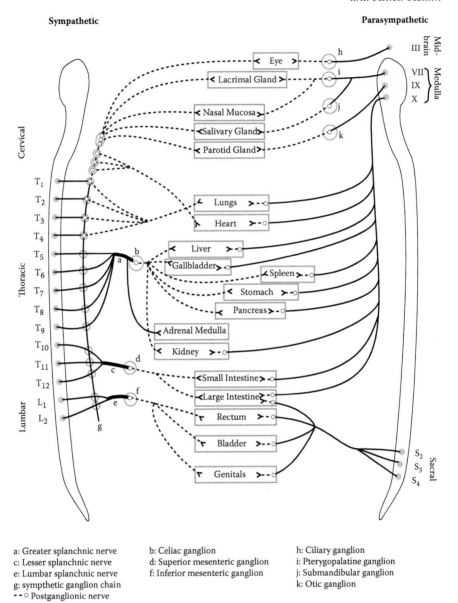

a: Greater splanchnic nerve
c: Lesser splanchnic nerve
e: Lumbar splanchnic nerve
g: sympthetic ganglion chain
- - ○ Postganglionic nerve

b: Celiac ganglion
d: Superior mesenteric ganglion
f: Inferior mesenteric ganglion

h: Ciliary ganglion
i: Pterygopalatine ganglion
j: Submandibular ganglion
k: Otic ganglion

Figure 14.1 Schematic representation of the autonomic nervous system and its effector organs. The efferent pathways of this system consist of two neurons that transmit impulses from the CNS to the effector tissue, the preganglionic neuron (solid line) and the postganglionic neuron (dashed line). As illustrated, most tissues receive nervous input from both divisions of the ANS, the sympathetic division and the parasympathetic division.

This divergence of the preganglionic neuron results in coordinated sympathetic stimulation to tissues throughout the body. The concurrent stimulation of many organs and tissues in the body is referred to as a *mass sympathetic discharge*.

Other preganglionic neurons exit the spinal cord and pass through the ganglion chain without synapsing with a postganglionic neuron. Instead, the axons of these neurons travel more peripherally and synapse with postganglionic neurons in one of the *sympathetic collateral ganglia* (see Figure 14.1). These ganglia are located about halfway between the CNS and the effector tissue.

Finally, the preganglionic neuron may travel to the *adrenal medulla* and synapse directly with this glandular tissue. The cells of the adrenal medulla have the same embryonic origin as neural tissue and, in fact, function as *modified postganglionic neurons*. Instead of the release of neurotransmitter directly at the synapse with an effector tissue, the secretory products of the adrenal medulla are picked up by the blood and travel throughout the body to all the effector tissues of the sympathetic system.

An important feature of this system, which is quite distinct from the parasympathetic system, is that the postganglionic neurons of the sympathetic system travel within each of the 31 pairs of spinal nerves (see Chapter 13). Interestingly, 8% of the fibers that constitute a spinal nerve are sympathetic fibers. This allows for the distribution of sympathetic nerve fibers to the effectors of the skin, including blood vessels and sweat glands. In fact, most innervated blood vessels in the entire body, primarily arterioles and veins, receive only sympathetic nerve fibers. Therefore, vascular smooth muscle tone and sweating are regulated by the sympathetic system only. In addition, the sympathetic system innervates structures of the head (eye, salivary glands, and mucus membranes of the nasal cavity), thoracic viscera (heart and lungs) and viscera of the abdominal and pelvic cavities (stomach, intestines, pancreas, spleen, adrenal medulla, kidneys, and urinary bladder) (see Figure 14.1).

The preganglionic neurons of the parasympathetic system arise from several nuclei of the brainstem and from the sacral region of the spinal cord (segments S_2-S_4) (see Figure 14.1). The axons of the preganglionic neurons are quite long compared with those of the sympathetic system and synapse with postganglionic neurons within *terminal ganglia*, which are close to or embedded within the effector tissues. The axons of the postganglionic neurons, which are very short, then provide input to the cells of that effector tissue.

The preganglionic neurons that arise from the brainstem exit the CNS through the cranial nerves. The oculomotor nerve (III) innervates the eyes; the facial nerve (VII) innervates the lacrimal glands, the salivary glands and the mucus membranes of the nasal cavity; the glossopharyngeal nerve (IX) innervates the parotid (salivary) glands; and the vagus nerve (X) innervates the viscera of the thorax and the abdomen (heart, lungs, stomach, pancreas, small intestine, upper half of the large intestine, and liver). The physiological significance of cranial nerve X in terms of the influence of the parasympathetic system is clearly illustrated by its widespread distribution and the fact that 75% of all parasympathetic fibers are in the vagus nerve. The preganglionic neurons that arise from the sacral region of the spinal cord exit the CNS and join to form the pelvic nerves. These nerves innervate the viscera of the pelvic cavity (e.g., lower half of the large intestine and organs of the renal and reproductive systems).

Because the terminal ganglia are located within the innervated tissue, there is typically little divergence in the parasympathetic system compared with the sympathetic system. In many organs, there is a 1:1 ratio of preganglionic fibers to postganglionic fibers. Therefore, the effects of the parasympathetic system tend to be more discrete and localized, with only specific tissues being stimulated at any given moment, compared with the sympathetic system where a more diffuse discharge is possible.

14.4   Neurotransmission

The two most common neurotransmitters released by neurons of the ANS are *acetylcholine (Ach)*, and *norepinephrine (NE)*. Neurotransmitters are synthesized in the axon varicosities and stored in vesicles for subsequent release. Several distinguishing features of these neurotransmitters are summarized in Table 14.3. Nerve fibers that release acetylcholine are referred to as *cholinergic* fibers. These include all preganglionic fibers of the ANS, both sympathetic and parasympathetic systems; all postganglionic fibers of the parasympathetic system; and some sympathetic postganglionic fibers innervating sweat glands (see Figure 14.2). Nerve fibers that release norepinephrine are referred to as *adrenergic* fibers. All other sympathetic postganglionic fibers release norepinephrine.

As previously mentioned, the cells of the adrenal medulla are considered modified sympathetic postganglionic neurons. Instead of a neurotransmitter, these cells release *hormones* into the blood. Approximately 20% of the hormonal output of the adrenal medulla is norepinephrine. The remaining 80% is *epinephrine (EPI)*. Unlike true postganglionic neurons in the sympathetic system, the adrenal medulla contains an enzyme that methylates norepinephrine to form epinephrine. The synthesis of epinephrine, also known as *adrenalin*, is enhanced under conditions of stress. These two hormones released by the adrenal medulla are collectively referred to as the *catecholamines*.

For any substance to serve effectively as a neurotransmitter, it must be rapidly removed or inactivated from the synapse or, in this case, the neuroeffector junction. This is necessary to allow new signals to get through

Table 14.3 Distinguishing features of the neurotransmitters of the autonomic nervous system

Feature	Acetylcholine	Norepinephrine	Epinephrine[a]
Site of Release	All preganglionic neurons of the autonomic nervous system; all postganglionic neurons of the parasympathetic system; some sympathetic postganglionic neurons innervating sweat glands (alpha motor neurons innervating skeletal muscle)[b]	Most sympathetic postganglionic neurons; adrenal medulla (20% of secretion)	Adrenal medulla (80% of secretion)
Receptor	Nicotinic, muscarinic (cholinergic)	α_1, α_2, β_1 (adrenergic)	α_1, α_2, β_1, β_2 (adrenergic)
Termination of Activity	Enzymatic degradation by acetylcholinesterase	Reuptake into nerve terminals; diffusion out of synaptic cleft and uptake at extraneuronal sites; metabolic transformation by monoamine oxidase (within nerve terminal) or catechol-O-methyltransferase within the liver	Metabolic transformation by catechol-O-methyltransferase within the liver

[a] Although epinephrine is not a direct neurotransmitter for the autonomic nervous system, its release from the adrenal medulla supplements the effects of a mass sympathetic discharge.
[b] Alpha motor neurons, a component of the somatic nervous system, also release acetylcholine as a neurotransmitter.

and influence effector tissue function. Neurotransmitter activity may be terminated by three mechanisms:

- Enzymatic degradation
- Reuptake into the neuron
- Diffusion away from the synapse

The primary mechanism used by cholinergic synapses is *enzymatic degradation.* *Acetylcholinesterase* hydrolyzes acetylcholine to its component choline and acetate. It is one of the fastest acting enzymes in the body, and acetylcholine removal occurs in less than 1 ms. The most important mechanism for

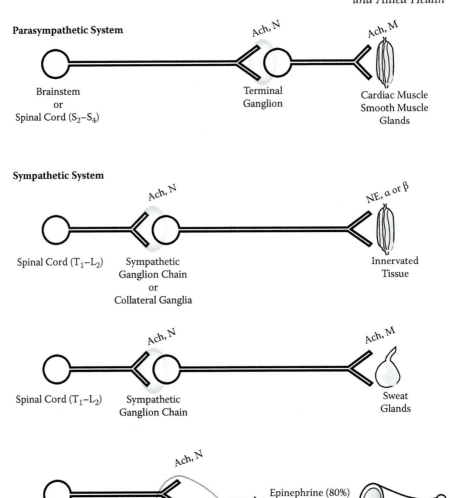

Figure 14.2 Autonomic nerve pathways. All preganglionic neurons release acetylcholine (Ach), which binds to nicotinic receptors (N) on the postganglionic neurons. All postganglionic neurons in the parasympathetic system and some sympathetic postganglionic neurons innervating sweat glands release Ach, which binds to muscarinic (M) receptors on the cells of the effector tissues. All the remaining postganglionic neurons of the sympathetic system release norepinephrine (NE), which binds to α or β receptors on the cells of the effector tissues. The cells of the adrenal medulla, which are modified postganglionic neurons in the sympathetic system, release epinephrine (EPI) and NE into the circulation.

the removal of norepinephrine from the neuroeffector junction is the *reuptake* of this neurotransmitter into the sympathetic postganglionic neuron that released it. Norepinephrine may then be metabolized intraneuronally by *monoamine oxidase (MAO)*. The circulating catecholamines, epinephrine and norepinephrine, are inactivated by *catechol-O-methyltransferase (COMT)* in the liver. Of lesser importance in terms of the termination of neurotransmitter activity, is the diffusion of the neurotransmitter away from the synapse. The neurotransmitter is then eliminated by extraneuronal sites.

14.5   Receptors

As discussed in the previous Section 14.4, Neurotransmission, all the effects of the ANS in tissues and organs throughout the body, including smooth muscle contraction or relaxation, alteration of myocardial activity and increased or decreased glandular secretion, are carried out by only three substances, acetylcholine, norepinephrine and epinephrine. Furthermore, each of these substances may stimulate activity in some tissues and inhibit activity in others. How can this wide variety of effects on many different tissues be carried out by so few neurotransmitters or hormones? The effect caused by any of these substances is determined by the receptor distribution in a particular tissue and the biochemical properties of the cells in that tissue, specifically, the second messenger and enzyme systems present within the cell.

The neurotransmitters of the ANS and the circulating catecholamines bind to specific receptors on the cell membranes of the effector tissue. All adrenergic receptors and muscarinic receptors are coupled to *G proteins*, which are also embedded within the plasma membrane. Receptor stimulation causes activation of the G protein and the formation of an intracellular chemical, the *second messenger*. (The neurotransmitter molecule, which cannot enter the cell itself, is the *first messenger*.) The function of the intracellular second messenger molecules is to elicit tissue-specific biochemical events within the cell that alter the cell's activity. In this way, a given neurotransmitter may stimulate the same type of receptor on two different types of tissue and cause two different responses due to the presence of different biochemical pathways within each tissue. (This signal transduction/second messenger mechanism is discussed in more detail in Chapter 11.)

Acetylcholine binds to two types of *cholinergic receptors*:

- Nicotinic receptors
- Muscarinic receptors

Nicotinic receptors are found on the cell bodies of all postganglionic neurons in the ganglia of the ANS, both sympathetic and parasympathetic divisions. Acetylcholine released from the preganglionic neurons binds to these nicotinic receptors and causes a rapid increase in the cellular permeability to Na^+ ions and Ca^{++} ions. The resulting influx of these two cations causes depolarization and excitation of the postganglionic neurons the ANS pathways.

Muscarinic receptors are found on the cell membranes of the effector tissues and are linked to G proteins and second messenger systems that carry out the intracellular effects. Acetylcholine released from all parasympathetic postganglionic neurons and some sympathetic postganglionic neurons traveling to sweat glands binds to these receptors. Muscarinic receptors may be either inhibitory or excitatory, depending on the tissue upon which they are found. For example, muscarinic receptor stimulation in the myocardium is inhibitory and decreases heart rate, whereas stimulation of muscarinic receptors in the lungs is excitatory and causes contraction of airway smooth muscle and bronchoconstriction.

There are two classes of *adrenergic receptors* for norepinephrine and epinephrine:

- Alpha (α)
- Beta (β)

Furthermore, there are at least two subtypes of receptors in each class: α_1, α_2, β_1, and β_2. These receptors are linked to G proteins and second messenger systems that carry out the intracellular effects.

Alpha receptors are the more abundant of the adrenergic receptors. Of the two subtypes, α_1 receptors are more widely distributed on the effector tissues. Alpha one receptor stimulation leads to an increase in intracellular calcium. As a result, these receptors tend to be excitatory. For example, stimulation of α_1 receptors causes contraction of vascular smooth muscle, resulting in vasoconstriction as well as increased glandular secretion by way of exocytosis.

PHARMACY APPLICATION: ALPHA ONE ADRENERGIC RECEPTOR ANTAGONISTS

Hypertension, or a chronic elevation in blood pressure, is a major risk factor for coronary artery disease, congestive heart failure, stroke, kidney failure and retinopathy. An important cause of hypertension is excessive vascular smooth muscle tone or vasoconstriction. Prazosin, an α_1-adrenergic receptor antagonist, is very effective in the management of hypertension. Because α_1-adrenergic receptor antagonist drugs include Terazosin™, Doxazosin™, Trimazosin™. α_1-receptor stimulation causes vasoconstriction, drugs that block these receptors result in vasodilation and a decrease in blood pressure (see Table 14.4).

Table 14.4 Agonists and antagonists of autonomic receptors

Receptor	Neurotransmitter/ Catecholamine	Agonist	Antagonist
Nicotinic	Acetylcholine	Nicotine	Mecamylamine
Muscarinic	Acetylcholine	Bethanechol	Atropine, Scopolamine
Alpha one	NE, EPI	Phenylephrine	Prazosin
Alpha two	NE, EPI	Clonidine	Yohimbine
Beta 1 (selective)	NE, EPI	Dobutamine	Metoprolol
Beta 2 (selective)		Albuterol	
Beta (nonselective)	EPI	Isoproterenol, Epinephrine	Propranolol, Carvedilol

Compared with α_1 receptors, α_2 receptors have only moderate distribution on the effector tissues. Alpha two-receptor stimulation causes a decrease in cAMP within the tissue's cells and, therefore, results in inhibitory effects such as smooth muscle relaxation and decreased glandular secretion. However, α_2 receptors have important presynaptic effects. Whereas α_1 receptors are found on the effector tissue cells at the neuroeffector junction, the α_2 receptors are found on the varicosities of the postganglionic neuron. Norepinephrine released from this neuron binds to not only the α_1 receptors on the effector tissue to cause some physiological effect; it also binds to the α_2 receptors on the postganglionic neuron itself. Alpha two receptor stimulation results in *presynaptic inhibition* or in a decrease in the release of norepinephrine. (Although it is the *postganglionic* neuron, at the neuroeffector junction this neuron is considered *presynaptic*). In this way, norepinephrine inhibits its own release from the sympathetic postganglionic neuron and controls its own activity. Both α_1 and α_2 receptors have equal affinity for norepinephrine released directly from sympathetic neurons as well as circulating epinephrine released from the adrenal medulla.

Stimulation of each type of *β receptor* leads to an increase in intracellular cAMP. Whether this results in an excitatory or an inhibitory response depends upon the specific cell type. As with α receptors, β receptors are also unevenly distributed with β_2 receptors being the more common subtype on the effector tissues. Beta-two receptors tend to be inhibitory. For example, β_2 receptor stimulation causes relaxation of vascular smooth muscle and airway smooth muscle resulting in vasodilation and bronchodilation, respectively. Beta-two receptors have a significantly greater affinity for epinephrine than for norepinephrine. Furthermore, terminations of sympathetic pathways are not found near these receptors. Therefore, β_2 receptors are stimulated only indirectly by circulating epinephrine instead of by direct sympathetic nervous activity.

Beta-one receptors are the primary adrenergic receptor on the heart (a small percentage of the adrenergic receptors on the myocardium are β_2).

Both subtypes of β receptors on the heart are excitatory, and stimulation leads to an increase in cardiac activity. Beta-one receptors are also found on certain cells in the kidney. Epinephrine and norepinephrine have equal affinity for β_1 receptors.

Beta-three (β_3) receptors are found primarily in adipose tissue. Stimulation of these receptors, which are innervated and have a stronger affinity for norepinephrine, causes lipolysis.

A summary of the autonomic receptors and their neurotransmitters, agonists and antagonists is found in Table 14.4.

PHARMACY APPLICATION: SYMPATHOMIMETIC DRUGS

Sympathomimetic drugs are those that produce effects in a tissue resembling those caused from stimulation by the sympathetic nervous system. An important use for these drugs is in the treatment of bronchial asthma, which is characterized by bronchospasm. As discussed, bronchodilation occurs following β_2-adrenergic receptor stimulation. Nonselective β receptor agonists, such as epinephrine and isoproterenol, can cause bronchodilation. However, a potential problem with these drugs is that they stimulate *all* β-receptors including β_1 receptors on the heart. Therefore, an undesirable side effect of treatment with these nonselective agents is an increase in heart rate. Instead, β_2-selective drugs, such as albuterol, are chosen for this therapy. They are equally effective in causing bronchodilation without the adverse cardiac effects of the nonselective agents (see Table 14.4).

14.6   Functions

The two divisions of the ANS are dominant under different conditions. As stated previously, the sympathetic system is activated during emergency "fight-or-flight" reactions and during exercise. The parasympathetic system is predominant during quiet, resting conditions. As such, the physiological effects caused by each system are quite predictable. In other words, all the changes in organ and tissue function induced by the sympathetic system work together to support strenuous physical activity and the changes induced by the parasympathetic system are appropriate for when the body is resting. Several of the specific effects elicited by sympathetic and parasympathetic stimulation of various organs and tissues are summarized in Table 14.5.

The "fight-or-flight" reaction elicited by the sympathetic system is essentially a whole-body response. Changes in organ and tissue function throughout the body are coordinated so that there is an increase in the delivery of well oxygenated, nutrient-rich blood to the working skeletal muscles.

Table 14.5 Effects of autonomic nerve activity on some effector tissues

Tissue	Sympathetic receptor	Sympathetic stimulation	Parasympathetic stimulation
Eye			
Radial muscle of iris	α_1	Contraction (dilation of pupil; mydriasis)	—
Sphincter muscle of iris		—	Contraction (constriction of pupil; miosis)
Ciliary muscle	β_2	Relaxation for far vision	Contraction for near vision
Heart	β_1, β_2	↑ Heart rate ↑ Force of contraction ↑ Rate of conduction	↓ Heart rate ↓ Rate of conduction
Arterioles			
Skin	α_1	Strong constriction	—
Abdominal viscera	α_1	Strong constriction	—
Kidney	α_1	Strong constriction	—
Skeletal muscle	α_1, β_2	Weak constriction	—
Spleen	α_1	Contraction	—
Lungs			
Airways	β_2	Bronchodilation	Bronchoconstriction
Glands	α_1, β_2	↓ Secretion	↑ Secretion
Liver	α_1, β_2	Glycogenolysis Gluconeogenesis	↑ Secretion of bile
Adipose Tissue	β_3	Lipolysis	—
Sweat Glands	Muscarinic	Generalized sweating	—
	α_1	Localized sweating	—
Piloerector Muscles	α_1	Contraction [erection of hair (goose bumps)]	—
Adrenal Medullae	Nicotinic	↑ Secretion of epinephrine, norepinephrine	—
Salivary Glands	α_1, β_2	Small volume K^+ and water secretion	Large volume K^+ and water secretion; amylase secretion

(Continued)

Table 14.5 (*Continued*)   Effects of autonomic nerve activity on some effector tissues

Tissue	Sympathetic receptor	Sympathetic stimulation	Parasympathetic stimulation
Stomach			
Motility	α_1, β_2	Decreased	Increased
Sphincters	α_1	Contraction	Relaxation
Secretion			Stimulation
Intestine			
Motility	α_1, β_2	Decreased	Increased
Sphincters	α_1	Contraction	Relaxation
Secretion			Stimulation
Gallbladder	β_2	Relaxation	Contraction
Pancreas			
Exocrine	α	↓ Enzyme secretion	↑ Enzyme secretion
Endocrine (pancreatic islets β cells)	α	↓ Insulin secretion	↑ Insulin secretion
Urinary Bladder			
Detrusor muscle (bladder wall)	β_2	Relaxation	Contraction
Urethra sphincter		Contraction	Relaxation
Kidney	β_1	↑ Renin secretion	—

Both heart rate and myocardial contractility are increased so that the heart pumps more blood per minute. Sympathetic stimulation of vascular smooth muscle causes widespread vasoconstriction, particularly in the organs of the gastrointestinal system and in the kidneys. This vasoconstriction serves to redirect or redistribute the blood away from these metabolically inactive tissues and toward the contracting muscles. Bronchodilation in the lungs facilitates the movement of air in and out of the lungs so that the uptake of oxygen from the atmosphere and the elimination of carbon dioxide from the body are maximized. An enhanced rate of glycogenolysis (breakdown of glycogen into its component glucose molecules) and gluconeogenesis (formation of new glucose from noncarbohydrate sources) in the liver increases the concentration of glucose molecules in the blood. This is necessary for the brain because glucose is the only nutrient molecule that it can utilize to form metabolic energy. An enhanced rate of lipolysis in adipose tissue increases the concentration of fatty acid molecules in the blood. Skeletal muscles then utilize these fatty acids to form metabolic energy for contraction. Generalized sweating elicited by the sympathetic system enables the individual to thermoregulate during these conditions of increased physical activity and heat production. Finally, the eye is adjusted such that the pupil dilates letting more light in toward the retina (*mydriasis*) and the lens adapts for distance vision.

The parasympathetic system decreases heart rate, which helps to conserve energy under resting conditions. Salivary secretion is enhanced to facilitate the swallowing of food. Gastric motility and secretion are stimulated to begin the processing of ingested food. Intestinal motility and secretion are also stimulated to continue the processing and to facilitate the absorption of these nutrients. Both exocrine and endocrine secretion from the pancreas is promoted. Enzymes released from the exocrine glands of the pancreas contribute to the chemical breakdown of the food in the intestine, and insulin released from the pancreatic islets promotes the storage of nutrient molecules within the tissues once they are absorbed into the body. Another bodily maintenance type of function caused by the parasympathetic system is contraction of the urinary bladder, which results in urination. Finally, the eye is adjusted such that the pupil contracts (*miosis*) and the lens adapts for near vision.

PHARMACY APPLICATION: CHOLINOMIMETIC DRUGS

Cholinomimetic drugs are those that produce effects in a tissue resembling those caused by parasympathetic nervous system stimulation. These drugs have many important uses including the treatment of gastrointestinal and urinary tract disorders that involve depressed smooth muscle activity without obstruction. For example, postoperative ileus is characterized by a loss of tone or paralysis of the stomach or bowel following surgical manipulation. Urinary retention may also occur postoperatively or it may be secondary to spinal cord injury or disease (neurogenic bladder). Normally, parasympathetic stimulation of the smooth muscle in each of these organ systems causes contraction to maintain gastrointestinal motility as well as urination. There are two different approaches in the pharmacotherapy of these disorders. One type of agent would be a muscarinic receptor agonist, which would mimic the effect of the parasympathetic neurotransmitter, acetylcholine, and stimulate smooth muscle contraction. One of the most widely used agents in this category is bethanechol, which can be given subcutaneously (see Table 14.4). Another approach is to increase the concentration and, therefore, activity of endogenously produced acetylcholine in the neuroeffector junction. Administration of an acetylcholinesterase inhibitor prevents the degradation and removal of neuronally released acetylcholine. In this case, neostigmine is the most widely used agent. Neostigmine may be given either subcutaneously or orally.

PHARMACY APPLICATIONL MUSCARINIC
RECEPTOR ANTAGONISTS

Inspection of the retina during an ophthalmoscopic examination is greatly facilitated by mydriasis, or the dilation of the pupil. Parasympathetic stimulation of the circular muscle layer in the iris causes contraction and a decrease in the diameter of the pupil. Administration of a muscarinic receptor antagonist, such as atropine or scopolamine, prevents this smooth muscle contraction. As a result, sympathetic stimulation of the radial muscle layer is unopposed. This causes an increase in the diameter of the pupil. These agents are given in the form of eye drops, which act locally and limit the possibility of systemic side effects (see Table 14.4).

A mass sympathetic discharge, which typically occurs during the "fight-or-flight" response and during exercise, involves the simultaneous stimulation of organs and tissues throughout the body. Included among these tissues are the *adrenal medullae*, which release epinephrine and norepinephrine into the blood. In large part, the indirect effects of these catecholamines are similar and, therefore, reinforce those of direct sympathetic stimulation. However, there are some important differences in the effects of the circulating catecholamines and those of norepinephrine released from sympathetic nerves including:

- Duration of activity
- Breadth of activity
- Affinity for β_2 receptors

The *duration of activity* of the catecholamines is significantly longer than that of neuronally released norepinephrine. Therefore, the effects on the tissues are more prolonged. This difference has to do with the mechanism of inactivation of these substances. Norepinephrine is immediately removed from the neuroeffector junction by way of reuptake into the postganglionic neuron. This rapid removal limits the duration of the effect of this neurotransmitter. In contrast, there are no enzymes in the blood to degrade the catecholamines. Instead, the catecholamines are inactivated by COMT in the liver. As one might expect, the hepatic clearance of these hormones from the blood would require several passes through the circulation. Therefore, the catecholamines are available to cause their effects for a comparatively longer period (minutes as opposed to milliseconds).

Because they travel in the blood, organs and tissues throughout the body are exposed to the catecholamines. Therefore, they are capable of stimulating tissues that are not directly innervated by sympathetic nerve fibers such as airway smooth muscle, hepatocytes, and adipose tissue. Catecholamines have a much wider *breadth of activity* compared with norepinephrine released from sympathetic nerves.

The third important feature that distinguishes the catecholamines from neuronally released norepinephrine involves epinephrine's *affinity for β_2 receptors*. Norepinephrine has a very limited affinity for these receptors. Therefore, circulating epinephrine causes effects that differ from those of direct sympathetic innervation including:

- Greater stimulatory effect on the heart
- Relaxation of smooth muscle
  - Vascular
  - Bronchial
  - Gastrointestinal
- Genitourinary

Epinephrine and norepinephrine have equal affinity for β_1 receptors, the predominant adrenergic receptor on the heart. However, the human heart also contains a small percentage of β_2 receptors, which, like β_1 receptors, are excitatory. Therefore, epinephrine can stimulate a greater number of receptors, causing a *greater stimulatory effect on the myocardium*.

Beta-two adrenergic receptors are also found on smooth muscle in several organ systems. These receptors tend to be inhibitory and cause *relaxation of the smooth muscle*. Vascular smooth muscle in skeletal muscle contains both α_1 and β_2 receptors. Norepinephrine, which stimulates only the excitatory α_1 receptors, causes strong vasoconstriction. However, epinephrine, which stimulates both types of receptors, causes only weak vasoconstriction. The vasodilation resulting from β_2 receptor stimulation opposes and, therefore, weakens the vasoconstriction resulting from α_1 receptor stimulation. Given that skeletal muscle may account for 40% of an adult's body weight, the potential difference in vasoconstriction, blood pressure and the distribution of blood flow could be quite significant.

Another noteworthy example of the relaxation of smooth muscle by way of β_2 receptor stimulation involves the airways. Bronchodilation, or the opening of the airways, facilitates airflow in the lungs. Any direct sympathetic innervation to the lungs is irrelevant in this respect, as only circulating epinephrine can stimulate these receptors on airway smooth muscle.

Medical terminology

adrenergic (ăd-rĕn-ĕr′jĭk): Refers to nerve fibers that release norepinephrine, receptors that bind with norepinephrine or epinephrine, or a substance that has catecholamine-like activity

affinity (ă-fĭn′ĭ-tē): Attraction; ability to bind with a specific receptor

cholinergic (kō″lĭn-ĕr′jĭk): Refers to nerve fibers that release acetylcholine, receptors that bind with acetylcholine or a substance that has acetylcholine-like activity

gap junction: Minute pore between muscle cells that allows for intercellular communication

miosis (mī-ō′sĭs): Contraction of the pupil

mydriasis (mĭd-rī′ă-sĭs): Dilation of the pupil

tonic (tŏn′ĭk): Refers to a pattern of continuous, prolonged activity

vagus (vā′gŭs): Cranial nerve X, the major parasympathetic nerve, it innervates structures in the thoracic and abdominal cavities

varicosity (văr″ĭ-kŏs′ĭ-tē): Swelling at the terminal of a postganglionic axon from which neurotransmitter is released

Bibliography

Bear, M. F., Connors, B. W., and Paradiso, M. A., *Neuroscience, Exploring the Brain,* 3rd ed., Lippincott Williams & Wilkins, Philadelphia, PA, 2007.

Brown, J. H., and Taylor, P., Muscarinic receptor agonists and antagonists, in *Goodman and Gilman's: The Pharmacological Basis of Therapeutics,* 11th ed., Brunton, L. L., Lazo, J. S., and Parker, K. L., Eds. McGraw-Hill, New York, 2006, chap. 7.

Fox, S. I., *Human Physiology,* 9th ed., McGraw-Hill, Boston, MA, 2006.

Guyton, A. C., and Hall, J. E., *Textbook of Medical Physiology,* 11th ed., Elsevier/Saunders, Philadelphia, PA, 2006.

Hoffman, B. B., Adrenoceptor-activating & other sympathomimetic drugs, in *Basic and Clinical Pharmacology,* 8th ed., Katzung, B. G., Ed., Lange Medical Books/McGraw-Hill, New York, 2001, chap. 9.

Hoffman, B. B., Adrenoceptor antagonist drugs, in *Basic and Clinical Pharmacology,* 8th ed., Katzung, B. G., Ed., Lange Medical Books/McGraw-Hill, New York, 2001, chap. 10.

Iversen, S., Iversen, L., and Saper, C., The autonomic nervous system and the hypothalamus, in *Principles of Neuroscience,* 4th ed., Kandel, E. R., Schwartz, J. H., and Jessell, T. M., Eds., McGraw-Hill, New York, 2000, chap. 49.

Katzung, B. G., Introduction to autonomic pharmacology, in *Basic and Clinical Pharmacology,* 8th ed., Katzung, B. G., Ed., Lange Medical Books/McGraw-Hill, New York, 2001, chap. 6.

Naftel, J. P., and Hardy, S. G. P., Visceral motor pathways, in *Fundamental Neuroscience for Basic and Clinical Applications,* 3rd ed., Haines, D. E., Ed., Churchill Livingstone/Elsevier, Philadelphia, PA, 2006, chap. 29.

Pappano, A. J., Cholinoceptor-activating & cholinesterase-inhibiting drugs, in *Basic and Clinical Pharmacology,* 8th ed., Katzung, B. G., Ed., Lange Medical Books/McGraw-Hill, New York, 2001, chap. 7.

Pappano, A. J., Cholinoceptor-blocking drugs, in *Basic and Clinical Pharmacology,* 8th ed., Katzung, B. G., Ed., Lange Medical Books/McGraw-Hill, New York, 2001, chap. 8.

Rhoades, R., and Pflanzer, R., *Human Physiology,* 4th ed., Thomson Learning, Pacific Grove, CA, 2003.

Sherwood, L., *Human Physiology from Cells to Systems,* 5th ed., Brooks/Cole, Pacific Grove, CA, 2004.

Silverthorn, D., *Human Physiology: An Integrated Approach*, 4th ed., Prentice Hall, Upper Saddle River, NJ, 2007.

Taber's Cyclopedic Medical Dictionary, 20th ed., F. A. Davis Co., Philadelphia, PA, 2005.

Taylor, P., Agents acting at the neuromuscular junction and autonomic ganglia, in *Goodman and Gilman's: The Pharmacological Basis of Therapeutics*, 11th ed., Brunton, L. L., Lazo, J. S., and Parker, K. L., Eds., McGraw-Hill, New York, 2006, chap. 9.

Westfall, T. C., and Westfall, D. P., Neurotransmission: The autonomic and somatic motor nervous systems, in *Goodman and Gilman's: The Pharmacological Basis of Therapeutics*, 11th ed., Brunton, L. L., Lazo, J. S., and Parker, K. L., Eds., McGraw-Hill, New York, 2006, chap. 6.

Westfall, T. C., and Westfall, D. P., Adrenergic agonists and antagonists, in *Goodman and Gilman's: The Pharmacological Basis of Therapeutics*, 11th ed., Brunton, L. L., Lazo, J. S., and Parker, K. L., Eds., McGraw-Hill, New York, 2006, chap. 10.

Widmaier, E. P., Raff, H., and Strang, K. T., *Vander's Human Physiology, The Mechanisms of Body Function*, McGraw-Hill, Boston, MA, 2006.

chapter fifteen

Pain

Study objectives

- Describe the three types of nociceptors and the stimuli that activate them
- Distinguish between A-delta fibers and C fibers
- Compare and contrast fast pain and slow pain
- Distinguish between primary hyperalgesia and centrally-mediated hyperalgesia
- Discuss the functions of the neurotransmitters, glutamate, and substance P
- Describe the pain pathway and the role that each stimulated region of the brain plays in the response to pain
- Explain how the endogenous analgesic system suppresses pain
- Describe the gate control theory and its contribution to the suppression of pain
- Distinguish between cutaneous pain and deep visceral pain
- Describe the mechanisms by which tissue ischemia and muscle spasm lead to pain
- Discuss the potential causes of visceral pain
- Describe the mechanism of referred pain
- Explain how phantom pain occurs
- List the properties of an ideal analgesic medication
- List and discuss the effects of nonnarcotic analgesic medications
- Discuss the effects of opioid analgesic medications
- Discuss the effects of adjuvant medications

Sensations interpreted as *pain*—including burning, aching, stinging and soreness—are the most distinctive forms of sensory input to the central nervous system (CNS). Pain serves an important protective function because it causes awareness of actual or potential tissue damage. Furthermore, it stimulates an individual to react to remove or withdraw from the source of the pain. Unlike other forms of sensory input—such as vision, hearing and smell—pain has an urgent, primitive quality. This quality is responsible for the behavioral and emotional aspects of pain perception.

15.1   Nociceptors

Nociceptors (Latin *nocere*, "to hurt") are bare or free nerve endings. Therefore, they do not adapt, or stop responding, to sustained or repeated stimulation. This is beneficial, in that, it keeps the individual aware of the damaging stimulus for as long as it persists. Nociceptors are widely distributed in the skin, dental pulp, bone, joints, muscle, blood vessels, meninges, and some internal organs. Stimulation of nociceptors involves the activation, or opening, of ion channels that alter membrane potential.

There are three major classes of nociceptors:

- Thermal nociceptors
- Mechanical nociceptors
- Polymodal nociceptors

Thermal nociceptors are activated by extreme temperatures, especially heat. One group of these receptors is stimulated by noxious heat (>45°C). Heat-sensitive ion channels on these nociceptors are activated at this temperature, causing depolarization and the generation of an action potential. A second group of thermal nociceptors is stimulated by noxious cold (<5°C). These are the temperatures at which the tissues begin to be damaged.

Mechanical nociceptors are activated by mechanical damage, such as cutting, pinching, or tissue distortion. They are also activated by intense pressure applied to the skin. The simple distortion of the nociceptor membrane activates mechanically gated ion channels, which results in depolarization and the generation of an action potential. Their firing rates increase with the destructiveness of the mechanical stimulus.

Most nociceptors in the human body are *polymodal nociceptors*, which are activated by all types of damaging stimuli (thermal, mechanical, chemical), including irritating exogenous substances that may penetrate the skin. Endogenous substances that may stimulate these receptors to elicit pain include potassium released from damaged cells; bradykinin; histamine; substance P; acids; and proteolytic enzymes (see Table 15.1). With the polymodal nociceptors, it is the chemicals that may activate ion channels on the nociceptors to cause depolarization and generate an action potential. Stimulation of polymodal nociceptors elicits sensations of slow, burning pain.

There are two types of afferent neurons associated with nociceptors:

- A-delta fibers
- C fibers

Thermal nociceptors and mechanical nociceptors are associated with *A-delta fibers*. These are small, myelinated fibers that transmit impulses at a

Table 15.1 Endogenous chemicals activating or sensitizing nociceptors

Chemical	Source	Enzyme Involved in Synthesis	Effect on First-Order Sensory Neuron	Pharmacological Intervention
Potassium	Damaged cells		Activation	
Serotonin	Platelets	Tryptophan hydroxylase	Activation	
Bradykinin	Plasma kininogen	Kallikrein	Activation	
Histamine	Mast cells		Activation	H1 receptor antagonists (e.g., diphenhydramine. chloride, Benadryl)
Prostaglandins	Arachidonic acid/ damaged cells	Cyclooxygenase	Sensitization	Nonsteroidal anti-inflammatory drugs (e.g., aspirin, ibuprofen)
Leukotrienes	Arachidonic acid/ damaged cells	Lipoxygenase	Sensitization	
Substance P	First-order sensory neurons		Sensitization	Opioid receptor agonists (e.g., morphine)

rate of 5–30 m/s. Polymodal nociceptors are associated with *C fibers*. These are small, unmyelinated fibers that transmit impulses at a rate generally less than 1.0 m/s (range of 0.5–2.0 m/s).

There are two types of pain:

- Fast pain
- Slow pain

Fast pain may be described as sharp or prickling pain (see Table 15.2). This pain is perceived first (within 0.1 s) because it is carried by the more rapidly conducting A-delta fibers. Because fast pain is elicited by the stimulation of specific thermal or mechanical nociceptors, it is easily localized. This type of pain is not felt in most of the deeper tissues of the body.

Slow pain may be described as dull, aching or throbbing pain. This pain is perceived second (only after 1 s or more) because it is carried by

Table 15.2 Characteristics of fast and slow pain

Fast pain	Slow pain
Occurs first	Occurs second, persists longer
Sharp, prickling sensation	Dull, aching, throbbing sensation; more unpleasant
A-delta fibers	C fibers
Thermal or mechanical nociceptors	Polymodal nociceptors
Easily localized	Poorly localized

C fibers. Slow pain persists longer and it is typically more unpleasant. In fact, this pain tends to become greater over time. Slow pain is typically associated with tissue destruction. Noxious chemicals released from damaged cells or activated in the interstitial fluid can spread in the tissue, causing a relatively diffuse stimulation of polymodal receptors. As a result, slow pain is poorly localized and may occur in the skin as well as in almost any deep tissue or organ.

15.2 Hyperalgesia

An injured area is typically more sensitive to subsequent stimuli and painful stimuli, or even normally non-painful stimuli, may cause an excessive pain response.

There are two types of hyperalgesia:

- Primary hyperalgesia
- Centrally mediated hyperalgesia

An increase in the sensitivity of nociceptors is referred to as *primary hyperalgesia*. A classic example of primary hyperalgesia is a burn. Even light touch of a burned area may be painful.

The sensitization of nociceptors following tissue damage or inflammation results from a variety of chemicals released or activated in the injured area (see Table 15.1). These substances decrease the threshold for activation of the nociceptors. One such substance that seems to elicit more pain than the others is *bradykinin*. Activated by enzymes released from damaged cells, bradykinin causes pain by several mechanisms including:

- Direct activation of A-delta and C fibers
- Along with histamine, it contributes to the inflammatory response to tissue injury
- Promotes the synthesis and release of prostaglandins from nearby cells.

The *prostaglandins* sensitize all three types of pain receptors, which in turn will enhance the response to a noxious stimulus. In other words, it hurts more when prostaglandins are present. Aspirin and nonsteroidal anti-inflammatory drugs (NSAIDs) inhibit the synthesis of prostaglandins, which accounts, in part, for their analgesic effects.

Centrally mediated hyperalgesia involves the hyperexcitability of the second-order sensory neurons in the dorsal horn of the spinal cord. In the case of severe or persistent tissue injury, C fibers fire action potentials repetitively and the response of the second-order sensory neurons increases progressively. The mechanism of this enhanced response, also referred to as *"wind-up,"* depends on the release of the neurotransmitter *glutamate* from the C fibers. An excitatory neurotransmitter, glutamate stimulates the opening of calcium channels gated by the *N*-methyl-D-aspartate (NMDA)-type glutamate receptor. Calcium influx ultimately leads to long-term biochemical changes and hyperexcitability of the second-order neuron.

15.3   Neurotransmission

There are two neurotransmitters released by the nociceptive afferent fibers in the dorsal horn of the spinal cord. These neurotransmitters, which stimulate the second-order sensory neurons, include:

- Glutamate
- Substance P

The amino acid, *glutamate*, is the major neurotransmitter released by both A-delta fibers and C fibers. Glutamate binds to the AMPA-type glutamate receptor on the second-order sensory neuron to elicit action potentials and continue the transmission of the signal to higher levels of the CNS.

Substance P is released primarily from C fibers. Levels of this neurotransmitter increase significantly under conditions of persistent pain. Substance P also stimulates ascending pathways in the spinal cord. Furthermore, it appears to enhance and prolong the actions of glutamate.

15.4   Pain pathways

Stimulation of a nociceptor in the periphery of the body elicits action potentials in the *first-order neuron*. The signal is transmitted by this neuron to the *second-order neuron* in the dorsal horn of the spinal cord. From the spinal cord, the signal is transmitted to several regions of the brain. The more prominent ascending nociceptive pathway is the *spinothalamic tract*. Axons of the second-order sensory neurons immediately project to the contralateral (opposite) side of the spinal cord and ascend in the white matter, terminating in the *thalamus* (see Figure 15.1). The thalamus contributes to the basic

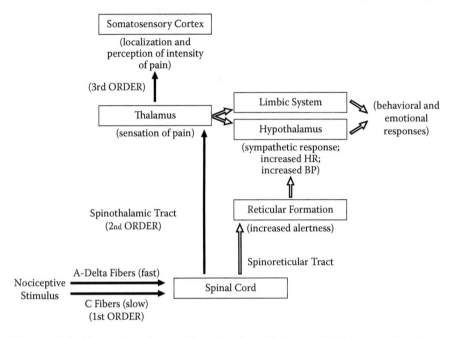

Figure 15.1 The pain pathway. The pain signal is transmitted to several regions
of the brain including the thalamus, the reticular formation, the hypothalamus,
the limbic system and the somatosensory cortex. Each region carries out a specific
aspect of the response to pain.

sensation or awareness of pain only. The source of the painful stimulus cannot be determined by the thalamus.

The thalamus houses the cell bodies of *third-order sensory* neurons. These
neurons transmit the pain signal to the *somatosensory cortex*. The function of
this region of the brain is to localize and perceive the intensity of the painful stimulus. Further transmission of the signal to the *association areas* of the
cerebral cortex is important for the perception and the meaningfulness of
the painful stimulus.

Other nerve signals are transmitted simultaneously from the spinal cord
to the *reticular formation* of the brainstem by way of the *spinoreticular tract*.
The reticular formation plays an important role in the response to pain. First,
it facilitates avoidance reflexes at all levels of the spinal cord. Second, it is
responsible for the significant arousal effects of pain. Signals from the reticular formation cause an increase in the electrical activity of the cerebral cortex
associated with increased alertness. Furthermore, it sends nerve impulses to
the *hypothalamus* to influence its functions associated with sudden alertness,
such as increased heart rate and blood pressure. These responses are mediated by the sympathetic nervous system.

Nerve signals from the thalamus and the reticular formation are transmitted to the *limbic system*, which may be involved with the mood-altering and attention-narrowing effect of pain, as well as the hypothalamus. Together, these regions of the brain are responsible for the behavioral and emotional responses to pain.

The *endogenous analgesic system* is a built-in neuronal system that suppresses the transmission of nerve impulses in the pain pathway. It functions by way of the following neurotransmitters produced in the CNS:

- Endorphins
- Enkephalins
- Dynorphin

Endorphins are found primarily in the limbic system, the hypothalamus and the brainstem. *Enkephalins* and *dynorphin* (in smaller quantities) are found primarily in the *periaqueductal gray matter (PAG)* of the midbrain, the limbic system and the hypothalamus. These endogenous substances mimic the effects of morphine and other opiate drugs (narcotics) at many points in the analgesic system, including in the dorsal horns of the spinal cord.

Opiate receptors are highly concentrated in the PAG area of the midbrain. Stimulation of this region produces long-lasting analgesia with no effect on the level of consciousness. For these reasons, the PAG area is often referred to as the *endogenous analgesia center*. The PAG area receives input from many regions of the CNS, including the cerebral cortex, hypothalamus, reticular formation of the brainstem and the spinal cord by way of the spinothalamic tracts. This region is also interconnected with the limbic system, which is responsible for the emotional response to pain.

There are three major components of the endogenous analgesic pathway:

- Periaqueductal gray area
- Nucleus raphe magnus
- Pain inhibitory complex in the dorsal horns of the spinal cord

The endogenous analgesic pathway begins in the PAG area. Neurons of the PAG area descend to the *nucleus raphe magnus (NRM)* in the medulla (see Figure 15.2). Neurons of the NRM then descend to the dorsal horn of the spinal cord where they synapse with local spinal interneurons. The interneurons then synapse with the incoming pain fibers. Many of the neurons derived from the PAG area secrete enkephalin from their axon terminals in the NRM. The neurons derived from the NRM secrete serotonin from their axon terminals in the spinal cord. The serotonin stimulates the local cord interneurons to secrete enkephalin. The enkephalin then causes presynaptic inhibition of the incoming pain fibers. Binding of enkephalin to opiate receptors on these pain fibers blocks the calcium channels in the axon terminals.

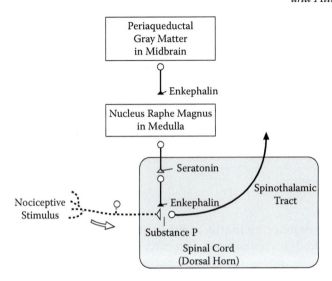

Figure 15.2   The endogenous analgesic system. The three major components of the endogenous analgesic system include the periaqueductal gray matter in the midbrain, the nucleus raphe magnus in the medulla and the pain inhibitory complex in the dorsal horns of the spinal cord. This system causes presynaptic inhibition of the pain fibers entering the spinal cord. The binding of enkephalin to opiate receptors on the pain fibers prevents the release of the neurotransmitter, substance P and the pain signal is terminated in the spinal cord and does not ascend to higher centers in the central nervous system.

Because the influx of calcium is necessary for the exocytosis of neurotransmitters, blocking these channels prevents the release of substance P. Thus, this system interrupts the pain signal at the level of the spinal cord.

The endogenous analgesic system is normally inactive. It remains unclear as to how this system becomes activated. Potential activating factors include exercise, stress, acupuncture, and hypnosis.

The transmission of nerve impulses in the pain pathway may also be inhibited by the activity of *A-beta neurons* by way of a mechanism referred to as the *gate control theory*. Under normal conditions, activity in the second-order neurons of the pain pathway is blocked by tonically active *inhibitory interneurons* in the dorsal horn of the spinal cord (see Figure 15.3a). When a painful stimulus results in the transmission of action potentials to the spinal cord along the C fibers, the activity of the inhibitory interneuron ceases. By way of divergence, C fibers directly inhibit the inhibitory interneurons. Therefore, the C fibers not only stimulate the second-order neurons, they prevent the inhibitory effect exerted upon those neurons and a strong pain signal is transmitted to the brain (see Figure 15.3b).

A-beta fibers are large-diameter fibers that transmit impulses at a rate of 30–70 m/s. Like the C fibers, they are activated by mechanical stimuli, such

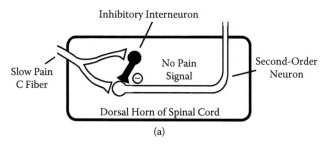

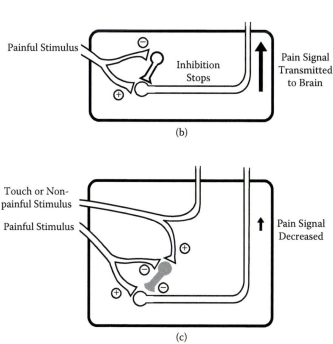

Figure 15.3 The gate control theory. The mechanism proposed by this theory involves the inhibition of the second-order neuron in the pain pathway. Cell bodies of these neurons are found in the dorsal horn of the spinal cord. (a) Under normal conditions, tonically active inhibitory interneurons in the dorsal horn of the spinal cord block the stimulation of the second-order neurons. This activity prevents the perception of pain. (b) When a strong pain stimulus reaches the spinal cord by way of the C fibers, the second-order neurons are stimulated. In addition, the C fibers block the activity of the inhibitory interneuron. As a result, the pain stimulus continues along the pain pathway to the brain. (c) The perception of pain may be reduced by simultaneous somatosensory input. The sensation of touch is transmitted by A-beta fibers. These fibers stimulate the inhibitory interneurons and activity of the second-order neurons is reduced. The signals to the brain are decreased and the perception of pain is decreased.

as touch. A-beta fibers also synapse with the inhibitory interneurons in the dorsal horn of the spinal cord. However, in contrast to the C fibers, which block activity in the inhibitory interneurons, A-beta fibers stimulate these interneurons (see Figure 15.3c). The inhibitory effect that these neurons exert upon the second-order neurons in the pain pathway is renewed. Therefore, the inhibitory interneurons modulate, or reduce, the activation of the second-order neurons and the pain signal transmitted to the brain becomes weaker.

The gate control theory explains the phenomenon that occurs by rubbing an injured body part. The rubbing activates the A-beta fibers and the perception of pain is reduced.

15.5   Types of pain

Cutaneous pain is felt in superficial structures such as the skin and subcutaneous tissues. A pinprick or a paper cut are examples of cutaneous pain. It is a sharp pain with a burning quality that may be easily localized. This pain may be abrupt or slow in onset.

As its name implies, *deep somatic pain* is generated in deep body structures, such as the periosteum, muscles, tendons, joints, and blood vessels. This type of pain is more diffuse than cutaneous pain. It may be elicited by strong pressure, ischemia and tissue damage.

15.5.1   Tissue ischemia

When blood flow to a tissue is decreased, or interrupted, the tissue becomes painful within a few minutes. In fact, the greater the rate of metabolism in the tissue, the more rapid is the onset of pain. The causes of pain due to *tissue ischemia* include:

- Accumulation of *lactic acid* due to the anaerobic metabolism that occurs during ischemia
- *Release and activation of noxious chemicals* in the area of tissue ischemia due to tissue damage (see Table 15.1)

The lactic acid and other noxious chemicals stimulate polymodal nociceptors.

15.5.2   Muscle spasm

The pain induced by *muscle spasm* results partially from the direct effect of tissue distortion on mechanical nociceptors. Muscle spasm also causes tissue ischemia. The increased muscle tension compresses blood vessels and decreases blood flow. Furthermore, the increased rate of metabolism associated with the spasm exacerbates the ischemia. As discussed Section 15.5.1, ischemia leads to the stimulation of polymodal nociceptors.

15.5.3   Visceral pain

Visceral pain occurs in the organs and tissues of the thoracic and abdominal cavities. This type of pain has several interesting characteristics including the following:

- Not all tissues evoke visceral pain (e.g., liver, lung parenchyma)
- It is diffuse and poorly localized
- It often generates referred pain (discussed in the Section 15.5.4 of this chapter)
- It is typically accompanied by autonomic nervous system responses (e.g., nausea, vomiting, sweating, pallor, increased blood pressure)

Visceral pain may be caused by several factors including:

- Inflammation
- Chemical stimuli
- Spasm of a hollow organ
- Overdistension of a hollow organ

Inflammation of the appendix (appendicitis) and the gallbladder (cholecystitis) are common examples of visceral pain. Mechanical receptors are activated by the tissue distension associated with inflammation. In addition, inflammatory mediators, such as histamine and bradykinin, may activate polymodal nociceptors.

Chemical stimuli may include gastric acid (gastroesophageal reflux disease [GERD], gastric ulcer, duodenal ulcer) or those substances associated with tissue ischemia, tissue damage and inflammation.

Spasm of the smooth muscle in the wall of a hollow organ causes pain due to the direct stimulation of mechanical nociceptors as well as ischemia-induced stimulation of polymodal nociceptors. This type of pain often occurs in the form of *cramps*. In other words, the pain increases to a high intensity and then subsides. This process occurs rhythmically, once every few minutes. Cramping pain frequently occurs in gastroenteritis, menstruation, and parturition (labor).

Overdistension of a hollow organ causes pain by the excessive stretch of the tissue and the stimulation of mechanical nociceptors. Overdistension may also cause collapse of the blood vessels resulting in the development of ischemic pain.

15.5.4   Referred pain

Referred pain is felt in a part of the body that is different from the actual tissue causing the pain. Typically, the pain is initiated in a visceral organ or tissue and referred to an area of the body surface. Classic examples of referred pain include *headache* and *angina*. Interestingly, the brain itself does not contain nociceptors. Therefore, the pain perceived as a headache originates in other tissues, such as the eyes, sinuses, muscles of the head and neck, and the meninges. Angina, or chest pain, is caused by coronary ischemia. It may be accompanied by pain referred to the neck, left shoulder and left arm.

Referred pain most likely results from the convergence of visceral and somatic afferent fibers on the same second-order neurons in the dorsal horn of the spinal cord (see Figure 15.4). Therefore, the brain has no way of identifying the original source of the pain. Because superficial inputs normally predominate over visceral inputs, higher centers may incorrectly attribute the pain to the skin instead of the deeper tissue.

Phantom pain is pain that appears to arise from an amputated limb or body part. As many as 70% of amputees experience phantom pain. This pain may begin with sensations of tingling, heat, cold, or heaviness; followed by burning, cramping, or shooting pain. Phantom pain may disappear spontaneously or persist for many years.

The exact cause of phantom pain is not clearly understood. One proposed mechanism involves stimulation of the sensory pathway that had once originated in the amputated body part. An important point is that the sensory pathway originating in each body part transmits impulses to the region of the somatosensory cortex devoted to that body part regardless of amputation. Stimulation at any point along this pathway results in the same sensation that would be produced by stimulation of the nociceptor in the

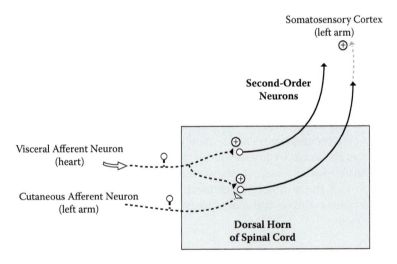

Figure 15.4 Referred pain. The mechanism of referred pain involves the convergence of visceral afferent neurons and cutaneous afferent neurons with the same second-order neurons in the dorsal horn of the spinal cord. In this example, the pain of angina that originates in the heart is referred to the left arm.

body part itself. Following amputation of a body part, the ends of the first-order afferent nerves arising from that body part become trapped in the scar tissue of the stump. These afferent nerve endings exhibit increased sensitivity and are easily stimulated. Therefore, action potentials are generated at these nerve endings and are transmitted to the area of the somatosensory cortex devoted to the amputated body part. This results in the perception of pain arising from the amputated portion of the body.

A second theory of phantom pain suggests that the second-order neurons in the dorsal horn of the spinal cord become hyperactive. Spontaneous firing of these neurons causes the transmission of nerve impulses to the brain and the perception of pain.

15.6   Treatment of pain

An *analgesic drug* acts on the nervous system to suppress or eliminate pain without causing loss of consciousness. As such, an ideal analgesic would exhibit the following qualities:

- Potent
- Nonaddictive
- Minimal adverse effects
- Effective without altering the patient's state of awareness
- Does not cause tolerance
- Inexpensive

Pain medications may be divided into three categories:

- Nonnarcotic analgesics
- Opioid analgesics
- Adjuvant analgesics

15.6.1   Nonnarcotic analgesics

The *nonnarcotic analgesics* include aspirin, NSAIDs and acetaminophen. *Aspirin* acts peripherally to block the transmission of pain impulses. Furthermore, it reduces fever (antipyretic effects) and inflammation and inhibits the synthesis of the prostaglandins (which increase the sensitivity of the nociceptors).

The *NSAIDs* exert their analgesic effects primarily through the inhibition of cyclooxygenase, the rate-limiting enzyme for prostaglandin synthesis. Typical nonselective NSAIDs inhibit both cyclooxygenase 1 (COX-1; constitutive) and cyclooxygenase 2 (COX-2; induced in areas of inflammation). More recently, medications specific for COX-2, such as celecoxib (Celebrex®) have been developed. (Other medications, such as rofecoxib

(Vioxx®) and valdecoxib (Bextra®) have been withdrawn from use due to adverse cardiovascular events reported in many patients.) The U.S. Food and Drug Administration (FDA) is strengthening an existing label warning that non-aspirin nonsteroidal anti-inflammatory drugs (NSAIDs) increase the chance of a heart attack or stroke.

The advantage of the COX-2 agents is that they reduce pain, fever and inflammation without a high risk of unwanted gastric side effects that accompany COX-1 inhibition, particularly those leading to gastrointestinal irritation and gastric ulcers. (The protective effects of the COX-1 produced prostaglandins in the stomach are discussed in Chapter 9, *The Digestive System*.)

Acetaminophen, another alternative to aspirin, is an effective analgesic and fever-reducing agent. However, at usually administered doses, this medication has no effect on inflammation.

15.6.2   Opioid Analgesics

Medications with morphine-like actions are referred to as *opioid* or *narcotic agents*. Opioid drugs exert their effects through three major categories of opioid receptors: mu (μ), kappa (κ), and delta (Δ). Analgesia appears to involve μ receptors (largely at supraspinal sites) and κ receptors (principally within the spinal cord). *Morphine* produces analgesia through interaction with μ receptors. In fact, most clinically used opioids are relatively selective for μ receptors. Morphine can stimulate μ_2 receptors spinally or μ_1 receptors supraspinally. When given systemically, it acts predominantly through supraspinal μ_1 receptors. Other effects of μ receptor activation include respiratory depression, reduced gastrointestinal motility (leading to constipation), and feelings of well-being or euphoria.

Morphine may be administered orally, intravenously or epidurally. An advantage of epidural administration is that it provides effective analgesia while minimizing the central depressant effects associated with systemic administration. The mechanism of action with the epidural route of administration involves the opiate receptors on the cell bodies of the first-order sensory neurons in the dorsal root ganglia as well as their axon terminals in the dorsal horn. Stimulation of these receptors inhibits the release of substance P and interrupts the transmission of the pain signal to the second-order sensory neuron.

Although opioid analgesics are very effective in relieving pain, they are also highly addictive. Furthermore, when needed for long-term use, there may be the development of tolerance. When this occurs, larger and larger doses of the narcotic agent are needed to elicit the same degree of pain relief.

15.6.3 *Adjuvant analgesics*

Adjuvant analgesics include medications such as *antidepressants* and *antiseizure medications*. The effectiveness of these agents may be due to the existence of nonendorphin synapses in the endogenous analgesic pathway. For example, the neurotransmitter, serotonin, has been shown to play a role in producing analgesia. Tricyclic antidepressant medications, such as imipramine, that block the removal of serotonin from the synapse, suppress pain in some individuals. Certain antiseizure medications, such as carbamazepine and phenytoin, have specific analgesic effects that are effective under certain conditions. For example, these medications, which suppress spontaneous neuronal firing, are particularly effective in the management of pain following nerve injury. Other agents, such as the *corticosteroids*, reduce pain by decreasing inflammation and the nociceptive stimuli responsible for the pain.

Medical terminology

Analgesia (ăn-ăl-jē′zē-ă): No perception of pain
Analgesic (ăn-ăl-jē′sĭk): Medication that relieves pain
Hyperalgesia (hī″pĕr-ăl-jē′zē-ă): Increased sensitivity to painful stimuli
Ischemia (ĭs-kē′mē-ă): Temporary blood flow deficiency to an organ or tissue
Narcotic (năr-kŏt′ĭk): Any drug derived from opium or opiumlike compounds; analgesic drug that depresses the central nervous system
Nociceptor (nō″sē-sĕp′tor): A free nerve ending responsive to painful stimuli
Opioid (ō′pē-oyd): A synthetic narcotic not derived from opium that binds to and stimulates an opiate receptor (e.g., morphine)
Spasm (spăzm): An involuntary muscle contraction

Bibliography

Basbaum, A. I. and Jessell, T. M., The perception of pain, in *Principles of Neuroscience*, 4th ed., Kandel, E. R., Schwartz, J. H. and Jessell, T. M., Eds., McGraw-Hill, New York, 2000, chap. 24.

Bear, M. F., Connors, B. W., and Paradiso, M. A., *Neuroscience, Exploring the Brain*, 3rd ed., Lippincott Williams & Wilkins, Philadelphia, PA, 2007.

Burke, A., Smyth, E. M., and Fitzgerald, G. A., Analgesic-antipyretic and antiinflammatory agents; pharmacotherapy of gout, in *Goodman and Gilman's: The Pharmacological Basis of Therapeutics*, 11th ed., Brunton, L. L., Lazo, J. S., and Parker, K. L., Eds., McGraw-Hill, New York, 2006, chap. 26.

Devine, E., Somatosensory function, pain, and headache, in *Pathophysiology, Concepts of Altered Health States*, 7th ed., Porth, C. M., Ed., Lippincott-Raven Publications, Philadelphia, PA, 2005, chap. 50.

FDA strengthens warning that non-aspirin nonsteroidal anti-inflammatory drugs (NSAIDs) can cause heart attacks or strokes. (January 1, 2016) Retrieved from https://www.fda.gov/Drugs/DrugSafety/ucm451800.htm

Gardner, E. P., Martin, J. H., and Jessell, T. M., The bodily senses, in *Principles of Neuroscience*, 4th ed., Kandel, E. R., Schwartz, J. H., and Jessell, T. M., Eds., McGraw-Hill, New York, 2000, chap. 22.

Guyton, A. C., and Hall, J. E., *Textbook of Medical Physiology*, 11th ed., W. B. Saunders, Philadelphia, PA, 2006.

Rhoades, R. and Pflanzer, R., *Human Physiology*, 4th ed., Brooks/Cole, Pacific Grove, CA, 2003.

Sherwood, L., *Human Physiology from Cells to Systems*, 5th ed., Brooks/Cole, Pacific Grove, CA, 2004.

Silverthorn, D. U., *Human Physiology, an Integrated Approach*, 4th ed., Prentice Hall, Upper Saddle River, NJ, 2007.

Stedman, T. L., *Stedman's Medical Dictionary for the Health Professions and Nursing*, 5th ed., Lippincott Williams & Wilkins, Baltimore, MD, 2005.

Venes, D. *Taber's Cyclopedic Medical Dictionary*, 20th ed., F. A. Davis Co., Philadelphia, PA, 2005.

chapter sixteen

Muscle

Study objectives

- Describe the morphological differences between skeletal muscle and smooth muscle
- Explain how contraction and relaxation of smooth muscle occurs
- Explain why smooth muscle contraction is slow and prolonged
- Describe the latch state condition
- Distinguish between multiunit smooth muscle and single-unit smooth muscle
- Compare and contrast pacemaker potentials and slow-wave potentials
- List the factors that may alter smooth muscle contractile activity
- Explain how intracellular calcium concentration may be increased
- Describe the stress–relaxation response
- Describe the length–tension relationship in smooth muscle
- Discuss hyperplasia in smooth muscle
- Explain the functions of skeletal muscle
- Distinguish between origin and insertion; flexion and extension; and agonist, antagonist and synergist muscles
- Distinguish between isometric and isotonic contractions
- Distinguish between concentric and eccentric contractions
- Describe the components of the thick filaments and the thin filaments
- Explain the functions of the following: myosin cross bridges, troponin, tropomyosin, sarcomeres, Z lines, neuromuscular junction, transverse tubules, and sarcoplasmic reticulum
- Describe the Sliding Filament Theory of skeletal muscle contraction
- Explain how creatine phosphate, oxidative phosphorylation and glycolysis provide energy for skeletal muscle contraction
- List the factors that influence the onset of muscle fatigue
- Describe the factors that lead to the development of muscle fatigue
- Describe the metabolic processes that lead to oxygen debt
- Distinguish between the three types of muscle fibers: slow-twitch oxidative, fast-twitch oxidative and fast-twitch glycolytic
- Explain how the percentage of a muscle fiber type, in a given muscle, is determined

- Describe the factors that influence the strength of skeletal muscle contraction including multiple motor unit summation, asynchronous motor unit summation, frequency of nerve stimulation, the length–tension relationship and the diameter of the muscle fiber
- Distinguish the major features for the various metabolic disorders associated with skeletal muscle
- Understand the genetic basis for the most common forms of muscular dystrophy
- List the major symptoms associated with the various forms of muscular dystrophy
- Describe the underlying causes of cerebral palsy. With what symptoms do patients commonly present?
- Discuss the mechanism by which myasthenia gravis occurs
- List the major symptoms associated with myasthenia gravis. Discuss why each occurs.

16.1   Smooth muscle

Although skeletal muscle comprises the bulk of the muscle tissue in the body, *smooth muscle* tissue is far more involved in terms of homeostasis. Most smooth muscle is found in layers or sheets within the walls of tubes and hollow organs. Contraction and relaxation of the smooth muscle in these structures regulates the movement of substances within them. For example, contraction of the smooth muscle in the wall of a blood vessel narrows the diameter of the vessel and leads to a decrease in blood flow. Contraction of the smooth muscle in the wall of the stomach exerts pressure on its contents and pushes these substances forward into the small intestine.

Smooth muscle functions at a subconscious level and is *involuntary*; it is innervated by the *autonomic nervous system*, which regulates its activity.

16.1.1   Structure of smooth muscle

Smooth muscle cells are small and spindle-shaped (thin and elongated) (see Table 16.1). Typically, these cells have a diameter of 5–10 μm and are 30–200 μm in length. In contrast, skeletal muscle fibers may be 10 times wider and thousands of times longer.

The contractile apparatus in smooth muscle is similar to skeletal muscle in that it consists of thick filaments composed of *myosin* and thin filaments composed of *actin*. However, in contrast to skeletal muscle, these filaments are not organized into sarcomeres. As such, there are no striations in this muscle, resulting in a "smooth" appearance, thus the name.

Because there are no sarcomeres in smooth muscle, there are no Z lines. Instead, the actin filaments are attached to structures called *dense bodies*. These structures, which contain the same protein as the Z lines, are

Table 16.1 Comparison of skeletal and smooth muscle

Feature	Skeletal muscle	Multiunit smooth muscle	Single-unit smooth muscle
Location	Attached to bones; openings of some hollow organs (sphincters)	Large blood vessels; eyes; hair follicles	Walls of hollow organs of digestive, reproductive, and urinary tracts; small blood vessels
Thick filaments	Myosin	Myosin	Myosin
Thin filaments	Actin, troponin, tropomyosin	Actin, tropomyosin	Actin, tropomyosin
Filament arrangement	Sarcomeres	Diamond-shaped lattice	Diamond-shaped lattice
Microscopic appearance	Striated	Smooth	Smooth
Control	Voluntary	Involuntary	Involuntary
Innervation	Somatic nervous system	Autonomic nervous system	Autonomic nervous system
Contraction	Neurogenic	Neurogenic	Myogenic
Role of nervous system	Initiate contraction	Initiate contraction	Modify contraction
Morphology	Large, cylindrical	Small, spindle shaped	Small, spindle shaped
Transverse tubules	Yes	No	No
Sarcoplasmic reticulum	Well developed	Very little	Very little
Source of calcium	Sarcoplasmic reticulum	Extracellular fluid (most); sarcoplasmic reticulum (some)	Extracellular fluid (most); sarcoplasmic reticulum (some)
Site of calcium binding	Troponin	Calmodulin	Calmodulin
Function of calcium	Reposition troponin/ tropomyosin to uncover myosin binding sites on actin	Phosphorylate and activate myosin to bind with actin	Phosphorylate and activate myosin to bind with actin
Regulation of tension development	Alter number of contracting motor units; frequency of nerve stimulation	Alter number of contracting cells; alter intracellular Ca^{++} concentration	Alter intracellular Ca^{++} concentration
Length-tension development	Narrow	Broad	Broad

positioned throughout the cytoplasm of the smooth muscle cell as well as attached to the internal surface of the plasma membrane. Myosin filaments are associated with the actin filaments forming contractile bundles that are oriented in a diagonal manner. This arrangement forms a *diamond-shaped lattice* of contractile elements throughout the cytoplasm. Consequently, the interaction of actin and myosin during contraction causes the cell to become shorter and wider.

As with skeletal muscle, an action potential is required for the contraction of smooth muscle. Based on its design and size, an action potential easily penetrates all regions of these small cells and, thus, smooth muscle does not require the use of *transverse tubules* to deliver the action potential throughout the cell. Furthermore, there is scant amount of *sarcoplasmic reticulum* in smooth muscle cells. Consequently, the intracellular storage of calcium is limited. Instead, the calcium needed for contraction is obtained primarily from the extracellular fluid. The cell membrane has multiple pouch-like infoldings referred to as *caveolae*. These caveolae are filled with extracellular fluid containing a high concentration of calcium. The influx of Ca^{++} ions through their channels in the cell membrane stimulates the release of a small amount of Ca^{++} ions from the sarcoplasmic reticulum.

16.1.2   Calcium and the mechanism of contraction

You should recall that in skeletal muscle, calcium binds to troponin and causes the repositioning of tropomyosin and the myosin binding sites on the actin become uncovered and cross bridge cycling takes place. Although an increase in cytosolic calcium is also needed in smooth muscle, its role in the mechanism of contraction is very different. There are three major steps involved in *smooth muscle contraction*:

- Calcium binding with calmodulin
- Activation of myosin light-chain kinase
- Phosphorylation of myosin

Upon entering the smooth muscle cell, Ca^{++} ions bind with *calmodulin*, an intracellular protein with a chemical structure similar to troponin. The resulting Ca^{++}–calmodulin complex binds to and activates the enzyme *myosin light-chain kinase*. This activated enzyme then *phosphorylates* myosin. Cross bridge cycling in smooth muscle only takes place when myosin has been phosphorylated.

Relaxation of smooth muscle involves two steps:

- Removal of Ca^{++} ions
- Dephosphorylation of myosin

Once a contraction is completed, Ca^{++} ions are actively pumped back into the extracellular fluid as well as into the sarcoplasmic reticulum by Ca^{++}-ATPase. When the concentration of calcium falls below a certain level, steps one and two of the contractile process are reversed. Calcium no longer binds with calmodulin and myosin light-chain kinase is no longer activated.

The dephosphorylation of myosin requires the activity of another enzyme, *myosin phosphatase*. This enzyme, found within the cytoplasm of the smooth muscle cell, splits the phosphate group from the myosin molecule. Because dephosphorylated myosin is inactive, cross bridge cycling no longer takes place and the muscle relaxes.

PHARMACY APPLICATION: ACHALASIA

Achalasia is a condition in which the lower esophageal sphincter leading into the stomach fails to relax. This esophageal spasm is also referred to as "nutcracker" esophagus. Achalasia results in considerable difficulty in swallowing, or *dysphagia*. Swallowed food remains lodged in the distended esophagus and passes into the stomach slowly over time. Of significant concern is the possibility of the aspiration, or the inhalation into the airways, of the esophageal contents when the patient lies down.

Pharmacotherapy may involve the administration of calcium channel antagonists. These medications facilitate the relaxation of the lower esophageal sphincter and the passage of food into the stomach.

16.1.3   Smooth muscle contraction is slow and prolonged

Contraction of smooth muscle is significantly slower than that of skeletal muscle. Furthermore, contraction in smooth muscle is quite prolonged (3,000 ms) compared to that in skeletal muscle (100 ms). The slow onset of a contraction as well as its sustained nature is due to the slowness of attachment and detachment of the myosin cross bridges with the actin. Two factors are involved:

- Myosin ATPase activity
- Rate of calcium removal

In smooth muscle, the myosin cross bridges have less *myosin ATPase activity* than the cells of skeletal muscle and the splitting of ATP that provides the energy to "prime" the cross bridges, preparing them to interact with actin, is markedly reduced. This results in a slower rate of cross bridge cycling and a slower rate of tension development. Furthermore, a slower *rate of calcium removal* causes the muscle to relax more slowly.

Interestingly, the reduction in myosin ATPase activity causes smooth muscle to be more *economical*. In other words, smooth muscle can maintain a contraction with significantly less ATP consumption; it can maintain the same degree of tension for prolonged periods with only 1% of the energy that would be required by skeletal muscle. This is of benefit in many tissues, such as the blood vessels, which maintain tonic contraction all day, every day, with little energy consumption and without developing fatigue. Furthermore, the prolonged attachment of the myosin cross bridges to actin results in an equal, if not greater, *force of contraction*. Smooth muscle can develop a force of 4–6 kg/cm² cross-sectional area compared to 3–4 kg/cm² in skeletal muscle.

In some smooth muscles, when stimulation is sustained and the cytosolic calcium levels remain elevated, the rate of myosin ATPase activity in the cross bridges declines although tension is maintained. This condition is referred to as the *latch state*. It occurs when a phosphorylated myosin cross bridge becomes dephosphorylated while it is still attached to the actin. Dissociation of dephosphorylated cross bridges from the actin occurs at a much slower rate than does the dissociation of phosphorylated cross bridges. Therefore, as previously stated, smooth muscle can maintain tension for long periods of time with very little ATP consumption.

16.1.4   Types of smooth muscle

There are two major types of smooth muscle (it should be noted that many smooth muscles exhibit properties of each type):

- Multiunit smooth muscle
- Single-unit smooth muscle

Multiunit smooth muscle is found within the large blood vessels, the eyes (iris and ciliary muscle of the lens), and the piloerector muscles at the base of hair follicles. Multiunit smooth muscle consists of discrete smooth muscle cells or units that function independently. Each of these units is innervated by the autonomic nervous system. In fact, like skeletal muscle, this type of smooth muscle *must* be stimulated by a neuron for a contraction to be initiated. Therefore, this muscle is referred to as *neurogenic*. Unlike skeletal muscle, action potentials do not occur in multiunit smooth muscle and nerve stimulation elicits graded potentials only. The amount of ion flux that occurs in a single smooth muscle cell is inadequate to depolarize the cell to threshold. However, the graded potentials are sufficient to cause smooth muscle contraction. The contractile response of the whole muscle results from the sum of the responses of the multiple individual units.

Most smooth muscle is *single-unit smooth muscle,* also referred to as *visceral smooth muscle,* and is found within the walls of small blood vessels and the walls of tubes and hollow organs of the digestive, reproductive, and urinary systems. The cells of this type of smooth muscle are connected electrically by *gap junctions,* which allow the spreading of electrical activity from one cell to the next, forming a *functional syncytium.* Any change in electrical activity in one region of single-unit smooth muscle quickly spreads throughout the muscle layer, such that the cells of the muscle function as one, or a "single-unit."

Action potentials are generated in single-unit smooth muscle. The simultaneous depolarization of 30–40 smooth muscle cells is required to generate a propagated action potential. The presence of the gap junctions allows this to occur readily.

Single-unit smooth muscle is *self-excitable* and capable of generating action potentials without any input from the autonomic nervous system. Therefore, this type of smooth muscle is referred to as *myogenic,* and the function of the autonomic nervous system is to modify contractile activity only. Input is not needed to elicit contraction.

The ability to spontaneously depolarize is related to the unstable resting membrane potentials in single-unit smooth muscle. There are two types of spontaneous depolarizations that may occur:

*   Pacemaker potentials
*   Slow-wave potentials

A *pacemaker potential* involves the gradual depolarization of the cell membrane to threshold. The subsequent generation of an action potential causes smooth muscle contraction. This type of spontaneous depolarization is referred to as a "pacemaker potential" because it creates a regular rhythm of contraction.

Slow-wave potentials also involve the gradual depolarization of the cell membrane. However, these depolarizations do not necessarily reach threshold. Therefore, the depolarization may simply be followed by a repolarization back to the initial membrane potential. These slow "wave-like" potentials occur rhythmically and do not lead to smooth muscle contraction. The peak-to-peak amplitude of the slow-wave potential is in the range of 15–30 mV. Therefore, under the appropriate conditions, the depolarization phase of the slow-wave potential may, in fact, reach threshold. When this occurs, a burst of action potentials is generated, resulting in muscle contraction.

The mechanism of the slow-wave potential is unclear. One hypothesis is that the rate at which sodium is actively transported out of the cell rhythmically increases and decreases. A decrease in the outward movement of Na^+ ions allows positive charges to accumulate along the internal surface of the cell membrane and depolarization takes place. This is followed by an increase in the outward movement of Na^+ ions, which causes the internal surface of the cell membrane to become more negative and repolarization takes place.

16.1.5 Factors influencing the contractile activity of smooth muscle

Many factors influence the contractile activity of smooth muscle. The strength of contraction of multiunit smooth muscle may be enhanced by the *stimulation of a greater number of cells*, or contractile units. This mechanism is directly comparable to motor-unit recruitment employed by skeletal muscle. As the number of contracting muscle cells increases, so does the strength of contraction. However, this mechanism is of no value in single-unit smooth muscle. Due to the presence of gap junctions, all the muscle cells in the tissue are activated at once.

Other factors that influence contractile activity include:

- Autonomic nervous system
- Hormones and blood-borne substances
- Locally produced substances
- Intracellular calcium concentration

The autonomic nervous system (ANS) modifies the contractile activity of both types of smooth muscle. As discussed in Chapter 9, the ANS innervates the smooth muscle layer in a very diffuse manner, such that neurotransmitter is released over a wide area of the muscle. Typically, the effects of sympathetic stimulation and parasympathetic stimulation in a given tissue oppose each other: One system enhances contractile activity, whereas the other system inhibits it. The specific effects (excitatory or inhibitory) that the two divisions of the ANS have on a given smooth muscle depend upon its location.

Many *hormones and other blood-borne substances* (including drugs) also alter the contractile activity of smooth muscle. Some of the more important substances include epinephrine, norepinephrine, angiotensin II, vasopressin, oxytocin, and histamine. *Locally produced substances* that may alter contraction in the tissue in which they are synthesized include nitric oxide, prostaglandins, leukotrienes, carbon dioxide, and hydrogen ion. It is important to note that smooth muscle cells are typically exposed to more than one of these substances at a time and the magnitude of contraction at any given moment is determined by the sum of the effects of the entire range of agents to which the muscle is exposed.

Factors (i.e., ANS stimulation and blood-borne and locally produced substances) that alter smooth muscle contractile activity do so by altering the *intracellular concentration of calcium*. An increase in cytosolic calcium leads to an increase in cross bridge cycling and an increase in tension development. There are several mechanisms by which the concentration of calcium within the cytoplasm of the smooth muscle cell may be increased, including:

- Voltage-gated Ca^{++} channels
- Ligand-gated Ca^{++} channels
- IP_3-gated Ca^{++} channels
- Stretch-activated Ca^{++} channels

Voltage-gated Ca^{++} channels open when the smooth muscle cell is depolarized. Calcium then enters the cell down its electrochemical gradient. *Ligand-gated Ca^{++} channels* are associated with various hormone or neurotransmitter receptors. The binding of a given substance to its receptor causes the ligand-gated Ca^{++} channel to open and, once again, Ca^{++} ions enter the cell. This process, which occurs without a significant change in membrane potential (due to a simultaneous increase in Na^+ ion removal from the cell), is referred to as *pharmacomechanical coupling*.

Inositol triphosphate *(IP$_3$)-gated channels* are also associated with membrane-bound receptors for hormones and neurotransmitters. In this case, binding of a given substance to its receptor causes the activation of another membrane-bound protein, phospholipase C. This enzyme promotes the hydrolysis of phosphatidylinositol 4,5-diphosphate (PIP_2) to IP_3. The IP_3 then diffuses to the sarcoplasmic reticulum and opens its calcium channels to release Ca^{++} ions from this intracellular storage site.

Finally, an increase in volume or pressure within a tube or hollow organ causes stretch or distortion of the smooth muscle in the organ wall that may cause activation of *stretch-activated Ca^{++} channels*. The subsequent influx of calcium initiates contraction of the smooth muscle. This process is referred to as *myogenic contraction*, although the increased tension is only temporary as the smooth muscle cells adapt to their new length and then relax. This is referred to as the *stress–relaxation response*. It allows a hollow organ to fill or expand slowly to accommodate a greater volume without developing strong contractions that would expel its contents. This is beneficial in organs such as the stomach and the urinary bladder whose functions include the temporary storage of food and urine, respectively.

16.1.6 Length–tension relationship

The length of the smooth muscle prior to stimulation has little effect on subsequent tension development. This is in marked contrast to skeletal muscle, which exhibits a strong length–tension relationship. The influence of the resting muscle length on the tension developed in skeletal muscle is based upon the arrangement of the thick and thin filaments into sarcomeres. Any change in muscle length alters the degree of overlap of these filaments and, therefore, the number of cross bridges cycling and the amount of tension developed.

The contractile elements in smooth muscle are not organized into sarcomeres. Furthermore, the resting length of smooth muscle is much shorter than its optimal length. In other words, this muscle can be significantly stretched and the amount of tension developed may increase as the muscle becomes closer to its optimal length. Finally, the thick filaments are longer in smooth muscle than they are in skeletal muscle: There is still overlap of the thick and thin filaments, even when the muscle has been markedly stretched.

This very broad length–tension relationship in smooth muscle is physiologically advantageous. Tubes and hollow organs may be stretched considerably as substances pass through them. For example, in the urinary bladder, the smooth muscle cells may be stretched up to 2.5 times their resting length. By the end of pregnancy, the smooth muscle cells of the uterus may be stretched up to eight times their resting length. Regardless, the smooth muscle must retain its ability to contract forcefully and regulate the movement of these substances through the organs.

16.1.7   Hyperplasia

All types of muscles may become larger by way of *hypertrophy* or an increase in cell size. Indeed, this is the only mechanism by which skeletal muscles enlarge because skeletal muscle fibers are incapable of mitosis. However, certain smooth muscles may also become larger by way of *hyperplasia*, or an increase in cell numbers. For example, uterine smooth muscle is responsive to estrogen. At puberty, when a female's estrogen levels rise, the synthesis of smooth muscle is stimulated, which enables the uterus to grow to adult size. Furthermore, during pregnancy, the high levels of estrogen result in both hypertrophy and hyperplasia of the uterine smooth muscle so that the uterus may accommodate the growing fetus.

16.2   Skeletal muscle

Under voluntary control, skeletal muscle is innervated by the somatic nervous system and comprises the largest tissue group in the human body. It accounts for up to 40% of the total body weight and perform several important functions in the body including:

- Movement of body parts
- Heat production
- Respiration
- Vocalization

Skeletal muscles are the organs of the muscular system and are attached to bones, which act as levers and enable the muscles to *control body movements* such as walking, making facial expressions, chewing, swallowing, and breathing. Skeletal muscles are also responsible for the manipulation of objects, such as writing with a pencil or eating with a fork. Furthermore, movement of the eyes is carried out by several pairs of skeletal muscles. Finally, the contractions of certain groups of muscles, referred to as "anti-gravity" muscles, are needed to maintain posture and provide body support.

Of the nutrient energy consumed during skeletal muscle activity, approximately 20%–30% is converted into purposeful work with the remaining 70%–80% of the nutrient energy being released as *heat*. Therefore, because of its large mass, skeletal muscle is the tissue most responsible for maintaining and increasing body temperature.

Although it typically occurs subconsciously, breathing *is* a voluntary activity. The diaphragm and the other muscles of inspiration and expiration are skeletal muscles, which, as previously mentioned, are under voluntary control of the somatic nervous system. As such, breathing can be voluntarily controlled to some extent (see Chapter 8). Last, *speaking*, and other forms of vocalization, depend upon the coordinated contraction of several skeletal muscles.

16.2.1 Muscle tension and movement

When a muscle contracts, it develops *tension*. This tension is what enables the muscle to perform work such as body movement. Skeletal muscles are typically attached by way of *tendons* to at least two different bones across a joint. The proximal end of the muscle that is attached to a relatively stationary part of the skeleton is referred to as the *origin*. The distal end of the muscle that is attached to a part of the skeleton that moves more freely is referred to as the *insertion*. When the muscle develops tension, and shortens, it pulls the insertion toward the origin. For example, the *biceps brachii* originates (O) at two areas of the scapula (shoulder), crosses the elbow joint and inserts (I) on the radius (one of the bones of the forearm). When this muscle contracts, the radius (I) is pulled toward the scapula (O).

Movement that decreases the angle of a joint, or bends the joint, and brings the bones toward each other is referred to as *flexion*. For the above example, the biceps brachii *flexes* the forearm. In contrast, movement that increases the angle of the joint and straightens the joint is referred to as *extension*. In the previously mentioned example, the *triceps brachii* acts as an opposing muscle to the biceps brachii. Located on the posterior surface of the arm, the triceps brachii originates on the scapula and the upper portion of the humerus (arm), and inserts on the ulna (the other bone of the forearm), and crosses the elbow joint. However, when it develops tension and shortens, the triceps *extends* the forearm and straightens the elbow joint. Thus, the triceps brachii causes a movement opposite to that of the biceps brachii. A muscle that works in opposition to another muscle is referred to as an *antagonist* muscle. An *agonist* muscle, or *prime mover*, provides the force for a specific movement. In this case, the agonist muscle is the biceps brachii. *Synergist muscles* work *with* the prime movers to achieve the movement. In this case, the synergist muscle is the *brachialis* muscle of the arm.

16.2.1.1   Isometric versus isotonic contraction

There are two primary types of muscle contraction:

- Isometric contraction
- Isotonic contraction

Isometric contraction occurs when the muscle develops tension and exerts force on an object, but does not shorten. In other words, it refers to muscle contraction during which the length of the muscle remains constant. For example, supporting an object in a fixed position, such as carrying a book or a backpack, requires isometric contraction. This type of contraction also occurs when attempting to move an object that is too heavy to shift or reposition. In this case, the muscle may exert maximal force against the object; however, because the object does not move, the length of the contracting muscle does not change. Finally, the anti-gravity muscles of the back and legs perform submaximal isometric contractions while maintaining posture and for body support.

Isotonic contraction occurs when the muscle changes length under a constant load. For example, when lifting an object, the muscle contracts and becomes shorter while the weight of the object remains constant. Because shortening of the muscle occurs, this is referred to as *concentric contraction*. When placing the object back down, once again, the muscle is generating tension. However, in this case, the muscle is lengthening. This is referred to as *eccentric contraction*. In addition to moving external objects, isotonic contractions are performed for movement of the body, such as moving the legs when walking.

Many activities require both types of contractions by the muscles. An example is running. When one of the legs hits the ground, isometric contraction of the muscles within this limb keep it stiff and help to maintain body support. At the same time, isotonic contractions in the opposite leg move it forward to take the next stride.

16.2.2   Structure of skeletal muscle

A whole muscle is composed of muscle cells, also called *muscle fibers*. Muscle fibers are elongated, cylindrical cells packed with protein strands. Due to the fusion of many smaller fibers during embryonic development, muscle fibers are the largest cells in the body and are multinucleated, containing several nuclei close to the inner surface of the cell membrane. Muscle fibers lie parallel to one another and extend along the entire length of the muscle. These fibers may be a few millimeters in length (muscles of the eyes) or up to two or more feet in length (muscles of the legs). Let us recap the relationship between muscle fibers and muscles: muscle fibers (muscle cells) make up muscles (organs).

Muscle fibers are incapable of mitosis. Research indicates the number of muscle fibers per muscle is likely determined by the second trimester of fetal development. Therefore, enlargement of a whole muscle is not due to an increase in the number of fibers in the muscle. Instead, it is due to the hypertrophy of the existing fibers.

There are no gap junctions between skeletal muscle fibers, so that electrical activity cannot spread from one cell to the next. Therefore, each muscle fiber must be innervated by a branch of an alpha motor neuron. A *motor unit* is defined as an alpha motor neuron and all the muscle fibers it innervates.

Internally, muscle fibers are highly organized. Each fiber contains numerous protein fibers called *myofibrils*. These cylindrical structures also lie parallel to the long axis of the muscle. The myofibrils are composed of *thick filaments* and *thin filaments*. It is the arrangement of these filaments that creates the alternating light and dark bands observed microscopically along the muscle fiber. Hence, skeletal muscle is also referred to as *striated muscle* due to the banding of the muscle fibers.

16.2.2.1 Sarcomeres

The thick filaments and thin filaments are organized into repeating segments referred to as *sarcomeres*, which are the functional units of skeletal muscle fibers. (In other words, the sarcomere is the smallest contractile unit within a skeletal muscle fiber.) Each myofibril is composed of hundreds or thousands of sarcomeres arranged end to end along the fiber's length. When a muscle fiber is stimulated, each of these sarcomeres shorten, resulting in the shortening of the entire muscle fiber, which results in the contraction of the muscle. Therefore, it is the function of the sarcomere that determines whole muscle contraction.

A sarcomere is the area between two Z *lines* (see Figure 16.1, panel c). The function of the Z line is to anchor the thin filaments in place at either end of the sarcomere. The thick filaments are found in the central region of the sarcomere. Ultimately, it is the interaction between the thick filaments and the thin filaments that causes shortening of the sarcomere.

16.2.2.2 Thick filaments

Thick filaments are long polymer strands comprised of protein molecules called *myosin*. There are approximately 200–300 myosin molecules

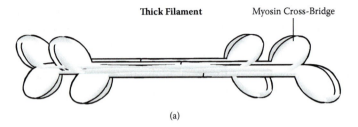

(a)

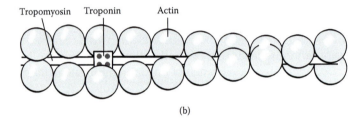

(b)

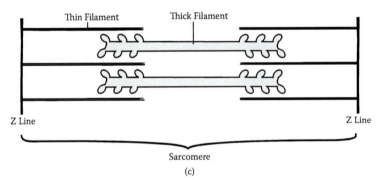

(c)

Figure 16.1 Components of the sarcomere. (a) Thick filament. The thick filament is composed of myosin molecules. These molecules are shaped like golf clubs and consist of a long shaft with a globular portion at one end. The myosin is arranged so that the shafts are in the center of the thick filament and the globular portions, or myosin cross bridges, protrude from each end of the thick filament. The myosin cross bridges bind to the actin of the thin filament. (b) Thin filament. The thin filament consists of three types of proteins. Globular actin molecules join together to form two strands of fibrous actin that twist around each other. Tropomyosin is a filamentous protein found on the surface of the actin, physically covering the binding sites for the myosin cross bridges. Troponin molecules stabilize the tropomyosin filaments in position on the actin. (c) Sarcomere. The thick filaments and thin filaments are highly organized. They are arranged to form a sarcomere, which is the functional unit of skeletal muscle. The sarcomere is the region between two Z lines.

in a thick filament. Each myosin molecule is made up of two identical subunits that are shaped like golf clubs: two long shafts that are wound together with a *myosin head*, or *cross bridge*, on the end of each of them. These molecules are arranged so that the shafts are bundled together and oriented toward the center of the thick filament. The myosin heads project outward from either end of the thick filament (see Figure 16.1, panel a).

16.2.2.3 Thin filaments

The thin filaments are composed of three types of proteins:

- Actin
- Tropomyosin
- Troponin

The predominant protein, *actin*, consists of spherical subunits (globular actin) arranged into two chains twisted around each other (fibrous actin). (Imagine two strands of pearls twisted around each other.) *Tropomyosin* is a long, thread-like protein found on the outer surface of the actin chain. Each tropomyosin molecule is associated with 6–7 actin subunits. The function of tropomyosin is to cover the binding sites for myosin on the actin subunits when the muscle is in the resting state. This prevents the interaction between actin and myosin that causes muscle contraction. *Troponin* is a smaller protein consisting of three subunits. One subunit binds to actin, another binds to tropomyosin and the third binds with calcium. When the muscle is relaxed, troponin holds the tropomyosin in its blocking position on the surface of the actin (see Figure 16.1, panel b).

A summary of the structural organization in skeletal muscle is as follows:

Muscle → Muscle fiber → Myofibril → Thick filaments (Myosin)
→ Thin filaments (Actin, Troponin, Tropomyosin)

16.2.3 Neuromuscular junction

Each muscle fiber is innervated by a branch of an alpha motor neuron. The synapse between the somatic motor neuron and the muscle fiber is referred to as the *neuromuscular junction*. Action potentials in the motor neuron cause the release of the neurotransmitter, *acetylcholine*. The binding of acetylcholine to its receptors on the muscle fiber causes an increase in the permeability to Na^+ ions and K^+ ions. The ensuing depolarization generates an action potential that travels along the surface of the muscle fiber in either direction. This is referred to as a *propagated action potential*. It is this action potential that elicits the intracellular events that lead to muscle contraction.

PHARMACY APPLICATION: MYASTHENIA GRAVIS

Myasthenia gravis is an autoimmune disorder that involves the neuromuscular junction. The peak incidence occurs in patients between 20 and 30 years of age, and it is approximately three times more common in women than it is in men.

Myasthenia gravis is characterized by progressive muscle weakness. It is caused by an antibody-mediated loss of acetylcholine receptors in the neuromuscular junction. As the number of receptors decreases, it becomes less likely that the acetylcholine released from the alpha motor neuron will bind to and stimulate a functioning receptor. The decrease in receptor stimulation leads to a decrease in the electrical activity in the muscle fiber and weaker muscle contractions.

A common approach in the pharmacotherapy of myasthenia gravis is to increase the concentration of acetylcholine in the neuromuscular junction. As the concentration of neurotransmitter increases, the likelihood that functioning receptors will be located and stimulated also increases and muscle function is therefore improved. Drugs of choice for this method of treatment include pyridostigmine and neostigmine. These reversible anticholinesterase drugs inhibit the breakdown of acetylcholine.

16.2.4   Mechanism of contraction

As mentioned previously, skeletal muscle fibers are very large cells with a wide diameter. The action potential is readily propagated, or transmitted, along the surface of the muscle fiber. However, a mechanism is needed to transmit the electrical impulse into the central region of the muscle fiber as well. The *transverse tubules* (*T-tubules*) are invaginations of the cell membrane that penetrate deep into the muscle fiber and surround each myofibril. (Imagine poking one's fingers into an inflated balloon.) As the action potential travels along the surface of the fiber, it is also transmitted into the T-tubules, resulting in the stimulation of all the regions of the muscle fiber.

All types of muscle require *calcium* for contraction. In skeletal muscle, Ca^{++} ions are stored within an extensive membranous network referred to as the *sarcoplasmic reticulum*. This network is found throughout the muscle fiber and surrounds each myofibril. Furthermore, segments of the sarcoplasmic reticulum lie adjacent to each T-tubule. The T-tubule with a segment of sarcoplasmic reticulum on either side of it is referred to as a *triad*. As the action potential is transmitted along the T-tubule, it stimulates the release of Ca^{++} ions from the sarcoplasmic reticulum through the Ca^{++}-release channels. The sarcoplasmic reticulum is the only source of calcium in skeletal muscle.

The mechanism of skeletal muscle contraction is described by the *Sliding Filament Theory* (see Figure 16.2). This mechanism begins with the *"priming"*

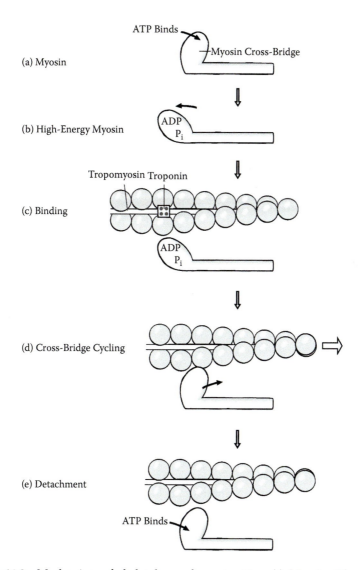

Figure 16.2 Mechanism of skeletal muscle contraction. (a) Myosin. The myosin cross bridge has a binding site for ATP. (b) High-energy myosin. Within the cross bridge, myosin ATPase splits ATP into ADP and inorganic phosphate (P_i). As a result, the cross bridge swivels outward and energy is stored. (c) Binding. In the presence of calcium, which binds to troponin, tropomyosin is repositioned into the groove between the two strands of actin and the binding sites for myosin on the actin are uncovered and the cross bridges attach to actin. (d) Cross bridge cycling. The energy stored within the myosin cross bridge is released and the cross bridge swivels inward, pulling the actin inward. The ADP and P_i are released. (e) Detachment. The binding of a new molecule of ATP to the myosin cross bridge allows the myosin to detach from the actin and the process begins again.

of the myosin cross bridge, a process that requires energy. This energy is supplied by adenosine triphosphate (ATP). Each myosin cross bridge contains an enzyme, *myosin ATPase*. When ATP attaches to its binding site on the myosin cross bridge, it is split by myosin ATPase to yield adenosine diphosphate (ADP) and inorganic phosphate (P_i). The ADP and P_i remain tightly bound to the myosin cross bridge. The energy released by this process causes the myosin cross bridge to swivel outward toward the end of the thick filament. When the myosin cross bridge is in this conformation, it is "primed" and is referred to as the *high-energy form of myosin*. It is the high-energy form of myosin that is capable of binding to actin. However, this interaction is prevented by tropomyosin, which physically covers the binding sites for myosin on the actin subunits. To uncover these binding sites, calcium is needed.

In a stimulated muscle fiber, Ca^{++} ions are released from the sarcoplasmic reticulum. These Ca^{++} ions bind to troponin, causing the troponin–actin linkage to become weakened, which allows the troponin and the tropomyosin to be repositioned. The troponin–tropomyosin complex moves away from the surface of the actin chains such that the myosin binding sites are uncovered. The primed myosin cross bridges now bind to the actin. Binding to actin causes the energy previously stored within the myosin to be discharged, and the cross bridge swivels inward toward the center of the thick filament. This process is referred to as *cross bridge cycling* or the *power stroke*. As the myosin cross bridge swivels inward, it pulls the actin inward as well. It is important to note that the interaction between the actin and the myosin causes the thin filaments to slide inward over the thick filaments toward the center of the sarcomere. Consequently, the sarcomeres shorten and, therefore, the whole muscle shortens or contracts. This is why this process is referred to as the sliding filament theory of muscle contraction.

When the myosin cross bridge binds with actin, the ADP and P_i are released from the myosin. This opens the binding site to another molecule of ATP. In fact, the myosin remains attached to the actin until another ATP molecule binds to the myosin. The binding of a new ATP causes the myosin to release the actin. This ATP is split by the ATPase and the myosin cross bridge swivels outward once again, returning the myosin to its high-energy state. As long as Ca^{++} ions are present and the binding sites on the actin are uncovered, cross bridge cycling continues. The cross bridges of the thick filament pull the thin filaments inward incrementally such that the sarcomeres become shorter and the muscle contracts further. The major events of muscle contraction are summarized in Table 16.2.

Interestingly, the myosin cross bridges do not all cycle at the same time. At any given moment, some cross bridges remain attached to the actin and others are in the process of releasing the actin to cycle once again. In other words, myosin cross bridge cycling is staggered. This process maintains the shortening of the sarcomere and prevents the thin filaments from slipping back to their original positions between cycles.

Table 16.2   Major events of muscle contraction

- ATP binds to the myosin cross-bridge and is split by myosin ATPase
- Energy released by this reaction causes the myosin cross-bridge to swivel outward toward the end of the thick filament forming the "primed" or high-energy form of myosin which is capable of binding with actin
- Nerve impulse is generated by the alpha motor neuron
- Acetylcholine is released from the axon terminal into the neuromuscular junction and binds to receptors on the muscle fiber
- The resulting increased permeability to Na+ ions and K+ ions elicits an action potential in the muscle fiber
- The action potential is propagated along the surface of the muscle fiber as well as into the transverse tubules
- The action potential in the transverse tubules triggers the release of calcium from the sarcoplasmic reticulum
- Calcium binds to troponin
- The troponin linkage with actin is weakened
- Troponin and tropomyosin are repositioned such that the binding sites on actin for the myosin cross-bridges are uncovered
- Myosin cross-bridges bind to actin and swivel inward (cross-bridge cycling or the power stroke)
- Cross-bridge cycling pulls actin inward toward the center of the sarcomere such that the sarcomere becomes shorter and tension is developed
- ATP binds to the myosin cross-bridge and is split by myosin ATPase
- The energy released allows the cross-bridges to release actin and swivel outward
- As long as calcium is present and the binding sites are uncovered, cross-bridges continue binding to actin and continue cycling so that the sarcomere becomes shorter and tension is maintained

---

In the absence of ATP, the myosin cross bridges are unable to release the actin. As a result, the sarcomeres and, therefore, the muscle, remain contracted. This phenomenon is referred to as *rigor mortis*. Following death, the concentration of intracellular calcium increases. This calcium allows the contractile process between the previously formed high-energy myosin and the actin to take place. However, the muscle stores of ATP are rapidly depleted, the myosin remains attached to the actin and stiffness ensues. Rigor mortis begins 3 to 4 hours after death and becomes complete in about 12 hours. It subsides during the next several days as the contractile proteins begin to degrade.

When the action potentials in the alpha motor neuron cease, stimulation of the muscle fiber is ended. The Ca^{++} ions are actively pumped back into the sarcoplasmic reticulum and, troponin and tropomyosin return to their original positions, resulting in the myosin binding sites on the actin being covered once again. The thin filaments return passively to their original positions, resulting in muscle relaxation.

16.2.4.1   Sources of ATP for muscle contraction

Skeletal muscle uses only ATP as a source of energy for contraction. However, intracellular stores of ATP are quite limited. In fact, the amount of ATP normally found in skeletal muscle is enough to sustain only a few seconds of contraction. Therefore, metabolic pathways to form additional ATP are needed. These pathways include:

- Creatine phosphate
- Oxidative phosphorylation
- Glycolysis

Energy may be transferred from *creatine phosphate* to ADP by way of the following reaction:

$$\text{Creatine phosphate} \overset{ck}{+} \text{ADP} \leftrightarrow \text{Creatine} + \text{ATP}$$

The enzyme, creatine kinase (CK), facilitates the transfer of phosphate and energy to a molecule of ADP to form ATP. There are sufficient stores of creatine phosphate to sustain approximately 15 more seconds of muscle contraction. Because this is a single-step process, it provides ATP very rapidly, and it is the first pathway for the formation of ATP to be accessed.

The second pathway to be utilized in the formation of ATP is *oxidative phosphorylation*. This process involves the metabolic breakdown of glucose and fatty acids. Because it requires oxygen (*aerobic* metabolism), oxidative phosphorylation provides energy at rest and under conditions of mild (walking) to moderate (jogging) exercise. This pathway is advantageous because it produces a large amount of energy (36 molecules of ATP) from each molecule of glucose. However, oxidative phosphorylation is comparatively slow because of the number of steps involved. Finally, this process requires enhanced blood flow to the active muscles for the continuous delivery of oxygen as well as nutrient molecules. Although glucose may be obtained by way of glycogenolysis within the skeletal muscle fibers, these glycogen stores are limited. Glycogenolysis in the liver and lipolysis in the adipose tissues yield additional molecules of glucose and fatty acids for energy formation. As exercise is sustained, skeletal muscle relies more upon fatty acids as a source of fuel for the oxidative phosphorylation pathway. In this way, glucose is spared for the brain.

During intense exercise, when the oxygen supply cannot keep pace with the oxygen demand, skeletal muscle produces ATP *anaerobically* by way of *glycolysis*. Although this pathway provides ATP more rapidly, it produces much less energy (two molecules of ATP) from each molecule of glucose. Furthermore, glycolysis results in the production of lactic acid in the muscle tissue. The accumulation of lactic acid may lead to pain as well as muscle fatigue.

16.2.5 Muscle fatigue

Muscle fatigue is defined as the inability of a muscle to maintain a particular degree of contraction over time. The onset of fatigue is quite variable and is influenced by several factors including:

- Intensity and duration of contractile activity
- Utilization of aerobic versus anaerobic metabolism for energy
- Composition of the muscle
- Fitness level of the individual

Although the exact mechanisms leading to muscle fatigue remain somewhat unclear, several factors have been implicated:

- Depletion of energy reserves
- Conduction failure
- Accumulation of lactic acid
- Increase in inorganic phosphate

Depletion of glycogen stores within the contracting skeletal muscles fibers is associated with the onset of fatigue. Interestingly, this occurs even though the muscle is utilizing fatty acids as its primary energy source.

The build-up of potassium in the T-tubules as the result of repetitive stimulation may result in *conduction failure*. Excess K^+ ions in the fluid within the T-tubules leads to a persistent depolarization and, consequently, the inactivation of sodium channels. As a result, action potentials are no longer conducted into the muscle fiber along the T-tubules and the release of Ca^{++} ions from the sarcoplasmic reticulum is interrupted. Recovery occurs rapidly upon the removal of the K^+ ions by way of the Na^+-K^+ pump.

The *accumulation of lactic acid* lowers the pH within the muscle. The change in pH may ultimately alter the activity of enzymes involved with energy production as well as cross bridge cycling.

The breakdown of creatine phosphate causes an *increase in the concentration of inorganic phosphate*. Fatigue associated with elevated inorganic phosphate may be due to a slowed release of P_i from myosin and, therefore, a decreased rate of cross bridge cycling. It may also involve a decreased sensitivity of the contractile proteins to calcium, which would also impair cross bridge cycling.

16.2.6 Oxygen debt

Hyperventilation persists for a period following the cessation of exercise. This hyperventilation is due to the *oxygen debt* incurred during the exercise. Specifically, oxygen is needed for the following metabolic processes:

- Restoration of creatine phosphate reserves
- Metabolism of lactic acid
- Replacement of glycogen stores

During the recovery period after exercise, ATP, newly produced by way of oxidative phosphorylation, is first needed to replace the *creatine phosphate reserves*. This process may be completed within a few minutes. Second, the *lactic acid* produced during glycolysis must be metabolized. In the muscle fiber, lactic acid is converted into pyruvic acid. Some of this pyruvic acid is then used as a substrate in the oxidative phosphorylation pathway to produce ATP. The remainder of the pyruvic acid is converted into glucose in the liver. This glucose is then stored in the form of *glycogen* in the liver and in the skeletal muscles. These later metabolic processes require several hours for completion.

16.2.7 Types of muscle fibers

There are two major differences between the types of muscle fibers:

- Speed of contraction
- Metabolic pathway used to form ATP

As such, there are three types of muscle fibers (see Table 16.3):

- Slow-twitch oxidative
- Fast-twitch oxidative
- Fast-twitch glycolytic

In humans, most skeletal muscles contain a mixture of all three types of muscle fibers. The dominant type of fiber in a given muscle is determined largely by the type of activity for which the muscle is specialized.

Fast-twitch muscle fibers develop tension two to three times faster than slow-twitch muscle fibers. This is due to the more rapid splitting of ATP by *myosin ATPase*. This enables the myosin cross bridges to cycle more rapidly. Another factor influencing the speed of contraction involves the rate of *removal of calcium* from the cytoplasm. Muscle fibers remove the Ca^{++} ions by pumping them back into the sarcoplasmic reticulum. Fast-twitch muscle fibers remove Ca^{++} ions more rapidly than slow-twitch muscle fibers. This results in quicker twitches that are useful in fast, precise movements.

Table 16.3   Features of skeletal muscle fiber types

Feature	Slow-twitch oxidative	Fast-twitch oxidative	Fast-twitch glycolytic
Myosin ATPase activity	Slow	Fast	Fast
Speed of contraction	Slow	Fast	Fast
Removal of calcium	Slow	Fast	Fast
Duration of contraction	Long	Short	Short
Mitochondria	Many	Many	Few
Capillaries	Many	Many	Few
Myoglobin content	High	High	Low
Color of fiber	Dark red	Red	Pale
Diameter of fiber	Small	Intermediate	Large
Source of ATP	Oxidative phosphorylation	Oxidative phosphorylation; glycolysis	Glycolysis
Glycogen content	Low	Intermediate	High
Onset of fatigue	Delayed	Intermediate	Rapid

The contractions generated in slow-twitch muscle fibers may last up to 10 times longer than those of fast-twitch muscle fibers. Therefore, these twitches are useful in sustained, more powerful movements.

Muscle fibers also differ in their ability to resist fatigue. Slow-twitch muscle fibers rely primarily on oxidative phosphorylation to produce ATP. Accordingly, these muscle fibers have a greater number of *mitochondria*, the organelles where these metabolic processes are carried out. These fibers also have an *extensive capillary network* for the delivery of oxygen and nutrient molecules. Furthermore, the *high myoglobin content* within slow-twitch muscle fibers facilitates the diffusion of oxygen into the cells from the extracellular fluid. It is the myoglobin that imparts the characteristic red color to these muscle fibers. Hence, these muscles are referred to as *"red muscles."*

Finally, slow-twitch muscle fibers have a *small diameter*. This facilitates the diffusion of oxygen through the fiber to the mitochondria where it is utilized. Taken together, each of these characteristics enhances the ability of these fibers to utilize oxygen. Therefore, in slow-twitch oxidative muscle fibers *oxidative phosphorylation predominates* and *fatigue is delayed*. Examples of these muscles include the anti-gravity muscles of the back, which are active and maintain posture for much of the day.

Fast-twitch muscle fibers fall into two categories. Fast-twitch, *glycolytic* muscle fibers have fewer mitochondria, fewer capillaries, less myoglobin, and larger diameters. These fibers rely primarily on glycolysis for the production of ATP. The resulting accumulation of lactic acid and decrease in pH hastens the onset of fatigue. Because this type of muscle fiber has less myoglobin, it has a much paler appearance than the slow-twitch oxidative muscle fibers. Therefore, these muscles are referred to as *"white muscles."* Examples of these muscles are the muscles of the hands and of the eyes.

Fast-twitch *oxidative* muscle fibers have many mitochondria, many capillaries, a significant amount of myoglobin and intermediate-sized diameters. These muscle fibers utilize a combination of oxidative and glycolytic metabolisms to produce ATP. Thus, fast-twitch oxidative muscle fibers are more fatigue-resistant than fast-twitch glycolytic muscle fibers. Examples of these muscles include the muscles that move the limbs.

The percentage of the different types of muscle fibers in each muscle may also be influenced by heredity. An individual with a high percentage of fast-twitch glycolytic muscle fibers would be better suited for power and sprint events. The individual with a high percentage of slow-twitch oxidative muscle fibers would be better suited for endurance events. For example, elite sprinters may have less than 20% slow-twitch muscle fibers in their *quadriceps femoris* muscles of the thighs, where marathon runners may have as high as 95% slow-twitch muscle fibers in these same muscles.

Finally, exercise training may cause fast-twitch muscle fibers of one type to convert to the other type. For example, fast-twitch glycolytic fibers may be converted to fast-twitch oxidative muscle fibers as the result of regular endurance training such as running. On the other hand, fast-twitch oxidative muscle fibers may be converted to fast-twitch glycolytic muscle fibers by resistance training such as weight lifting. Interestingly, fast-twitch and slow-twitch muscle fibers are not interconvertible. Whether a muscle fiber is fast-twitch or slow-twitch is determined by its nerve supply. Fast-twitch muscle fibers are innervated by motor neurons that exhibit intermittent, rapid bursts of electrical activity. Conversely, slow-twitch muscle fibers are innervated by motor neurons that exhibit a low-frequency pattern of electrical activity. It is important to note that all the muscle fibers within a given motor unit are of the same type.

16.2.8   Muscle mechanics

A *muscle twitch* is a brief, weak contraction produced in a muscle fiber in response to a single action potential. Although the action potential lasts 1–2 ms, the resulting muscle twitch lasts approximately 100 ms. However, a muscle twitch in a single muscle fiber is too brief and too weak to be useful or to perform any meaningful work. In fact, hundreds or thousands of muscle fibers are organized into whole muscles. In this way, the fibers may work together to produce muscle contractions that are strong enough and of sufficient duration to be productive. Furthermore, muscles must be able to generate contractions of variable strengths. Different tasks require different degrees of contraction or tension development within the whole muscle. The *strength of skeletal muscle contraction* depends on two major factors:

• Number of muscle fibers contracting
• Amount of tension developed by each contracting muscle fiber

16.2.8.1   *Number of muscle fibers contracting*

As the *number of contracting muscle fibers* increases, then the strength of skeletal muscle contraction increases. Two major factors determine the number of muscle fibers that are activated at any given moment:

• Multiple motor unit summation
• Asynchronous motor unit summation

A *motor unit* is defined as an alpha motor neuron and all the skeletal muscle fibers it innervates. The number of muscle fibers innervated by an alpha motor neuron varies considerably, depending upon the function of the muscle. For example, the muscles of the eyes and the hands have very small motor units. In other words, each alpha motor neuron associated with these muscles synapses with only a few muscle fibers but each of these muscles is innervated by a comparatively large number of alpha motor neurons. Densely innervated muscles can carry out more precise, complex motor activities. On the other hand, anti-gravity muscles have very large motor units. For example, the gastrocnemius muscle of the calf has about 2,000 muscle fibers in each motor unit. Muscles with large motor units tend to be more powerful and more coarsely controlled.

Multiple motor unit summation involves the recruitment of motor units. As the number of motor units stimulated at any given moment increases, the strength of contraction increases.

Asynchronous motor unit summation refers to the condition where motor unit activation within a muscle is alternated. In other words, at one moment, some of the motor units within the muscle are activated, while other motor units are relaxed. This is followed by the relaxation of previously activated motor units and the activation of previously relaxed motor units. Consequently, only a fraction of the motor units within the muscle generate tension at any given moment. Therefore, this type of summation may generate submaximal contractions only.

An advantage of asynchronous motor unit summation is that the onset of muscle fatigue is significantly delayed. This is because each motor unit has alternating periods of relaxation in which there is time for the restoration of energy supplies. The anti-gravity muscles of the back and of the legs employ asynchronous motor unit summation. These muscles are required to generate sustained, submaximal contractions to maintain posture and body support over the course of the day.

16.2.8.2   *Amount of tension developed by each contracting muscle fiber*

As the amount of tension developed by each individual muscle fiber increases, then the overall strength of skeletal muscle contraction increases. Three major factors determine the amount of tension that may be developed by a contracting muscle fiber:

- Frequency of nerve stimulation
- Length of the muscle fiber at the onset of contraction
- Diameter of the muscle fiber

As mentioned previously, a single action potential lasting only 2 ms causes a muscle twitch that lasts approximately 100 ms. If the muscle fiber has adequate time to completely relax before it is stimulated by another action potential, the subsequent muscle twitch will be of the same magnitude as the first. However, if the muscle fiber is restimulated before it has completely relaxed, then the tension generated during the second muscle twitch is added to that of the first (see Figure 16.3). In fact, the *frequency of nerve impulses* to a muscle fiber may be so rapid that there is no time, whatsoever, for relaxation in between stimuli. In this case, the muscle fiber attains a state of smooth, sustained, maximal contraction referred to as *tetanus*.

The amount of tension developed by a muscle fiber during tetanic contraction can be as much as three to four times greater than that of a single muscle twitch. The mechanism involved with this increased strength of contraction involves the concentration of cytosolic calcium. Each time the muscle fiber is stimulated by an action potential, Ca^{++} ions are released from the sarcoplasmic reticulum. However, as soon as the Ca^{++} ions are released, a

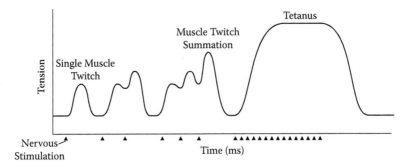

Figure 16.3   Muscle twitch summation and tetanus. A single action potential (represented by ▲) generates a muscle twitch. Because the duration of the action potential is so short, subsequent action potentials may restimulate the muscle fiber before it has completely relaxed. This leads to muscle twitch summation and greater tension development. When the frequency of stimulation becomes so rapid that there is no relaxation between stimuli, tetanus occurs. Tetanus is a smooth, sustained, maximal contraction.

continuously active calcium pump begins returning the Ca^{++} ions to the sarcoplasmic reticulum. Consequently, fewer Ca^{++} ions are available to bind with troponin and only a portion of the binding sites on the actin become available to the myosin cross bridges. Each subsequent stimulation of the muscle fiber results in the release of more Ca^{++} ions from the sarcoplasmic reticulum. In other words, as the frequency of nerve stimulation increases, the rate of Ca^{++} ion release exceeds the rate of Ca^{++} ion removal. Therefore, the cytosolic concentration of calcium remains elevated. A greater number of Ca^{++} ions bind with troponin, resulting in a greater number of binding sites on the actin that become available to the myosin cross bridges. As the number of cycling cross bridges increases, the amount of tension that is developed increases.

The amount of tension developed by a stimulated muscle fiber is highly dependent upon the *length of the muscle fiber at the onset of contraction*. This association between the resting length of the muscle fiber and tension development is referred to as the *length–tension relationship*. The sarcomere length at which maximal tension can be developed is termed the *optimal length* (L_o). In skeletal muscle, optimal length is between 2.0 and 2.2 µm. At this point, the actin filaments have overlapped all the myosin cross bridges on the thick filaments (see Figure 16.4, point a). In other words, the potential for cross bridge cycling and tension development upon stimulation has been maximized.

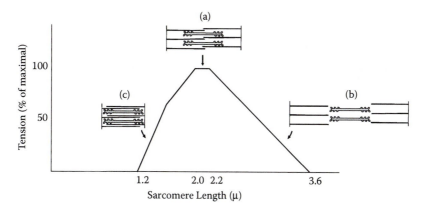

Figure 16.4 The length–tension Relationship. The length of the sarcomere prior to stimulation influences the amount of tension that may be developed in the muscle fiber. (a) The optimal length of the sarcomere is between 2.0 and 2.2 µm. At this length, actin overlaps all the myosin cross bridges. The potential for cross bridge cycling and the tension that may be developed upon stimulation of the muscle fiber are maximized. (b) When the sarcomere is overstretched so that the actin does not overlap the myosin cross bridges, then cross bridge cycling cannot take place and tension cannot be developed in the muscle fiber. (c) When the sarcomere is shortened prior to stimulation, then the thin filaments oveslap each other and the thick filaments about the Z lines. Further shortening and tension development upon stimulation is markedly impaired.

If the muscle fiber is stretched prior to stimulation such that the actin filaments have been pulled out to the end of the thick filaments, then there is no overlap between actin and the myosin cross bridges (see Figure 16.4, point b). In this case, there is no cross bridge cycling and tension development is zero.

Tension development is also impaired when the muscle fiber is allowed to shorten prior to stimulation (see Figure 16.4, point c). First, if the actin filaments overlap each other, there are fewer binding sites available for the myosin cross bridges. Second, if the thick filaments are forced up against the Z lines, further shortening cannot take place.

Interestingly, the range of resting sarcomere lengths is limited by the attachment of the skeletal muscles to the bones. Because of this fixed orientation, skeletal muscles cannot overstretch or over-shorten prior to stimulation. Typically, these muscles are within 70% to 130% of their optimal length. In other words, attachment to the bones ensures that the overlap of actin and myosin is such that cross bridge cycling always approaches maximum ability. As the number of cycling cross bridges increases, then the strength of muscle contraction increases.

The *diameter of the muscle fiber* is influenced by two major factors:

- Resistance training
- Testosterone

Repeated bouts of anaerobic, high-intensity *resistance training*, such as weight lifting, causes muscle hypertrophy and an increase in the diameter of the muscle fiber. This form of training promotes the synthesis of actin and myosin filaments, resulting in an increase in the number of cross bridges available to cycle and develop tension. Hence, larger muscles are capable of developing more powerful contractions.

Muscle fibers in males are thicker than those found in females. Therefore, their muscles are larger and stronger, even without the benefit of resistance training. This enlargement is due to the effects of *testosterone*, a sex hormone found primarily in males. Testosterone promotes the synthesis of actin and myosin filaments in muscle fibers.

16.3   Disorders of skeletal muscle

16.3.1   Metabolic disorders of skeletal muscle

Skeletal muscles rely heavily on glucose/glycogen and fatty acids for their energy needs. Several genetic disorders may occur in which the enzymes necessary for muscle energy metabolism are lacking or deficient.

16.3.1.1   McArdle's disease
- The disease effects approximately 1 in 100,000 individuals.
- Autosomal recessive disorder characterized by a defect on chromosome 11 for the enzyme *myophosphorylase* that is responsible for the breakdown of stored glycogen in skeletal muscle. As a result, the disease is also classified as a *Type V Glycogen Storage Disease*.

16.3.1.1.1   Symptoms
- Muscle fatigue
- Exercise intolerance
- Muscle cramps
- Muscle wasting is possible in elderly patients
- Creatinine kinase levels are often elevated in the majority of patients even at rest
- *Myoglobinuria*—the presence of dark myoglobin in the urine. May occur after periods of strenuous exertion

16.3.1.1.2   *Diagnosis*   In addition to the physical symptoms and presentation, diagnosis may be confirmed by histochemical analysis of myophosphorylase activity from muscle biopsies.

16.3.1.1.3   *Treatment*   McArdle's disease is generally a benign condition that is managed by lifestyle changes and adaption. Although strenuous exertion should be avoided, regular aerobic exercise can be beneficial for muscle function and overall health.

16.3.1.2   Pompei disease
- A rare autosomal recessive disorder caused by defect in the gene for the lysosomal *acid alpha-glucosidase* enzyme that is involved in the breakdown of glycogen in muscle.
- Also called *Glycogen Storage Disease Type II*
- The severity of the disease can vary greatly depending upon the percentage of active enzyme that is produced. Infantile forms tend to have the most severe presentation because 1% or less of the affected enzyme may be normal. In childhood and adult forms, the presentation can be milder because up to 40% of the normal enzyme may be produced. Progression of the disease tends to be worse in individuals who present with the disorder earlier in life.

16.3.1.2.1 Symptoms

- Hypertrophy and damage of muscle due to the accumulation of glycogen. Cardiac hypertrophy and liver enlargement can occur in infants as a result of glycogen accumulation.
- Muscle weakness, pain and cramping. The respiratory muscles can be affected in severe cases and lead to difficulty in breathing with exertion.
- Difficulty chewing and swallowing.

16.3.1.2.2 Diagnosis   A definitive diagnosis for Pompe disease can be made by measuring levels of the acid alpha-glucosidase enzyme, which are always reduced in patients with Pompe disease. This enzyme assay may be done through a simple blood test and does require a muscle biopsy.

16.3.1.2.3 Treatment   Enzyme replacement therapy is available for patients with Pompe disease including those with the infantile form. Supportive therapies may include physical therapy and respiratory therapy.

16.3.2   Cerebral palsy

Cerebral palsy is a neurologic disorder that primarily affects motor function and muscle coordination. The condition is caused by a brain injury or malformation that occurs while a child's brain is developing. The brain damage that occurs may be the result of ischemia, trauma, infection genetic defects, or abnormal brain development.

16.3.2.1 Symptoms

- Symptoms will vary depending upon the location and extent of CNS injury that occurred
- Typical symptoms may include abnormal muscle tone, ataxia, involuntary muscle movements, hemiplegia or quadriplegia, cognitive impairment
- Diagnosis is often made through brain scans and EEG

16.3.2.2 Treatment

- Physical, occupational, speech therapy
- Muscle relaxants may be helpful with muscle spasms
- Selected neurologiic, orthopedic and musculoskeletal surgeries may be needed for symptomatic relief

16.3.3   Muscular dystrophy (MD)

The muscular dystrophies are a group of more than 30 disorders that are associated with progressive weakness and degeneration of skeletal muscles. The muscular dystrophies have a genetic basis and it is believed that each form of MD has a unique genetic defect. Some forms of MD present in infancy or early childhood, whereas others do not manifest until adulthood. Duchenne MD is the most common and severe form of MD and is the condition we will focus on here.

16.3.3.1 Duchenne muscular dystrophy

Duchenne MD is an X-linked disease caused by single-gene defect. The disease primarily affects boys with an incidence of approximately 1 in 3,300 live male births. The defective gene codes for a protein called *dystrophin*, which is present in normal skeletal muscle but lacking in the skeletal muscle of affected patients. The dystrophin protein appears to play an important structural role in anchoring muscle proteins. When dystrophin is lacking, the skeletal muscle fibers function poorly and may become damaged during the contraction process (Figure 16.5).

16.3.3.1.1 Symptoms

- Symptoms begin to manifest in early childhood as progressive muscle weakness and wasting along with significant developmental motor delays
- Muscle weakness normally begins in the pelvic girdle. This weakness affects normal walking. Hypertrophy of calf muscles is often present as a result of abnormal muscle and the accumulation of scar tissue
- Children often require the use of a wheelchair by 7–10 years of age
- The lack of dystrophin may also weaken the myocardium and lead to *cardiomyopathy* in the teenage years

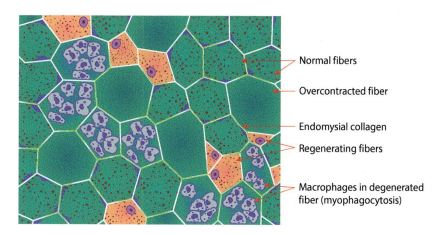

Figure 16.5 Cross-section of skeletal muscle fibers in Duchenne muscular dystrophy.

- The diaphragm and respiratory muscle begin to weaken in later childhood, placing the patient at risk for respiratory infections and respiratory failure
- The majority of patients succumb to the disease by their late teens or early twenties

16.3.3.1.2   Diagnosis
- Presentation of symptoms
- Family history
- Elevations of serum *creatinine kinase*, an enzyme released from damaged muscle tissue
- Genetic testing for mutations in dystrophin genes
- Muscle biopsy for dystrophin expression

16.3.3.1.3 *Treatment* Current therapies are mainly supportive. Although there is no cure, research continues into therapies that might one day modify or reverse the effects of the disease.

16.3.3.2   Becker muscular dystrophy
Also called *benign Duchenne muscular dystrophy* because the symptoms and presentation are similar, but much milder. The incidence of Becker MD is significantly rarer than that of Duchenne MD. In Becker MD, patients still produce a mutated dystrophin protein but one that is still somewhat functional in anchoring muscle proteins. Affected patients often remain ambulatory well into their twenties and with proper care they can live well into adulthood. Treatment is mainly supportive.

16.3.3.3   Facioscapulohumeral muscular dystrophy
Mild, progressive autosomal dominant condition. Mainly presents with weakness and atrophy of the muscle of the face and shoulder. Life expectancy is normal; treatment is mainly supportive and often includes physical and occupational therapy.

16.3.3.4   Limb girdle muscular dystrophy
Presentations usually begin when patients are 20–30 years of age. Both males and females are affected at equal rates. The underlying cause is uncertain, but it may actually be a group of different conditions, all of which affect skeletal muscle. Symptoms usually include weakness of the pelvic girdle, arms and shoulder. Individuals may have elevated creatinine kinase levels and marked abnormalities of skeletal muscle fibers seen with biopsy. Patients usually remain ambulatory well into adulthood. The progression and severity of the disease is often more severe in cases with earlier presentation.

16.3.4 Myasthenia gravis

Myasthenia gravis is a condition that affects the neuromuscular junction. It is an autoimmune condition in which antibodies are produced against the post-synaptic acetylcholine receptors in the neuromuscular junction. When activated by acetylcholine, the postsynaptic acetylcholine receptors are associated with sodium channels that open and lead to depolarization of skeletal muscle. Immune-mediated destruction of these receptors results in an inability to contract skeletal muscles. Although myasthenia gravis can affect individuals of any age, it is more common in women under 40 years of age and men older than 60 years of age.

A variant of myasthenia gravis called *Lambert-Eaton myasthenic condition* may occur in patients with certain cancers such as small cell lung cancer. This condition may be a component *paraneoplastic syndrome* that is seen in cancer patients and is likely related to circulating substances released from growing malignant tumors.

16.3.4.1 Symptoms
- Initial symptoms often involve weakness of the eye muscle and include drooping of the eyelids (*ptosis*) and diplopia (see Figure 16.6)
- Muscles of the head and neck may also be involved and this can lead to difficulty speaking, chewing, and swallowing
- Weakness of muscles in the arms, neck, and legs may also occur
- In severe cases, respiratory muscles may also be affected

16.3.4.2 Diagnosis
- Neurologic exam and muscle strength tests
- Electromyography and repetitive nerve stimulation to determine if skeletal muscles fatigue prematurely

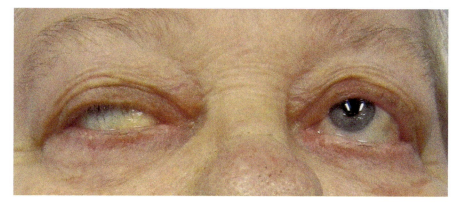

Figure 16.6 Difficulty controlling eye muscles in myasthenia gravis.

- Blood tests for abnormal antibodies
- *Edrophonium (tensilon) test* – a short acting acetylcholinesterase inhibitor is administered. This drug rapidly increases levels of acetylcholine by inhibiting its breakdown in the neuromuscular junction. If myasthenia gravis is present, the injection of edrophonium will result in a dramatic and rapid reversal of symptoms related to muscle weakness.

16.3.4.3   Treatment

There is no cure for myasthenia gravis. Treatment involves the regular administration of long-acting acetylcholinesterase inhibitors such as pyridostigmine. Corticosteroids and immunosuppressant drugs may also be helpful in reducing the production of abnormal antibodies. Approximately 15% of patients with myasthenia gravis have a benign tumor (myoma) in their thymus gland. Removing this tumor often helps symptoms but may not completely eliminate the condition. The long-term prognosis of patients with myasthenia gravis is generally favorable and most patients live relatively normal lives with the correct treatment.

Medical terminology

Agonist (ăg′ŏn-ĭst): Prime mover; muscle directly engaged in contraction and causing a movement

Antagonist (ăn-tăg′ō-nĭst): Muscle that opposes the action of the prime mover

Caveola (kăv-ē-ō′lă): Small pit or pouch formed on the cell surface

Extension (ĕks-tĕn′shŭn): The act of straightening a joint

Flexion (flĕk′shŭn): The act of bending a joint

Hyperplasia (hī″pĕr-plā′zē-ă): Increase in the number of cells in an organ or tissue

Hypertrophy (hī-pĕr′trŏ-fē): Increase in size of an organ, tissue or cell

Insertion (ĭn-sĕr′shŭn): The more movable attachment at the distal end of a muscle

Isometric (ī″sō-mĕ′trĭk): Regarding the maintenance of a constant length during muscular contraction

Isotonic (ī″sō-tŏn′ĭk): Regarding the maintenance of a constant force during muscular contraction

Ligand (lī′gănd, lĭg′ănd): Any chemical that binds to a specific receptor

Motor unit: Somatic motor neuron and all the muscle fibers it innervates

Myogenic (mī-ō-jĕn′ĭk): Originating in muscle

Myoglobin (mī″ō-glō′bĭn): Iron-containing protein within muscle cells that binds with and stores oxygen

Neurogenic (nū-rō-jĕn′ĭk): Resulting from nerve impulses

Origin (or'ĭ-jĭn): The relatively fixed attachment of a muscle

Oxygen debt: The oxygen required during the recovery period following strenuous physical activity

Phosphorylation (fŏs"for-ĭ-lā'shŭn): The addition of a phosphate to an organic compound

Rigor mortis (rĭg'or mŏr'tĭs): Stiffness that occurs in a dead body

Sarcomere (săr'kō-mēr): Unit of contraction in muscle consisting of thick and thin filaments

Synergist (sĭn'ĕr-jĭst): Muscle that assists the prime mover in producing a movement

Syncytium (sĭn-sĭt'ē-ŭm): Group of cells in which the cytoplasm of one cell is continuous with that of the adjacent cells

Tendon (tĕn'dŭn): Fibrous connective tissue that attaches muscles to bones

Tension (tĕn'shŭn): Force; muscle contraction that performs work and produces heat

Tetanus (tĕt'ă-nŭs): Smooth, sustained muscle contraction

Bibliography

Costanzo, L., *Physiology*, 3rd ed., W. B. Saunders Company, Philadelphia, PA, 2006.

Fox, S. I., *Human Physiology*, 9th ed., McGraw Hill, Boston, MA, 2006.

Guyton, A. C., and Hall, J. E., *Textbook of Medical Physiology*, 11th ed., Elsevier/ Saunders, Philadelphia, PA, 2006.

Lombard, J. H. and Rusch, N. J., Cells, nerves and muscles, in *Physiology Secrets*, Raff, H., Ed., Hanley and Belfus, Inc., Philadelphia, PA., 1999, chap.1.

Marieb, E. N., and Hoehn, K., *Anatomy & Physiology*, 3rd ed., Pearson Benjamin Cummings, San Francisco, CA, 2008.

McArdle, W. D., Katch, F. I., and Katch, V. L., *Exercise Physiology, Energy, Nutrition and Human Performance*, 5th ed., Williams & Wilkins, Baltimore, 2001.

Pasricha, P. J., Prokinetic agents, antiemetics, and agents used in irritable bowel syndrome, in *Goodman & Gilman's The Pharmacological Basis of Therapeutics*,10th ed., Hardman, J. G. and Limbird, L. E., Eds., McGraw Hill, New York, 2001.

Porth, C. M., *Pathophysiology, Concepts of Altered Health States*, 7th ed., Lippincott, Williams & Wilkins, Philadelphia, PA, 2005.

Rhoades, R., and Pflanzer, R., *Human Physiology*, 4th ed., Thomson Learning, Pacific Grove, CA, 2003.

Robergs, R. A., and Roberts, S. O., *Exercise Physiology, Exercise, Performance, and Clinical Applications*, Mosby, St. Louis, MO, 1997.

Sherwood, L., *Human Physiology from Cells to Systems*, 5th ed., Brooks/Cole, Pacific Grove, CA, 2004.

Silverthorn, D., *Human Physiology: An Integrated Approach*, 4th ed., Prentice Hall, Upper Saddle River, NJ, 2007.

Taber's Cyclopedic Medical Dictionary, 20th ed., F. A. Davis Co., Philadelphia, PA, 2005.

Sperelakis, N., *Essentials of Physiology*, 2nd ed., Sperelakis, N., and Banks, R. O., Eds., Little, Brown and Company, Boston, 1996.

Weisbrodt, N. W., Swallowing, in *Gastrointestinal Physiology*, 7th ed., Johnson, L. R., Ed., Mosby, St. Louis, MO, 2007, chap. 3.

Widmaier, E. P., Raff, H., and Strang, K. T., *Vander's Human Physiology, The Mechanisms of Body Function*, McGraw Hill, Boston, MA, 2006.

chapter seventeen

The skeletal system

Study objectives

- List the function of the human skeletal system
- Explain how the skeletal system helps the body maintain homeostasis
- Distinguish between bone as a tissue and an organ
- Discuss the role of bones in regulating blood calcium and phosphate levels

The *skeletal system* comprises a system of bones and associated cartilages, and performs important functions necessary for survival. These functions include:

- *Support*: The hard framework of the skeletal system supports and anchors the soft organs of the body
- *Protection*: Bones enclose and protect soft organs of the body, such as the brain, heart, spinal cord, and lungs
- *Movement*: Bones act as levers for the body's skeletal muscles
- *Storage*: Bones function in the storage of inorganic minerals, such as calcium and potassium. In addition, several long bones store lipids in the form of yellow bone marrow
- *Blood cell formation*: Red bone marrow is responsible for the production of blood cells and platelets
- *Electrolyte balance*: Storage of calcium and phosphate ions used to maintain blood levels needed for homeostasis
- *Acid-base balance*: Bone tissue buffers the blood during excessive pH changes
- Describe the process of osteoporosis in terms of bone resorption and deposition. What role might osteoclasts play in the process?
- List risk factors for osteoporosis. Include the use of certain drugs that might increase an individual's risk for developing the disease
- Describe the etiology of Paget's disease and osteomalacia
- Compare and contrast rheumatoid arthritis with osteoarthritis in terms of their etiology, manifestations, long-term complications, and treatment
- Discuss the etiology of systemic lupus erythematosus. Why is it often referred to as the "great imitator"?
- What is gout? Why might it occur? What are some of the possible long-term complications of poorly treated gout? Discuss strategies to treat gout

17.1   Bone as a tissue and an organ

Bone, or *osseous* tissue, is a connective tissue in which the extracellular environment, called the matrix, is hardened due to the presence of calcium phosphate and other minerals. The hardening process of the matrix is called *calcification*, or mineralization. Osseous tissue is only one of the tissues that make up bones, the organs of the skeletal system. Also present are blood, bone marrow, cartilage, adipose tissue, nervous tissue, and fibrous connective tissue.

17.2   Hemopoiesis

Hemopoiesis is the process of blood cell formation and occurs primarily in the red bone marrow. It starts with undifferentiated cells called hemocytoblasts. These stem cells give rise to the many different cellular components found within the blood: red blood cells, white blood cells, and platelets.

Several hormones and growth factors, known as colony stimulating factors (CSFs), regulate the differentiation of hemocytoblasts into myeloid or lymphoid cell lines. Myeloid cells lines give rise to red blood cells and platelets, as well as some white blood cells.

Hemopoiesis along the myeloid cell line follows one of three pathways: erythropoiesis, the formation of erythrocytes; thrombopoiesis, the production of thrombocytes; and leukopoiesis, the formation of leukocytes.

17.2.1   Erythropoiesis

Erythrocytes, red blood cells (RBCs), live an average of 120 days, starting at the time they are produced within the red bone marrow until they are destroyed by the spleen or liver. In a homeostatic state, the birth and death of RBCs amount to about 1 million cells per second, nearly 100 billion cells per day, or a packed cell volume of 20 mL/day.

The process of erythropoiesis takes 3–5 days and involves four major developments:

- A reduction in cell size
- An increase in cell number
- Synthesis of hemoglobin
- Loss of the nucleus and other organelles

One of the major CSFs controlling erythropoiesis is erythropoietin (EPO), a hormone secreted by the kidneys (see Chapter 5).

17.2.2   Thrombopoiesis

Thrombocytes, or platelets, are not cells; they are small fragments of marrow cells called megakaryocytes and are the second most abundant of the formed elements after RBCs. A normal platelet counts from a fingerstick ranges from

130,000 to 400,000 platelets/μL (average about 250,000). Thrombopoietin is a major CSF involved in platelet formation (see Chapter 5).

17.2.3 Leukopoiesis

Leukopoiesis, the production of leukocytes, or white blood cells (WBCs), begins with the same hemopoietic stem cells as erythropoiesis and is regulated by several CSFs (see Chapter 5).

17.3 Mineral deposition

Mineral deposition, or mineralization, is a crystallization process in which calcium and phosphate ions are taken from the blood plasma and deposited in bone tissue as needlelike crystals of hydroxyapatite.

   The process of mineralization starts with osteoblasts, the bone forming cells. Hydroxyapatite crystals form when the product of calcium and phosphate concentration in the tissue fluids, represented as $[Ca^{2+}] \bullet [PO_4^{3-}]$, reaches a critical value called the solubility product. The first few crystals to form act as "seed crystals" that attract more calcium and phosphate from solution. The more hydroxyapatite that forms, the more it attracts additional minerals from the tissue fluid. This positive-feedback mechanism continues until the matrix is thoroughly calcified.

PHARMACY APPLICATION: HETEROTOPIC OSSIFICATION

Osseous tissue sometimes forms in the lungs, eyes, muscles, tendons, arteries, and other organs. Such abnormal calcification of tissues is called heterotopic ossification. An example of this is arteriosclerosis, or hardening of the arteries, which results from calcification of an arterial wall. A calcified mass in an otherwise soft organ such as the lungs is called a *calculus*.

   Anti-platelet medications, such as aspirin, reduce the likelihood that platelets will clump in narrowed arteries, form a blood clot and cause further blockage.

   PCSK9 inhibitors are a relatively new class of drugs used to lower cholesterol and have been shown to reduce heterotopic ossification.

17.4 Mineral resorption

Mineral resorption is the process of dissolving bone tissue. It releases minerals into the blood, making them available for bodily functions. The bone cells responsible for resorption are osteoclasts. Bone resorption can be triggered by parathyroid hormone (PTH) in response to hypocalcemia.

17.5   Calcium homeostasis

Calcium levels are strictly maintained within the body in the range of 9–11 mg per 100 mL. The parathyroid gland releases PTH when blood levels of ionic calcium decline below normal. It stimulates osteoclasts to begin resorption, releasing calcium into the bloodstream. When the calcium concentration in the blood returns to the normal level, the stimulus for PTH release ends. When blood calcium levels rise above normal, calcitonin is released by the thyroid gland. Calcitonin stimulates the deposition of calcium in bone, by osteoblasts, and inhibits the action of osteoclasts. Calcium homeostasis is a negative-feedback mechanism.

17.6   Disorders of the skeletal system

This section begins with a focus on metabolic diseases of bone and includes conditions such as osteoporosis, Paget's disease, osteomalacia and rickets. These conditions are metabolic in that they are caused by abnormalities of minerals, vitamins or bone mineralization. The second portion of the chapter focuses on rheumatic and degenerative conditions that affect the joints and skeleton such as rheumatoid arthritis, systemic lupus erythematous, ankylosing spondylitis, and osteoarthritis. The chapter concludes with a discussion of gout.

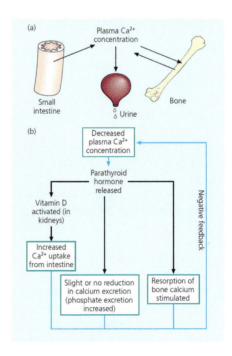

17.6.1 Osteoporosis

Osteoporosis is a disease characterized by decreased bone density. It most commonly occurs as a result of aging and is likely related to an imbalance between bone *resorption* (breakdown) and bone formation. With aging, the activity of bone forming cells called *osteoblasts* decreases. Decreased physical activity associated with aging may also play a role because mechanical forces on bone are important for maintaining normal bone density. Excess activity of *osteoclasts*, cells that demineralize bone, may also play a factor in the etiology of osteoporosis. Because estrogen plays an important role in maintaining bone density in females, post-menopausal women are at an increased risk for osteoporosis. A number of other factors can also put an individual at an increased risk for osteo-porosis (see Table 17.1).

Table 17.1   Risk factors for osteoporosis

Non-modifiable Risk Factors
- White or Asian race
- Advancing age
- Postmenopausal
- Female sex
- Family history of osteoporosis

Modifiable Risk Factors
- Sedentary lifestyle
- Deficiency of calcium or vitamin D
- Smoking
- Excess protein intake
- Excess alcohol or caffeine intake

Drugs
- Corticosteroids
- Dilantin, phenobarbital
- Aluminum-containing antacids
- Chemotherapy agents
- Heparin
- Excess thyroid hormone

Diseases
- Rheumatoid arthritis
- Lupus
- Celiac disease
- Inflammatory bowel disease
- Gastrectomy
- Diabetes
- Cushing syndrome
- Hyperthyroidism
- Hyperparathyroidism

17.6.1.1 Manifestations of osteoporosis

- Demineralization of bone that leads to an increased risk of fractures. Fractures most commonly occur in the long bones such as the femur and humerus. Vertebral fractures are also possible.
- Falls are more likely to result in broken hipbones, which require a long recovery period and are associated with a high secondary mortality rate.
- Degenerative changes in the vertebral column can lead to *kyphosis* or hunchback.

17.6.1.2 Diagnosis of osteoporosis

Osteoporosis is diagnosed through the use of a bone mineral density (BMD) test. The most common BMD test utilizes dual energy X-ray absorptiometry (DXA) that is capable of detecting even small amounts of bone mineral loss. The World Health Organization (WHO) has established a reference scale for determining the severity of osteoporosis in an individual. Their scale is based on the bone density measurement of a population of healthy young adults and is called a T-score. A normal T-score for hipbone density is −1 or greater. Osteoporosis is present if a T-score is −2.5 or below. The U.S. Preventative Services Task Force currently recommends that all women 65 years of age and older be screened for osteoporosis.

17.6.1.3 Treatment of osteoporosis

- Bisphosphonates (e.g., Alendronate)—suppress the activity of bone demineralizing osteoclast cells. These agents have been shown to increase bone density and reduce the risk for fractures.
- Hormones such as estrogen can help prevent osteoporosis but have been shown to increase the risk for heart attacks and certain cancers. Selective estrogen receptor modulators (SERMs) such as raloxifene may provide the benefits of estrogen with reduced risks of cancer in breast and endometrial tissues.
- Denosumab—a monoclonal antibody that prevents activation of osteoclasts. Must be given by injection.
- Teriparatide—recombinant human PTH. Stimulates the formation of new bone.

17.6.2 Paget's disease

Paget's disease is also called *osteitis deformans* and is a condition characterized by excess bone remodeling. The resorption of normal bone is accompanied by the rapid replacement with bone that is abnormally formed. Although the actual cause of Paget's disease is uncertain, Alterations in genes encoding for RANK protein appear to be associated with development of the disease. RANK stands for "receptor activator of NF-kappaβ" signaling pathways.

17.6.2.1 Clinical manifestations of Paget's disease

- Clinical features may be highly variable and the disease is rarely diagnosed before 40 years of age

- Abnormal distortions of the face, jaw, and skull are often noticed first
- Thickening of the skull may cause frequent headaches and impair brain function. Sensory defects, and altered motor function is possible
- The vertebrae of the spine may also be affected, which can lead to spinal deformities
- Evaluation is usually made by radiographic findings
- Most individuals do not require treatment. If treatment is needed, bisphosphonates and calcitonin can be administered

17.6.3   Osteomalacia

Osteomalacia is a condition in which bone does not properly mineralize in adults. It is most commonly caused by a dietary deficiency of calcium, vitamin D or phosphate. A similar condition called *rickets* can affect the developing bones of infants. Although nutritional deficiency is rarely a cause of osteomalacia in developed countries, it can still occur in patients who have intestinal diseases that affect nutrient absorption or in patients with significant renal disease due to abnormalities in calcium and phosphate regulation or vitamin D activation.

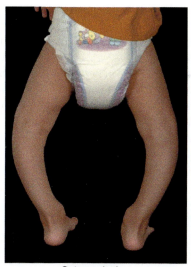

Osteomalacia

17.6.3.1   Clinical manifestations of osteomalacia

- Skeletal pain
- Increased risk for bone fractures
- Skeletal deformation and abnormal growth in children
- Treatment for nutritional osteomalacia includes dietary supplementation with calcium, phosphorus and vitamin D

17.6.4   Rheumatoid arthritis (RA)

RA is a systemic autoimmune disorder that is associated with pain and swelling in joints. RA is more common in women than men and usually presents before 40 years of age. Although the etiology of RA is uncertain, a key feature is the immune system inappropriately targeting the *synovium*, which is the membrane surrounding the joint capsule. The majority of patients with RA have circulating autoantibodies (IgGs) called *rheumatoid factors* that play a key role in the abnormal immune response. A second antibody called *anti-cyclic citrullinated peptide (ACPA)* antibody is also found in patients with RA. A genetic predisposition to RA has been identified, and individuals with certain HLA variants (HLA-DRB1, HLA-DR4) have an increased risk for developing the disease. There is also evidence that infection with certain microorganisms in susceptible individuals can act as a trigger for initiating the inappropriate immune response that is seen in RA through activation of the T-cells. In addition to joint symptoms, RA also causes a number of systemic manifestations related to an excessive inflammatory response. An overview of the disease process is shown in Figure 17.1

17.6.4.1   Manifestations of rheumatoid arthritis

- Progressive destruction of joints that over time can lead to joint instability and deformation (*subluxation*) (see figure below)
- Joint pain
- Morning stiffness
- *Rheumatoid nodules*—firm subcutaneous areas of swelling that occur in approximately 20% of patients with RA. The nodules are composed of inflammatory tissue and most commonly arise in the exposed joints of the fingers and elbows. On rare occasions, rheumatoid nodules may also form in the heart, lungs, and spleen where they can interfere with organ function.
- Systemic symptoms include fatigue, fever, and weight loss
- Extra-articular complications may include vasculitis, pulmonary fibrosis, and pericarditis

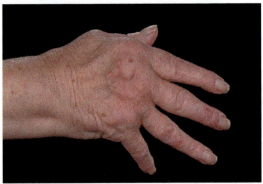

Rheumatoid arthritis in the hand

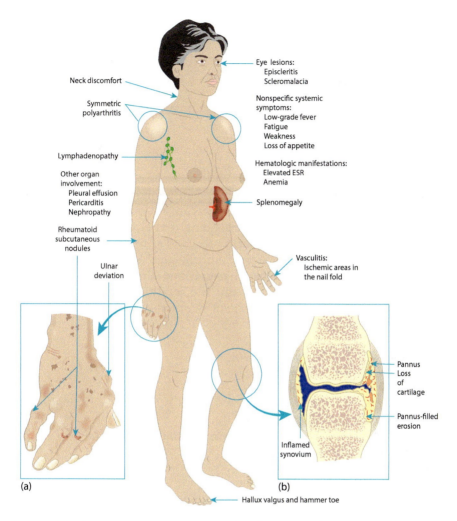

Figure 17.1 Manifestations of rheumatoid arthritis. (a) Subcutaneous rheumatoid nodules; (b) Damage to synovium in knee joint. (Adapted from *Porth's Pathophysiology: Concepts of Altered Health States* by Grossman, Lippincott Williams and Wilkins, 2013.)

17.6.4.2 Diagnosis of rheumatoid arthritis

- Blood tests may reveal an elevated *erythrocyte sedimentation rate (ESR)*, which is indicative on an ongoing inflammatory process somewhere in the body. The presence of rheumatoid factor and other autoimmune antibodies such as ACPA may also be detected by a blood test.
- X-rays and other diagnostic imaging tests are useful for assessing inflammatory or degenerative changes in the joints.

17.6.4.3   Treatment of rheumatoid arthritis

Treatment for RA involves the use of nonsteroidal anti-inflammatory drugs (NSAIDs) and corticosteroids to reduce pain and swelling. A number of drugs called *disease modifying anti-rheumatic drugs* (e.g., methotrexate) are used to slow the progression of joint destruction. *Biologic agents* may also be used to prevent immune cell activation or the activity of inflammatory cytokines such as TNF-α.

17.6.5   Systemic Lupus Erythematosus

Systemic lupus erythematosus (SLE) is an autoimmune condition in which the immune system produces antibodies against a number of cell components including nucleic acids, phospholipids, and ribonucleoproteins. The joint tissues are often affected and arthralgia and arthritis are the most common manifestations. The deposition of antigen–antibody complexes can also cause inflammatory lesions in blood vessels and affect organs such as the kidney, heart, spleen, lungs, and brain. The condition has been called the *great imitator* due to the diverse range of symptoms that may be present in numerous tissues and organs.

17.6.5.1   Manifestations of SLE
- Facial (butterfly-shaped) rash
- Joint stiffness and pain
- Skin lesions
- Vasospasm in fingers and toes
- CNS symptoms—headache, impaired memory, confusion
- Dyspnea, chest pain
- Complications may include:
  - Kidney damage
  - Anemia, neutropenia, thrombocytopenia
  - Pleuritis, pericarditis, vasculitis

17.6.5.2   Diagnosis and treatment of SLE

The diagnosis of SLE may be difficult initially due to the wide range of possible symptoms and the varying presentation from patient to patient. Some diagnostic findings associated with SLE include alterations in the complete blood count (CBC), ESR (which is an indicator of an ongoing inflammatory process), and the presence of antinuclear antibodies (ANA). Treatment for SLE includes the use of NSAIDs, corticosteroids, and immunosuppressants.

17.6.6   Ankylosing spondylitis

Ankylosing spondylitis (AS) is a systemic inflammatory condition that affects joint tissue. Although the exact etiology of AS is uncertain, patients with the HLA-B27 gene have a significantly increased risk for developing the condition. The hallmark feature of AS is inflammation of the fibrocartilage in the joints. The most commonly affected joints include those of the spine and vertebrae as well as the hip and shoulder.

Symptoms of AS include pain and stiffness that worsen with periods of inactivity. The most common complications of AS are osteoporosis of the spine and joints, which predisposes patients to compression fractures. Treatment includes the use of NSAIDs and anti-TNF-α therapies.

17.6.7   Osteoarthritis

Osteoarthritis (OA) is a condition associated with progressive degeneration of the joint tissues. A main feature of OA is degeneration of the articular cartilage that cushions the ends of the bones. This loss of protective cartilage may eventually lead to bones rubbing upon bones within the joint. OA is mainly caused by wear and tear of the joint tissues over the course of many years. However, there is a genetic tendency for OA to run within families. Women are at a greater risk for developing OA than men. The joints most commonly affected include the hands, knees, hip, and spine. Risk factors for OA include:

- Increasing age
- Obesity
- Female sex
- Family history of OA
- Occupations with high joint stresses
- Presence of other bone or rheumatic diseases

17.6.7.1   Manifestations of OA

- Joint pain and inflammation
- Joint swelling and stiffness
- Decreased range of motion in affected joints
- Bone spurs or *osteophytes* that often occur at the edges of the bone
- The diagnosis of OA may be confirmed through X-rays and MRI

OA in joints of the hands and feet

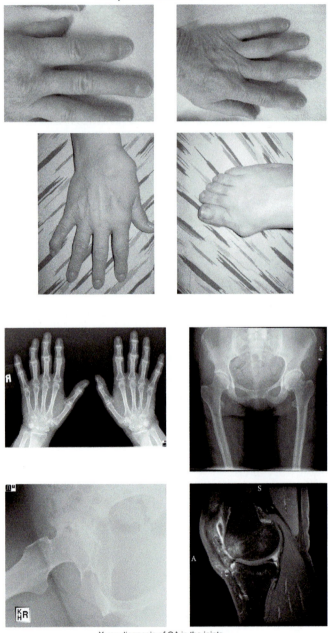

X-ray diagnosis of OA in the joints

17.6.7.2   Treatment of OA

- There is no cure for OA and treatment focuses mainly on the management of symptoms
- Pharmacologic therapy includes NSAIDs, and acetaminophen. Corticosteroid injections may also help relieve joint inflammation. The injection of lubricating substances such as *hyaluronic acid* may also be useful by providing some additional cushioning in the joint
- Physical therapy is helpful for strengthening the muscles around the joints and to help maintain flexibility

17.6.8   Gout

Gout is a condition that occurs when crystals of urate/uric acid accumulate in joint tissues and cause inflammation. Uric acid is a by-product of purine metabolism in the body. The purines adenine and guanine are derived from the breakdown of DNA and RNA. The majority of uric acid produced in the body is eliminated by the kidneys in the urine. The accumulation of uric acid can occur as a result of uric acid overproduction or a decreased elimination of uric acid by the kidneys. Uric acid crystals tend to precipitate in peripheral joint tissues because the temperature there is somewhat cooler and the synovial fluid is a poor solvent. Immune cell attack on precipitated uric acid crystals can cause marked inflammation of the joints. The accumulation of uric acid also leads to the formation of hard uric acid nodules called *tophi*.

Risk factors for the development of gout include:

- Increasing age
- Male sex
- Obesity
- Diets high in meat, and seafood
- Kidney disease
- Family history of gout
- Use of thiazide diuretics, aspirin

17.6.8.1   Manifestations of gout

- Severe joint pain
- Joint swelling and inflammation
- Limited range of joint motion
- Complications include an increased risk for the formation of uric acid kidney stones and tophi (see Figure 17.2)
- The diagnosis of gout may be made by testing of blood and synovial fluids for excess uric acid levels. Ultrasound and computed tomography scans may be used to detect the presence of uric acid crystals in the joints.

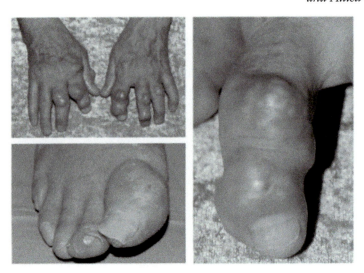

Figure 17.2   Tophi formed from uric acid deposits.

17.6.8.2   Treatment of Gout

NSAIDs are a mainstay for treating the inflammation associated with gout. Drugs called *uricosuric agents* (e.g., probenecid) may be used to enhance the elimination of gout by the kidneys. Agents such as allopurinol and febuxostat may be used to inhibit *xanthine oxidase,* a key enzyme involved in the production of uric acid.

chapter eighteen

Cancer

Study objectives

- List the main characteristics of benign and malignant tumors
- Describe the nomenclature used for various types of tumors
- Discuss tumor metastasis. How do tumors facilitate their own spread? What are some common sites of metastasis for tumors?
- Define oncogenesis. Discuss some of the theories as to how it might occur. List some viruses that are oncogenic along with the cancers they may cause
- What is a carcinogen? List some substances that are carcinogenic
- List the local and systemic effects of cancer
- Define cancer cachexia. Why might it occur?
- Describe the system by which tumors are "staged"
- What are tumor cell markers? How are they used clinically?
- Discuss the various treatment options for cancer, including the drawbacks of each

18.1 Introduction

Cancer is the second leading cause of death in the United States (see Table 18.1). The most common sites for cancer development are the prostate, breast, lung, and colon. Although cancer can arise at any age, the incidence of cancer increases proportionally with increasing age. Cancer is a disease that results from abnormal growth and differentiation of tissues.

18.2 Cancer terminology

The word "cancer" is from the Greek word for crab and reflects the finger-like projections that malignant tumors use to invade adjacent tissues. Malignant tumor cells may also produce *growth factors* that stimulate the formation of new blood vessels (a process called *angiogenesis*) that in turn support the rapid growth of tumor cells.

Table 18.1   Estimated number of new cancer cases for 2008 in the United States

Male		Female	
Prostate	164,690	Breast	266,120
Lung & bronchus	121,680	Lung & bronchus	112,350
Colon & Rectum	75,610	Colon & rectum	64,640
Urinary Bladder	62,380	Uterine	63,230
Melanoma	55,150	Thyroid	40,900
Kidney	42,680	Melanoma	36,120
Non-Hodgkin lymphoma	41,730	Non-Hodgkin lymphoma	32,950
Oral cavity & pharynx	37,160	Pancreas	26,240
Leukemia	35,030	Leukemia	25,270
Liver	30,610	Kidney	22,660
All Sites	**856,370**	**All sites**	**878,980**

Tumor or *neoplasm*: a mass of tissue in which the growth rate is excessive and uncoordinated when compared with normal tissues (see Table 18.2).

Benign neoplasm: tumor cells that tend to be clustered in a single mass and are not malignant. Benign tumors usually will not cause death unless they interfere with vital function.

Malignant neoplasm: tumors that have the ability to *"metastasize"* or break loose and spread to other areas of the body. Can cause great suffering and death if not treated.

Specific names end with *"oma."* For example, a hepatoma is a benign tumor of the liver, whereas a hepatocarcinoma would be a malignant tumor.

Table 18.2   Characteristics of neoplasia

Benign	Malignant
• Slow growth rate	• Rapid growth rate
• Encapsulated	• Nonencapsulated
• Well-differentiated cells	• Poorly differentiated
• Cells resemble tissue of origin	• Cells do not resemble tissue of origin
• Grow by expansion	• Loss of contact inhibition
• Do not metastasize	• Grow by invasion
• Rarely fatal unless they impinge upon a vital organ	• Metastasize, fatal if untreated
	• Abnormal gene expression
	• Express foreign antigens

18.2.1 Specific nomenclature examples

Carcinoma: malignant tumor of *epithelial cell origin.*
Sarcoma: malignant tumor of *skeletal or connective tissue origin.*
Lymphoma: malignant tumor of lymphatic tissue.
Glioma: malignant tumor of the glial support cells in the central nervous system.
Adenoma: benign tumor of glandular tissue.
Adenocarcinoma: malignant tumor of glandular tissue

Metastasis: the ability of tumor cells to spread to other parts of the body and establish secondary tumors. Malignant tumor cells can break off and utilize blood vessels or lymphatic vessels to spread to other areas of the body. Tumor cells enhance their potential for local invasion and metastatic spread by releasing *protease* enzymes that digest the extracellular matrix surrounding adjacent cells. Certain organs such as the lungs are prime locations for the formation of metastasis due to the large amount of blood flow they receive from the body. The liver is also a common site of metastasis for tumors originating in the gastrointestinal tract because blood draining the intestines must first pass through the liver via the hepatic portal system. Some common sites of metastasis for various cancers are listed in Table 18.3.

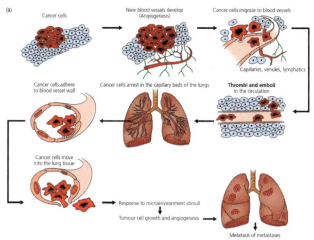

Process of cancer cell invasion and metastasis

Table 18.3   Common sites of metastasis for selected cancers

- Breast cancer—bones, lymph nodes (axillary), brain
- Lung cancer—many organs including liver, brain and bone
- Prostate cancer—bones, lungs, liver, endocrine glands
- Colon cancer—liver
- Testicular cancer—lungs, liver
- Ovarian cancer—peritoneum, liver, lungs, diaphragm

18.3   Theories of oncogenesis

Oncogenesis is the process by which normal cells are transformed into cancer cells.

Abnormalities of tumor suppressor/inducer genes (see Figure 18.1). Several proteins produced within cells such as the *p53* protein are known to limit cellular division by regulating certain parts of the normal cell cycle. The genes that code for these proteins are referred to as *anti-oncogenes* because they suppress cell growth. Failure of these anti-oncogenes may lead to the unregulated cellular division that is characteristic of cancer cells. In contrast, other groups of genes are classified as *proto-oncogenes* because they produce proteins and substances that enhance cellular growth and proliferation. Excessive activity of these genes (or a lack of their regulation) may likewise cause excessive cellular division and growth.

18.3.1   Mutation of DNA

Numerous chemical, physical and biologic agents have been shown to be *carcinogenic*, meaning they can induce the formation of cancers (see Table 18.4).

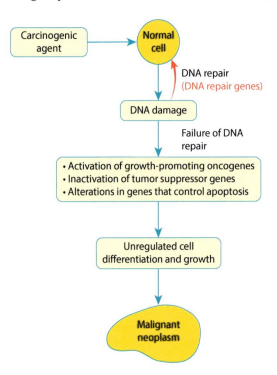

Figure 18.1 Oncogenesis and the mutation of tumor-suppressor genes. (Adapted from *Porth's Pathophysiology: Concepts of Altered Health States* by Grossman, Lippincott Williams and Wilkins, 2013.)

Table 18.4 Possible cancer-causing agents (carcinogens)

- Chemicals—many such as benzene, vinyl chloride, cigarette smoke, aromatic hydrocarbons
- Radiation, radon gas, radioactive materials, ultraviolet radiation
- Occupational exposure—asbestos, coal dust, uranium, solvents
- Oncogenic viruses
- Dietary factors—high-fat diet, excessive alcohol intake, nitrosamine preservatives, grilled, charred foods
- Hormones—estrogens, progesterone

Table 18.5 Oncogenic viruses

A number of DNA and RNA viruses have been shown to be "oncogenic," meaning they can cause cancers in the hosts they infect.
Viruses that may be oncogenic in humans include:
- *Human Papillomavirus*—cervical carcinoma
- *Hepatitis B and C Virus*—liver cancer
- *Epstein–Barr Virus*—Burkett lymphoma, nasopharyngeal cancer
- *HIV Virus*—Kaposi sarcoma

Many of these agents can damage cellular DNA, either directly, or though the production of toxic intermediates such as free radicals. Certain viruses are also *oncogenic* in that they may induce mutations in host cell DNA or alter rates of cellular transcription (see Table 18.5). Mutations of cellular DNA can lead to the formation of cells with abnormal growth and differentiation patterns.

18.3.2   Hereditary

A genetic predisposition has been observed for a number of cancers including colon cancer, breast cancer, retinoblastoma and certain forms of leukemia and lymphoma. A great deal of research has recently focused on identifying certain genetic markers in individuals that might pinpoint them as being at risk for the development of certain types of cancer.

18.4   Local effects of cancer

Many cancers may be asymptomatic in the early stages. As the tumor(s) continue to grow, they have effects on local tissues as well as systemic effects on the body.

- Compression of blood vessels
- Ischemia
- Pain
- Bleeding
- Infection
- Altered tissue function

18.5   Systemic effects of cancer

- Fatigue
- Cachexia (see Box)
- Paraneoplastic syndrome (see Box)
- Bleeding and hemorrhage
- Anemia due to chronic bleeding or bone marrow destruction. This anemia may be exacerbated by chemotherapy
- Altered organ function
- Abnormal hormone production from an affected gland or directly from certain types of hormone producing tumors

---

CACHEXIA

A complex syndrome characterized by anorexia, weight loss, and lean body (muscle) wasting seen in a significant percent of cancer and AIDS patients. A number of metabolic abnormalities have been demonstrated in patients with cachexia that lead to poor utilization of nutrients and overall malnutrition. A key factor in cachexia appears to be the production of *cytokines* such as *tumor necrosis factor* and *interleukins* in response to the presence of cancer. These substances are produced by many cells within the body and appear to be protective against bacterial and viral infections as well as against malignant cells. Unfortunately, these substances also appear to be responsible for many of the effects of cachexia including anorexia and lean body wasting.

PARANEOPLASTIC SYNDROME

Paraneoplastic syndrome is a group of symptoms that may occur in patients with cancer that are distant to the site of the growing cancers such. It is believed that these symptoms are produced by substances released from the growing cancer cells and from cytokines released in response to the growing cancer. Typical symptoms of paraneoplastic syndrome include:

- *Dermatologic*—itching, flushing, rashes
- *Endocrine*:
  - Cushing syndrome from tumor adrenocorticotropic hormone (ACTH) production
  - Water and electrolyte imbalance from tumor antidiuretic hormone (ADH) release
  - Hypercalcemia due to parathyroid hormone (PTH) release by tumor cells

(Continued)

PARANEOPLASTIC SYNDROME (Continued)

- *Neurologic:*
    - Neuropathies
    - *Lambert–Eaton syndrome*—myasthenia-like syndrome associated with skeletal muscle weakness. Caused by IgG antibodies that attack motor neurons impair acetylcholine release in the neuromuscular junction.
- *Rheumatologic*—polyarthritis, polymyalgia

Table 18.6   Staging of tumors

T—Primary Tumor: (Is there a tumor and if so, how big is it?)
   TX—primary tumor cannot be assessed
   T0—no evidence of primary tumor
   Tis—carcinoma *in situ*
   T1–T4—increasing size of tumor
N—Involvement of Lymph Nodes: (Has the tumor spread to the lymph nodes?)
   NX—regional lymph nodes cannot be assessed
   N0—no evidence that the tumor has metastasized to lymph nodes
in the region of the primary tumor
N1–N3—progressive involvement of regional lymph nodes
M—Distant Metastasis: (Has the tumor spread to distant sites in the body?)
   Mx—distant metastasis cannot be assessed
   M0—no evidence of distant metastasis
   M1–M4—single or multiple sites of metastasis have been located

---

18.6   Tumor staging

Tumors are classified or "staged" based upon the "TNM" system that includes a description of tumor size (T), involvement of lymph nodes (N) and metastasis (M). The TNM system for staging tumors is explained in Table 18.6.

18.7   Cancer detection

18.7.1   Tumor cell markers

- Tumor markers are usually substances produced by or found on the surface of tumor cells.
- Tumor cell markers may be used clinically to screen for the presence of tumor cells in the body.
- Drawbacks to the use of tumor markers in cancer diagnosis include the fact that they may not be specific for a certain type of cancer and the

Table 18.7   Examples of tumor cell markers

Alpha-fetoprotein:
- Secreted by embryonic liver cells
- High levels seen in liver, ovarian and testicular cancer
- May also be observed with viral hepatitis

Prostate-specific antigen (PSA):
- Markedly increased in prostatic cancer
- Slightly elevated in benign prostatic hypertrophy

CA (Cancer Antigen) 15-3:
- Elevated in breast cancer
- High levels often indicate advanced or metastatic breast cancer
- May be elevated in benign breast disease or liver disease

CA 19-9:
- Elevated in cancers of the gastrointestinal tract and pancreas
- May also be elevated in gall bladder disease and pancreatitis

CA 27-29:
- Elevated in breast cancer as well as a number of other cancers
- May also be elevated in benign breast disease as well as disease of the kidney and liver

CA 125:
- Elevated in ovarian cancer
- May be elevated in pregnancy and with pelvic inflammatory disease

Calcitonin:
- Thyroid cancer

Carcinoembryonic antigen (CEA):
- Colorectal, lung and pancreatic cancers

Human Chorionic Gonadotrophin:
- Used as a marker for a number of different cancers
- Elevated in pregnancy

Prostate-specific antigen (PSA):
- Prostate cancer

possibility that by the time tumor cell markers are detected, the particular cancer may be well progressed. Certain noncancerous conditions may also be associated with the appearance of some of these markers in the blood (see Table 18.7).

18.7.2   Tumor grading

Tumors may be examined microscopically to determine their degree of differentiation. The greater the degree of differentiation in a tumor, the more closely it will resemble its normal tissue. Tumors with a high degree on *anaplasia* are very poorly differentiated, do not resemble normal cells and tend to be very aggressive. In general, the higher the degree of anaplasia a tumor exhibits, the poorer the prognosis. Tumors are grades on a scale from I to IV, with I being more differentiated (less aggressive growth) and IV being the least differentiated (most aggressive growth)

18.7.3 Visualization

- X-rays, computer tomography (CT scans), magnetic resonance imaging may all be used to identify the presence of a tumor or tumors. Can also be used to evaluate metastasis
- *Endoscopy* may also be utilized to visually detect tumors in the bronchi and gastrointestinal tract

18.7.4 Biopsy

- Removal of a piece of suspect tissue for detailed histological or histochemical analysis as well as for tumor grading
- May be accomplished surgically, by a needle biopsy, by scraping cells from a surface (Pap smear) or by endoscopic biopsy

18.8 Rationale for cancer therapy

Cancer treatment can be multifaceted and may include surgical removal of tumors, as well as chemotherapy and/or radiation therapy to kill or arrest rapidly growing tumor cells. A number of immune-based treatments are currently under investigation as alternatives to toxic chemotherapy and radiation therapy. Treatment with specific hormones has also been shown to inhibit the growth of certain types of cancers.

18.8.1 Treatment of cancer

Surgical removal of tumors is often a first step in treating cancer if the tumors are accessible and are isolated masses. Surgery is normally accompanied by chemotherapy or radiation therapy to kill any cancer cells that are not removed or have metastasized.

Chemotherapy agents are drugs used to treat cancer. They fall into one of several general categories (see Table 18.8).

18.8.2 Hormonal therapy

Sex hormones are routinely used to inhibit tumor growth in breast, prostate and uterine cancer. The estrogen inhibitor *tamoxifen* has also been shown to be effective in the treatment of breast cancer and may be used as a prophylactic agent in women who are at a high risk for developing breast cancer. The androgen inhibitor *flutamide* has been approved for the treatment of prostate cancer.

Table 18.8   Chemotherapy drugs

Alkylating Agents and Nitrosoureas (e.g., cyclophosphamide, carmustine):
- Cytotoxic to cancer cells due to alkylation of cancer cell DNA
- Major toxicities include nausea and vomiting and bone marrow suppression

Antimetabolites (e.g., methotrexate, fluorouracil):
- Inhibit synthesis of essential nucleotides and nucleic acids in cancer cells
- Major toxicities include myelosuppression, nausea, vomiting, oral and gastrointestinal ulceration

Plant Alkaloids (e.g., vinblastine, vincristine):
- Disrupt mitosis in cancer cells by interfering with formation of the mitotic spindle
- Numerous toxicities including cardiotoxicity, bone marrow depression, neurologic and muscle effects as well as alopecia

Antibiotics (e.g., doxorubicin, bleomycin):
- Bind directly to cancer cell DNA to block the formation of new RNA or DNA
- Major toxicities include bone marrow suppression, alopecia

18.8.3   Radiation therapy

Utilizes ionizing or particle beam radiation to destroy cancer cells that are highly mitotic and most susceptible to the lethal effects of radiation. Radiation therapy can have a number of localized and systemic side effects including alopecia, diarrhea, tissue irritation, and organ inflammation.

18.8.4   Immune-based therapies ("biologic response modifiers")

Agents such as *interferons, immunomodulators, tumor antigens,* and *lymphokines/cytokines* are being investigated as means of enhancing the immune system response of individuals with cancer. *Monoclonal antibodies* have also been studied as a highly specific means of delivering chemotherapeutic drugs directly to cancer cells or as a means of blocking specific pathways in cancer cells that might be essential for replication or survival. Two monoclonal antibodies currently used for the treatment of cancer are, bevacozumab™ (Avastin™, an angiogenesis receptor inhibitor), and cetuximab™ (Erbitux™, a growth factor receptor inhibitor).

chapter nineteen

HIV

Study objectives

- Describe the structure of HIV. What is HIV reverse transcriptase enzyme and why is it essential for HIV replication?
- List the three stages of HIV infection, and give the key characteristics for each
- Define the term "opportunistic infection," and provide some examples of opportunistic infections in AIDS
- Describe the mechanism by which the HIV virus infects a human cell
- List ways in which the HIV virus is transmitted. What steps can be taken to prevent its transmission?
- Describe the various tests that are used to diagnose HIV infection
- Define "viral load." What is its clinical utility?
- Describe the mechanism of action for each of the various antiretroviral drug groups. List common adverse effects for each of these drug classes
- What does HAART stand for? How is it used in the treatment of HIV?
- Discuss the problem of HIV drug resistance. Why might it occur and what can be done to combat it?

19.1   Introduction

The syndrome of AIDS was first identified in the 1981 in a small group of gay men in the San Francisco area who presented with unusual opportunistic infections. In 1983, the human immunodeficiency virus (HIV) responsible for AIDS was first isolated. It is estimated that nearly 22 million persons have died since the epidemic began. Today, just over 1 million Americans are living with HIV infection. Recent news in the United States is encouraging because the annual rate of HIV infections decreased nearly 18% between 2008 and 2014. In addition, highly effective antiretroviral therapy has greatly improved the quality of life and life expectancy for patients infected with HIV. Although there are positive trends worldwide with regard to overall infection rates and treatment availability, developing countries are still especially hard hit by the HIV epidemic. It is estimated that 95% of people with HIV infection now live in developing countries. Globally only 46% of individuals infected with HIV are receiving antiretroviral therapy.

19.2   HIV structure and lifecycle

The HIV virus is an RNA virus that belongs to a family of viruses called *retroviruses*. The flow of genetic information in these viruses is the reverse of that normally occurring in mammalian cells (RNA to DNA instead of DNA to RNA). In order for these retroviruses to replicate in infected host cells, they must utilize a special enzyme called *reverse transcriptase*, which allows the viral RNA genome to be first copied into a DNA/RNA hybrid and then into mRNA, which can be translated into new viral proteins by host cell *DNA* and *RNA polymerase*. The HIV genome also contains codes for two other important enzymes, *HIV* integrase, and *HIV protease*, which are essential for successful HIV infection of the host cell. Structurally, HIV has an inner protein *core* containing a double strand of identical (+/+ RNA) (see Figure 19.1). The inner protein core of HIV is surrounded by a second protein layer called the protein *shell*. The protein shell in turn is encased in a lipid bilayer called the lipid *envelope*. This lipid bilayer is taken from host cell membranes when new HIV particles "bud" or *exocytose* from host cells. Protruding from the lipid envelope are numerous glycoprotein *spikes* or *peplomers*, which serve as organs of attachment to host cell membranes.

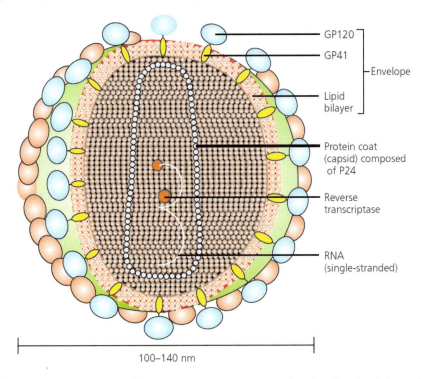

Figure 19.1   Structure of HIV Figure 6.1 in essentials of pathophysiology for pharmacy—third party source. (Adapted from *Porth's Pathophysiology: Concepts of Altered Health States* by Grossman, Lippincott Williams and Wilkins, 2013.)

HIV peplomers comprise two distinct glycoproteins, *gp41*, and *gp120*. The gp41 serves to anchor the peplomer in the HIV lipid envelope, whereas the gp120 serves as a specific binding site for the human cellular proteins called *CD4* (CD stands for cluster of differentiation). These CD4 proteins are found in greatest concentration on the surfaces of *helper T-cells* (CD4+ lymphocytes, or CD4 cells) and in lesser concentrations on *monocytes* and *macrophages*. When HIV encounters a CD4-bearing cell, the glycoprotein gp120 part of the peplomer binds specifically to it at the CD4 site. This binding uncovers the gp41 glycoprotein on the HIV peplomer, which now embeds itself in the host cell membrane (see Figure 19.2). Effective HIV binding to CD4 cells requires that HIV also attach to a second set of receptors on the surface of CD4 cells called *chemokine* receptors. Once *fusion* of the HIV has occurred with the host cell, the viral core (containing the HIV genome) is injected into the host cell. Inside the host cell, the viral core breaks down and the HIV genome is released into the host cell cytoplasm. This step is called *uncoating*. The free HIV RNA is copied into a DNA/RNA hybrid molecule with the assistance of HIV reverse transcriptase. The single strand of viral DNA is then released from the DNA/RNA hybrid and copied into a double strand of viral DNA by cellular polymerases. The double strand of HIV DNA becomes integrated into the host cell DNA through the actions of the HIV integrase enzyme. Then, each time the cellular DNA is expressed, viral DNA is also expressed. New HIV viruses are formed as the viral proteins are translated by the host cell from mRNA. These newly replicated viruses can leave the host cell by *budding* or exocytosis. The newly formed HIV viruses, however, are not fully "mature" or functional until they are enzymatically modified by HIV protease enzymes to the fully active and infectious state. A number of genetically different yet related HIV viruses have thus far been identified. Some of these variants appear to be particularly virulent because the progression of disease in patients infected with these strains is quite rapid. Other strains appear to be somewhat more "benign" because disease progression occurs more slowly.

CHEMOKINE MUTATION AND
RESISTANCE TO HIV INFECTION

It has long been observed that certain untreated individuals infected with HIV may progress very slowly in the course of their disease if at all. These "slow progressors" or "nonprogressors" may have a natural mutation in the chemokine proteins (CCR5) on the surface of their CD4 cells that are used by HIV for attachment. This mutation prevents HIV from fully attaching to their CD4 cells and makes viral entry more difficult. This finding led to development of the HIV drug maraviroc, which impairs HIV entry into CD4 cells by blocking CCR5 chemokine proteins on the surface of CD4 cells.

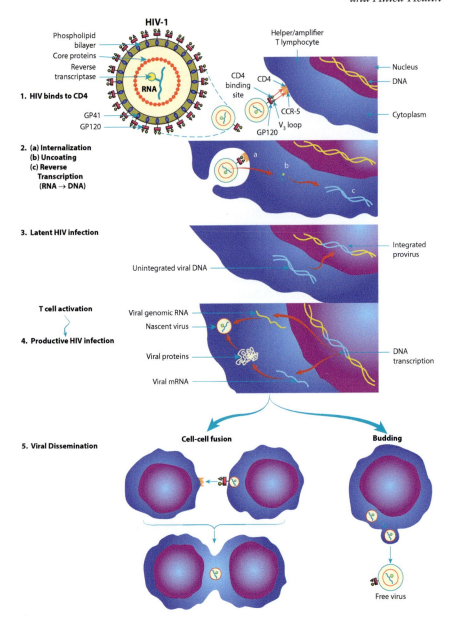

Figure 19.2 HIV life cycle. (Adapted from Clancy, John, and Andrew McVicar. *Physiology and Anatomy for Nurses and Healthcare Practitioners*, CRC Press, 2009.)

19.3   Stages in an HIV infection

Clinically, HIV infection presents in several distinct stages:

19.3.1   Acute illness stage

- Generally occurs several weeks after infection with the virus.
- Manifestations are very nonspecific and include acute-onset fever, headache, malaise, lymphadenopathy, sore throat, and skin rash.
- Symptoms usually subside within several weeks and the patient becomes asymptomatic.
- During the acute illness phase, there is a transient reduction in circulating CD4+ and CD8+ lymphocytes.

19.3.2   Asymptomatic stage

- Following the acute illness stage, most patients go into a prolonged period in which there are no symptoms of the infection. Patients generally remain in relatively good health for a period of 5–10 years. This asymptomatic period may be highly variable in duration.
- During this period, there is slow but persistent destruction of immune cells, particularly CD4 cells. Toward the end of this period, circulating levels of CD4 cells decline significantly from a normal range of approximately 500–1,500 cells/μL to less than 500 cells/μL. Levels of CD8 cells may also show moderate decreases.

19.3.3   Symptomatic or AIDS stage

- When circulating levels of CD4 cells fall below a critical level (generally 200 cells/μL), the infected individual becomes symptomatic.
- A number of symptoms falling under the heading of *AIDS-related complex* (ARC) may occur. These symptoms include fever, night sweats, diarrhea, and *opportunistic infections* (see Table 19.1). "Opportunistic" organisms are those that take advantage of the patient's weakened immune status to infect their system. Infections with many of these organisms are unique to AIDS or immunocompromised patients.
- As levels of CD4 cells continue to fall, levels of HIV in the blood can increase markedly.
- Malignant cancers may also appear as levels of CD4 cells continue to decline. The most common of these is *Kaposi sarcoma*, a malignant neoplasm that can occur in skin, oral mucosa, lymph nodes and viscera. The development of Kaposi sarcoma may be associated with infection by the human herpes virus 8 (HHV-8).
- Neurologic manifestations are common in the late stages of HIV infection and can include *AIDS dementia complex* in which the patient suffers loss of memory, personality changes and loss of control over motor functions. The American Academy of Neurology currently recognizes three categories of HIV-associated neurocognitive disorders (HANDs) based on their varying severity.

Table 19.1   Opportunistic infections in AIDS

- *Pneumocystis jiroveci*—a fungal parasite that can cause a severe pulmonary infection and pneumonia
- *Candida*—a fungus that can infect the oral cavity (oral "thrush") as well as the trachea and bronchi
- *Cryptococcosis*—a fungus that can cause pneumonia but can also spread to the brain
- *Cryptosporidium*—a gastrointestinal protozoal parasite that can cause severe, chronic diarrhea
- *Cytomegalovirus*—Herpes virus that can infect the eye, intestine, esophagus, lungs, or brain
- *Histoplasmosis*—fungal infection (*Histoplasma capsulatum*) that can enter the lungs and cause a pneumonia-like syndrome
- *Mycobacterium avium complex*—bacteria found in bird droppings, water and soil. Benign to healthy individuals but can be life threatening in the immunocompromised patient
- *Toxoplasmosis*—a parasite (*Toxoplasma gondii*) that can infect many tissues including the brain
- *Tuberculosis*—bacteria (*M. tuberculosis*) that primarily infects the lungs

---

- The AIDS stage is also associated with the development of *wasting syndrome*, or cachexia, characterized by marked weight loss, anorexia, metabolic changes and endocrine dysfunction.

19.4   Epidemiology of HIV infection

The HIV virus is a blood-borne pathogen that is transmitted via contact with contaminated body fluids. Unprotected sexual intercourse (vaginal or anal) with an infected individual currently accounts for the vast majority of new HIV infections. The virus may also be spread through contaminated blood products (blood and blood factor transfusions) as well as though sharing of contaminated needles. Transmission of the HIV virus from infected mothers to their fetus currently account for approximately 10% of all HIV infections. Because the HIV virus appears in breast milk, breastfeeding is not recommended in HIV-infected mothers. The HIV virus may also be detected in trace amounts in the saliva of infected individuals; however, there is no current evidence that the virus can be transmitted by casual contact.

19.5   Laboratory of diagnosis of HIV

Enzyme immunoassay (EIA) is used to detect HIV antibodies. A positive EIA must be confirmed by Western blot or immunofluorescence assay (IFA) to detect specific HIV proteins. HIV core protein p24 is the most abundant protein produced by HIV. Other HIV proteins such as p55, p40, gp120, and gp41 may also be part of the analysis. *Polymerase chain reaction (PCR)* is a technique used to measure HIV DNA levels (viral load).

19.6 Rationale for treatment of HIV

- Prevent viral replication in infected cells by inhibiting various steps in the HIV life cycle. Treatment should begin immediately upon diagnosis for all patients and regardless of their CD4 cell counts.
- Treat opportunistic infections when they arise and prophylactically.
- Provide nutritional, medical and emotional support for a chronic illness.

19.6.1 Treatment of HIV

- The most effective way to limit the occurrence of HIV infection is through proper prevention (see Table 19.2).
- The effectiveness antiretroviral therapy is determined be measuring CD4 counts and plasma HIV RNA (viral load).
- Currently available drugs for the treatment of HIV target various phases of the HIV life cycle (see Table 19.3). These agents are always used in combination to enhance effectiveness and reduce the possibility of drug resistance. The current *HAART* or *highly active antiretroviral therapy* regimen involves the use of three different antiretroviral drugs from at least two different drug classes.
- Considerable research is currently being conducted on developing an HIV vaccine that would protect individuals from HIV infections even after exposure to the virus.

Table 19.2 Prevention of HIV infection

- Practice safe sex
- Prevent sharing of used needles among intravenous drug abusers
- Implement effective screening of blood products in all countries
- Increase voluntary HIV screening in high-risk individuals
- Increase counseling on AIDS awareness and prevention
- Effective antiretroviral therapy has the potential to reduce or even stop the spread of HIV from person to person and from mother to infant
- *Preexposure prophylaxis (PrEP)*—individuals at high risk for HIV may reduce their risk of becoming infected if they take daily HIV medications. PrEp may reduce the risk of contracting HIV through sex by 90% and through intravenous drug use by 70%

Table 19.3   HIV drug therapy

---

1. Nucleoside Reverse Transcriptase Inhibitors (e.g., Abacavir, Zidovudine (AZT):
   - Competitive inhibitors of HIV reverse transcriptase enzyme
   - Side effects may include rash, nausea, diarrhea, and peripheral neuropathy
2. Non-nucleoside Reverse Transcriptase Inhibitors (e.g., Nevirapine, Efavirenz):
   - Bind directly to HIV reverse transcriptase to inhibit it
   - Side effects may include severe skin rashes, nausea, diarrhea, central nervous system effects
3. Protease Inhibitors (e.g., Atazanavir, Saqiunavir):
   - Inhibit HIV protease enzymes that are essential for enzymatic modification and activation of newly synthesized HIV proteins
   - Side effects may include abnormal fat distribution ("buffalo hump"), hyperlipidemia, diarrhea, gastrointestinal disturbances, paresthesia
4. Integrase Inhibitors (e.g., Elvitegravir, Raltegravir):
   - Inhibits the HIV integrase enzyme that is necessary for integration of HIV DNA into the host cell genome
   - Side effects may include nausea, diarrhea, headache
5. Entry Inhibitors (e.g., Maraviroc):
   - Blocks chemokine receptors (CCR5 protein) on the surface of CD4 cells that is used by HIV for attachment
   - Side effects may include nausea, diarrhea, fatigue, increased upper respiratory infections
6. Fusion Inhibitors (e.g., Enfuvirtide (T-20):
   - Inhibits gp41-mediated HIF fusion with the CD4 cell membrane
   - Side effects may include injection site reactions

HIV DRUG RESISTANCE

Emerging resistance of HIV to current drug therapies is a cause of great concern. The low fidelity of reverse transcriptase coupled with high rates of HIV replication and genetic recombination lead to the emergence of numerous HIV variants, many of which are resistant to currently used antiretroviral drugs. The problem of HIV drug resistance may be partially offset by using several antiretroviral drugs in combination with one another. These HIV drug "cocktails" are highly effective in reducing detectable levels of HIV and have become a mainstay of antiretroviral therapy. *Genotypic* and *phenotypic* testing of HIV viruses for specific drug resistance is also gaining widespread acceptance as a possible tool for aiding clinicians in choosing the best drug to treat a particular strain of HIV (see HIV Resistance Testing Box).

HIV DRUG RESISTANCE TESTING

Genotypic Resistance Testing:

- More than 100 drug-resistant HIV mutants have thus far been identified along with many of the specific genetic mutations that confer the resistance.
- Genotypic testing looks for one or more of these specific resistant mutations in a particular HIV.
- Testing is generally rapid and relatively simple but can only detect a single or a few mutations in any one virus and may not detect new mutations that have arisen.

Phenotypic Resistance Testing:

- Directly measures the ability of a particular HIV to grow in the presence of a specific drug or drugs.
- Can be a direct measure of drug susceptibility for a specific virus.
- Expensive and technically more difficult and time consuming than genotypic testing.

Index

Note: Page numbers in italic and bold refer to figures and tables respectively.

absolute refractory period (ARP) 19, *22*
absorption atelectasis 346
accessory digestive organs 357
ACE (angiotensin-converting enzyme)
         inhibitors 56, 154, 187
acetylcholine 212, 225
achalasia 385
acidosis 33, 148
acquired/conditioned reflex 364
ACTH (adrenocorticotropic hormone) 484
action potentials 17–20, *21–2*; conduction 20,
         22, *23*, 24–5; generation 17; graded
         potentials *versus* **16**
activation gate 18–19
active immunity 72
active transport 11
acute chest syndrome 124
acute coronary syndromes 248–50
acute pericarditis 234
acute respiratory distress syndrome (ARDS)
         348–9, **349**
AD *see* Alzheimer's disease (AD)
adaptive immune system 65–6; active *versus*
         passive immunity 72–4; antibodies
         see antibodies; clonal selection
         theory 70–1, *71*; MHC molecules
         77–8; primary *versus* secondary
         responses 71–2; T cells types and
         actions 74–5
Addison's disease 509–10
adenocarcinoma 331
adenohypophysis: ACTH 484; GH 485–6;
         gonadotropins 483–4; PRL 484–5;
         TSH 484
adenomatous polyps 398
ADH (antidiuretic hormone) 427, 479–81
adrenal androgens 495

adrenal cortex 491
adrenal glands: adrenal cortex 491; adrenal
         medulla 491; mineralocorticoid
         491–3
adrenal glands disorders: Addison's disease
         509–10; CAH 507–9; Cushing
         syndrome 510–12, *511*; physiologic
         effects **508**
adrenal medulla 491;
         pheochromocytoma 512
adrenal medullae 640
adrenergic receptors 634, 641
adrenocorticotropic hormone (ACTH) 484
ADS (anatomical dead space) 283, 300–1
adult respiratory distress syndrome
         (ARDS) 194
aerobic metabolic processes 281
afferent arteriole resistance 439
afferent arterioles 417
afferent division 561
afferent neuronal pathways 53–4
afferent neurons 561, *561*, *583*, 584–6, 591
affinity 635–6, 641
after-hyperpolarization 19
afterload 231, 250, 259
agglutination 69, 103
agonist 6, 34
agranulocytes 106
AIDS 721; *see also* human immunodeficiency
         virus (HIV)
airway obstruction 294–5
airway resistance 293–4; airway obstruction
         294–5; bronchial smooth muscle
         tone 295; lung volume 294
airways 282
alanine aminotransferase (ALT) 399
albumin 100

albuterol 34
alkalization 4
alkalosis 33
allergies and autoimmune diseases 60
alpha receptors 634–5
ALS *see* amyotrophic lateral sclerosis (ALS)
ALT (alanine aminotransferase) 399
alternative pathway 64
alveolar dead space 301, 308
alveolar ducts 283
alveolar pressure 287
alveolar ventilation 300–1, **301**
alveolar wall 282
alveoli 281
Alzheimer's disease (AD) 29; APP 611, 613;
        clinical manifestations 613–14;
        diagnosis 614; etiology 611, 613;
        treatment 614
amenorrhea 549
amine hormones 468–9
amphipathic molecules 3
amplification 474–5
AMP second-messenger system *473*
amyloid precursor protein (APP) 611
amyotrophic lateral sclerosis (ALS) 608;
        complications 617; diagnosis
        617; management 617; symptoms
        616–17
anaphylactic shock 191, **191**, *192*
anaphylaxis 78–80
anaplasia 718
anastomoses 247
anatomical dead space (ADS) 283, 300–1
androgenic 495
anemia 102, 312–13, *313*; blood loss 120–1;
        causes 119; classification **121**;
        feature 119; hemolytic 120;
        inherited 121–8
anesthesia: epidural 589–90; spinal 587
aneurysm: clinical manifestations 175–6;
        treatment 176; types *176*
angina 155
angina pectoris 247
angiotensin-converting enzyme (ACE)
        inhibitors 56, 154, 187
angiotensin II 150–1, 154, 262, 441–2
angiotensin receptor blockers (ARBs) 187
ankylosing spondylitis (AS) 707
annuli fibrosi 205
antagonism 471
antagonist 6, 34
anterior pituitary gland disorders
        499–502

anti-arrhythmic drugs 217–18, 244
antibiotic agents 73–4
antibiotics 73
antibodies 103; actions 68–70, *69*;
        classification 66; structure 67–8, *68*
antibody-mediated immunity 66
anticipatory adjustments 322
anticoagulant drugs **101**, 113, 179
anti-cyclic citrullinated peptide (ACPA) 704
antidiuretic hormone (ADH) 427, 479–81
antigenic drift 324
antigenic portion 72
antigens 5, 65, 102–4
antihistamines 80
antihypertensive drugs 153–4
anti-inflammatory drugs 337
anti-oncogenes 714
antiphospholipid syndrome 116
antiplatelet drugs **101**, 109
antipsychotic drugs 34
antipyretic 109
antrum 367, 534
aortic stenosis 242
aortic valve 205
aphasia 572
aplastic anemia 126–7
apolipoprotein 170
apoptosis 41, 528
APP (amyloid precursor protein) 611
aquaporins 9, 427
arachidonic acid 95
ARP (absolute refractory period) 19, *22*
arrhythmia 217, 239
arterial baroreceptors 53
arterial pressure, regulation: baroreceptors
        146–8; blood pressure **142**;
        cardiovascular principles **142**;
        chemoreceptors 148–9;
        hypertension 141; hypotension 141;
        low-pressure receptors 149–50;
        MAP 141–4; sympathetic system
        144–5; vasoconstrictors 150–4;
        vasodilators 154–5; vasomotor
        center 145–6
arteries 134–5; arterial disease 168–9;
        inflammatory disease 173–4
arterioles 135
arthus reaction 83
ascending tracts, spinal cord 586, *586*, **589**
ascites 403
aspartate aminotransferase (AST) 399
aspirin **101**, 109, 179
association tracts 564, 566

asthma 333, 474–5; and chronic bronchitis 295; clinical classification **336**; complications 335–6; manifestations 335; pharmacological treatment 296–7; staging **336**; treatment 336–7; triggers **333**
astrocytes 577–8
ataxia 576
atelectasis 346–7
atherosclerosis 246–7; familial dyslipidemias **171**; lipoprotein 169–71; risk factors for 169, **169**; steps 172
atopic asthma 333–5
atresia 535
atria 205–6, 217
atrial arrhythmia 270–1
atrial fibrillation 270–1, 599
atrial flutter 270
atrial natriuretic peptide (ANP) 155
atrial septal defects 246
atrial stretch receptors *see* low-pressure receptors
atrial tachycardia 270
atrioventricular (AV) valves 203–4; bundle 213
atrium 202, 219
atrophy 36–7
atypical pneumonia 328
autoimmune diseases 84, **85**; genetic factors 84; infection 84–5; sequestered antigens expression 85
autonomic nervous system (ANS) 208, 224, *225*; divisions 626–30, **627**, *628*; on effector tissues **637–8**; features **624**; functions 636–41, **637–8**; neurotransmission 630–3, **631**, *632*; pathways 625–6; receptors 633–6, **635**; regulation 624–5
autonomic reflexes 625
autoregulation 437
axon 20
axon hillock 20
axon terminal 20

bacteria 61
bacterial STDs 553
baroreceptors: aorta 146; carotid sinus 146; reflex 146–8, *147*, 159; stretch receptors 146
Barrett's esophagus *386*, 386–7
basal ganglia 572
basement membrane 136

basic electrical rhythm (BER) 378
basophils 62, 106
B cells (B lymphocytes) 62, 65, 107
benign neoplasm 712
benign prostatic hyperplasia (BPH) 541–3
BER (basic electrical rhythm) 378
berry aneurysm *176*
β_2-adrenergic receptor 153
β-blockers 186
bicarbonate ions 314–15
bicuspid valve 204
bile salt deficiency 397
bile secretion 375
bilirubin 374, 401
2,3-bisphosphoglycerate (2,3-BPG) 312
bisphosphonates 702
bladder cancer 461
blood: erythrocytes 101–4; hematopoiesis 100, 118–19; leukocytes 105–7; plasma 100–1; platelets 107–8; pooling 159; total blood volume 118; viscosity 139–40; volume 100, 157
blood-brain barrier 578–80
blood coagulation: activated factor X 111; anticoagulant drugs 113; clot dissolution 112; clot formation 112; coagulation pathways *110*; extrinsic pathway 111–12; fibrinogen into fibrin, conversion 111; hypercoagulability 116–17; intrinsic pathway 111–12; prevention 112–13; process 374; prothrombin into thrombin, conversion 111; tissue thromboplastin 111
blood doping 102
blood flow: active hyperemia 160; autoregulation 161; capillaries 163–4; hematocrit 140; Ohm's law 139; Poiseuille's law 141; pressure gradient 139; thermoregulation 133; tissues 133; vascular resistance 139; vessel radius 140
blood-gas interface 281
blood loss anemia 120–1
blood pressure: blood volume 157; centrally acting agents 187; disorders of 180–8; hypertension 180–7; hypotension 187–8; mean arterial pressure 137–8; pulse pressure 137
blood reservoirs *see* veins, disease

blood vessels 201; arteries 134; arterioles 135;
    basement membrane 136; chronic
    hypertension 184–5; diffusion
    136; direct-acting vasodilators
    187; disease of 168–80; elastic
    connective tissue 133; endothelium
    134; fibrous connective tissue 133;
    smooth muscle 134; stroke volume
    134; valves 137; vasodilation 134;
    veins 136–7; venules 136
B lymphocytes (B cells) 62, 65, 107
Bohr effect 312
bone mineral density (BMD) 702
bone resorption 699
bone tissue 698
Bowman's capsule 418
BPH (benign prostatic hyperplasia) 541–3
bradycardia 217
brain: adult brain structures **564**; association
    tracts 564, 566; basal ganglia 572;
    brainstem **565**; Broca's area 572;
    cerebellum **565**, 575–6; cerebrum
    564; commissural tracts 566;
    disorders *see* brain disorders;
    expressive aphasia 572; forebrain
    565; gray matter 564, *566*;
    hypothalamus 573–4; language
    processing 571; limbic multimodal
    association 570; lobes *see* lobes;
    medulla 574–5; multimodal
    sensory association 569; posterior
    multimodal association area 570;
    posterior parietal cortex 569;
    prefrontal multimodal association
    area 570; primary motor cortex
    571; projection tracts 564; receptive
    aphasia 572; somatosensory cortex
    569; thalamus 573; unimodal
    association area 569; white matter
    564, *566*
brain disorders: coma 598, **598**; increased
    intracranial pressure 596; injury
    593; intracranial hematoma 594–5,
    595; ischemia and hypoxia 597;
    traumatic injury 594
brain injury 593
brain ischemia and hypoxia 597
brainstem 563, **563**, **565**, 574
breast cancer: diagnosis 552; fibrocystic
    changes 551; mastitis 550;
    prognosis 552; proliferative
    changes 551; risk factors 551;
    treatment 552

breathing mechanics 284; expiration 285;
    inspiration 284–5; lung volume
    285–6; pulmonary pressures *286*,
    286–92; thoracic volume 284
Broca's area 572
bronchial asthma 296
bronchial smooth muscle tone 295
bronchiectasis *347*, 347–8
bronchiolar smooth muscle 308
bronchioles 282
bronchitis 337–8
bronchoconstriction 295
bronchodilation/bronchodilators
    295, 336–7
Brugada syndrome 267
Buerger's disease *see* thromboangiitis
    obliterans
bulbourethral glands 531
bundle branch block 273
Bundle of His 213

C3b protein 93, *93*
cachexia/lean tissue 406
calcification 698
calcitonin 489
calcium channel blockers 154, 187
calcium homeostasis 700
calcium levels 700
calcium release mechanism 207
calculus 699
cancer 711; hormonal therapy 719;
    immune-based therapy
    720; local effects 715;
    radiation therapy 720;
    systemic effects 716;
    treatment 719
cancer detection 717–19; biopsy 719; tumor
    cell markers 717; tumor grading
    718–19; visualization 719
capillary exchange: blood flow through
    163–4; bulk flow 164, 167;
    diffusion 164; edema formation
    167–8; filtration 164; lymphatic
    system 167; precapillary
    sphincter 164; reabsorption 164;
    Starling principle *165*, 165–6;
    transcytosis 164
caput medusae 405
carbaminohemoglobin 314
carbon dioxide, transport 314–15, *316*
carbonic anhydrase (CA) 315
carbon monoxide (CO) *313*, 313–14
cardiac action potentials *211*

cardiac arrhythmia 266; diagnosis 273, **274**; factors 267; heart block 272, 272–3; inherited arrhythmias 267; mechanisms 267–8, *268*; treatment 273–5; types 269–72

cardiac biomarkers **253**

cardiac cycle 218–19; ejection 221; events during **220**; isovolumetric contraction 219, 221; isovolumetric relaxation 221–2; ventricular filling 219

cardiac function curve 228, *229*

cardiac glycosides 232; and CO 232; and myocardial contractility 207

cardiac index 223

cardiac muscle cells 208; *versus* skeletal muscle 206, **206**

cardiac output (CO) 222–4; cardiac glycosides and 232; diuretics and 229–30; exercise effect on 232–3, **233**; heart rate 227–8

cardiac reserve 223

cardiac tamponade 234, *235*

cardiogenic shock 193–4, 491

cardiomyopathies 236; cardiac hypertrophy 237–8; dilated 236–7; hypertrophic 237; restrictive 239; treatment 239

cardiovascular system 201

carotid sinus 146

carrier molecules 5

cartilage 282–3

caseous necrosis 329

caspases 41

catabolism 493, 514

catecholamines 226–7

catechol-O-methyltransferase (COMT) 633

cauda equina 582

CD4 proteins 723

CD 39 113

celiac disease 397

cell(s): adaptive changes in 37; electrical signals 15–26; injury 35–47; membrane potential 11–15; plasma membrane 2–11; synaptic transmission 26–35

cell death: apoptosis 41; gangrene 41–3; necrotic 41

cell injury 35–6; causes **39**; cell death 41–3; cellular adaptation 36–8; manifestations 40–1; mechanisms 38–40; tissue repair 43–7

cell-mediated immunity 74

cell-to-cell attachment 6

cellular accumulations 41

cellular adaptation 36; atrophy 36–7; dysplasia 38; hyperplasia 38; hypertrophy 37; metaplasia 38

cellular necrosis, types 41, **42**

cellular swelling 40

central chemoreceptors 319

centrally acting drugs 576–7

central nervous system (CNS) 22, 53–4; brainstem 563, **563**; cerebrum and cerebral cortex 563, **563**; glial cells 577; infections *see* CNS infections; spinal cord 562–3, **563**; tumors *see* CNS tumors

centriacinar emphysema 340

cephalic phase 371–2, 376

cerebellum **565**, 575–6

cerebral cortex 322; electrical impulses transmission *568*

cerebrocerebellum 576

cerebrospinal fluid (CSF) 319, *566*, 580

cerebrum and cerebral cortex 563, **563**

cervical lesions and cancer 545

cervix 482

chemical receptors 5

chemical synapse mechanism 27, *27*

chemokine 97, 723

chemoreceptor response: to decreased arterial PO_2 319–20; to increase arterial PCO_2 320–1; increase in arterial hydrogen ion 321

chemoreceptors 148–9, 318–19, 360

chemotaxis 65, 70, 92

chemotherapy agents 719

chief cells 370

chloride reabsorption 427

chloride shift 315

cholecystokinin 376

cholesterol 4

cholinergic 630–1

cholinergic receptors 633

cholinomimetic drugs 639

chordae tendineae *204*, 204–5

christmas disease (type C hemophilia) 114

chronic bronchitis 295

chronic gastritis 388

chronic obstructive pulmonary disease (COPD) 337; bronchitis 337–8; emphysema 338–41

chronic venous insufficiency 180

chronotropic effect 224

chylomicron lipoprotein **170**

chyme 366, 369

cigarette smoking 326
circulatory system 52; acute exercise on
          161–3, **163**; arterial pressure,
          regulation 141–55; blood flow
          139–41, 160–1; blood pressure
          137–8, 180–8; blood vessels
          133–7, 168–80; capillary exchange
          163–8; functions 133; gravitational
          forces 159; resistance vessels 135;
          schematic diagram *135*; shock
          188–95; venous regulation 155–8
cirrhosis 403
cirrhosis alcoholic 403; treatment 405;
          types **404**
classical pathway 64
class II MHC glycoproteins 78
class I MHC glycoproteins 77
clonal selection theory 70–1, *71*
closed/spontaneous pneumothorax 346
Clostridium tetani 33
clot-dissolving drugs 179
CNS infections: diagnosis 602; encephalitis
          601; meningitis 601; symptoms 602;
          treatment 602
CNS tumors: diagnosis 604; manifestations
          603; treatment 604; type 603
coagulation *see* blood coagulation
cobalamin-deficiency anemia 120–1
cold shock 191
collapsing pressure 289, 291
colony stimulating factor (CSF) 698
colorectal cancer 398
coma 598, **598**
commissural tracts 566
common cold and rhinosinusitis 323–4
compensated heart failure 259
compensatory homeostatic mechanisms 54
complement system 64
complete AV block 273
complete blood count (CBC) **103**
compliance 288
compressions atelectasis 346
computed tomography (CT) 399
concentric hypertrophy 231
conditioned reflex 322
conducting airways 282
conduction, velocity 24, **24**
congenital adrenal hypoplasia (CAH):
          manifestations 508; treatment
          508–9
congenital heart defects 245, *245*; atrial/
          ventricular septal defects 246;
          patent ductus arteriosus 245–6

congestive heart failure 258
constipation 396–7
constrictive carditis 235
convergence 32
COPD *see* chronic obstructive pulmonary
          disease (COPD)
coronary artery bypass grafting (CABG) 256
coronary blood flow 246
cor pulmonale 338
corpus luteum 535, 538–9
cortical nephron 418
corticosteroids 95, 296, 494–5
corticotropin-releasing hormone (CRH) 494
Coxsackie B 235
creatinine 435
Crohn's disease (CD) 391, *392*
cromolyn sodium 337
crossed-extensor reflex 593
CSF *see* cerebrospinal fluid (CSF)
cushing syndrome *511*; diagnosis 510;
          manifestations 510–11; treatment
          511–12
cushing ulcers 389
cyclic adenosine monophosphate (cAMP) 472
cystic fibrosis 342; diagnosis 343;
          manifestations 342; treatment
          343–4
cystic fibrosis transmembrane conductance
          regulator (CFTCR) protein 342
cytokines 75, 335; actions **98**; interferons 97;
          interleukins 96
cytotoxic T cells 74–5, *76*

Dalton's Law 303
dawn phenomenon 516
dead space 301
decompensated heart failure 260
deep vein thrombosus (DVT) 177–8
deficient neurotransmitter, replacement 35
dementia complex 725
dendrite 20
denervated heart 226
denosumab 702
depolarization process 16–18
dermatome 581
descending tracts, spinal cord *586*, 587–8, **589**
desmosomes 208
diabetes insipidus 482, 502–3
diabetes mellitus: diabetic nephropathy
          520–1; diabetic neuropathy
          519–20; diabetic retinopathy 521;
          diagnosis and monitoring **520**;
          endocrine pancreas **513**, 513–14;

impaired healing 521; infections
risk 521–2; oral hypoglycemic
agents **519**; pregnancy 522; risk
factors **513**; tissue injury **520**; type 1
514–16; type 2 517, 518; vascular
disease 521
diabetic ketoacidosis (DKA) 515, **515**
diabetic nephropathy 520–1
diabetic neuropathy 519–20
diabetic retinopathy 521
diapedesis 92
diaphragm 284
diarrhea 396
diastasis phase 219
diastole phases 218, **218**, 227
diastolic failure 257
DIC (disseminated intravascular
coagulation) 117–18, 194
diffusion 7, 7–8, 302–4; ions 8; rate 7, **7**
digestive system 356, **362**; accessory
digestive organs 357;
gastrointestinal tract 357, 363
digestive tract 357; mucosa 357–8; muscularis
externa 358–9; serosa 359–60;
submucosa 358
digoxin 207
dilated cardiomyopathy 236–7
disease modifying anti-rheumatic
drugs 706
disorders, female reproductive system:
breast 550–2; menstrual cycle
549–50; ovaries 547–9; vagina,
cervix, and uterus 544–7
disorders, male reproductive system: penis
539–40; prostate 541–4; testis and
scrotum 540–1
disproportionate 568, 571
dissecting aneurysm 175–6, 176
disseminated intravascular coagulation
(DIC) 117–18, 194
distributive shock: symptoms 191; treatment
191, 193; types of **191**
diuretics 56, 186; and CO 229–30;
drug 153
diurnal 484, 486, 494
divergence 32–3
diverticular disease 395, 395
dorsal respiratory group (DRG) 317
dorsal root 582
down-regulation 488, 498
drug-induced hypoventilation 302
dry gangrene 41, 42, 43
dry mouth 365

ductus arteriosus 245
duodenum, chyme receptors 368
DVT (deep vein thrombosus) 177–8
dynamic equilibrium 7
dynamic exercise 231
dynamic steady state 51–2
dyslipidemias 170–2, **171**
dysmenorrhea 549
dysphagia, swallowing disorders 384
dysplasia 38
dyspnea 341, 344
dysrhythmia 266

eccentric hypertrophy 233
ECF (extracellular fluid) 2, 7, 319
ECG (electrocardiogram) 215–18, 216
echocardiography 234, 240
ectopic pacemakers 267–8
edema 80, 167–8, 303
effective rate of plasma flow (ERPF) 436
effector tissues 54
efferent arteriole 417
efferent division 561
efferent neuronal pathways 54
efferent neurons 561, 562, 583, 591
efflux 7
ejaculation 530
ejaculatory ducts 530
ejection 221
ejection fraction 230
elastic connective tissue 289
elastic recoil 288
electrical gradient 8
electrical signals by neurons 15;
action potentials 17–20;
conduction of action
potential 20, 22, 24–5;
graded potentials 15–17, **16**
electrocardiogram (ECG) 215–18, 216
embolism 179
emission 530
emphysema 338–41, 339, **341**
end-diastolic volume (EDV) 219
endocardium layer 205, 239; infectious
endocarditis 239–40; rheumatic
heart disease 240–1
endocrine disorders: adrenal glands
507–12, **508**, 511; adrenal
medulla 512; anterior pituitary
gland 499–502; hypothalamus/
pituitary glands 498–9; posterior
pituitary 502–3; thyroid function
503–7

endocrine system 54, 466; adenohypophysis 483–6; adrenal glands 491–5; diabetes *see* diabetes mellitus; disorders *see* endocrine disorders; hormones *see* hormones; negative feedback control 479, *480*; neurohypophysis 479–83; pancreas 495–8; parathyroid glands 489–90; pituitary gland *476*, 476–9, **478**; thyroid gland 486–9
endometrial cancer 546–7
endometriosis 545–6
endometrium 533, *536*, 538–9
endoplasmic reticulum 66, 71
endoscopy 719
endothelial cells **134**, 282
endothelin 151
endothelium 205, 246; physiological functions 134; TxA$_2$ 151–2
end-systolic volume (ESV) 221
endurance training effect 223, 232
enteric nervous system 360
enterogastric reflex 361, 368
enterohepatic circulation 375
enzymes 5, 639
eosinophils 62, 106
ependymal cells 578
epicardium layer 202, 205
epididymis 529–30
epidural anesthesia 589–90
epidural space 589–90
epinephrine 155, 295
epithelium 283–4
epoetin alfa 102
equilibrium potential 14
erectile dysfunction (ED) 531
erection 530–1
ERPF (effective rate of plasma flow) 436
erythema marginatum 241
erythroblastosis fetalis 104
erythrocytes 698; aged cells 102; analysis **103**; anemia based on **121**; antibodies 103; antigen types 102–3; average life span 102; erythropoietin 102; globin proteins 102; hematocrit 101; heme portion 102; hemoglobin 102; Rh factor 103–4; sedimentation rate **103**; shape 101; Sickle cell disease 121–4; thalassemia 125–8
erythrocyte sedimentation rate (ESR) 705
erythropoietin (EPO) 102, 118–19, 415, 698
esophageal cancer 398

esophageal diverticula 385
esophagus 366
estrogen 534–5, **536–8**, 550
excitatory postsynaptic potential (EPSP) 29–31
excitatory synapse 28–9
exocytosis process 27
exogenous pulmonary surfactants 292
expanding pressure 287
expiration, breathing mechanics 285
expiratory neurons 317
expiratory reserve volume (ERV) 297
expressive aphasia 572
external intercostal muscles 285
extracellular fluid (ECF) 2, 7, 319
extravasation 495
extrinsic autonomic nerves 361
eyes, chronic hypertension 185

facilitated diffusion 11
fallopian tubes 533
fatty liver 402
favism, G6PD 126
female reproductive system: disorders *see* disorders, female reproductive system; fallopian tubes 533; follicular phase 534–5; hormonal regulation, ovarian cycle 535–6, *536*; luteal phase 535, 538–9; ovaries 532; sex hormones **536–7**; uterus 533; vagina 533–4
ferritin 374
fertilization 528, 535
fever 98
fibrinogen 101
fibrinolysis 112
fibrinolytic drugs 179
fibrocystic changes 551
Fick's Law of Diffusion 136, 281, 306
"fight-or-flight" reaction 636, 640
first-degree heart block 272
fissure 566
flutamide 719
flux 7
foam cells 172
folate-deficiency anemia 120–1
follicles 486
follicle-stimulating hormone (FSH) 483–4
follicular phase 534–5
foramen magnum 581
forebrain **565**
Frank-Starling Law of the Heart 228
Frank-Starling mechanism 208

Frank-Starling principle graph *261*
free radical injury 38–40
FSH (follicle-stimulating hormone) 483–4
F-type sodium channels 210
functio laesa 89
functional residual capacity (FRC) 298
fundus 366

galactopoeisis 484
gallbladder 375–6; cholecystitis 407;
        disorders 406
gametes 483, 528
gametogenesis 528
gamma amino butyric acid (GABA) 34–5
gamma globulins 66
ganglion 586
gangrene 41, *42*, 43
gap junctions 208, **624**, 626
gas exchange 281
gas transport 309; carbon dioxide, transport
        314–15, *316*; oxygen, transport
        309–14
gastric phase 372, 376
gastrin 371
gastritis 387
gastroesophageal reflux disease (GERD)
        6, 385
gastroileal reflex 361
gastrointestinal hormones 361
gastrointestinal motility 359
gastrointestinal sphincters 359
gastrointestinal tract 52, 357
genital herpes 554
genitalia 529, 554
gestational diabetes 522
gestational hypertension **184**
GFR (glomerular filtration rate) 419–21
GH *see* growth hormone (GH)
GHIH (growth hormone-inhibiting
        hormone) 486
Ghon focus 329
Ghon's complex 329
GHRH (growth hormone-releasing
        hormone) 486
giant cell temporal arteritis 174
glial cells in CNS: astrocytes 577–8;
        ependymal cells 578; microglia
        578; oligodendrocytes 578
globin proteins 102
globulins 100–1
glomerular capillary pressure (P_{GC}) 421
glomerular filtration rate (GFR) 419–21
glomerulus 428

glucagon 497–8
glucocorticoids 94, 493–4
gluconeogenesis 493, 497, 516
glucose-6-phosphate dehydrogenase (G6PD)
        deficiency 126
glucose-dependent insulinotropic peptide
        (GIP) 368
glycogenesis 496
glycogenolysis 497
gonad 467, 483
gonadotropins 483–4
goodpasture disease 80
gout 709–10
G protein 472
graafian follicle 534
graded potentials 15–17
granulation tissue 46
granulocytes 105
granulomatous inflammation 391
granulosa cells 534–5
granzymes 75
Graves' disease 80, 82
gray matter 583–5
great imitator 706
growth factors 711
growth hormone (GH) 485–6; gigantism and
        acromegaly 500–1; hypersecretion
        501–2; hyposecretion 499–500;
        manifestation 500; measurement
        499; treatment 500
growth hormone-inhibiting hormone
        (GHIH) 486
growth hormone-releasing hormone
        (GHRH) 486
guanosine triphosphate (GTP) 472
gyrus 566, 568, 571

half-life 469
Hashimoto's thyroiditis 505
HDL (high density lipoprotein) 170, **170, 171**
headache 607–8
heart 199–202; autonomic nerves effects on
        225; blood flow through *203*; body
        temperature 227; cardiac cycle
        218–22; chronic hypertension 185;
        CO 222–4, **223**; diseases 233–46;
        ECG 215–18, *216*; ejection fraction
        230; electrical activity 209–15;
        excitation/conduction in *213*;
        fibrous skeleton 212; functional
        anatomy 202–9; heart rate control
        224–7, **226**, 231–2; myocardium 228;
        SV control 227–32

heart block condition *272*, 272–3
heart failure 232, 256; circulatory
　　　　disturbances in *257*; classification
　　　　256–7; diagnosis 264–5; left 257–8,
　　　　258; physiologic compensation for
　　　　259–64, *261*; rationale for treatment
　　　　265–6; right 258–9, *260*
heart valves disorders 241–2; congenital
　　　　heart defects 245–6; mitral valve
　　　　prolapse 243–5; treatment 244
helper T-cells 74–5, **77**
hemagglutinin protein 324
hematocrit 101, **103**, 140
hematopoiesis 100, 118–19
heme protein 119
hemocytoblasts 698
hemoglobin 102; molecule 309–10
hemolysis 103, 120, 124
hemolytic anemia 120, 126
hemophilia 114
hemopoiesis 698
hemostasis: alterations in 114–18; antiplatelet
　　　　drugs 109; blood coagulation
　　　　110–12; drug-induced alterations in
　　　　116; platelet plug, formation 108–9;
　　　　vascular constriction 108
heparin 101, 106, 113, 179
hepatic encephalopathy 405
hepatitis alcoholic 403
Hepatitis A Virus (HAV) 400
Hepatitis B Virus (HBV) 400
Hepatitis C Virus (HCV) 400
Hepatitis D Virus (HDV) 401
Hepatitis E Virus (HEV) 401
hepatobiliary disorders 398–9
hepatoma 712
hepatorenal syndrome 404
hepatosplenomegaly 403
hereditary 715
Hering-Breuer reflex 318
heterotopic ossification 699
high density lipoprotein (HDL) 170, **170**, **171**
Hirschsprung disease 396
histamine 95, 106, 371
HIV *see* human immunodeficiency virus (HIV)
homeostasis 51–4; functions of drugs 56;
　　　　negative feedback 54–5, *55*; organ
　　　　systems to **52**; positive feedback
　　　　55–6
homeostatic state 698
horizontal osmotic gradient 430
hormonal regulation, ovarian cycle
　　　　535–6, *536*

hormone action: gene activation 475;
　　　　hormone-receptor complex 475;
　　　　HRE 475; second-messenger
　　　　systems 472, *473*; signal
　　　　transduction 472
hormone response elements (HRE) 475
hormones: biochemical categories
　　　　467–9; hypothalamus **467**;
　　　　interactions 471; mechanisms
　　　　471–5; nontrophic 470; target
　　　　tissues 467; transport 469;
　　　　trophic 470
HPV (human papillomavirus) 553–4
HRE (hormone response elements) 475
human immunodeficiency virus (HIV)
　　　　721–2; acute illness stage
　　　　725; asymptomatic stage 725;
　　　　epidemiology 726; inner protein
　　　　core 722; intergrase 722; laboratory
　　　　726–7; lifecycle 722–4, *724*; protease
　　　　722; rationale for treatment 727;
　　　　stages 725–6; structure *722*,
　　　　722–4; symptomatic stage 725–6;
　　　　treatment 727
human papillomavirus (HPV) 553–4
Huntington's disease: diagnosis 616;
　　　　manifestations 615–16;
　　　　treatment 616
hyaluronic acid 709
hydrocephalus 596
hydrochloric acid (HCl) 370
hydrogen ions secretion 434
hydronephrosis 459
hydrophilic 3, 6
hydrophobic fatty acid chains 3
hydrostatic pressure 9, 159
hydroureter 459
hydroxyapatite crystals 699
hydroxyurea drug 126
hypercalcemia 489
hypercapnia 148
hypercapnic failure 351
hypercoagulability 116–17
hyperemia, active 160
hyperglycemia 516
Hyperglycemic-Hyperosmolar-Nonketotic
　　　　Syndrome (HHNKS) **518**
hyperkinesias 573
hyperplasia 38
hyperpolarization process 16, 29
hypersensitivity reactions 78; type I 78, 80, *81*;
　　　　type II 80, 82, *82*; type III 83;
　　　　type IV 83, *84*

hypertension 141, 153; cardiovascular disease 181; CDC estimation 180; chronic **184**, 184–5; diagnosis 185; isolated systolic hypertension 181; JNC 8 report **186**; malignant 183; in pregnancy 183–4; prehypertension 180–1; primary 181–2; secondary 182; treatment 185–7

hyperthyroidism: Graves' disease 506; manifestations 506; thyroid storm 506–7; treatment 507

hypertrophic cardiomyopathy 237

hypertrophy 37, 485, 490, 504–5

hypoglycemia 516

hypokinesia 573

hypopituitarism 499

hypotension 141, 187–8

hypothalamus **467**, 478, **478**, 573–4

hypothyroidism 488; congenital 505; Hashimoto's thyroiditis 505; manifestations 505; treatment 506

hypotonia 576

hypovolemic shock: baroreceptors 189; causes 188–9; stages 190; treatment 190–1

hypoxemia 148, 308, 312, 319

hypoxemic failure 351

hypoxia 33, 319

hypoxic cell injury 40

IBD *see* inflammatory bowel disease (IBD)

IBS (irritable bowel syndrome) 390

ICF (intracellular fluid) 2, 7

idiopathic 234

ileogastric reflex 361

immune function: alterations in 78–85; overview 59–78

immune reactions 6

immune responses 62

immune surveillance 60

immune system 59–85, 283–4; adaptive 65–78; effector cells 62; innate 63–5; types 62

immune thrombocytopenia purpura 116

immunity 59

immunoglobulins 66

implantable cardioverter-defibrillator (ICD) 275

implantable pacemakers 275

implantation 533, 535

impotence 540

incentive spirometer 291

incompetent/regurgitant valves 242

increased intracranial pressure (ICP) 596

infant respiratory distress syndrome 291–2

infectious disease, agents 60–1

infectious endocarditis 239–40

inferior vena cava 202

inflammatory bowel disease (IBD) 390–1; diagnosis 394; systemic manifestations 394–5

inflammatory disease of arteries 173–5

inflammatory mediators: chemokines 97; cytokines 96–7; fever 98; leukotrienes 95; nitric oxide 98; prostaglandins 95

inflammatory response: anti-inflammatory drugs 94; chemotaxis 92; diapedesis 92; increased capillary permeability 91; localized edema 91; macrophages 91; margination 92; opsonization 92–3, *93*; phagocytes, infiltration 91; phagocytosis 93; purpose 89; steps *90*; symptoms 89; vasodilation 91

inflammatory stage 44–6

influenza pneumonia 326

influenza virus 324; structure *325*; symptoms 325–6; treatment 326, **326**

influx 7

inherited anemia: sickle cell disease 121–4; thalassemia 125–8

inherited arrhythmias 267

inhibitory postsynaptic potential (IPSP) 29

inhibitory synapse 29

innate immune system 63–5

inspiration, breathing mechanics 284–5

inspiratory capacity (IC) 298–9

inspiratory neurons 317

inspiratory reserve volume (IRV) 297–8

insulin 496–7

insulin therapy 516

intention tremors 576

interatrial conduction pathway 212

intercalated discs 208

interdependence 293

interferons 63–4, 97, **98**

interleukins 96, **98**

intermediate density lipoprotein (IDL) **170**

internal environment 51–2

interneurons *561*, 562, 585, *591*, 592–3

internodal conduction pathway 212

interstitial cells of Cajal (ICC) 358

interstitial lung diseases 350–1, **351**

interstitial tissue 529

interstitium 282

interventricular septum 212–13
intestino-intestinal reflex 361
intracellular fluid (ICF) 2, 7
intracranial hematoma 594–5, *595*
intranasal 482
intrapleural pressure 287
intratract reflexes 361
intravenous solutions 9–10
intrinsic asthma 333
inulin 435
ipratropium 296
iron-deficiency anemia 120
irritable bowel syndrome (IBS) 390
irritant receptors 318
isolated systolic hypertension 181
isovolumetric contraction process 219, 221
isovolumetric relaxation 221–2
ivacaftor drug 344

jaundice 124, 401
juxtamedullary nephron 418

kaposi sarcoma 725
keloid scars 46
kidney and urinary tract, disorders 448; acute glomerulonephritis 449; Berger's disease 449–50; IgA nephropathy 449–50; nephrotic syndrome 450–1; pyelonephritis 451; renal function evaluation 448; stones 452–3; tumors 453; urinary tract infections 451–2
kidneys: chronic hypertension 185; enzymes 415; functional anatomy 415–17; renal system 413; tubular component 418; vascular component 417
Kupffer cells 373

lactase deficiency 397
lactogenesis 484
lamina propria 357–8
large cell lung carcinoma 332
large intestine 382–3; GERD 384–7; motility 383–4; secretion 384
larvacidal 106
laryngeal cancer 331
LDL (low density lipoprotein) **170**, 170–2, **171**
lectin pathway 64
left circumflex artery 250
left-heart failure 257–8, *258*
left-ventricular assist devices 266

left-ventricular end-diastolic volume (LVEDV) 260
leiden mutation 116
LES (lower esophageal sphincter) 358
leukocytes 62; agranulocytes 106; basophils 106; eosinophils 106; granulocytes 105; inflammatory/immune functions 105; lymphocytes 107; macrophage 107; monocytes 106–7; neutrophils 105–6; WBC differential count **103**
leukopoiesis 699
leukotrienes 95; modifiers 337
levodopa (L-dopa) 35
leydig cell 529, 531
LH (luteinizing hormone) 483–4
limbic multimodal association 570
lingual lipase 364
lipid bilayer 3
lipid envelope 722
lipid solubility and drug elimination 4
lipid-soluble substances 164
lipogenesis 486, 496
lipolysis 493, 497
lipophilic 3
lipoprotein: apolipoprotein 170; and functions **170**; structure *169*
liver 373–5
liver cancer 405–6
liver disease 115
lobar bronchi branch 282
lobes: cerebral cortex **567**, *567*; frontal 567–8; functions **567**; occipital 568; parietal 568; temporal 568
local anesthetics 26
local current flow 17
long QT syndrome (LQTS) 267
Loop of Henle 418; ascending limb 430; descending limb 429; proximal tubule and 426
low density lipoprotein (LDL) **170**, 170–2, **171**
lower esophageal sphincter (LES) 358
low-pressure receptors 149–50
LQTS (long QT syndrome) 267
lung cancer 331–2
lung volume 294; airway resistance 294; breathing mechanics 285–6
luteal phase 535
luteinization 538
luteinizing hormone (LH) 483–4
lymphatic system 167
lymphocytes 62, 65–6, 107
lysozyme 364

macrophages 107, 172
mad cow disease 602
malabsorption 397
male reproductive system: bulbourethral
        glands 531; disorders *see* disorders,
        male reproductive system;
        ED 531; ejaculatory ducts 530;
        epididymides 529–30; penis 530;
        prostate 530; seminal vesicles 530;
        testes 529; testosterone **532**; vas
        deferens 530
malignant hypertension 183
malignant neoplasm 712
malignant tumor cell 713
Mallory-Weiss Syndrome 385
mammogenesis 484
mannose-binding lectin (MBL) 64
MAP *see* mean arterial pressure (MAP)
Marfan's syndrome 175
mass sympathetic discharge 629
mast cells 91, 95; allergic reactions 106
mastication 363
mastitis 550
matrix 698
maturation and remodeling stage 44–6
mean arterial pressure (MAP) 423; arterial
        pressure, regulation 141–4; blood
        pressure 137–8
mean corpuscular hemoglobin concentration
        (MCHC) **103**
mean corpuscular volume (MCV) **103**
mechanoreceptors 360, 368
mediated transport process 10;
        characteristics 10–11; forms 11
medulla 574–5
medullary respiratory center 315, 317–18
megakaryocytes 107, 698
meiosis 528
membrane attack complex (MAC) 64
membrane fluidity 4
membrane potential 11–12; *see also* plasma
        membrane; changes in *16*; resting
        12, 12–15, *13*
menopause 550
menstrual disorders 549–50
menstruation 535, 539, 546, 549–50
mesentery 360
metabolic acidosis 321
metabolic processes 374
metabolic syndrome 182
metabolic vasodilation 162
metaplasia 38
metastasis 713

metastasize 712
MHC molecules 77–8
microbe components 72
microglia 578
mineral deposition 699
mineralization 698–9
mineralocorticoid 491–3
mineral resorption 699
miosis 639
mitosis 528
mitral stenosis 242
mitral valve 204
mitral valve prolapse 243; heart valve
        disease treatment 244–5;
        manifestations 244; valvular heart
        disease, diagnosis 243
mitral valvotomy 244
mixed venous blood 306–7, 311
Mobitz II 272
Mobitz I/Wenckebach 272
modified postganglionic neurons 629
monoamine oxidase (MAO) 633
monoclonal antibodies 719
monocytes 62, 106–7
motor cortex 322
mouth 363–4
mucociliary escalator 283
mucosa 357–8
mucus 366, 370
mucus glands 283
multidrug-resistant TB (MDR-TB) 331
multimodal sensory association 569
multiple organ dysfunction syndrome
        (MODS) 194
multiple sclerosis (MS) 25, 617–18
muscarinic receptor antagonist 640
muscarinic receptors 634
muscular activity 359
muscularis externa 358–9
Mycobacterium tuberculosis 329
mydriasis 639–40
myelin 22, 25
myocardial infarction 250; clinical
        manifestations 252; compensatory
        mechanisms for 252–3;
        complications 254; coronary blood
        flow and 250–2; rationale for
        therapy 254–6; treatment for 255–6
myocardial ischemia 246–7; acute coronary
        syndromes 248–50; diagnosis **248**;
        manifestations 247–8; rational for
        treatment 248; treatment 249–50
myocardial oxygen balance *253*

myocardial wall 205–9
myocardium 205, 228; cardiomyopathies
236–9; contractility 230; diseases
235; myocarditis 235–6
myogenic 161, 208, 212, 437
myometrium 533

naïve lymphocyte 70, *71*
natural killer (NK) cells 62, 64, 70
nausea 364
nebulizer 296, 336
necrotic 107
necrotic cell death 41
negative chronotropic effect 224
negative feedback 54–5, *55*
negative feedback control 479, *480*
negative inotropic effect 230
neonate 292
neoplasm 712
nervous system 52; blood-brain barrier 578–80;
brain *see* brain; cerebrospinal
fluid 580; CNS *see* central nervous
system (CNS); components 53, *53*;
disorders *see* nervous system
disorders; integrative portion
53–4; motor division 54; neurons
561–2; PNS *see* peripheral nervous
system (PNS)
nervous system disorders: brain 593–8; CNS
infections 600–2; CNS tumors
602–4; degenerative disorders
608–18, *610*; headache 607–8;
seizure 604–7; spinal injury 618–19;
stroke 598–600, **599**
net diffusion 7
neuraminidase protein 324
neurodegenerative diseases: AD 611–14;
ALS 616–17; Huntington's disease
615–16; MS 617–18; Parkinson's
disease 608–10, *610*
neurogenic 208
neurogenic bladder 460
neurogenic shock **191**
neurohypophysis: antidiuretic hormone
479–81; oxytocin 482–3
neurologic manifestations 725
neurons 33; afferent 561, *561*; axon 20; axon
hillock 20; axon terminal 20;
cell body 20; convergence 32;
divergence 32–3; efferent *561*, 562;
functions 15; interconnections
between 32–3; interneurons
561, 562

neurosecretory cells *476*, 477–9, 481
neurotransmission: autonomic nerve
pathways *632*; catecholamines 630;
EPI 630; features **631**; hormones
630; MAO and COMT 633;
mechanism 631
neurotransmitter 26–7; altered release
33–4; deficient 35; interaction
with receptor 34–5; molecules 28;
removal from synaptic cleft 35
neutralization 69, 376
neutrophilia 105
neutrophils 62, 105–6
New York Heart Association (NYHA)
functional 264, **264**
nicotinic receptors 633–4
nitroglycerin 155
NK (natural killer) cells 62, 64, 70
nodes of Ranvier 24
nonciliated cuboidal epithelial cells 284
non-small cell lung cancer 331–2
nonsteroidal anti-inflammatory drugs
(NSAIDs) 94, **101**
nontrophic hormone 470
norepinephrine 212
nutrients categories 368–9

OA *see* osteoarthritis (OA)
obstructive disorders 322
obstructive pulmonary disorders 332;
asthma 333–7
oligodendrocytes 578
oncogenesis 714
oogenesis 528
open/communicating pneumothorax 345
opsonization *69*, 70, *82*, 92–3, *93*
oral contraceptives 539
orthopnea 257–8
orthostatic hypotension 187
osmoreceptors 360; stimulation 369
osmosis 9
osmotic pressure 9–10
osmotic regulator 100
osseous tissue 698
osteitis deformans 702–3
osteoarthritis (OA) 707–9; manifestations
707; risk factors 707;
treatment 709
osteoblasts 485, 489, 699, 701
osteoclasts 489–90, 701
osteomalacia 703, *703*
osteoporosis 697, 701, **701**, 702
ovarian cancer 548–9

ovarian cycle regulation: follicular phase 535, 538; hormone levels/changes, correlation *536*; luteal phase 538–9; sex hormones **536–7**
ovarian follicle 528
ovaries 532
ovaries disorders: ovarian cancer 548–9; polycystic ovary syndrome 547
ovulation 535, 538
ovum 482–3
oxygen, transport: 2,3-BPG 312; anemia 312–13, *313*; in blood 309; CO *313*, 313–14; PCO_2, pH and temperature 312
oxyhemoglobin dissociation curve 310, *311*
oxyntic gland area 369
oxytocin 482–3

pacemaker potential 210
Paget's disease 702–3
pain receptors 318
panacinar emphysema 340, *341*
pancreas 376; cancer 408; clinical manifestations 409; disorders 407; glucagon 497–8; insulin 496–7; islets of Langerhans 496
pancreatic juice 376
pancreatitis **408**
papillary muscles *204*, 204–5
para-aminohippuric acid (PAH) 436
paraneoplastic syndrome 332
parasympathetic innervation 361
parasympathetic nervous system 295
parasympathetic stimulation 212, 225, 375
parasympathetic system *628*; features **627**; preganglionic neurons 629; resting conditions 639
parathyroid glands 489–90
Parkinson's disease 35; clinical manifestations 609; diagnosis 609; etiology *610*; treatment 609–10
paroxysmal atrial tachycardia 270
partial pressure of carbon dioxide (PCO_2) 304, **304**, *305*; alveolar process 305; arterial blood 306; chemoreceptors to increase arterial 320–1; mixed venous blood 306–7; venous blood leaving 306
partial pressure of oxygen (PO_2) 303, **304**, *305*; alveolar gas 305; arterial 313; blood 306, 310;

chemoreceptors to decreased arterial 319–20; in conducting airways 304; mixed venous blood 306–7; venous blood leaving 306
parturition 483, 533
passive diffusion 7
passive immunity 73
patent ductus arteriosus 245–6
pathophysiology 56
PCI (percutaneous coronary intervention) 256
PCR (polymerase chain reaction) 727
PCSK9 inhibitors 699
penis 530
penis disorders: impotence 540; peyronie's disease 539; priapism 539
peplomers 722, *723*
pepsinogen 370
peptic ulcer 388
percutaneous coronary intervention (PCI) 256
perforin molecules 70, 75
perfusion 164, 188, 190
pericardial effusion 234
pericardial fluid 202
pericardial friction rub 234
pericardiocentesis 235
pericardium 202
pericardium, disorders 233; acute pericarditis 234; constrictive carditis 235; pericardial effusion 234; treatment 235
perimetrium 533
peripheral chemoreceptors 318–19
peripheral nervous system (PNS) 22, 560, 578, 582
peristalsis 359, 367
peritoneum 359
peritubular capillaries 417, 433
permeability barrier 2
permissiveness 471
pernicious anemia 371
peyronie's disease 539
phagocytosis 62–3, 93, 106
pharyngeal stage 365
pharyngitis 324
pharynx 365
phenobarbital 4
pheochromocytoma 512
phospholipids molecules 3
phrenic nerve 284–5, 317
physiological dead space 301
physiology 51

pituitary gland: adenohypophysis *476*, 477; and hypothalamus *476*, 477–9; neurohypophysis *476*, 477
placenta 533
plasma 428; albumin 100; antiplatelet and anticoagulant drugs **101**; fibrinogen 101; globulins 100–1
plasma clearance 434–6
plasma colloid osmotic pressure 100, 165, *422*, *422*
plasma membrane 2; carbohydrate 5; cellular functions 5; components 2; mechanisms by 7; structure and function 2–6, *3*; transport 6–11
plasma osmolarity 415
plasmin 112
plasminogen 112
platelets 107–8; antiphospholipid syndrome 116; immune thrombocytopenia purpura 116; plug 108–9; thrombocytopenia 115
pleura 284, 344
pleural cavity 288, 344
pleural effusion 344
pleuritis 344
pneumonia 327; atypical 328; community acquired 327; hospital/healthcare acquired 327; in immunocompromised patients 328; risk for **327**; treatment 329; typical 327–8
pneumothorax 288, 336, 344; closed/spontaneous 346; manifestations 346; open/communicating 345; tension 345; treatment 346; types *345*
PNS *see* peripheral nervous system (PNS)
polyarteritis nodosa 174
polyclonal 73
polycystic kidney disease 454
polycystic ovary syndrome 547
polycythemia 127–8
polydipsia 515
polymerase chain reaction (PCR) 727
polymorphonuclear leukocytes (PMNs) *see* neutrophils
polyphagia 515
polyuria 515
portal hypertension 405
portal vein *476*, 478–9, 496
positive chronotropic effect 224
positive feedback 55–6
positive inotropic effect 230

posterior multimodal association area 570
posterior parietal cortex 569
postmenopausal osteoporosis *489*
postural hypotension *see* orthostatic hypotension
potassium ions secretion 434
potent 492, 494
precapillary sphincter 164
predisposing factors 239
preeclampsia **184**
prefrontal multimodal association area 570
preganglionic neuron 625
pregnancy, hypertension in 183–4
prehypertension 180–1
pre-infarct angina 247
preload 228
premature atrial contractions 270
premature beats/extrasystole 270
priapism 539
primary capillary plexus 478–9
primary headache 607–8
primary motor cortex 571
primary oocytes 528
procainamide 218
progesterone 535, **537**, 538
prognosis 552
projection tracts 564
prolactin (PRL) 484–5
prolactin-releasing factor (PRF) 485
proliferative changes 551
proliferative stage 44–6
prolific 71
proprioceptors 318, 322
prostacyclin 154
prostaglandins 95, 442
prostate 530
prostate cancer 543–4
prostate disorders: BPH 541–3; prostatitis 541
prostatitis 541
protease 713
protein/peptide hormones 468
proteins 4–5
protein shell 722
proteinuria 168, **184**
proteolysis 513
proton pump 370
proto-oncogenes 714
proximal tubule 418, 428
puberty 528
pulmonary capillaries 281
pulmonary compliance 288
pulmonary pressures *286*, 286–92
pulmonary stretch receptors 318

pulmonary surfactant 290
pulmonary valve 205
pulmonary vascular smooth muscle 308
pulsatile 137–8
pulse pressure (PP) 137
pulsus paradoxus 234
Purkinje fibers 214
P wave 216, *216*
pyloric gland area 369
pyloric sphincter 366
pyrogenic 98

QRS complex *216*, 216–17
quantum 28

RA (rheumatoid arthritis) *704*, 704–6
Raynaud's disease 174–5
RBCs (red blood cells) 698
RBF *see* renal blood flow (RBF)
receptive aphasia 572
receptive relaxation 367
receptor agonist 6
receptors 6; adrenergic 634; Alpha 634–5;
        Beta 635–6; cholinergic 633;
        G proteins 633
red blood cells (RBCs) 698; *see also*
        erythrocytes
reentry impulses 268
relative refractory period (RRP) 19, *22*
renal blood flow (RBF) 422–3, 436–7;
        afferent arteriole resistance
        439; angiotensin II 441–2;
        autoregulation 437; myogenic
        mechanism 437; prostaglandins
        442; sympathetic nerves 439–40;
        tubuloglomerular feedback 438–9
renal system 52, 413; chronic failure
        455–6, **457**; failure 454–5; foreign
        compounds 415; GFR 419;
        hemodialysis 458–9; kidneys 414;
        nephron 419; vicious cycle 458
renin-angiotensin system, activation 262
repolarization 16
reproductive system: female reproductive
        system 532–9, *536*, **536–7**;
        gametogenesis 528; male
        reproductive system 529–31, **532**
reservoir 469
residual volume (RV) 297
resistance exercise 231
resorption 489–90
respiratory bronchioles 283
respiratory disease 322, **323**, **334**

respiratory distress syndrome in newborn
        349–50
respiratory failure 351–2, **352**
respiratory infections 323; lower respiratory
        tract 326–31; upper respiratory
        tract 323–6
respiratory system 52, 281, 415; airway
        resistance 293–7; airways
        282–4; blood-gas interface 281–2;
        breathing mechanics 284–92;
        defenses **323**; disorders 322–52;
        interdependence 293; the pleura
        284; ventilation 297–302
respiratory zone 283
resting membrane potential **12**, 12–15, *13*, 210
restrictive cardiomyopathy 239
restrictive disorders 322
restrictive pulmonary disorders 332, 344–8
reticular formation 575
retropropulsion 367
retroviruses 722
reverse transcriptase 722
rheumatic heart disease 240–1
rheumatoid arthritis (RA) *704*, 704–6
rheumatoid factors 704–5
Rh factor 103–4
rhinitis 324
rhinosinusitis 323–4
rickets 703
right coronary artery 250
right-heart failure 258–9, *260*
Rosenthal's disease (type C hemophilia) 114
RRP (relative refractory period) 19, *22*

salivary glands 363–4
saltatory conduction 24, *24*
SA (sinoatrial) node 208, 210, 224
saturation 10
scar tissue 234
scopolamine 365
scrotum 529, 540–1
secondary capillary plexus 478–9
secondary headache 608
second-degree heart block 272
secretin 375
seed crystals 699
seizure disorders: diagnosis 606; epilepsy
        604; focal 604–5; generalized
        605–6; treatment 607; type 604
seizures 20
self-antigens 77–8
semen 530
semilunar valves 205

seminal vesicles 530
seminiferous tubules 529
semipermeable barrier 3
semipermeable membrane 9
sensory receptors 53
septic shock 191, **191**, *192*
septum 237
serosa 359–60
serous fluid 233, 344
sertoli cells 528–9, **532**
serum sickness 83
sexually transmitted diseases (STDs) 552;
        see also human immunodeficiency
        virus (HIV); bacterial 553;
        diagnosis 553, 555; long-term
        consequences 555; risk factors 553;
        treatment 555; trichomoniasis 555;
        viral 554
shock: cardiogenic 193–4; complications 194;
        distributive 191–3; hypovolemic
        188–91
shunt 307, *307*
sickle cell disease *122*; deoxygenation
        123; heterozygous form 121;
        homozygous form 121; and
        malaria 124; manifestations 124;
        mutation in 122
silent ischemia 248
simple/unconditioned reflex 364
single-unit smooth muscle 358
sinoatrial (SA) node 208, 210, 224
sinusitis 324
sinus node arrhythmia 270
skeletal muscle cells 208; *versus* cardiac
        muscle 206, **206**; pump 158–9
skeletal system 697
SLE *see* systemic lupus erythematosus (SLE)
slow-wave potentials 358
small cell lung cancer 332
small intestine 377; carbohydrates 378,
        380; digestion and absorption
        378; digestive enzymes **379**;
        motility 378
smooth muscle 134; precapillary
        sphincter 164
sodium 229
sodium excretion, control 443–5
sodium reabsorption 425–7
solubility product 699
somatic nervous system **624**
somatomedins 485
somatosensory cortex 568
Somogyi effect 516

spatial summation 30–1, *32*
sperm 482–3
spermatocele 540
spermatogenesis 528
spermatozoa 528–30
Sphincter of Oddi 375, 377
spinal anesthesia 587
spinal cord 562–3, **563**, *583*; anesthesia 587;
        ascending tracts 586, *586*, **589**;
        cervical and thoracic level 581;
        dermatome 581; descending
        tracts *586*, 587–8, **589**; dorsal root
        582; epidural anesthesia 589–90;
        foramen magnum 581; gray matter
        583–5; lumbar and sacral region
        581; spinal reflexes 590–3; ventral
        root 582; vertebral magnum 581;
        white matter 585–6
spinal injury 619
spinal reflexes 590; crossed-extensor reflex
        593; reflex arcs *591*; withdrawal
        reflex 591–3, *592*
spinocerebellum 576
splenomegaly 124
squamous cell carcinoma 332
standard lung volumes/capacities 297–300,
        298, **299**
Starling principle *165*, 165–6
STDs *see* sexually transmitted diseases
        (STDs)
steatorrhea 397
steatosis alcoholic 402
stem cell 118
stenosis 242
steroid hormones 468
Stokes-Adams syndrome 273
stomach cancer 398
stratified squamous epithelium 363
stretch receptors 146
strokes 598–9; complications 600; diagnosis
        600; occlusive 599; risk factors
        599; symptoms 599–600;
        TIAs/"mini-strokes" 599;
        treatment 600
stroke volume (SV) control 227–32
subcutaneous nodules 241
submucosa 358
summation 30–2
superior vena cava 202
suppressor T cells 74
suprathreshold stimulus 17
supraventricular tachycardia 217
surface tension (ST) 289

surfactant 290–1
surgical removal 719
sutures 44
sweat chloride test 343
sympathetic collateral ganglia 629
sympathetic innervation 361
sympathetic stimulation 212, 224
sympathetic system 144–5, 158, *628*; affinity
    for β_2 receptors 641; breadth of
    activity 641; bronchodilation 638;
    catecholamines 640; duration of
    activity 640; features **627**; "fight-
    or-flight" reactions and exercise
    626; preganglionic neurons **627**;
    vasoconstriction 638
sympatholytics drug 153
sympathomimetic drugs 636
synapse 15, 26; chemical 26–30; excitatory
    28–9; inhibitory 29
synaptic cleft 26, 35
synaptic knob 27–8
synaptic transmission 26; characteristics 28;
    chemical synapses 26–30; factors
    affecting 33–5; interconnections
    between neurons 32–3; summation
    30–2; types 28
syncope 159
syncytiums 208, 358
syndenham chorea 241
syndrome of inappropriate ADH
    (SIADH) 502
synergism 471
synovium 704
systemic lupus erythematosus (SLE) 83, 706;
    diagnosis 706; manifestations 706;
    treatment 706
systole phases 218, **218**
systolic failure 256–7

tachycardia 217
tamoxifen 719
TB (tuberculosis) 329–31, **330**, *330*
T cells *see* T lymphocytes (T cells)
temporal summation 30, *31*
tension pneumothorax 345
testes 529
testicular cancer 540–1
testis and scrotum disorders: spermatocele
    540; testicular cancer 540–1;
    varicocele 540
testosterone 531, **532**
tetanus 215
thalamus 573

thalassemia: aplastic anemia 126–7;
    diagnosis 125; forms 125; G6PD
    deficiency 126; hydroxyurea drug
    126; hypoxia 125; polycythemia
    127–8; treatment 125–6
thecal cells 534, **536**, 538
therapeutic agents 230
third-degree heart block 273
thoracic volume 284
threshold potential 17
thromboangiitis obliterans 173–4
thrombocytes 698; *see also* platelets
thrombocytopenia 115
thrombolytic drugs 179–80
thrombomodulin 113
thrombopoietin 699
thrombosis 109, 117
thromboxane A_2 (TxA_2) 151–2
thrombus 176–9
thyroid gland: calcitonin 489; hormones
    486–8; hyperthyroidism 506–7;
    hypothyroidism 504–6; tests 503
thyroid-stimulating hormone (TSH) 80, 484
tidal volume (V_T) 297
tissue plasminogen activator 113
tissue repair 43; by connective tissue
    replacement 43; by regeneration 43;
    stages 44–5; steps in 44
tissue thromboplastin 111
T lymphocytes (T cells) 62, 65, 107; actions 75;
    types 74
toll-like receptors (TLRs) 63
tonic activity 626
tophi 710, *710*; manifestations 709; risk
    factors 709; treatment 710
Torsades de Pointes 271
total lung capacity (TLC) 299
toxic megacolon 394
trachea 282
training-induced bradycardia 224
transcription 63
transcytosis 164
translation 63
translocates 475
transmural infarcts 251
transplacental 73
transpulmonary pressure 287
traumatic brain injury 594
trichomoniasis 554
tricuspid valve 204
trophic hormone 470
true aneurysms 175
trypsin 380

T-score 702
TSH (thyroid-stimulating hormone) 80, 484
T-type calcium channels 210
tuberculosis (TB) 329–31, **330**, *330*
tubular reabsorption 423–4
tubular secretion 433–4
tubuloglomerular feedback 438–9
tumor 89, 712
tumor cells 64–5, 332, 713
tumor necrosis factor-alpha (TNF-α) 97, **98**
tumor staging 717
T wave *216*, 216–17
type 1 diabetes mellitus 56; dawn
        phenomenon 516; DKA 515;
        manifestations 514–15; Somogyi
        effect 516; treatment 515
type 2 diabetes: etiology *517*; HHNKS **518**;
        manifestations 518; treatment 518
type I hypersensitivity reactions 78, 80, *81*
type II hypersensitivity reactions 80, 82, *82*
type III hypersensitivity reactions 83
type IV hypersensitivity reactions 83, *84*
typical pneumonia 327–8

UES (upper esophageal sphincter) 365
ulcerative colitis *393*, 393–4
unimodal association area 569
universal donors/recipients 103
unstable angina 247
upper esophageal sphincter (UES) 365
uric acid 709
uricosuric agents 710
urinary incontinence 461
urine reflux 459–60, *460*
uterine fibroids/prolapse 547
uterus 533

vagina 533–4
vagina, cervix, and uterus disorders: cervical
        lesions and cervical cancer
        544–5; endometrial cancer 546–7;
        endometriosis 545–6; uterine
        fibroids 547; uterine prolapse 547;
        vaginitis 544
vaginitis 544
vagus 624, 629–30
valvular heart disease, diagnosis 243
valvular incompetence 180
valvuloplasty 244
variant angina 247–8
varicocele 540
varicose veins 180
varicosities 625–6

vasa recta/straight vessels 418, 433
vascular constriction 108
vascular disease 521
vas deferens 530
vasoactive substances 149, **150**, 494
vasoconstrictors: angiotensin II 150–1;
        catecholamines 150; endothelin
        151; serotonin 152, **152**;
        vasopressin 151
vasodilation/vasodilators 134, 153–5, 244, 255
vasogenic shock *see* distributive shock
vasomotion 164
vasomotor center 145–6
vasomotor tone 145
vasopressin 151, 427; *see also* antidiuretic
        hormone (ADH)
veins, disease: anticoagulant drugs 179;
        chronic venous insufficiency 180;
        embolism 179; thrombolytic drugs
        179–80; varicose veins 180; venous
        thrombosis 176–9
venous regulation: blood volume 157;
        compliance 156–7; distensibility
        155–6; respiratory activity 158;
        skeletal muscle pump 158;
        sympathetic stimulation 158
venous return 228
venous thrombosis: DVT 177–8; factors **178**;
        prevention 179; treatment 179
ventilation 297; alveolar ventilation 300–1,
        301; dead space 301; by medullary
        respiratory center 317; regulatory
        system for 315–21; standard
        lung volumes 297–300, *298*; total
        ventilation 300
ventilation-perfusion (V:Q) matching
        306–8, *307*
ventilatory response to exercise 321–2
ventral respiratory group (VRG) 317
ventral root 582
ventricular arrhythmia 271
ventricular fibrillation 271
ventricular filling process 219
ventricular hypertrophy 263
ventricular premature contractions
        (VPCs) 271
ventricular septal defects 246
ventricular tachycardia 218, 271
verapamil 217
vertical osmotic gradient 428
very low density lipoprotein (VLDL) **170**
vessel radius 140
vestibulocerebellum 576

viral core 723
viral hepatitis 399–402, **400**
viral STDs 554
virulent portion 72–3
viruses 61
visceral pleura 284
vital capacity (VC) 299
vitamin K deficiency 115
VLDL (very low density lipoprotein) **170**
voltage-gated K+ channel 19
voltage-gated Na+ channels 18
von Willebrand disease 114–15
von Willebrand factor (vWF) 109
VPCs (ventricular premature contractions) 271
VRG (ventral respiratory group) 317

warfarin therapy **101**, 113, 179
warm shock 191

water and electrolytes 382
water excretion, control 445–7
water reabsorption 427–8
water-soluble substances 164
wet gangrene 42, 43
white blood cell (WBC) 699; *see also* leukocytes
white matter 585–6
withdrawal reflex 562, 591–3, *592*
World Health Organization (WHO) 329, 337
wound healing process 46, **47**

xanthine drugs 337

Zollinger-Ellison syndrome 389
zona pellucida 534
zone of ischemia 252
zone of necrosis 251–2